Health Assessment *for* Nursing Practice

5th Edition

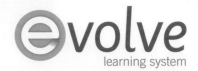
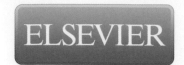
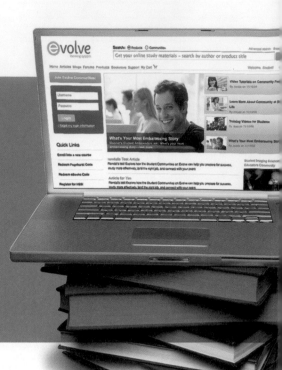

Health Assessment
for Nursing Practice

5th Edition

Susan Fickertt Wilson, PhD, RN, CNE
Associate Professor
School of Nursing
College of Health
University of Alaska Anchorage
Anchorage, Alaska;
Emeritus Associate Professor
Harris College of Nursing and Health Sciences
Texas Christian University
Fort Worth, Texas

Jean Foret Giddens, PhD, RN, FAAN
Professor and Executive Dean
College of Nursing
University of New Mexico
Albuquerque, New Mexico

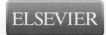

3251 Riverport Lane
St. Louis, Missouri 63043

Notices

Knowledge and best practice in this field are constantly changing. As new research and experience broaden our understanding, changes in research methods, professional practices, or medical treatment may become necessary.

Practitioners and researchers must always rely on their own experience and knowledge in evaluating and using any information, methods, compounds, or experiments described herein. In using such information or methods they should be mindful of their own safety and the safety of others, including parties for whom they have a professional responsibility.

With respect to any drug or pharmaceutical products identified, readers are advised to check the most current information provided (i) on procedures featured or (ii) by the manufacturer of each product to be administered, to verify the recommended dose or formula, the method and duration of administration, and contraindications. It is the responsibility of practitioners, relying on their own experience and knowledge of their patients, to make diagnoses, to determine dosages and the best treatment for each individual patient, and to take all appropriate safety precautions.

To the fullest extent of the law, neither the Publisher nor the authors, contributors, or editors, assume any liability for any injury and/or damage to persons or property as a matter of products liability, negligence or otherwise, or from any use or operation of any methods, products, instructions, or ideas contained in the material herein.

Executive Content Strategist: Kristin Geen
Content Manager: Laurie Gower
Senior Content Development Specialist: Jamie Horn
Associate Content Development Specialist: Sarah Hembree
Content Coordinator: Laura Goodrich
Publishing Services Manager: Deborah L. Vogel
Senior Project Manager: Jodi M. Willard
Design Direction: Brian Salisbury

Printed in Canada

Last digit is the print number: 9 8 7 6 5 4 3 2 1

To my daughter, Megan, for her continued love, patience, and support; and to the faculty, colleagues, and students who have challenged me through the years.
SFW

To my husband, Jay, for his unconditional support; to my mentors and role models for their guidance throughout my career; and to our nursing students, the future of our profession.
JFG

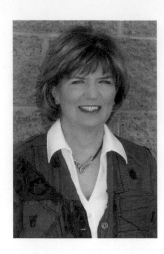

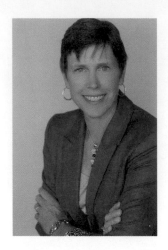

Susan Fickertt Wilson has over 40 years of teaching experience, including 30 years teaching health assessment. She has cared for adult patients in critical care, general care, and rehabilitation units. Dr. Wilson has taught undergraduate and graduate students about the care of patients in a variety of settings. This text is a synthesis of all she has learned about performing health assessment and teaching health assessment, as well as how to meet the challenges she knows students experience in learning health assessment.

Jean Foret Giddens is a professor and Executive Dean at the College of Nursing at the University of New Mexico in Albuquerque. Dr. Giddens earned a Bachelor of Science in Nursing from the University of Kansas, a Master of Science in Nursing from the University of Texas at El Paso, and a doctorate in Education and Human Resource Studies from Colorado State University. Dr. Giddens has been involved with nursing education since 1984. Her teaching experience includes associate, baccalaureate, and master's degree programs in New Mexico, Texas, and Colorado. Her content areas in nursing education include adult health nursing, health assessment, nursing process, curriculum development, and innovative educational strategies.

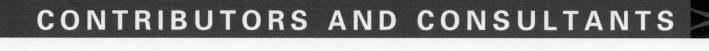

CONTRIBUTORS AND CONSULTANTS

Clinical Reasoning Special Consultant
for previous editions
Christine A. Tanner, PhD, RN
A.B. Youmans-Spaulding Distinguished Professor
Oregon Health & Science University
School of Nursing
Portland, Oregon

Chapter 20
Joanne Bartram, RN, MSN, FNP
Clinical Educator, Family Nurse Practitioner
University of New Mexico
Albuquerque, New Mexico

Carolyn Montoya, RN, MSN, PNP
Academic Coordinator, Advanced Practice
Concentrations
University of New Mexico
Albuquerque, New Mexico

Special thanks to the Chamberlain College of Nursing
in St. Louis, Missouri, for providing a state-of-the-art
facility in which to take several of the photos for the
fifth edition. Their hospitality and collaboration were
most appreciated.

Ancillary Writers
Case Studies
Scharmaine Lawson-Baker, DNP, FNP-BC
Family Health Nurse Practitioner
Associate Professor, School of Nursing
Southern University
Baton Rouge, Louisiana

Case Studies, Review Questions
Maria E. Lauer, MSN, RN, CNE
Instructor, School of Nursing
Thomas Edison State College
Trenton, New Jersey

PowerPoint Slides
Darlene D. Brink, MSN, RN, CCM, NE-BC
Manager, Resource Center
Sentara Healthcare
Virginia Beach, Virginia

Test Bank
Susan Fickertt Wilson, PhD, RN, CNE
Associate Professor
School of Nursing
College of Health
University of Alaska Anchorage
Anchorage, Alaska;
Emeritus Associate Professor
Harris College of Nursing and Health Sciences
Texas Christian University
Fort Worth, Texas

Test Bank Review
Anne F. Meyer, RN, MS, FNP-BC
Instructor, Nursing Department
Fitchburg State University
Fitchburg, Massachusetts

REVIEWERS

Anthony J. Brunello, RN, MS, TNS, PHRN
Clinical Leader and Stroke Coordinator
Cardiovascular Services
Provena St. Mary's Hospital
Kankakee, Illinois

Sharon M. Forney, MSN, RN, MSHCA
Faculty
Associate Degree Nursing
North Central Texas College
Gainesville, Texas

Rebecca A. Fountain, PhD, RN
Assistant Professor
College of Nursing
University of Texas at Tyler
Tyler, Texas

Colleen J. Hewes, DC, MSN, RN
Director of Nursing Programs
Nursing
Lake Washington Technical College
Kirkland, Washington

Pamela Newland, RN, PhD
Assistant Professor
School of Nursing
Southern Illinois University Edwardsville
Edwardsville, Illinois

Kit Sebrey Schafer, DNP, BSN, MSN, NP
Clinical Associate Professor
School of Nursing
Purdue University
West Lafayette, Indiana

Mary Shelkey, PhD, ARNP
Post-Doctoral Fellow
School of Nursing
Biobehavioral Nursing and Health Systems
University of Washington
Seattle, Washington

Donna Walls, PhD, RN
Associate Clinical Professor
Nursing
Texas Woman's University
Dallas, Texas

If a teacher is indeed wise, he does not bid you enter the house of his wisdom, but rather leads you to the threshold of your own mind.

KAHLIL GIBRAN *The Prophet*

Following this teaching we have revised this text *Health Assessment for Nursing Practice* to retain the strong features and add others. The underlying principles of the previous editions are steadfast. As with the previous editions, the fifth edition is based on the assumption that every patient—from neonate to older adult—is an interactive, complex being who is more than a collection of his or her parts. Each patient's health status depends on the interactions of physiological, psychological, sociocultural, and spiritual factors. These interactions occur within their physical environments (what they eat, drink, and breathe; what type of activity and work they participate in and where they live), their social environments and health beliefs (friends, family, and support systems; when and how they seek health care), and their internal environments (what they eat and drink, how they sleep, and how often they exercise).

As faculty, we are challenged with several responsibilities toward our students:

1. Demonstrate caring and compassion when we interact with patients to act as role models for students.
2. Help students become knowledgeable and skilled in history-taking and physical assessment.
3. Model for students as well as teach them how to be objective and nonjudgmental.
4. Assist students to mobilize their resources to apply health assessment knowledge and skills to patients of all ages and from a multitude of cultures and ethnic groups.

We know that students will need this content for the remainder of their professional lives. This textbook is a toolbox of information and techniques. As a wise teacher, you lead students to the threshold.

ORGANIZATION

Health Assessment for Nursing Practice is organized into four units to assist students and faculty efficiently to find their areas of interest. Unit 1, entitled **Foundations for Health Assessment,** provides a strong foundation for students, covering issues pertinent to nursing practice with all age-groups, such as *Importance of Health Assessment, Interviewing to Obtain a Health History, Techniques and Equipment for Physical Assessment,* and *General Inspection and Vital Signs.* Also included are chapters on *Ethnic, Cultural, and Spiritual Considerations; Pain Assessment; Mental Health and Abusive Behavior Assessment;* and *Nutritional Assessment.*

Unit 2, entitled **Health Assessment of the Adult,** is organized by body system. Several chapters in Unit 2 begin with a **Concept Overview** that features concepts in the context of health assessment. These concepts include pain, oxygenation, perfusion, tissue integrity, motion, sensory perception, and intracranial regulation. The concept and interrelated concepts are shown along with an explanation of how these concepts are linked.

Each chapter includes a review of **Anatomy and Physiology**. This is found at the beginning of the chapter because physical assessment techniques allow the student to answer the question, "How does this patient's anatomy and physiology compare with that expected for his or her age-group and ethnic group?"

The **Health History** section instructs the student on history data to collect by providing sample questions to ask patients along with the reasons for asking those questions. The text below each question describes the variances that the student may find. Included in the Health History section are headings for **Present Health Status**, **Past Medical History**, **Family History**, **Personal and Psychosocial History,** and **Problem-Based History**. Descriptions of how to assess patients with special needs and how to teach patients to improve their health and reduce their risk for illness or injury are retained from the fourth edition.

The **Examination** section begins with a table that outlines procedures performed routinely and in special circumstances or in advanced practice. A list of the appropriate **Equipment** needed for these procedures is included in the table. This section sequentially guides the student in the techniques routinely performed during the physical assessment of an adult, telling what to do, how to do it, and what to expect. Photographs are provided to enhance learning. The subsequent section describes the examination procedures performed in special circumstances or in advanced practice. The indication for performing each procedure is followed by expected and abnormal findings. The left column, **Procedures and Techniques with Expected Findings**, details the techniques of the assessment and the expected findings, and the right column describes **Abnormal Findings**. When applicable, a section on **Patients with Situational Variations** may include examinations of patients who are hearing impaired or paralyzed.

The **Clinical Application and Clinical Reasoning** section at the end of each chapter contains Review Questions, and answers are provided in Appendix D. **Case Studies** give subjective and objective data about a patient and ask the student to use clinical reasoning skills to answer questions. Answers for these questions are included in Appendix D to facilitate self-study.

Health Promotion for Evidence-Based Practice boxes outline new *Healthy People 2020* objectives and include thorough discussions of recommendations for health promotion and reducing health risks. These special feature boxes follow the Health History section so that data are collected at the time of history taking. The **Common Problems and Conditions** section toward the end of each chapter has been updated. It now includes **Risk Factors** boxes for disorders in each body system to remind students to discuss these behaviors with patients to help them maintain health and reduce the risk of disease. The areas of risk factor identification and health promotion are unique to this text. These areas indicate our commitment to not only teaching students how to gather data from patients and examine their bodies to detect health and disease, but also to teaching students how to attain and maintain a higher level of health. Special **Ethnic, Cultural, and Spiritual Variations** boxes throughout the body systems chapters contain racial, cultural, and religious variations the nurse should consider when assessing patients.

Unit 3, entitled **Health Assessment Across the Life Span**, begins with an overview of growth and development and continues with chapters on *Assessment of the Infant, Child, and Adolescent; Assessment of the Pregnant Patient;* and *Assessment of the Older Adult.* These chapters describe how to individualize the examination for patients of different ages and in pregnancy. Each chapter includes a box that lists the differences in anatomy and physiology pertinent to those patients. Health history and examination follow along with procedures and techniques and expected and abnormal findings. The Common Problems and Conditions section toward the end of each chapter has been retained in these chapters as they pertain to the patients described.

Unit 4, entitled **Synthesis and Application of Health Assessment**, contains *Conducting a Head-to-Toe Examination, Documenting the Comprehensive Health Assessment,* and *Adapting Health Assessment to the Hospitalized Patient* (**new to the fifth edition**). These chapters provide guidelines and photographs for combining the body system assessments into one comprehensive examination, for communicating the findings to other health care professionals, and for adapting the comprehensive assessment to patients in a hospitalized setting.

A **Glossary** at the end of the book provides definitions to enhance student comprehension of key concepts and terms.

Chapters were updated and revised based on feedback from both faculty and students. Consider each chapter a different type of tool from the toolbox. Collectively they provide all that students need to perform a comprehensive health assessment.

SUMMARY OF SPECIAL FEATURES

- Updated **Health Promotion for Evidence-Based Practice** boxes outline new *Healthy People 2020* objectives and include thorough discussions of recommendations for health promotion and reducing risk.
- The **Examination** section in each body system chapter has a table that outlines procedures performed routinely, in special circumstances, or in advanced practice.
- **Advanced Practice Skills** are distinguished from basic skills and are identified with a special icon. This feature bridges the gap between undergraduate and advanced practice education. Advanced content is denoted with a symbol to highlight this material for advanced practice students without being obtrusive for undergraduate students.
- Special **Risk Factors** boxes are found at the beginning of each Common Problems and Conditions section in the body system chapters and highlight information specific to various body systems and disorders.
- Unique and revised **Clinical Reasoning: Thinking Like a Nurse** boxes walk students through the thought process of how an experienced nurse or nurse practitioner makes decisions and includes examples of how experts notice, interpret, and respond to clinical situations.
- **Frequently Asked Questions** boxes answer common questions students have as they are learning health assessment. These "FAQs" appear throughout Unit 2.
- Near the end of each chapter is a section on **Clinical Application and Clinical Reasoning**. Included are the Case Studies and Review Questions, and answers to these exercises are provided in Appendix D to help students evaluate their learning.
- New **Quality Improvement Competencies for Nurses** tables provide assessment related to selected Quality and Safety Education for Nurses (QSEN) competencies, including patient-centered care, teamwork and collaboration, safety, and informatics.
- Reformatted **Ethnic, Cultural, and Spiritual Variations** boxes anticipate the unique needs of a multicultural patient population.

TEACHING AND LEARNING AIDS

The **Evolve website** for this book contains extensive student and instructor resources and can be accessed at http://evolve. elsevier.com/Wilson/assessment. This dynamic educational component allows students and faculty to access the most current information and resources for further study and research. The comprehensive **Evolve Instructor Resources** include **TEACH for Nurses**, a resource that ties together every chapter resource necessary for the most effective class presentations. TEACH for Nurses incorporates objectives, key terms, nursing curriculum standards (including QSEN, BSN Essentials, and Concepts), student and instructor chapter resources, in-class/online case studies, and teaching strategies consisting of student activities, online activities, and discussion topics. The ExamView **Test Bank** has been updated and includes approximately 650 test questions. Also included is a comprehensive **Image Collection**, which contains hundreds of full-color images that can be imported into the **PowerPoint Lecture Slides** for use in classroom lectures. **Audience Response Questions** and **Case Studies** are also provided for the PowerPoint lecture slides.

Evolve Student Resources include animations, case studies, content updates, examination techniques, lab guides, key points, heart and lung sounds, review questions, skills checklists, and video clips.

Visit http://evolve.elsevier.com/Wilson/assessment to access these resources.

CONTENTS

UNIT 2
Health Assessment of the Adult

CHAPTER 11
Lungs and Respiratory System, 191

CHAPTER 12
Heart and Peripheral Vascular System, 223

CHAPTER 16
Breasts and Axillae, 366

CHAPTER 17
Reproductive System and the Perineum, 386

UNIT 3
Health Assessment Across the Life Span

CHAPTER 18
Developmental Assessment Throughout the Life Span, 439

CHAPTER 19
Assessment of the Infant, Child, and Adolescent, 455

CHAPTER 20
Assessment of the Pregnant Patient, 495

CHAPTER 21
Assessment of the Older Adult, 515

UNIT 4
Synthesis and Application of Health Assessment

CHAPTER 22
Conducting a Head-to-Toe Examination, 531

CHAPTER 23
Documenting the Comprehensive Health Assessment, 538

CHAPTER 24
Adapting Health Assessment to the Hospitalized Patient, 542

APPENDIXES

Importance of Health Assessment

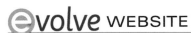 WEBSITE

http://evolve.elsevier.com/Wilson/assessment

Health assessment refers to a systematic method of collecting and analyzing data for the purpose of planning patient-centered care. The nurse collects health data from the patient and compares these to the ideal state of health, taking into account the patient's age, gender, culture, ethnicity, and physical, psychologic, and socioeconomic status. Data about the patient's strengths, weaknesses, health problems, and deficits are identified. The nurse incorporates the patient's knowledge, motivation, support systems, coping ability, and preferences to develop a plan of care that will help the patient maximize his or her potential.

One approach to developing a plan of care is using the American Nurses Association's (ANA) *Standards of Practice.*[1] The first six standards are based on the nursing process (i.e., assessment, diagnosis, outcome identification, planning, implementation, and evaluation) (Box 1-1). The first and foundational step is assessment, defined as the collection of "comprehensive data pertinent to the patient's health and/or situation."[1 p.32] The assessment and subsequent analysis of data are performed by nurses in all settings.

Quality improvement competencies are applied in all areas of nursing practice, including health assessment. The Institute of Medicine identified five core competencies as essential for health care professionals to demonstrate so they might respond effectively to patient care needs: (1) provide patient-centered care, (2) work in interdisciplinary teams, (3) use evidenced-based practice, (4) apply quality improvements, and (5) use informatics.[2]

COMPONENTS OF HEALTH ASSESSMENT

Components of health assessment include conducting a health history (collecting subjective data), performing a physical examination (collecting objective data), and documenting the findings. The amount of information collected by the nurse during a health history and the extent of the physical examination depend on the setting, the situation, the patient's needs, and the nurse's experience.

Health History

A health history consists of subjective data collected during an interview. This history includes information about patients' current state of health, medications they take, previous illnesses and surgeries, and family history and a review of systems. Patients may report feelings or experiences associated with health problems. These reports from patients are called *symptoms* and are considered subjective data (Box 1-2). Subjective data acquired directly from the patient are considered *primary source data.* If data are acquired from another individual (such as a family member), they are referred to as *secondary source data.* More information about conducting a health history is presented in Chapter 2.

Physical Examination

A physical examination involves the collection of objective data; these data are sometimes referred to as *signs* (see Box 1-2). During a physical examination, objective data are collected using the techniques of inspection, palpation, percussion, and auscultation. In addition, the patient's height, weight, blood pressure, temperature, pulse rate, and respiratory rate are measured. Specific physical examination skills and techniques are presented in chapters throughout this textbook.

Documentation of Data

Health assessment data are documented so the health status at the time of the interaction is recorded and so other health care team members can use the information. Complete,

---

BOX 1-1   STANDARDS OF NURSING PRACTICE

The Nursing Process

Standard 1: Assessment
The registered nurse collects comprehensive data pertinent to the health care consumer's health and/or the situation.

Standard 2: Diagnosis
The registered nurse analyzes the assessment data to determine the diagnoses or issues.

Standard 3: Outcome Identification
The registered nurse identifies expected outcomes for a plan individualized to the health care consumer or the situation.

Standard 4: Planning
The registered nurse develops a plan that prescribes strategies and alternatives to attain expected outcomes.

Standard 5: Implementation
The registered nurse implements the identified plan.
  5A: Coordination of Care—The registered nurse coordinates care delivery.
  5B: Health Teaching and Health Promotion—The registered nurse uses strategies to promote health and a safe environment.
  5C: Consultation—The graduate level–prepared specialty nurse or APRN provides consultation to influence the identified plan, enhance the ability of others, and effect change.
  5D: Prescriptive Authority and Treatment—The APRN uses prescriptive authority, procedures, referrals, treatments, and therapies in accordance with state and federal laws and regulations.

Standard 6: Evaluation
The registered nurse evaluates progress toward attainment of outcomes.

From American Nurses Association: *Nursing: scope and standards of practice,* ed 2, Washington, DC, 2010, American Nurses Association. Available at *nursesbooks.org.*
APRN, Advanced practice registered nurse.

BOX 1-2   CLARIFICATION OF TERMS

Signs and Symptoms
- *Signs* are objective data observed, felt, heard, or measured. Examples of signs include rash, enlarged lymph nodes, and swelling of an extremity.
- *Symptoms* are subjective data perceived and reported by the patient. Examples of symptoms include pain, itching, and nausea.

Occasionally data may fall into both categories. For example, a patient may tell the nurse that he "feels sweaty"—a symptom. At the same time the nurse may observe excessive sweating, or diaphoresis—a sign.

Clinical Manifestations
Clinical manifestation is a term often used to describe the presenting signs and symptoms experienced by a patient.

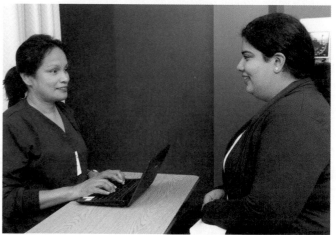

FIG. 1-1 The nurse may take notes while conducting a health assessment.

---

accurate, and descriptive documentation improves the plan of care. Documenting these data also prevents the patient from having to provide the same information to another health care provider. The health record serves as the legal permanent record of the patient's health status at the time of the health care visit. Thus it serves as a baseline to evaluate subsequent changes and decisions related to care. The format for documentation varies from agency to agency. Although some agencies still use paper-based documentation systems, most agencies have adopted an electronic health record (EHR) system. An EHR is a computerized version of data previously found in a paper chart (i.e., data from the history, physical examination, laboratory and diagnostic tests, and surgical procedures and progress and nursing notes) (Fig. 1-1). In the future, EHRs aim to integrate documentation of care across participating systems for a single patient.[3] Regardless of the format used, basic underlying principles of documentation are common to all. Data must be recorded accurately, concisely, and without bias or opinion. Health assessment documentation is discussed further in Chapter 23.

TYPES OF HEALTH ASSESSMENT

As mentioned previously, the amount of information gained during a health assessment depends on several factors, including the context of care, the patient's needs, and the nurse's experience.

Context of Care

The term *context* refers to circumstances or situations associated with an event or events. The phrase *context of care* refers to the circumstances or situations related to the health care

BOX 1-3   TYPES OF HEALTH ASSESSMENT

- **Comprehensive assessment:** This involves a detailed history and physical examination performed at the onset of care in a primary care setting or on admission to a hospital or long-term care facility. The comprehensive assessment encompasses health problems experienced by the patient; health promotion, disease prevention, and assessment for problems associated with known risk factors; or assessment for age- and gender-specific health problems.
- **Problem-based/focused assessment:** The problem-based or problem-focused assessment involves a history and examination that are limited to a specific problem or complaint (e.g., a sprained ankle). This type of assessment is most commonly used in a walk-in clinic or emergency department, but it may also be applied in other outpatient settings. Although the focus of data collection is on a specific problem, the potential impact of the patient's underlying health status also must be considered.
- **Episodic/follow-up assessment:** This type of assessment is usually done when a patient is following up with a health care provider for a previously identified problem. For example, a patient treated by a health care provider for pneumonia might be asked to return for a follow-up visit after completion of antibiotics. An individual treated for an ongoing condition such as diabetes is asked to make regular visits to the clinic for episodic assessment.
- **Shift assessment:** When individuals are hospitalized, nurses conduct assessments each shift. The purpose of the shift assessment is to identify changes in a patient's condition from baseline; thus the focus of the assessment is largely based on the condition or problem the patient is experiencing. Adapting an assessment to the hospitalized patient is discussed in Chapter 24.
- **Screening assessment:** A screening assessment, or screening examination, is a short examination focused on disease detection. A screening examination might be performed in a health care provider's office (as part of a comprehensive examination) or at a health fair. Examples include blood pressure screening, glucose screening, cholesterol screening, and colorectal screening.

delivery. Many such circumstances contribute to the context of care, including the setting or environment; the physical, psychological, or socioeconomic circumstances involving patients; and the expertise of the nurse. Because of these variables, different types of assessments are performed (e.g., a comprehensive health assessment, a problem-based or focused health assessment, an episodic assessment, a shift assessment, and a screening assessment) (Box 1-3). In some settings such as a hospital admission or a community-based primary care setting, a comprehensive history and examination are collected. In an urgent care or emergency department setting a problem-based or focused assessment is indicated, although additional subjective and objective data that may have direct or indirect impact on the management of the patient are collected. In addition, if it is determined that the patient is at risk or in need of further evaluation, the patient is referred to an appropriate agency so a comprehensive assessment might be completed.

Patient Need

The type of health assessment performed by the nurse is also driven by patient need. Because patient needs can vary widely, the nurse must be prepared to conduct the appropriate level of assessment. The patient's age, general level of health, presenting problems, knowledge level, and support systems are among many variables that impact patient need. For example, a healthy 17-year-old male presenting to a primary care clinic for a sports physical clearly has different needs than a 78-year-old, recently widowed patient with diabetes, presenting to the same clinic with increasing fatigue.

Nurse Expertise

The expertise of the nurse is another factor determining the type of assessment conducted. Experience affects what is done and how data are interpreted. For example, a nurse working in an adult intensive care unit has expertise in assessing a patient with hemodynamic instability; a family nurse practitioner working in a women's clinic has expertise in performing routine pelvic examinations. Such expertise is gained through experience and specialization within a given area of practice.

This textbook presents basic-to-advanced health assessment skills. Learning every assessment skill described in this book is not realistic for the beginning student; in fact, few providers apply all health assessment skills. Research involving the physical assessment skills used in clinical practice has shown that nurses incorporate some skills regularly and others less frequently. In a study representing a sample of 193 nurses across multiple areas of clinical practice, respondents reported performing only 30 of 124 examination skills on a routine basis; the remaining skills were reportedly performed occasionally or not performed at all.[4] Secrest, Norwood, and duMont[5] reported that 92.5% of physical assessment skills on a 120-item survey were taught and practiced in baccalaureate nursing programs, yet only 29% of nurses in clinical practice actually performed those skills on a regular basis. A survey of baccalaureate students in one nursing program found that fewer than half of the skills taught in the physical examination course were actually used in clinical practice.[6] In all three studies, the large majority of the skills routinely performed by nurses represented inspection and auscultation involving cardiovascular and respiratory systems. These findings suggest the need to clearly differentiate skills that are more likely to be used in practice from those that are used infrequently. Box 1-4 presents *core* physical assessment skills identified through research. Throughout this textbook techniques that are frequently performed by most nurses in most settings are differentiated from techniques that are less commonly performed by nurses or are indicated only in special situations. Furthermore, assessment techniques typically performed by an advanced practice nurse (such as a clinical nurse specialist, nurse practitioner, or certified nurse

---

BOX 1-4 CORE EXAMINATION SKILLS*

Skin
- Inspect skin.
- Inspect skin lesions and wounds.

Head, Eyes, Ears, Nose, Throat
- Inspect face.
- Inspect oral cavity.
- Assess hearing (based on conversation).
- Inspect external eyes.
- Inspect pupils and response to light and accommodation.

Chest and Lungs
- Inspect chest.
- Evaluate breathing effort.
- Auscultate lung sounds.

Cardiovascular
- Auscultate heart sounds and apical pulse.
- Palpate the distal pulses.
- Palpate and inspect the nails (capillary refill).
- Inspect and palpate extremities for edema.
- Palpate extremities for temperature.
- Inspect extremities for skin color and hair growth.

Musculoskeletal
- Inspect upper and lower extremities for size and symmetry.
- Palpate extremities for tenderness.
- Observe range of motion.
- Assess muscle strength.
- Inspect spine.
- Assess gait.

Abdomen
- Inspect abdomen.
- Auscultate bowel sounds; aortic vascular sounds.
- Palpate abdomen lightly (generalized tenderness and distention).

Neurologic
- Assess mental status and level of consciousness.
- Evaluate speech.

Genitalia
- Inspect male genitalia (penis/scrotum).
- Inspect female genitalia.

Data from Giddens JF: A survey of physical assessment techniques performed by RNs: lessons for nursing education, *J Nurs Educ* 46:83-87, 2007; Secrest JA, Norwood BR, and Dumont PM: Physical assessment skills: a descriptive study of what is taught and what is practiced, *J Prof Nurs* 21(2):114-118, 2005.
*Find related Skills Checklists for use in the laboratory or further study at *http://evolve.elsevier.com/Wilson/assessment/*.

---

midwife) are indicated with the following "Advanced Practice" symbol: ★.

CLINICAL REASONING AND JUDGMENT

The outcome of a health assessment is a portrait of patients' physical status, strengths and weaknesses, abilities, support systems, health beliefs, and activities to maintain health in addition to their health problems and lack of resources for maintaining health. The nurse must analyze and interpret these data before initiating a plan of care.

Data Organization

After collecting data, nurses organize or cluster them so the problems appear more clearly. This might be done based on a body system format (e.g., cardiovascular, musculoskeletal, auditory, visual) or conceptual formats (e.g., oxygenation, perfusion, mobility).

Data Analysis, Interpretation, and Clinical Judgment

After collecting and organizing data, nurses consider and analyze expected and abnormal findings to identify problems experienced by patients and initiate an appropriate plan of care. The term *clinical judgment* is defined as "an interpretation or conclusion about a patient's needs, concerns, or health problems and/or the decision to take action (or not), use or modify standard approaches, or improvise new ones as

deemed appropriate by the patient's response."[7, p 204] Although clinical judgment requires accurate collection of assessment data, it is the nurse's interpretation of data that impacts the decisions made. According to Tanner,[7] clinical judgment is influenced more by the nurse's experiences, knowledge, attitudes, and perspectives than the data alone. Consider the following situation:

A 50-year-old man arrives at a walk-in medical clinic reporting a gradual onset of cough over the course of the day. He states that his symptoms began while he was at work. He takes no medications and smokes one-half pack of cigarettes a day. His vital signs and oxygen saturation are within normal limits.

- A novice nurse seeing this patient is likely to collect and document these initial data, auscultate his lungs, and inform the primary care provider that a patient with a cough and wheezing is waiting to be seen.
- An experienced nurse seeing this patient notices that he is anxious and his skin is pale and moist. This nurse intuitively collects additional information and learns that he has been nauseated and was exposed to chemical fumes at work. Although vital sign data are in the "normal" range, this nurse recognizes that the respiratory rate and pulse are borderline high and the oxygen saturation is on the lower end of the expected range. This nurse suspects that the patient is becoming hypoxic and administers low-flow oxygen and informs the primary care provider that he is a priority for evaluation.

Both providers in the preceding scenario noted the same initial signs and symptoms; however, the analysis and interpretation of data differed, resulting in different nursing actions. These differences can partly be explained by clinical judgment. As described by Tanner,[7] the process of clinical judgment includes four components: noticing, interpreting, responding, and reflecting. Noticing involves recognizing that a situation is or is not consistent with what nurses anticipate or expect that they will see based on the context of the patient situation. Tanner describes this process as a perceptual grasp of the situation. Although assessment is linked to noticing, the process of assessment in itself does not automatically lead to noticing. Noticing is based on the nurse's expectations associated with multiple variables, including clinical experience, knowledge, and the clinical context. The next step, interpreting, is a process in which the nurse uses patterns of reasoning (involving analysis and intuition) to gain an understanding of the situation. Once an understanding is gained, the nurse determines appropriate actions and interventions to take (if any)—what Tanner refers to as responding. Reflecting is a critical component of the development of clinical judgment. Tanner differentiates reflection-*in*-action (in other words reflecting on past experiences while in the midst of another situation) from reflection *on* action (thinking about a situation that has occurred and developing a better understanding of what happened and the appropriateness of the patient outcomes). By reflecting nurses use what is learned from clinical experiences for future encounters (Fig. 1-2).

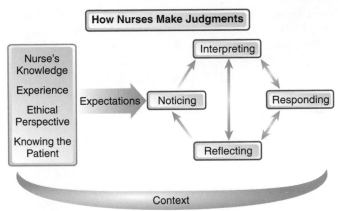

FIG. 1-2 Clinical Judgment Model. *Noticing* refers to the nurse's expectations and initial grasp of a situation. It triggers reasoning patterns that allow the nurse to interpret the situation and respond with interventions. *Reflection-in-action* specifically relates to evaluating outcomes of interventions, whereas *reflection-on-action* represents the contribution of an experience to a nurse's collective experiences. (From Tanner C: Thinking like a nurse: a research-based model of clinical judgment in nursing, *J Nurs Educ* 45:204-211, 2006.)

HEALTH PROMOTION AND HEALTH PROTECTION

A central component of health care is the promotion of health. Health promotion begins with health assessment; thus health promotion is found throughout this textbook. Through the process of health assessment, nurses assess patients' current health status, health practices, and risk factors. Interpretation of such data allows nurses' to target appropriate health promotion needs for patients. *Health promotion* is behavior motivated by the desire to increase well-being and actualize human health potential. *Health protection* is behavior motivated by a desire to actively avoid illness, detect it early, or maintain functioning within its constraints.[8]

Three levels of health promotion—primary prevention, secondary prevention, and tertiary prevention—address the promotion of health regardless of a patient's health status. Nurses are instrumental in providing education and care to help an individual meet his or her health promotion needs. The focus of *primary prevention* is to prevent a disease from developing through the promotion of healthy lifestyles. *Secondary prevention* consists of screening efforts to promote early detection of disease. *Tertiary prevention* is directed toward minimizing the disability from acute or chronic disease or injury and helping the patient to maximize his or her health. Table 1-1 clarifies these levels of health promotion further.

The framework for health promotion efforts in the United States is found in *Healthy People 2020* located on the Healthy People 2020 website found at http://www.healthypeople.gov/2020/. *Healthy People* is managed by the U.S. Department of Health and Human Services. This website contains the national health objectives that address the most significant preventable threats to health and national goals to reduce

TABLE 1-1	LEVELS OF HEALTH PROMOTION	
LEVEL OF PREVENTION	**FOCUS**	**EXAMPLES**
Primary prevention	Protection to prevent occurrence of disease	Immunizations, pollution control, nutrition, exercise
Secondary prevention	Early identification of disease before it becomes symptomatic to halt the progression of the pathologic process	Screening examinations and self-examination practices (e.g., colorectal screening, mammography, blood pressure screening)
Tertiary prevention	Minimize severity and disability from disease through appropriate therapy for chronic disease	Diabetes mellitus management Cardiac rehabilitation Hypertension management

such threats. There are four overarching goals of *Healthy People 2020:* (1) attain high-quality, longer lives free of preventable disease, disability, injury, and premature death; (2) achieve health equity, eliminate disparities, and improve the health of all groups; (3) create social and physical environments that promote good health for all; and (4) promote quality of life, healthy development, and healthy behaviors across all life stages.[9] These goals are supported by detailed objectives in 42 topic areas. The four foundational health measures that are used as indicators of progress toward goals are general health status, health-related quality of life and well-being, determinates of health, and disparities. Although a discussion of all of the *Healthy People 2020* objectives is beyond the scope of this textbook, selected areas are presented in health promotion boxes found throughout the text.

You are now challenged to study this health assessment textbook diligently. You need to be prepared to collect accurate health assessment data about patients, make accurate clinical judgments about their situation, and develop interventions that will improve their actual or potential health status. If you do this, patient health has a higher probability of improving. Accurate health assessment is one of the cornerstones of the art and science of professional nursing practice.

CLINICAL APPLICATION AND CLINICAL REASONING

See Appendix D for answers to exercises in this section.

REVIEW QUESTIONS

1. A 52-year-old male patient is admitted to the hospital with a new diagnosis of rectal cancer. The nurse conducts which type of assessment on his admission?
   1. A comprehensive assessment
   2. A problem-based health assessment
   3. An episodic assessment
   4. A screening assessment for colorectal cancer

2. The formation of a plan of care is initiated with:
   1. Analysis of data
   2. Collection of data
   3. Clustering of data
   4. Identification of nursing diagnoses

3. During an interview the nurse learns that a patient has a 5-year history of hypertension. Which health promotion intervention is most appropriate at this time?
   1. Teaching the patient how to relieve stress to prevent hypertension
   2. Monitoring and minimizing the progression of hypertension
   3. Establishing a screening schedule for detection of hypertension
   4. Advising the patient on the benefits of exercise to lower blood pressure

4. A patient reports painful urination for 2 days. The urine is pink tinged and cloudy. What type of data does this information represent?
   1. Subjective data
   2. Objective data
   3. Subjective and objective data
   4. Secondary source data

5. Which process does the clustering of data facilitate?
   1. Analyzing data
   2. Collecting data
   3. Implementing nursing care
   4. Evaluating nursing care

CASE STUDY 1

Sharon Faulkner is a 42-year-old woman admitted to the hospital with a diagnosis of acute cholecystitis. She tells the nurse the pain she is experiencing in her right upper abdomen feels like a knife and that it goes all the way to her shoulder. She is also very nauseated. She tells the nurse that she is exhausted and has not slept for three nights because the pain keeps her awake. The nurse observes dark circles under Sharon's eyes. Her vital signs are as follows: blood pressure (BP), 132/90 mm Hg; heart rate, 104 beats/min; respiratory rate, 22 per minute; temperature, 101.8° F (38.8° C). A complete blood count laboratory test reveals that Sharon has an elevated white blood cell count. She lies in her bed in a fetal position and tells the nurse that she hurts too much to get up and move.

1. List the subjective data described in this case study.
2. List the objective data described in this case study.

CASE STUDY 2

Mark Lyons is a 41-year-old man on the orthopedic unit. Listed in the next paragraph are data collected by the nurse during an interview and assessment.

Interview Data

Mark states, "I fell off my horse while riding. The horse stepped on my leg and crushed the bone in my upper leg." He complains of pain in his right leg and states that the pain medication helps only a little. He wants to move but cannot because of an external fixator device. Mark says, "My butt hurts because I can't move around." He tells the nurse, "I have not had a bowel movement for 3 days; the last time I had a bowel movement the stool looked like hard, dry rabbit turds. Normally at home I go every day." Mark has not been hungry either. He says that "the food is horrible." He also complains that he is so bored he can't stand it. "I'm used to being active; being stuck in bed is driving me crazy. Television shows aren't worth watching."

Examination Data

- *Vital signs:* BP, 108/72 mm Hg; pulse, 88 beats/min; respiration, 16 breaths/min; temperature, 98.1° F (36.7° C); height, 5 ft 5 in (165 cm); weight, 135 lb (61 kg).
- *Medication:* Percocet 1 or 2 by mouth every 4 to 6 hours as needed for pain. He has taken 2 every 6 hours over the last several days.
- *Diet:* Regular diet. Has eaten, on average, 30% of meals. Fluid intake has averaged 1000 mL/day.
- *Activity:* Patient is on complete bed rest.
- *Respiratory:* Breathing even/unlabored. Lungs clear to auscultation bilaterally.
- *Cardiovascular:* All distal pulses in lower extremities palpable. Heart rate and rhythm regular. No peripheral edema.
- *Abdomen:* Slightly distended. Bowel sounds auscultated throughout abdomen.
- *Musculoskeletal:* Right leg in skeletal traction. Reports sensation to foot/toes, rapid capillary refill. Other extremities: full range of motion. No pain over joints and muscles.
- *Integument:* Skin warm and dry. Pin sites for external fixation device without redness or drainage. 2 in–diameter redness over sacrum. Skin intact.

The following three problems are applicable to Mark. List data presented in this case study that support each problem. NOTE: Some data may be placed under more than one problem.

1. Pain
   a. Subjective data
   b. Objective data
2. Altered elimination (constipation)
   a. Subjective data
   b. Objective data
3. Risk for skin breakdown
   a. Subjective data
   b. Objective data

2

Interviewing Patients to Obtain a Health History

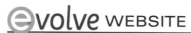 WEBSITE

http://evolve.elsevier.com/Wilson/assessment

When nurses first meet patients, they begin a database with a health history followed by a physical examination. The purpose of the health history is to obtain subjective data from patients so the nurse and patient can create a plan to promote health, prevent disease, resolve acute health problems, and minimize limitations related to chronic health problems. Information gathered includes how patients' define health and their beliefs about attaining and maintaining health such as how they view their responsibility for their health, which health behaviors they currently practice, and which unhealthy behaviors they are willing to change. The patient's expectations for health are based on their life experiences, the experiences of their families and friends, and the culture in which they live. The nurse has a broader view of health and compares a patient's current state of health to a standard needed to attain or maintain optimal health and then determines how far the patient is from the desired standard.

THE INTERVIEW

The health history is obtained through an interview process. During the interview the nurse facilitates discussion to collect and record data. An interview outline or electronic device may be used to prompt questions and take brief notes.

Nurses learn about patients' health concerns and the social, economic, and cultural factors that influence their health and their responses to illness. Data generated from an interview provide the foundation for personalized, safe, and effective health care for each individual. Incorporating quality improvement competencies during the interview process helps to minimize incorrect information and enhances the quality of the information recorded. Selected knowledge,

skills, and attitudes for achieving quality in the areas of patient-centered care, teamwork and collaboration, safety, and informatics are provided in Table 2-1.

In many settings patients are asked to complete a health history questionnaire. Questionnaires typically consist of a series of yes-or-no questions pertaining to specific problems or symptoms that they may have experienced. Although questionnaires are useful for collecting a health history, the information should only be considered adjunct data—they are never a substitute for an interview. Any past medical problems or symptoms identified by patients on a questionnaire should be investigated further.

Phases of the Interview

The interview consists of three phases: introduction, discussion, and summary (Box 2-1). To begin the introduction phase, the nurse introduces himself or herself and informs the patient about the nurse's role in the patient's care (Fig. 2-1). Address patients by their title (e.g., Mr., Mrs., Miss, or Ms.) and surname. Avoid using their first name unless they request it or when they are adolescents or children. Also avoid substituting their role for their name (e.g., referring to the patient as "mom" or "grandpa"). During the introduction the nurse should also explain to patients what to expect during the interview and how long the process should take.

Next the interview moves into the discussion phase. During this phase the nurse collects the health history by facilitating a discussion regarding various aspects of the patient's health. Although the role of the nurse is to facilitate the direction of conversation, ideally the conversation is *patient-centered,* meaning that patients are free to share their concerns, beliefs, and values in their own words.[1] During the

TABLE 2-1	QUALITY IMPROVEMENT COMPETENCIES FOR NURSES: OBTAINING A HEALTH HISTORY		
	KNOWLEDGE	**SKILLS**	**ATTITUDES**
Patient-Centered Care	Discuss principles of effective communication.	Elicit patient values, preferences, and expressed needs.	Value seeing health care situations "through the patient's eyes."
Teamwork and Collaboration	Describe impact of own communication style on others.	Demonstrate awareness of own strengths and limitations as a team member.	Value different styles of communication used by patients, families, and team members
Safety	Discuss effective strategies to reduce reliance on memory.	Use appropriate strategies to reduce reliance on memory such as checklists or computerized health history form.	Value the contributions of standardization/reliability to safety.
Informatics	Identify essential information that must be available in a common database to support patient care.	Navigate the electronic health record.	Protect confidentiality of protected health information in electronic health records.

www.qsen.org.

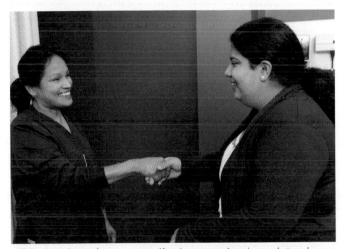

FIG. 2-1 Introduce yourself when you begin an interview.

BOX 2-1 PHASES OF AN INTERVIEW

Introduction Phase
Nurse:
• Introduces self to patient.
• Describes purpose of interview.
• Describes interview process.

Discussion Phase
Nurse:
• Facilitates and maintains patient-centered discussion.
• Uses various communication techniques to collect data.

Summary Phase
Nurse:
• Summarizes data with patient.
• Allows patient to clarify data.
• Validates to patient that he or she understands problems.

discussion phase a variety of communication skills and techniques are used to enhance the conversation and data collection.

The summary phase of the interview is a time for closure. Summarize with patients the main points and emphasize data that have implications for health promotion, disease prevention, or resolution of their health problems. The summary allows for clarification of data and provides validation to patients that the nurse has an accurate understanding of their health issues, problems, and concerns.

Communication Skills for Interviewing

Perhaps the single most important factor in the success of an interview is the communication skills of the nurse. Through the use of professional communication skills the nurse gains the patient's trust to share personal information. Numerous factors affect the interview and the communication process,

including the physical setting, the nurse's behaviors, the type of questions asked, and how they are asked. In addition, the personality and behavior of patients, how they are feeling during the interview, and the nature of information being discussed or the problem being confronted may affect the data revealed.

The Physical Setting

Before conducting an interview, consider the physical setting, which can impact the exchange of information. Ideally an interview is conducted in a private, quiet, comfortable room free from environmental distractions where the nurse and patient can sit face to face.

The importance of privacy, especially when discussing issues that are highly personal, cannot be overemphasized. Patients may not be willing to share sensitive information openly and honestly if they are fearful of being overheard or are in the presence of friends or family members. For example, consider the potentially compromising situation if the nurse asks patients about drug use or sexual activity in the presence of family members. Privacy is best gained by conducting an interview in an unoccupied room such as an examination room or a private hospital room. Unfortunately the physical layout of many health care facilities makes it difficult to find a completely private place to conduct an interview; thus you must take measures to allow for as much privacy as possible. If the interview occurs in an environment with multiple treatment areas or in a semiprivate hospital room, drawing the curtains helps provide some degree of privacy and blocks out visual distractions.

Patients should be physically comfortable during an interview. When possible, allow them to remain in street clothes during the interview and then have them change into a gown for the physical examination. The nurse and patient should sit at a distance from each other that provides a comfortable flow of conversation. The patient's comfort level is partly related to personal space (i.e., the area that surrounds the person's body). The amount of space the patient needs varies and is influenced by his or her culture and previous experiences in similar situations. Be attentive to how comfortable the patient appears; if you are not sure, ask, "Is this a comfortable seating arrangement for you?" Also, if possible, be sure that the room temperature is set at a comfortable level.

Finally the interview should be conducted in a quiet setting without distractions. Interruptions by other individuals should be avoided. Ensure that unnecessary noise is eliminated and unnecessary equipment is removed from the area or turned off if possible. Except for emergencies, cell phones and pagers should not be answered while conducting an interview.

Professional Behavior

The first impression nurses make start with their appearance. Dressing and grooming are important in establishing a positive first impression. Modest dress, clean fingernails, and neat hair are imperative. Avoid extremes in dress and manner so appearance does not become an obstacle or a distraction to the patient's responses.

Nurses' interpersonal skills are instrumental in a successful interview. They must convey a professional yet warm demeanor. A stiff, formal attitude may inhibit communication; yet being too casual or displaying a "laid-back" attitude may fail to instill confidence. Actively listen to patients and project a genuine interest in them and what they are saying. Patients have a need to feel understood; nurses should make every attempt to understand their point of view, communicate acceptance, and treat them with respect. Failure to do so jeopardizes the flow of information. Nurses must also avoid being careless with words. What may seem like an innocent comment to the nurse may be interpreted differently by patients. Finally nonverbal behavior is as important as words. Avoid extreme reactions (e.g., startle, surprise, laughter, grimacing) as patients provide information.

Patient-Related Variables

When conducting an interview, consider patient variables such as age and physical, mental, and emotional status. Ideally patients are mentally alert and in no physical or emotional discomfort. Conducting an interview with a patient in physical or emotional distress is difficult. In such a case, use a focused assessment to limit the number and nature of questions to those absolutely necessary for the given situation, and save additional questions for a later time.

The Art of Asking Questions

The art of obtaining information from patients and listening carefully to their responses is an essential competency. Questions must be clearly spoken and understood by patients. Define words patients may not understand, but do not use so many technical terms that the definitions become confusing. Use terms familiar to patients if possible. Slang words such as "pee" as opposed to "urinate" may be used if necessary to describe certain conditions. Adapt questions to a patient's developmental level, knowledge, and understanding. For example, the nurse might ask a young child where he or she hurts but would ask an adult more detailed questions such as onset, duration, and characteristics of the pain. Encourage patients to be as specific as possible. For example, if the nurse asks how many glasses of water the patient drinks each day and the patient says, "Oh, a few," the nurse clarifies what the patient means by asking, "How many is a few? Three? Four? Five?" This approach yields a more specific answer and provides the patient's interpretation of "a few."

Ask one question at a time and wait for the reply before asking the next question. If several questions are asked at a time, a patient may become confused about which question to answer, or the nurse may be uncertain about which question the patient is answering. For example, the nurse asks, "Have you had immunizations for tetanus, hepatitis B, and influenza?" If the patient answers yes, it is not clear if the patient means yes to all three or to one. If something a patient says is confusing, the nurse asks for clarification. The explanation may clear up the confusion, or it may indicate that the patient has misinformation or some underlying emotional or thought-processing difficulty that impairs understanding.

Be attentive to the feelings that accompany the patient's responses to some questions. These responses may signify that additional information is needed during the interview or that problems exist that need to be addressed in the future. For example, if the patient reports that her mother died of breast cancer and she begins to cry, this may indicate a future need to discuss coping or adjustment strategies with her.

Some areas of questioning (such as sexuality, domestic violence, and use of alcohol or drugs) may be more sensitive than others. What is perceived as sensitive may vary from patient to patient. When asking questions about sensitive issues, nurses explain that they need to ask personal or sensitive questions. Another technique is referred to as *permission giving*. For example, the nurse might say, "Many people have experimented with drugs; have you ever used street drugs?" or "Many young people your age have questions about sex.

What questions or concerns do you have?" With the permission-giving technique, the nurse communicates to the patient that it is safe to discuss such topics.

Patients may ask the nurse questions during the interview. The nurse can answer them using terms that patients understand but avoiding in-depth answers representing more information than necessary. If patients ask broad questions or questions that the nurse is unprepared to answer at the moment, it is acceptable to ask the patient for more information about the situation, "Tell me more about what you are thinking." This gives the nurse better direction in answering the broad questions or allows the nurse to refer patients to the appropriate resources.

Types of Questions to Ask

Begin the interview with *open-ended questions* such as, "How have you been feeling?" This broadly stated question encourages a free-flowing, open response. The aim of open-ended questions is to elicit responses that are more than one or two words. Patients might respond to this type of question by describing the onset of symptoms in their own words and at their own pace. However, the open-ended question should focus on the patient's health. A question that is too broad such as, "Tell me a little about yourself," may be too general to provide useful information. The risk of asking open-ended questions is that patients may be unable to focus on the specific topic of the question or may take excessive time to tell their story. In these cases the nurse needs to focus the interview. However, flexibility is necessary when using this type of question because patients' associations may be important and the nurse must allow them the freedom to pursue them.

To gain more precise details, nurses ask more direct, specific, *closed-ended questions* that require only one or two words to answer. For example, the nurse might ask, "Do you become short of breath?" or "Do you frequently get bruises?" Another reason for using this type of question is to give patients options when answering questions such as, "Is the pain in your stomach sharp, dull, or aching?" This type of question is valuable in collecting data, but it must be used in combination with open-ended questions because failure to allow patients to describe their health in their own words may lead to inaccurate conclusions. *Directive questions* lead patients to focus on one set of thoughts. This type of question is most often used in reviewing systems or evaluating an individual's functional capabilities. An example would be, "Describe the drainage you have had from your nose."

Techniques That Enhance Data Collection

The question-answer format is the essential tool used in obtaining a patient history. Data collection can be facilitated by using the following techniques.

Active Listening

Active listening involves listening with a purpose to spoken words as well as noticing nonverbal behaviors. This is performed by concentrating on what the patient is saying and the subtleties of the message being conveyed together with the facial expressions and body language observed. The nurse must pay full attention to the patient's response rather than predict how the patient will respond to the question or formulate the next question. When assumptions are made, the nurse may ask an illogical question; or, if the nurse is concentrating on how the next question will be worded, attention is shifted away from the information that the patient is providing.

Facilitation

Facilitation uses phrases to encourage patients to continue talking. These include verbal responses such as, "Go on," "Uh-huh," and "Then?" and nonverbal responses such as head nodding and shifting forward in your seat with increased attention.

Clarification

Clarification is used to obtain more information about conflicting, vague, or ambiguous statements. Examples might be, "What do you mean by 'you almost lost it'?" or "What do you think kept you from returning to work?"

Restatement

Restatement involves repeating what patients say to confirm the interpretation of what was said. For example, "Let me make sure I understand what you said. The pain in your stomach occurs before you eat and is relieved by eating. Is that correct?"

Reflection

Reflection asks patients a question to clarify a phrase or sentence. This encourages elaboration and indicates that you are interested in more information.

> *Patient:* "I got out of bed and I just didn't feel right."
> *Nurse:* "You didn't feel right?"
> *Patient:* "Uh huh, I was dizzy and had to sit back on the bed before I fell over."

Confrontation

Confrontation is used when inconsistencies are noted between what the patient reports and observations or other data about the patient. For example, "I'm confused. You say you're staying on your diet and exercising three times a week, yet your weight has increased since your last visit. Can you help me to understand this?" The nurse's tone of voice is important when using confrontation; use a tone that communicates confusion or misunderstanding rather than one that is accusatory and angry.

Interpretation

The nurse uses interpretation to share with patients the conclusions drawn from data they have given. After hearing the conclusion, patients can confirm, deny, or revise the interpretation. For example, "Let me share my thoughts about what you just told me. The week you were out of the office you exercised, felt no muscle tension, felt relaxed, and slept well. I wonder if your work environment is contributing to the anxiety that you're experiencing."

Summary

A summary condenses and orders data obtained during the interview to help clarify a sequence of events. This is useful when interviewing a patient who rambles or does not provide sequential data.

Techniques That Diminish Data Collection

The following communication techniques have been found to interrupt the flow of the interview, interfere with data collection, and possibly impair the patient-nurse relationship. These techniques can often be avoided by considering the interview from the patient's perspective.

Using Medical Terminology

Using medical terminology or abbreviations not known to patients interferes with the communication process. Some examples include saying "hypertension" instead of "high blood pressure," "dysphagia" rather than "difficulty in swallowing," "CVA" rather than "stroke," or "myocardial infarction" rather than "heart attack." Using medical jargon might confuse the patients, lead them to misunderstand the question, or cause them to feel too embarrassed to ask for clarification. Such a scenario can lead to inaccurate data collection.

Expressing Value Judgments

Value judgments expressed by the nurse have no place in an interview. For example, the nurse should ask, "What kind of protection do you use during intercourse, if any?" rather than saying, "You do use protection during intercourse, don't you?" The latter question forces the patient to respond in a way that is consistent with the nurse's values, or it might cause the patient to feel guilty or defensive when he or she must answer to the contrary.

Interrupting the Patient

Allow patients to finish sentences; do not become impatient and finish their sentences for them. The ending the nurse might add to a sentence may be different from that which the patient would have used. Associated with interrupting is changing the subject before a patient has finished giving information about the last topic discussed. Nurses may feel pressured for time and eager to move on to other topics, but they should allow patients an opportunity to complete their thoughts.

Being Authoritarian or Paternalistic

Nurses who use the approach, "I know what is best for you, and you should do what I say," risk alienating the patient. Despite personal beliefs held by the nurse, a patient's health is his or her responsibility. The patient may choose to follow or ignore advice and teaching offered by the nurse.

Using "Why" Questions

Using "why" questions can be perceived as threatening and may put patients on the defensive.[2] When patients are asked why they did something, the implication is that they must defend their choices. Instead of asking, "Why didn't you take

the entire antibiotic?" the nurse might say, "I noticed that you stopped taking the antibiotic before all the pills were gone," and wait to see if the patient offers an explanation. If no explanation is forthcoming, the nurse can follow up with, "I'm curious about the reason for not taking all of the antibiotics."

Managing Awkward Moments During an Interview
Answering Personal Questions

Patients may ask questions about nurses from time to time. They may be curious about the nurse and his or her personal life. A brief, direct answer usually satisfies their curiosity. Sharing personal experiences that may support patients may be helpful (such as parenting issues or how you handle stress) and may enhance the relationship with patients and increase your credibility.

Silence

Silence can be awkward. There is often an urge to break it with a comment or question. However, remember that patients may need the silence as time to reflect or gather courage. Some issues can be so painful to discuss that silence is necessary and should be accepted. It may indicate that they may not be ready to discuss this topic or that your approach needs to be evaluated. Nurses should become comfortable with silence; it can be useful.

Displays of Emotion

Crying is a natural emotion. Saying, "Don't cry" is not a therapeutic response. A therapeutic approach is to provide tissues and let patients know that it is all right to cry by giving a response such as, "Take all the time you need to express your feelings." Postpone further questioning until the patient is ready. Crying may indicate a need that can be addressed at a later time. Compassionate response to a crying patient demonstrates caring and may enhance the therapeutic relationship.

A patient's anger may be uncomfortable. One approach is to deal with it directly by first identifying its source. The nurse may say, "You seem angry; can you tell me the reason for your feelings?" If patients choose to discuss the anger, they may identify whether the anger is directed at themselves, someone else, or directly at the nurse. If patients are angry at someone else, discuss with them an approach for talking with that person about the reason for the angry feelings. When patients are angry with the nurse, encourage them to discuss their feelings. Acknowledge their feelings and, if appropriate, apologize. Nurses may be able to continue working with patients after the angry feelings are discussed; but, if patients would prefer to interact with another nurse, their request should be honored. Regardless of the outcome, nurses should model a healthy, appropriate approach to managing anger.

Challenges to the Interview
Managing the Overly Talkative Patient

Some patients are difficult to interview because they are overly talkative. They may feel a need to go into every detail of a problem or illness and become distracted as they tell their story. Some patients focus on remote past events with no apparent relevance to their present situation. Still others may want to discuss issues that do not relate directly to themselves such as other people or current world events. When interviewing overly talkative patients, the nurse might have difficulty determining what is actually bothering them. Although each situation is unique, ideally the nurse tactfully redirects the conversation. The use of closed-ended questions may help to maintain direction and flow of the conversation.

Others in the Room

Patients might be accompanied by other individuals. When this is the case, don't assume relationships among the people present. Ask the other people, "What is your relationship to the patient?" The parent or guardian of a child usually answers interview questions on behalf of the child. When adults are unable to answer questions for themselves, other persons might assist with the interview. However, all patients should be involved with the interview to the extent that their mental or physical ability allows. When adult or adolescent patients are able to speak for themselves, they should be interviewed directly and in private if possible. If other individuals are present, the nurse should obtain the patient's permission for them to remain in the room during the interview.

At times individuals who accompany patients are disruptive to an interview. For example, sometimes a parent, spouse, or friend answers questions for the patient. Usually these individuals are trying to be helpful, but it may also suggest a dominant personality. Such situations can adversely affect the accuracy of data collected, and the nurse must validate with patients that the information is correct. If others persist in answering for a patient, the nurse can specifically request them to allow the patient to answer or ask them to leave until the end of the interview.

A disruptive interview also occurs when attempting to talk with mothers with active children in the room causing constant distractions. If children are too young to wait in the waiting room, find developmentally appropriate activities for them while you complete the interview.

Language Barrier

A translator might be needed for accurate communication when patients speak a different language from the nurse. An objective observer who is the same gender as the patient is a better translator than a family member who may alter the meaning of what is said or describe what they think is wrong. Keep in mind that conducting an interview through a translator takes considerably more time than a typical interview because everything spoken must be repeated. For this reason, time must be used well; focus on collecting the most important data.

Cultural Differences

Nurses work with patients from many cultural backgrounds. Patient-centered care is provided when nurses develop cultural competence to identify cultural factors that may

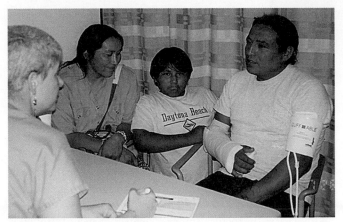

FIG. 2-2 Interact with the patient as a unique person and be sensitive to cultural diversities.

influence patients' beliefs about health and illness. The health care system places accountability for cultural competence with the nurse and others who give direct patient care.[3] Cultural competence refers to "the ability to communicate between and among cultures and to demonstrate skill outside one's culture of origin."[4] To deliver culturally competent care, nurses must interact with each individual as a unique person who is a product of past experiences, beliefs, and values that have been learned and passed down from one generation to the next (Fig. 2-2). However, remember that all individuals within a specific cultural group do not think and behave in a similar manner. Avoid stereotyping patients because of their culture or ethnicity. There may be as much diversity within a cultural group as there is across cultural groups. The nurse should ask patients about experiences that illustrate what has been of value to them and that characterize their culture. This increases the nurse's understanding and demonstrates interest in them as individuals. Further information about cultural considerations is presented in Chapter 5.

THE HEALTH HISTORY

Types of Health Histories

A health history is obtained from patients on every visit; the amount of data collected for a history depends largely on the setting and the purpose of the visit. A history is a component of all the types of health assessments described in Box 1-3, including a comprehensive assessment, a problem-based or focused assessment, and an episodic or follow-up assessment.

The *comprehensive health history* may be performed during a hospital admission, with an initial clinic or home visit, or when the patient's reason for seeking care is for relief of generalized symptoms such as weight loss or fatigue. A comprehensive health history requires more time than other types of histories because a complete database is being established. The admission process for many hospitals includes obtaining a comprehensive database. However, the patient's condition must be considered. For example, a critically ill patient is unable to participate in a comprehensive interview; thus it is inappropriate to pursue. Family members may be of assistance in providing important, essential information to the nurse while the patient is seriously ill. A comprehensive health history should be conducted once the patient is no longer critically ill. An example of a comprehensive health history for an adult is presented in Chapter 23.

The history for a *problem-based* or *focused health assessment* includes data that are limited in scope to a specific problem. However, it must be detailed enough that the nurse is aware of other health-related data that might affect the current problem. For example, the history for a patient with a lacerated foot should include information about the incident and symptoms and also medications that the patient is taking currently, medication allergies, other health problems that the patient has, and immunization status. Imagine the disastrous result that could occur if this patient had a history of diabetes mellitus and a severe allergy to penicillin and this information were not discovered. A focused interview is also used when the patient seeks help to address an urgent problem such as relief from asthma attacks or chest pain. Further data may be collected once the patient is stabilized, particularly if he or she requires ongoing care.

The history associated with an *episodic* or follow-up assessment generally focuses on the specific problem or problems for which a patient has already been receiving treatment. The nurse should assess for changes in the history since the last visit.

Components of the Health History

Because the scope of a health history varies with the type of health assessment to be conducted, the nurse can expect variations in history format. However, many components are found consistently in all health histories. A comprehensive health history includes the following components:

- Biographic data
- Reason for seeking care
- History of present illness
- Present health status
- Past health history
- Family history
- Personal and psychosocial history
- Review of systems

Biographic Data

Biographic data are collected at the first visit and updated as changes occur. These data begin to form a picture of the patient as a unique individual. Box 2-2 lists the data to be obtained.

Reason for Seeking Health Care

The reason for seeking care (also called the *chief complaint* [CC] or *presenting problem*) is a brief statement of the patient's purpose for requesting the services of a health care provider. The patient's reason for seeking care is often recorded in direct quotes. Some patients present for a routine examination or well visit and thus do not have a chief complaint or presenting problem. When multiple complaints or

---

> **BOX 2-2   BIOGRAPHIC DATA**
>
> - Name
> - Gender
> - Address, telephone number, and email address
> - Birth date
> - Birthplace (important when born in foreign country)
> - Race/ethnicity
> - Religion
> - Marital status
> - Occupation
> - Contact person
> - Source of data

problems are verbalized, list them all and ask patients to indicate the priority of the problems. Some patients initially may be uncomfortable giving the nurse the actual reason for seeking care. When this is the case, they may not divulge the true reason they came until the end of the visit, after they begin to feel more comfortable. The patient's condition dictates how the nurse proceeds. Urgency dictates expediency. Patients with severe pain, dyspnea, or injury should not be subjected to a prolonged history. Biographic data may be delayed to pursue the health concern. This approach enables the nurse to analyze the data quickly, identify the cause of the health concern, prioritize the patient's needs, and plan how to alleviate the signs or symptoms.

History of Present Illness

When patients seek health care for a specific problem, the nurse documents the present illness or problem as described previously but then should further investigate the history of the present problem. This is best accomplished by conducting a *symptom analysis* (a systematic way to collect data about the history and status of symptoms). Not all individuals seeking health care have a specific problem or illness; thus recording a history of present illness or a symptom analysis is not always indicated.

Several formats are used to conduct a symptom analysis, but it should include all of the following variables: onset of symptoms, location and duration of symptoms, characteristics, aggravating and alleviating factors, related symptoms, attempts at self-treatment, and severity of symptoms (Box 2-3). Patients may describe not only symptoms but also objective findings (or signs), as illustrated in the following example.

Jeff, a 23-year-old man, comes to an urgent care center after falling 9 feet while rock climbing the previous afternoon. The presenting problem is recorded as "injured foot." Jeff tells the nurse that his ankle and foot hurt quite a lot—an 8 on a scale of 0 to 10. Jeff also reports that his foot and ankle are swollen "twice the normal size" and he noticed that there is extensive bruising around the ankle. These data are included in the history because these are subjective data being reported by the patient. When the nurse observes edema and ecchymosis around the foot or ankle, these data are also recorded as objective data in the examination section of the medical record.

BOX 2-3 MNEMONIC FOR SYMPTOM ANALYSIS: OLD CARTS

Onset: When Did the Symptoms Begin?
- When did the symptom(s) begin?
- Did they develop suddenly or over a period of time? (Ask specific date, time, day of week if appropriate.)
- Where were you or what were you doing when the symptoms began?
- Does anyone else with whom you have been in contact have a similar symptom?

Location: Where Are the Symptoms?
- Are they located in a specific area?
- Are they vague and generalized?
- Does symptom radiate to another location?

Duration: How Long Do the Symptoms Last?
- Since they began, have the symptoms become worse? About the same?
- Are symptoms constant or intermittent (come and go)?
- If constant, does the severity of symptoms fluctuate?
- If intermittent, how many times a day, week, or month do the symptoms occur? How do you feel between episodes of the symptom?

Characteristics: Describe the Characteristics of the Symptoms
- Describe how the symptoms feel or look.
- Describe the sensation: stabbing, dull, aching, throbbing, nagging, sharp, squeezing, itching.
- If applicable, describe the appearance: color, texture, composition, and odor.

Aggravating and Alleviating Factors: What Affects the Symptoms?
- What makes the symptoms worse? Is symptom aggravated by an activity (e.g., walking, climbing stairs, eating, a body position)? Are there psychologic or physical factors in the environment that may be causing them (e.g., stress, smoke, chemicals)?
- What makes the symptoms better? Do certain body positions relieve the symptoms?

Related Symptoms: Are Other Symptoms Present?
- Have you noticed that other symptoms have occurred at the same time (e.g., fever, nausea, pain)?

Treatment: Describe Self-Treatment Before Seeking Care
- Which methods of self-treatment have you tried? Medications? (If so, ask the name of the medication, dosage, and time of last dose.) Heat applications? Cold applications?
- Have any of these methods been effective?
- Have you seen another health care provider for this same problem?

Severity: Describe the Severity of the Symptom
- Describe the size, extent, number, or amount.
- On a scale of 0 to 10, with 10 being most severe, how would you rate your symptom?
- Is the symptom so severe that it interrupts your activities (e.g., work, school, eating, sleeping)?

Present Health Status

The present health status focuses on the patient's conditions (acute and chronic), medications the patient is currently taking, and allergies the patient has experienced.

- *Health Conditions.* Examples include diabetes, hypertension, heart disease, sickle cell anemia, cancer, seizures, pulmonary disease, arthritis, mental illness. Ask patients how long they have had the condition(s) and the impact of the illness on their daily activities.
- *Medications.* Inquire about prescription, over-the-counter, and herbal preparations. Include the reason for taking the medication, how long the patient has been taking it, dose and frequency, any adverse effects, and the patient's perception of its effectiveness.
- *Allergies.* Ask patients about allergies to foods, medications, environmental factors, and contact substances. Be sure to ask specifically about substances to which patients could be exposed in the health care setting such as latex and iodine. The nurse should explain the term *allergy* to ensure that patients understand the question. Many people do not know the difference between an adverse effect (such as nausea) and a true allergic reaction (such as rash or difficulty breathing).

When patients indicate that they have an allergy to a medication or substance, ask them to describe what happens with exposure to determine if the reaction is an adverse effect or an allergic reaction.

Past Health History

The past health history is important because past and present conditions may have some effect on the patient's current health needs and problems. The following data categories are included:

- *Childhood illnesses:* measles, mumps, rubella, chickenpox, pertussis, *Haemophilus influenzae* infection, streptococcal throat infection, otitis media (Ask if there were complications in later years such as rheumatic fever or glomerulonephritis that can occur after streptococcal throat infection.)
- *Surgeries:* types, dates, outcomes
- *Hospitalizations:* illnesses, dates, outcomes
- *Accidents or injuries:* type (fractures, lacerations, loss of consciousness, burns, penetrating wounds), dates, outcomes
- *Immunizations:* tetanus, diphtheria, pertussis, mumps, rubella, poliomyelitis, hepatitis A or B, influenza,

pneumococcal pneumonia, and varicella; for foreign-born patients: bacille Calmette-Guérin (BCG)

- *Last examinations:* type (physical, dental, vision, hearing, electrocardiogram [ECG], chest radiograph, skin test for tuberculosis; for women: Papanicolaou [Pap] test, mammogram; for men: prostate examination), dates, and outcomes
- *Obstetric history:* number of pregnancies (gravidity), number of births (parity), and number of abortions/miscarriages if applicable (If working with a pregnant patient or woman in childbearing years, further information is recorded; see Chapter 20.)

Family History

A family history of the patient's blood relatives (biologic grandparents, parents, aunts, uncles, and siblings), spouse, and children is obtained to identify illnesses of genetic, familial, or environmental nature that might affect the patient's current or future health. As recommended in the Competencies of Genetic and Genomic Nursing, trace back at least three generations.[5] Specifically ask about the presence of any of the following diseases among family members: Alzheimer's disease, cancer (all types), diabetes mellitus (specify type 1 or type 2), coronary artery disease (including myocardial infarction), hypertension, stroke, seizure disorders, mental illness (including depression, bipolar, schizophrenia), substance abuse, endocrine diseases (specify), and kidney disease. The family history can be documented in narrative form, or it can be illustrated. A genogram is a tool consisting of a family-tree diagram depicting members within a family over several generations. This tool is useful in tracing diseases with genetic links. Symbols are used to indicate males and females and those who are alive and deceased. Include the current ages of those who are alive and the cause of and age at death of those who are deceased (Fig. 2-3).

Personal and Psychosocial History

The personal and social history explores a variety of topics, including information that affects and reflects the patient's physical and mental health.

Personal Status. Ask the patient for a general statement of feelings about self. Ask about cultural/religious affiliations and practices. Ask about education preparation; occupational history, satisfaction with work, and perception of adequate time for leisure and rest; and current hobbies and interests.

Family and Social Relationships. Ask about general satisfaction with interpersonal relationships, including significant others, persons with whom patient lives, and the patient's role within the family. Sometimes health information about significant others, sexual partners, and roommates is relevant to the patient's health. Ask about the current state of health for these family members. Ask about social interactions with friends, participation in social organizations (community, school, work), and participation in spiritual or religious groups. If interactions are limited, find out what keeps the patient from social interactions—perhaps this is by choice, or there could be an underlying problem. Be aware of issues associated with domestic violence; make a point to screen all patients (Box 2-4).

Diet/Nutrition. Patients should describe their appetite and a typical daily dietary intake for both food and fluids. Inquire about food preferences and dislikes, food intolerances, use of caffeine-containing beverages, dietary restrictions, and use of dietary supplements such as vitamins or protein drinks. Ask about recent changes in appetite or weight, changes in the taste of food, or problems with nutritional intake (e.g., indigestion, pain or difficulty associated with eating, heartburn, bloating, difficulty chewing or swallowing). Also ask about overeating, sporadic eating, or intentional fasting. Further information about a dietary history is presented in Chapter 8.

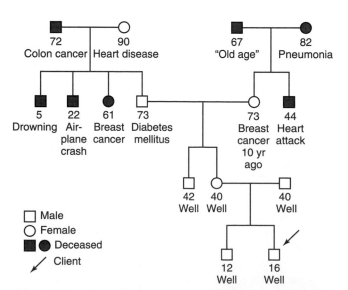

FIG. 2-3 Sample genogram identifying great-grandparents, grandparents, parents, aunts, uncles, and siblings.

BOX 2-4   DOMESTIC VIOLENCE

Recognizing Domestic Violence
- *What:* Domestic violence can be either physical or emotional and occurs within the home.
- *Victims:* Victims are usually women and children; men have been known to be victimized, although less frequently.
- *Perpetrators:* The perpetrator is most often an intimate partner or parent figure.
- *Contributing factors:* Domestic violence is often associated with drug or alcohol use (or both).

Screening Questions for Domestic Violence
Ask the patient:
- Have you been physically injured (hit, kicked, punched) by someone in your home in the last year?
- Many women are victims of domestic violence. Do you feel safe in your current relationship with your husband or significant other?
- Are you fearful of an individual with whom you have previously had a relationship?

Functional Ability. The functional ability (or functional assessment) focuses on a person's ability to perform self-care activities such as dressing, toileting, bathing, eating, and ambulating. Functional ability also includes a person's ability to perform skills needed for independent living such as shopping, cooking, housekeeping, and managing finances. Ask patients questions related to their perceived ability to complete these tasks. Assessment of functional ability is especially important for adults with physical or mental disabilities and for older adults.

Mental Health. Ask the patient about personal stress and sources of stress. Common causes of stress include recent life changes such as divorce, moving, family illness, new baby, new job, and finances. Also ask about feelings of anxiety or nervousness, depression, irritability, or anger. Explore with the patient personal coping strategies for stressful situations and previous counseling or mental health care in the past. Further information about obtaining a mental health history is presented in Chapter 7.

Tobacco, Alcohol, and Illicit Drug Use. The personal habits most detrimental to health include tobacco use, excessive intake of alcohol, and use of illicit street drugs. Obtain specific information, including the substance used, the amount of use, and the duration of the habit.

- *Tobacco:* identify type of tobacco used (cigarette, cigars, pipe, chewing tobacco) and frequency. For cigarette smokers, record the smoking history in *pack-years* (the number of packs per day times the number of years smoked). For example, a patient who has smoked one-half pack a day for 20 years has a 10 pack-year smoking history.
- *Alcohol:* identify the type and amount of alcohol consumed. Ask how many alcoholic drinks are consumed in a day; if not daily use, then weekly or monthly. Ask about driving under the influence of alcohol. Screening questionnaires such as the Alcohol Use Disorders Identification Test (AUDIT) screening test can be used to assess problem drinking and are discussed further in Chapter 7.
- *Illicit drug use:* specifically ask about use of marijuana, cocaine, crack cocaine, barbiturates, and amphetamines. Ask about high-risk behaviors such as sharing needles or driving under the influence of drugs.

Health Promotion Activities. Ask the patient which activities are regularly performed to maintain health. Specifically ask about exercise, stress management, usual sleep habits, use of seat belts, routine examinations, and self-examinations (such as breast self-examinations or testicular self-examinations). Health promotion practices can be assessed further when reviewing specific body systems.

Environment. The history also includes data related to environmental health. Obtain a general statement of the patient's assessment of environmental safety or concerns. Variables to consider include potential hazards within the home (lack of fire and smoke detectors, poor lighting, steep stairs, inadequate heat, open gas heaters, inadequate pest control, violent behaviors), hazards in the neighborhood or community (noise, water and air pollution, heavy traffic on surrounding streets, overcrowding, violence, firearms, sale/use of street drugs), and hazards associated with employment (inhalants, noise, heavy lifting, machinery, psychologic stress). Also ask patients about recent travel outside the United States (when and which countries visited, length of stay).

Review of Systems

Review of systems is conducted to inquire about the past and present health of each of the patient's body systems. Conduct a symptom analysis when the patient acknowledges the presence of symptoms (see Box 2-3). If sufficient data have been collected about a body system from the present illness/present health status section, these questions are not repeated. For example, if you completed a symptom analysis on "cough" when completing the present health status, you need not repeat questions about cough in the review of systems.

Symptoms listed in the review of systems are written in medical terms. A brief definition of each term is included as needed to facilitate patient understanding. For example, if the nurse wants to know if the patient has dyspnea, the nurse asks, "Do you become short of breath?" If the patient says, "No," the nurse documents "denies dyspnea" or "no dyspnea," but if the patient says, "Yes," questions from the symptom analysis are used, and findings documented. Therefore use medical terms for documentation and communication with other health care providers, but only use terms understood by the patient during the interview. Although some health promotion data are included in other sections of the health history, additional information is collected during the review of systems.

An outline of symptoms to ask the patient follows. This list, organized by body system or region, is not inclusive; rather it is an example of questions to ask. More detailed questions are presented in the chapters that follow. Remember that a comprehensive health assessment includes most of the questions; in a focused health assessment nurses only ask about systems related to the reason for seeking care. In an episodic or follow-up assessment, the questions are limited to asking the patient about changes since the last visit.

General Symptoms
- Pain; general fatigue, weakness; fever; problems with sleep; unexplained changes in weight

Integumentary System *(see Chapter 9)*
- *Skin:* skin disease, problems, lesions (wounds, sores, growths); excessive dryness, diaphoresis (sweating), or odors; changes in temperature, texture, or pigmentation; discoloration; rashes, pruritus (itching); frequent bruising
- *Hair* (refers to all body hair, not just head and pubic area): changes in amount, texture, character, distribution; alopecia (loss of hair); scalp itching
- *Nails:* changes in texture, color, shape
- *Health Promotion:* measures taken to limit sun exposure; use of sunscreen; skin self-examination; type and frequency of nail care

Head and Neck (see Chapter 10)

- *Head:* headaches; past significant trauma; vertigo (dizziness); syncope (brief lapse of consciousness)
- *Eyes:* discharge, redness, pruritus; excessive tearing; eye pain; changes in vision (generalized or vision field); difficulty reading; visual disturbances such as blurred vision, photophobia (sensitivity to light), blind spots, floaters, halos around lights, diplopia (double vision), or flashing lights; use of corrective or prosthetic devices; interference with activities of daily living
- *Ears:* pain; excessive cerumen (earwax); discharge; recurrent infections; changes in hearing (deceased hearing or increased sensitivity to environmental noises); tinnitus (ringing or crackling); use of prosthetic devices; change in balance; interference with activities of daily living
- *Nose, nasopharynx, and paranasal sinuses:* nasal discharge; frequent epistaxis (nosebleed); sneezing; obstruction; sinus pain; postnasal drip; change in ability to smell; snoring
- *Mouth and oropharynx:* sore throat; tongue or mouth lesion (abscess, sore, ulcer); bleeding gums; use of prosthetic devices (dentures, bridges); altered taste; dysphagia (difficulty swallowing); difficulty chewing; changes to voice or hoarseness
- *Neck:* lymph node enlargement; edema (swelling), or masses in neck; pain/tenderness; neck stiffness; limitation in movement
- *Health promotion:* use of protective headgear and eyewear; protection of ears from excessively loud noise; dental hygiene practices (brushing/flossing); dental care from dentist

Breasts (see Chapter 16)

- *General:* breast pain/tenderness; edema (swelling); breast lumps or masses, breast dimpling; nipple discharge; changes in nipples
- *Health promotion:* breast self-examination (frequency, method)

Respiratory System/Chest (see Chapter 11)

- *General:* cough (nonproductive or productive); hemoptysis (coughing up blood); frequent colds; dyspnea (shortness of breath); night sweats; wheezing; stridor (abnormal, high-pitched, musical sound); pain on inspiration or expiration; exposure to smoke or other respiratory irritants
- *Health promotion:* handwashing (reduction of respiratory infection); tuberculosis screening; wearing mask for occupational or environmental respiratory irritants or hazards; annual influenza immunizations (flu shots); smoking cessation; secondhand smoke

Cardiovascular System (see Chapter 12)

- *Heart:* palpitations; chest pain; dyspnea (shortness of breath); orthopnea (difficult to breathe unless sitting up); paroxysmal nocturnal dyspnea (periodic dyspnea during sleep)
- *Blood vessels:* coldness in extremities; numbness; edema (swelling); varicose veins; intermittent claudication (leg pain with exercise that ceases with rest); rest pain (leg pain with exercise that does not cease with rest); paresthesia (abnormal sensations); changes in color of extremities
- *Health promotion:* dietary practices to limit salt and fat intake; cholesterol screening; blood pressure screening; use of support hose if work involves standing; avoids crossing legs at the knees; exercise/activity

Gastrointestinal System (see Chapter 13)

- *General abdominal symptoms:* abdominal pain; heartburn, nausea/vomiting; hematemesis (vomiting blood); jaundice (yellowish color to skin and sclera); ascites (increase in size of abdomen caused by intraperitoneal fluid accumulation)
- *Elimination:* bowel habits (frequency, appearance of stool); pain or difficulty with defecation; excessive flatus, change in stools (color, consistency); problems with diarrhea or constipation; presence of blood in stool; hemorrhoids; use of digestive or evacuation aids (stool softener, laxatives, enemas)
- *Health promotion:* dietary analysis (compare diet to MyPlate); use of dietary fiber supplements; colon cancer screening

Urinary System (see Chapter 13)

- *General:* characteristics of urine (color, contents, odor); hesitancy; frequency; urgency; change in urinary stream; nocturia (excessive urination at night); dysuria (painful urination); flank pain (pain in back between ribs and hip bone); hematuria (blood in urine); dribbling or incontinence; polyuria (excessive excretion of urine); oliguria (decreased urination)
- *Health promotion:* measures to prevent urinary tract infections (females); Kegel exercises (performed to strengthen muscles of the pelvic floor to help prevent urine leakage)

Reproductive System (see Chapter 17)

- *Male genitalia:* presence of lesions; penis or testicular pain or masses; penile discharge; hernia
- *Female genitalia:* presence of lesions, pain, discharge, odor; menstrual history (date of onset, last menstrual period [LMP], length of cycle); amenorrhea (absent menstruation); menorrhagia (excessive menstruation); dysmenorrhea (painful menstruation); metrorrhagia (irregular menstruation); pelvic pain
- *Sexual history:* ask about current and past involvement in sexual relationships; nature of sexual relationship(s) (heterosexual, homosexual, bisexual); type and frequency of sexual activity; number of sexual partners (past and present); satisfaction with sexual relationships; method of contraception used (if applicable); changes in sex drive; problems with infertility; exposure to sexually transmitted infections; females: dyspareunia (pain during intercourse); postcoital bleeding (bleeding after intercourse); males: impotence; premature ejaculation
- *Health promotion:* methods to prevent unwanted pregnancy; protection from sexually transmitted infections; testicular or vulvar self-examination; Papanicolaou (Pap) test (females); prostate screening (males)

Musculoskeletal System (see Chapter 14)
- *Muscles:* twitching; cramping; pain; weakness
- *Bones and joints:* joint edema (swelling); pain; redness; stiffness; deformity; crepitus (noise with joint movement); limitations in range of motion; arthritis; gout; interference with activities of daily living
- *Back:* back pain; pain down buttocks and into legs; limitations in range of motion; reference with activities of daily living
- *Health promotion:* amount and kind of exercise per week; calcium intake; osteoporosis screening

Neurologic System (see Chapter 15)
- *General:* syncope (fainting episodes); loss of consciousness; seizures (which body parts moved, incontinence, characteristics); cognitive changes; changes in memory (short-term, recent, long-term); disorientation (time, place, person)

- *Motor-gait:* loss of coordinated movements; ataxia (balance problems); paralysis (partial versus complete inability to move); paresis (weakness); tremor; spasm; interference with activities of daily living
- *Sensory:* paresthesia (abnormal sensations, e.g., "pins and needles," tingling, numbness); pain (describe sensation and location)

Alternative Health History Formats

Not all health histories are organized in a body systems format as previously described. Alternative formats are based on a health status approach. Two examples include the North American Nursing Diagnosis Association Taxonomy II and Gordon's Functional Health Patterns.[6-7] These alternative approaches are used by nurses in many settings. An example of a health history based on Gordon's Functional Health Patterns is presented in Appendix A.

AGE-RELATED VARIATIONS

This chapter discusses principles of interviewing and conducting a health history with adult patients. Nurses will find that a health history may require a different approach and focus on different information, depending on the age of the patient.

INFANTS, CHILDREN, AND ADOLESCENTS

The pediatric health history is similar to that of the adult, with the addition of questions regarding pregnancy, prenatal care, growth and development, and behavioral and school status, as applicable. Most data are obtained from the adult accompanying the child, but the nurse should include the child as much as appropriate for his or her age. When obtaining a health history from an adolescent, the nurse determines if an adult or pediatric database and history format is more appropriate. In addition, a decision is made whether to interview the adolescent with the parent present or alone. Chapter 19 presents further information regarding conducting a health history from this age-group.

PREGNANCY

A comprehensive health history is obtained at the first prenatal visit to establish baseline data. This health history is similar to the information presented in this chapter, but with a special emphasis on data that could impact pregnancy outcomes. See Chapter 20 for further information.

OLDER ADULTS

The primary difference in conducting a health history with an older adult from that previously described is the incorporation of various age-related questions and questions involving functional status. Also, depending on the age of the older adult, data about childhood immunizations or developing a genogram may not be necessary. Remember that more time may be needed to conduct a comprehensive health history for many older adults because they may have multiple symptoms, conditions, and medications and a long past health history. Chapter 21 presents further information regarding the health history for an older adult.

SUMMARY

Collecting a thorough history accomplishes several goals. It establishes a therapeutic relationship with the patient. It also provides a picture of the patient and identifies problems mentioned by the patient that you can confirm or refute during the physical examination. Once data are collected, they must be organized, synthesized, and documented. When you collect health history data in an organized manner, documentation becomes easier.

CLINICAL APPLICATION AND CLINICAL REASONING

See Appendix D for answers to exercises in this section.

REVIEW QUESTIONS

1. The nurse is interviewing an adult Navajo woman. Which statement demonstrates cultural sensitivity and acceptance of the patient?
   1. "How often do you visit the medicine man for your health care?"
   2. "Tell me about your health care beliefs and practices."
   3. "Many Navajo people are afraid of hospitals. Are you afraid?"
   4. "Have you ever had a physical examination with a physician or a nurse practitioner?"

2. The nurse is conducting an interview with Jeremy, a 17-year-old accompanied by his mother. Which statement by the nurse is an age-appropriate adjustment when conducting a health history on an adolescent?
   1. "Jeremy, do you have a girlfriend, and if so are you sexually active yet?"
   2. "Mrs. Williams, is your son sexually active yet?"
   3. "Jeremy, how do you incorporate safe sex practices into your daily life?"
   4. "Mrs. Williams, would you mind waiting outside for a few minutes while I discuss a few things with Jeremy?"

3. During an interview an elderly patient tells the nurse that she has periodic problems keeping her balance. The nurse asks her what she is doing when the episodes occur. Which area of the symptom analysis is the nurse pursuing with this question?
   1. Severity
   2. Frequency
   3. Aggravating factors
   4. Location

4. Which communication technique conveys genuine interest in what the patient has to say?
   1. Active listening
   2. Sitting close to the patient
   3. Maintaining professional dress and conduct
   4. Holding the patient's hand during the interview

5. A 62-year-old patient tells the nurse that he is in excellent health and does not take any medications. What is the most appropriate response by the nurse to follow up on the patient's statement?
   1. "Do you avoid taking drugs because of bad experiences?"
   2. "Which medications have you taken in the past?"
   3. "That is hard to believe. Most men your age take medications."
   4. "Do you use over-the-counter medications or herbal preparations?"

CASE STUDY

During an interview Jean Reinhardt provides the following family history. She is 37 years old, married, and in good health. Her husband is 43, also in good health. The couple has a 12-year-old son, an 11-year-old daughter, and a 10-year-old son, all in good health. Jean has a 42-year-old brother and three sisters who are 32, 36, and 40 years old. All of her siblings are in good health. Both of Jean's parents are alive. Her 70-year-old father has mild emphysema and is an only child. Her mother is 66 and has hypertension. Jean's mother has three siblings. The oldest brother (Jean's uncle) is 74 and suffers from glaucoma. Another brother is 72 and is in good health. A sister is 69 and has osteoarthritis. All of Jean's grandparents are deceased. Her paternal grandfather died at age 89 of prostate cancer. Her paternal grandmother died of heart failure at age 91. Jean's maternal grandfather died at age 86 of prostate cancer; her maternal grandmother died of "old age" at age 96. Jean does not know anything about her great-grandparents.

Activity
Draw a genogram for Jean's family history with the information provided.

Techniques and Equipment for Physical Assessment

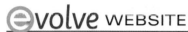

Before conducting an examination, you must become familiar with infection control practices, assessment techniques, optimal patient positions for examination, and equipment used to perform the examination. Safety measures are described throughout the chapter. Correct technique and proper use of equipment are essential for accurate data collection and patient safety.

INFECTION CONTROL PRACTICES

As health care providers, nurses are expected to incorporate infection control principles—referred to as *Standard Precautions*—in all aspects of practice. These precautions apply to all patients in all health care settings. Even though health assessment is a relatively safe activity, the potential for infection transmission exists. It can occur from patient to nurse, from nurse to patient, or from patient to patient via the hands of the nurse or equipment used by the nurse.

Hand Hygiene

Hand hygiene is considered to be the single most important action to reduce transmission of infection and is an essential element of Standard Precautions. Hands should be washed with soap and water when visibly dirty or contaminated, before eating, and after using the restroom. Use of an alcohol-based hand rub for hand hygiene is acceptable before and after direct contact with patients and contact with objects in the immediate vicinity of the patient (including medical equipment) and after removing gloves.[1]

Consensus recommendations for hand hygiene technique issued by the World Health Organization (WHO) include the following:

- When washing hands with soap and water, wet hands and apply enough soap to cover hands surfaces completely. Rub hands palm to palm, palms to back of hands with fingers interlocked, palm to palm with fingers interlocked, backs of fingers to opposing palms with fingers interlocked and rotating thumbs clasped in palms (Fig. 3-1). Rinse hands with water and dry thoroughly with a disposable towel. Turn faucet off using towel. When this process is done correctly, it takes 40 to 60 seconds.
- When decontaminating hands using alcohol-based hand rub, obtain a palmful of handrub and cover all surfaces of the hands. Rub hands in the same manner described previously until dry.

Personal Protective Equipment

Standard precautions guidelines for infection control include personal protective equipment (PPE) (e.g., gloves, masks, eye protection, face shields, and gowns) worn by the nurse. The Centers for Disease Control and Prevention Standard Precaution Guidelines[2] for personal protective equipment are presented in Box 3-1.

Latex Allergy

Occupational latex allergy has become a problem for many health care professionals because latex is found in gloves and many other types of medical equipment and supplies. A latex allergy is a reaction to proteins in latex rubber. The amount of exposure needed to produce a latex allergy reaction is unknown, but frequent exposure increases the risk of developing allergic symptoms.[3] Health care professionals are at risk for developing latex allergy because of their frequent exposure to latex. According to the American Latex Allergy

---

BOX 3-1   STANDARD PRECAUTION GUIDELINES

Personal Protective Equipment

Gloves

Gloves should be worn when contact with a patient's blood or other body fluid is possible or if handling equipment contaminated with blood or other body fluids.

Gloves are worn for three primary reasons:

1. To protect the health care worker from exposure to bloodborne pathogens carried by the patient
2. To protect the patient from microorganisms on the hands of the health care worker
3. To reduce the potential of infection transmission from one patient to another patient via the hands of the health care worker

The use of gloves does not reduce the frequency or importance of hand hygiene. Hands must be washed before performing a procedure even when gloves are worn and again immediately after removal of gloves. Gloves should be changed between procedures on the same patient if they have become contaminated to prevent cross-contamination. If a glove breaks during a procedure, it should be removed promptly and replaced with a new glove. Gloves should be discarded after all procedures; they should never be washed and reused.

Masks, Eye Protection, Face Shields

The nurse should wear a mask with eye protection or a face shield during procedures that may result in splashes or sprays of the patient's blood, body fluids, secretions, or excretions. Such equipment protects the mucous membranes of the eyes, nose, and mouth from contact, thus reducing the likelihood of pathogen transmission. Although not routinely needed for health assessment, situations may occur in which this equipment becomes necessary.

Gowns

A gown should be worn to protect the health care worker's arms and other exposed skin surfaces and to prevent contamination of clothing during procedures with the patient's blood or other body fluids or contact with other potentially infectious material.

From Siegel JD et al and the Healthcare Infection Control Practices Advisory Committee: *2007 Guideline for Isolation Precautions: Preventing Transmission of Infectious Agents in Healthcare Settings,* June 2007. Available at www.cdc.gov/ncidod/dhqp/pdf/isolation2007.pdf.

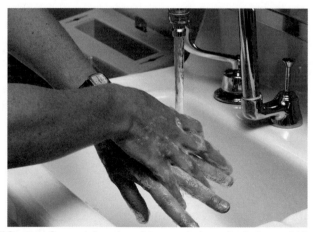

FIG. 3-1 Correct handwashing technique includes rubbing palms to back of hands with fingers interlocked.

BOX 3-2   PREVENTING LATEX ALLERGY

- Use nonlatex gloves for activities that are not likely to involve contact with infectious materials.
- If latex gloves are to be used, use a powder-free, low-allergen glove if possible.
- Do not use oil-based hand lotions when wearing latex gloves.
- Immediately after removing latex gloves, wash hands with mild soap and dry thoroughly.

From National Institute for Occupational Safety and Health: *NIOSH alert preventing allergic reactions to natural rubber latex in the workplace,* NIOSH publication no. 97-135, Cincinnati, 1997, NIOSH; National Institute for Occupational Safety and Health: *Latex allergy: a prevention guide,* NIOSH publication no. 98-113, Cincinnati, 1998, NIOSH.

Association, 8% to 17% of health care professionals have sensitivity to latex compared to 1% of the general population.[4] Latex reactions can range from a localized contact dermatitis of the skin, to contact dermatitis that involves the immune system, to a systemic reaction. Use of nonpowdered latex gloves and nonlatex gloves have been shown to reduce the incidence of latex allergy. The National Institute for Occupational Safety and Health recommendations to prevent latex allergy for nurses are summarized in Box 3-2.

Patients may also have a latex allergy; those particularly at risk are children with spina bifida and people who have had multiple medical procedures and surgeries, especially genitourinary surgery. For this reason nurses should routinely ask patients about latex allergy; if it exists they should protect the patient from coming in contact with latex gloves and other medical equipment made of latex such as urinary catheters and gastrostomy tubes.

Patient Care Equipment

Management of patient care equipment is another aspect of Standard Precautions.[2] The nurse should avoid touching equipment contaminated with blood or other body fluids unless gloves are worn. Multiple-use patient equipment that has been soiled with blood or other body fluids (e.g., a vaginal speculum) should not be reused until it has been adequately cleaned and reprocessed. Single-use items must be disposed of properly after patient use. The nurse must be cautious when handling contaminated sharp equipment. (Gloves do not provide protection from a sharp injury such as a needle-stick.) Appropriate handling of sharps includes the following principles:

- Never recap a needle after patient use.
- Never attempt to remove a needle from a disposable syringe by hand.
- After use, place disposable syringes and needles directly into a "sharps container" (i.e., a puncture-resistant container designated for contaminated sharp items).

TECHNIQUES OF PHYSICAL ASSESSMENT

Data for physical assessment are collected using four basic assessment techniques: inspection, palpation, percussion, and auscultation.

Inspection

Physical examinations begin with inspection. The term *inspection* refers to a visual examination of the body, including body movement and posture. Data obtained by smell are also a part of inspection. Examination of every body system includes the technique of inspection. For example, when inspecting the lungs and respiratory system, the nurse observes the shape of the chest, giving attention to breathing (noting the rate, depth, and effort of respirations); and notices the overall color of the skin, lips, and nail beds. During inspection the patient is draped appropriately to maintain modesty while allowing sufficient exposure for examination; adequate lighting is essential.

Inspection can be hindered when nurses have preconceived assumptions about the patient; thus thoroughly observing the patient with a critical eye becomes important. By concentrating on the patient without being distracted, the nurse notices potentially important data. Although inspection at first may seem like an easy assessment technique to master, practice is necessary to develop expertise.

Sometimes the use of equipment facilitates inspection of certain body systems. For example, a penlight may be used to increase the light on a specific location (looking in a mouth, looking at a skin lesion) or to create shadows by directing light at right angles to the area being inspected—a technique referred to as *tangential lighting* (Fig. 3-2). Other instruments such as an otoscope, an ophthalmoscope, or a vaginal speculum are used to enhance inspection for specific body systems. Equipment used to facilitate inspection is presented later in this chapter.

Palpation

Palpation involves using the hands to feel texture, size, shape, consistency, pulsations, and location of certain parts of the patient's body and also to identify areas the patient reports as being tender or painful. This technique requires the nurse to move into the patient's personal space. The nurse's touch is

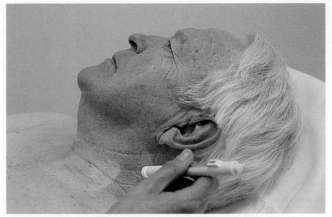

FIG. 3-2 Tangential light used to inspect jugular vein pulsation.

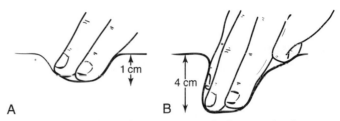

FIG. 3-3 A, Superficial palpation. **B,** Deep palpation.

gentle, hands are warm, and nails are short to prevent discomfort or injury to the patient. Touch has cultural significance and symbolism. Each culture has its own understanding about the uses and meanings of touch. Because of this, the nurse must tell the patient the purpose of and need for the touch (e.g., "I'm feeling for lymph nodes now") and manner and location of touch (e.g., "I'm going to press deeply on your abdomen to feel the organs"). Gloves are worn when palpating mucous membranes or any other area where contact with body fluids is possible.

The palmar surfaces of fingers and finger pads are more sensitive for palpation than the fingertips; thus they are better for determining position, texture, size, consistency, masses, fluid, and crepitus. The ulnar surface of the hands extending to the fifth finger is the most sensitive to vibration, whereas the dorsal surface (back) of the hands is more sensitive to temperature.

Palpation using the palmar surfaces of the fingers may be light or deep and is controlled by the amount of pressure applied. Light palpation is accomplished by pressing down to a depth of approximately 1 cm and is used to assess skin, pulsations, and tenderness (Fig. 3-3, *A*). Deep palpation is accomplished by pressing down to a depth of 4 cm with one or two hands and is used to determine organ size and contour (Fig. 3-3, *B*). A bimanual technique of palpation uses both hands, one anterior and one posterior, to entrap a mass or an organ (such as the uterus, kidney or large breasts) between the fingertips to assess size and shape. Light palpation should always precede deep palpation because palpation may cause

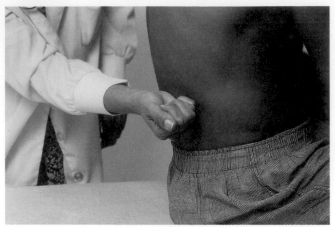

FIG. 3-4 Hand position for direct fist percussion of kidney.

tenderness or disrupt fluid, which could interfere with collecting data by light palpation.

Percussion

Percussion is performed to evaluate the size, borders, and consistency of internal organs; detect tenderness; and determine the extent of fluid in a body cavity. There are two percussion techniques: direct and indirect.

Direct Percussion

Direct percussion involves striking a finger or hand directly against the patient's body. The nurse may use direct percussion technique to evaluate the sinus of an adult by tapping a finger over the sinus or to elicit tenderness over the kidney by striking the costovertebral angle (CVA) directly with a fist (Fig. 3-4). How and where to strike the CVA is discussed in Chapter 13.

Indirect Percussion

Indirect percussion requires both hands and is done by different methods, depending on which body system is being assessed. It is an awkward technique at first but can be mastered with practice. For example, indirect fist percussion of the kidney involves placing the nondominant hand palm down (with fingers together) over the CVA and gently striking the fingers with the lateral aspect of the fist of the dominant hand.

Indirect percussion is performed by placing the distal aspect of the middle finger of the nondominant hand against the skin over the organ being percussed and striking the distal interphalangeal joint (between the cuticle and first joint) with the tip of the middle finger of the dominant hand. Placement of other fingers of the nondominant hand is important; they are spread apart and slightly elevated off the patient's skin so they do not dampen the vibrations (Fig. 3-5). The force of the downward snap of the striking finger comes from rapid flexion of the wrist. The wrist must be relaxed and loose while the forearm remains stationary. Rebound the striking finger as soon as it makes contact with the striking surface so the vibration is not muffled. Listen for the vibrations created by

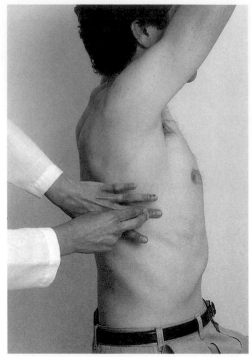

FIG. 3-5 Indirect percussion of lateral chest wall.

the percussion. The tapping produces a vibration 1.5 to 2 inches (4 to 5 cm) deep in body tissue and subsequent sound waves. Percuss two or three times in one location before moving to another. Stronger percussion is needed for obese or very muscular patients because thickness of tissue can impair the vibrations; the denser the tissue, the quieter the percussion tones.

Five percussion tones are described in Table 3-1. *Tympany* is normally heard over the abdomen. *Resonance* is heard over healthy lung tissue, whereas *hyperresonance* is heard in overinflated lungs (as in emphysema). *Dullness* is heard over the liver, and *flatness* is heard over bones and muscle. Detecting sound changes is easier when moving from resonance to dullness (e.g., from the lung to the liver).

Auscultation

Auscultation involves listening to sounds within the body. Although some sounds are audible to the ear without the use of special equipment (e.g., respiratory stridor, severe wheezing, and abdominal gurgling), a stethoscope is usually used to facilitate auscultation. The stethoscope blocks out extraneous sounds when evaluating the condition of the heart, blood vessels, lungs, and intestines (Fig. 3-6). Listen for the sound and its characteristics: intensity, pitch, duration, and quality (Box 3-3). Concentration is required because sounds may be transitory or subtle. Closing the eyes may improve listening because it reduces distracting visual stimuli. The isolation of specific sounds such as sounds of air during inspiration or a single heart sound is referred to as selective listening.

Precautions should be taken to optimize the quality of auscultation findings. Auscultation is best performed in a quiet room because environmental noise can interfere with

TABLE 3-1 PERCUSSION TONES

AREA PERCUSSED	TONE	INTENSITY	PITCH	DURATION	QUALITY
Lungs	Resonant	Loud	Low	Long	Hollow
Bone and muscle	Flat	Soft	High	Short	Extremely dull
Viscera and liver borders	Dull	Medium	Medium high	Medium	Thudlike
Stomach and gas bubbles in intestines	Tympanic	Loud	High	Medium	Drumlike
Air trapped in lung (emphysema)	Hyperresonant	Very loud	Very low	Longer	Booming

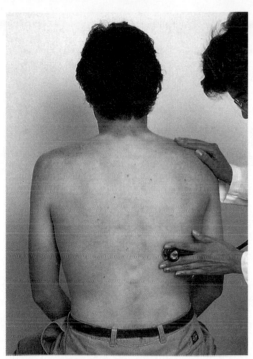

FIG. 3-6 The diaphragm of the stethoscope is stabilized between the index and middle fingers.

BOX 3-3 CHARACTERISTICS OF SOUNDS HEARD BY AUSCULTATION

- *Intensity* is the loudness of the sound, described as soft, medium, or loud.
- *Pitch* is the frequency or number of sound waves generated per second. High-pitched sounds have high frequencies. Expected high-pitched sounds are breath sounds, whereas cardiac sounds are low pitched.
- *Duration of sound vibrations* is short, medium, or long. Layers of soft tissue dampen the duration of sound from deep organs.
- *Quality* refers to the description of the sounds (e.g., hollow, dull, crackle).

hearing the sounds. The stethoscope must be placed directly on the skin because clothes obscure or alter sounds. Warm the head of the stethoscope before placing it on the patient. If the patient becomes cold and shivers, involuntary muscle contractions could interfere with normal sounds. The friction of body hair rubbing against the diaphragm of the stethoscope could be mistaken for abnormal lung sounds (crackles). Bumping the stethoscope tubing while auscultating produces a loud tapping sound that obscures underlying auscultation findings. Because the stethoscope diaphragm and bell are placed on a patient's skin, they must be cleaned between patients to prevent the spread of infection.

PATIENT POSITIONING

The patient may assume a number of positions during the examination; the positions depend on the type of examination to be performed and the condition of the patient. The sitting and supine positions are the most common. Various positions for examination are presented in Table 3-2. Draping

the patient appropriately is important to provide for patient modesty while allowing exposure needed for the examination. The inability of a patient to assume a position may be a significant finding about the patient's physical status and require the nurse to make necessary accommodations. For example, a patient who is short of breath may not be able to tolerate a supine position. In this situation the nurse elevates the head of the bed or examination table for certain aspects of the assessment (e.g., abdominal assessment).

EQUIPMENT USED DURING THE EXAMINATION

Examination equipment is used to facilitate the collection of data. Keep in mind that not all equipment presented in this chapter is used for all examinations. The type of equipment used varies, depending on the type of examination and the problem being assessed. Like a carpenter who chooses tools from a toolbox based on the job to be performed, the nurse chooses equipment based on the examination performed.

Thermometer

A thermometer is an instrument used to measure body temperature. Common thermometers used in health care settings are the electronic, tympanic, and temporal artery thermometers.

The electronic thermometer, used for measurement of oral, axillary, or rectal temperatures, consists of a

TABLE 3-2 POSITIONS FOR EXAMINATION

POSITION		AREAS ASSESSED	RATIONALE	LIMITATIONS
Sitting		Head and neck, back, posterior thorax and lungs, anterior thorax and lungs, breasts, axilla, heart, vital signs, and upper extremities	Sitting upright provides full expansion of lungs and better visualization of symmetry of upper body parts.	Physically weakened patient may be unable to sit. Nurse should use supine position with head of bed elevated instead.
Supine		Head and neck, anterior thorax and lungs, breasts, axilla, heart, abdomen, extremities, pulses	This is the most normally relaxed position. It provides easy access to pulse sites.	If patient becomes short of breath easily, nurse may need to raise head of bed.
Dorsal recumbent		Head and neck, anterior thorax and lungs, breasts, axilla, heart, abdomen	This position is used for abdominal assessment because it promotes relaxation of abdominal muscles.	Patients with painful disorders are more comfortable with knees flexed.
Lithotomy*		Female genitalia and genital tract	This position provides maximal exposure of genitalia and facilitates insertion of vaginal speculum.	Lithotomy position is embarrassing and uncomfortable; thus nurse minimizes time that patient spends in it. Patient is kept well draped.
Sims		Rectum and vagina	Flexion of hip and knee improves exposure of rectal area.	Joint deformities may hinder patient's ability to bend hip and knee.
Prone		Musculoskeletal system	This position is used only to assess extension of hip joint.	This position is poorly tolerated in patients with respiratory difficulties.
Lateral recumbent		Heart	This position aids in detecting murmurs.	This position is poorly tolerated in patients with respiratory difficulties.
Knee-chest*		Rectum	This position provides maximal exposure of rectal area.	This position is embarrassing and uncomfortable.

From Potter PA, Perry AG: *Basic nursing: essentials for practice,* ed 6, St Louis, 2006, Mosby.
*Patients with arthritis or other joint deformities may be unable to assume this position.

battery-powered display unit, a thin wire cord, and a temperature-sensitive probe (Fig. 3-7, *A*). The probe is covered with a disposable sheath before use and placed either under the tongue with the mouth closed, in the axilla with the upper arm held close to the chest, or in the rectum. The probe measures the temperature of the blood flowing near the tissue surface. The thermometer calculates and displays the temperature in either Fahrenheit or Celsius on a digital screen within 15 to 30 seconds.

The tympanic thermometer (Fig. 3-7, *B*) measures the temperature of the blood flowing near the tympanic membrane. The device works when the temperature-sensitive probe, covered with a disposable sheath, is inserted into the patient's ear; a temperature measurement in either

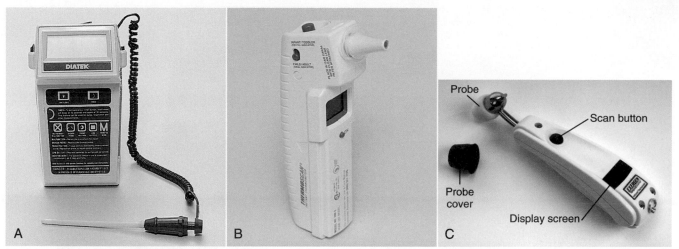

FIG. 3-7 A, Electronic thermometer. **B,** Tympanic thermometer. **C,** Temporal artery thermometer. (**B** from Seidel et al., 2011; **C** from Bonewit-West, 2012.)

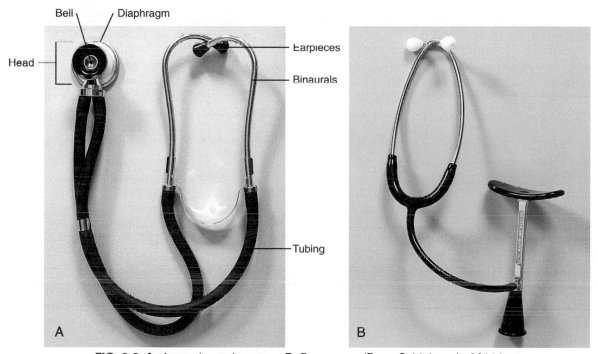

FIG. 3-8 A, Acoustic stethoscope. **B,** Fetoscope. (From Seidel et al., 2011.)

Fahrenheit or Celsius is displayed on the screen in less than 5 seconds. Multiple studies have evaluated the accuracy of tympanic thermometers with widely varied results[5-7]; thus the evidence for accuracy remains in question.

The temporal artery thermometer (Fig. 3-7, *C*) provides a temperature measurement from the temporal artery using infrared technology. Depress the scan button on the thermometer and slide it from one side of the patient's forehead to behind the ear. Heat emitted from the skin surface of the forehead and behind the ear is detected while scanning the temporal artery to record the temperature. The device is noninvasive and demonstrates a high level of accuracy in a study

involving children between ages 1 and 4 and among adults in a critical care setting.[8-9]

Stethoscope

A stethoscope is used to auscultate sounds within the body that are not audible with the naked ear. Although there are several types of stethoscopes (acoustic, magnetic, electronic, and stereophonic), the acoustic stethoscope is used routinely for health assessment (Fig. 3-8, *A*).

The acoustic stethoscope is a closed cylinder that transmits sound waves from the source through the tube to the ears. It does not magnify sounds but allows difficult-to-hear

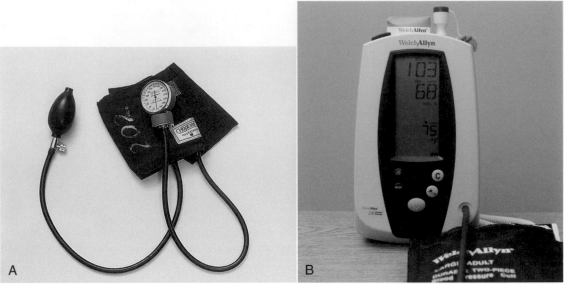

FIG. 3-9 A, Aneroid sphygmomanometer. **B,** Automated blood pressure device.

sounds to be heard more easily by blocking out extraneous room noise. The stethoscope consists of four components: the earpieces, the binaurals, the tubing, and the head. The earpieces, which may be hard or soft, should fit snugly and completely fill the ear canal. The binaurals are tubes of metal that connect the stethoscope tubing to the earpieces. They allow the earpieces to be angled toward the nose so sound is projected toward the tympanic membrane. The tubing is usually a firm polyvinyl material that is no longer than 12 to 18 inches (30 to 46 cm). If the tubing is longer than 18 inches (46 cm), the sounds may become distorted.

The head of the stethoscope consists of two components: the diaphragm and the bell. It should be heavy enough to lie firmly on the body surface without being held. This piece is configured by a closure valve so only the diaphragm or the bell may be activated at any one time. The diaphragm consists of a flat surface with a rubber or plastic ring edge. It is used to hear *high-pitched* sounds such as breath, bowel, and normal heart sounds. Its structure screens out low-pitched sounds. The nurse holds the diaphragm firmly against the patient's skin, stabilizing it between the index and middle fingers (see Fig. 3-6). The bell of the stethoscope is constructed in a concave shape. It is used to hear soft, *low-pitched* sounds such as extra heart or vascular sounds (bruit). When using the bell, the nurse presses it lightly on the skin with just enough pressure to ensure that a complete seal exists around it. If the bell is pressed too firmly on the skin, the concave surface is filled with skin, and the bell functions as a diaphragm and inhibits vibrations. Some stethoscopes have varying head sizes that are interchangeable. When assessing an infant or young child, the nurse uses a pediatric stethoscope, which has a small head. The diaphragm and bell should span one intercostal space of the patient's thorax.

A special type of acoustic stethoscope known as a fetoscope (Fig. 3-8, *B*) is used to auscultate the fetal heart. The fetoscope has a metal attachment that rests against the nurse's head. This metal piece aids in the conduction of sound so fetal heart tones are heard more easily.

Equipment to Measure Blood Pressure

Blood pressure is usually measured indirectly (noninvasively) using a manual sphygmomanometer or an electronic automated blood pressure device.

The sphygmomanometer consists of the gauge to measure the pressure (manometer), a blood pressure cuff that encloses an inflatable bladder, and a pressure bulb with valve used to manually inflate and deflate the bladder within the cuff (Fig. 3-9, *A*). A stethoscope is used in conjunction with the sphygmomanometer to auscultate the blood pressure.

The automated blood pressure device attaches to a blood pressure cuff (Fig. 3-9, *B*). It operates by sensing circulating blood flow vibrations through a blood pressure cuff sensor and converting these vibrations into electric impulses. These impulses are translated to a digital readout. The readout generally consists of blood pressure, mean arterial pressure, and pulse rate. The device is not capable of determining quality of the pulse such as rhythm or intensity. The device may be programmed to repeat the measurements on a scheduled basis and alarm if the measurements are outside of the desired limits. This feature is especially useful for patients requiring frequent blood pressure monitoring. A stethoscope is not required when the automated device is used. A study comparing the accuracy of manual and automated blood pressure measurements found that automated devices could be used with confidence to accurately measure systolic readings; caution was advised related to diastolic measurement.[10]

Blood pressure cuffs come in a variety of sizes and are either reusable (occlusive cloth shell) or disposable (a vinyl

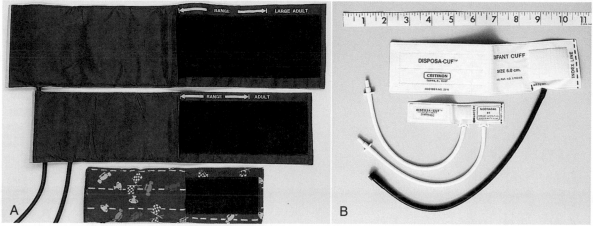

FIG. 3-10 Blood pressure cuffs in various sizes. **A,** Reusable cuffs in large adult *(top),* adult *(middle),* and child *(bottom)* sizes. Note the range lines above the Velcro material on the right side of each cuff. **B,** Disposable infant *(top)* and neonatal *(bottom)* cuffs. (**B** From Seidel et al., 2011.)

TABLE 3-3	SIZES FOR BLOOD PRESSURE CUFFS BASED ON ARM CIRCUMFERENCE
ARM CIRCUMFERENCE (MEASURED AT MIDDLE OF ARM)	**NAME AND SIZE OF CUFF**
5-7.5 cm	Newborn (4 × 8 cm)
7.5-13 cm	Infant (6 ×12 cm)
13-20 cm	Child (9 × 18)
22-26 cm	Small adult (12 × 22 cm)
27-34 cm	Adult (16 × 30 cm)
35-44 cm	Large adult (16 × 36 cm)
45-52 cm	Adult thigh (16 × 42 cm)

Based on American Heart Association Recommendations (Pinkering TG et al: Recommendations for blood pressure measurement in humans and experimental animals. Part 1: Blood pressure measurement in humans, *Hypertension* 45:142-161, 2005).

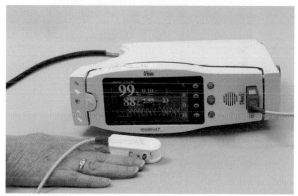

FIG. 3-11 Pulse oximeter shown with a clip and tape sensor probe. (From Potter et al., 2013.)

material) (Fig. 3-10). Both have a Velcro-type material on one end used to secure the cuff when wrapped around the arm. To obtain accurate results, the nurse must select a blood pressure cuff that is the correct size for the patient. If the cuff is too wide, it underestimates the blood pressure; if it is too narrow, it overestimates the blood pressure. Ideally the cuff width should be 40% of the circumference of the limb to be used. The bladder within the cuff should encircle at least 80% of the upper arm.[11] The American Heart Association recommends cuff sizes based on arm circumference (Table 3-3).[12] On most cuffs, range lines are indicated to assess proper size. When a correctly sized cuff is applied, the cuff edge should lie between the range lines (see Fig. 3-10). Adult cuffs are available in two widths. The standard cuff is adequate for most adults. If the adult is large or obese, an oversized cuff

may be used. If the adult has an extremely obese arm, the nurse uses a larger cuff designed to measure the blood pressure around a thigh. There are many different sizes of cuffs for children. The width of the cuff should cover two thirds of the child's or infant's upper arm. Only 43% of nurses participating in a study assessing their knowledge related to blood pressure measurement correctly answered questions regarding assessment of cuff size.[13] In another study, 22% of participants reported a lack of ability to regularly obtain the correct cuff size.[14]

Pulse Oximeter

The pulse oximeter, used to measure the oxygen saturation in arterial blood, consists of a light-emitting diode (LED) probe connected by a cable to a monitor (Fig. 3-11). The LED emits light waves that reflect off oxygenated and deoxygenated hemoglobin molecules circulating in the blood. This reflection is used to estimate the percentage of oxygen saturation in arterial blood and a pulse rate. The sensor probe is taped or clipped to a highly vascular area—typically a digit (finger or toe), an earlobe, or the bridge of the nose. Pulse oximetry

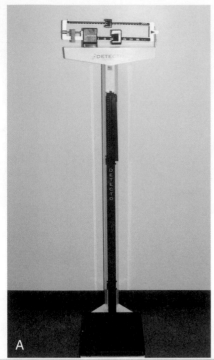

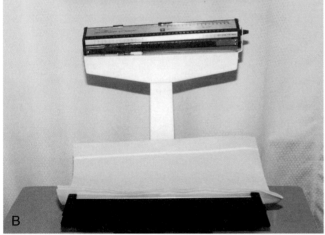

FIG. 3-12 A, Adult platform scale. **B,** Infant platform scale.

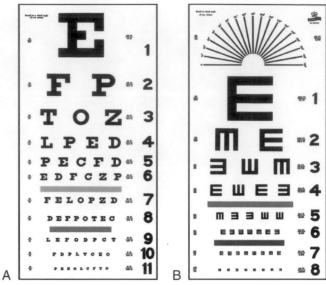

FIG. 3-13 A, Snellen visual acuity chart. **B,** "E" chart. (From Seidel et al., 2011.)

Electronic scales are also used in many health care facilities. When the patient steps on the scale, the weight is calculated, and a digital readout of the patient's weight (in either pounds or kilograms) is provided. Calibration of these scales occurs automatically with each use.

Infants are measured using an infant platform scale (Fig. 3-12, B). These work similarly to the adult platform scale but can measure weight in ounces or grams. The child may sit or lie on the platform while the weight is measured. Because the infant platform scale does not have a height attachment, height (length) is measured using a mat or board. This is discussed further in Chapter 4.

Visual Acuity Charts

Visual acuity or eye charts are used as a screening examination for visual acuity, color perception, and field perception. Several types of charts may be used.

Snellen Chart

The Snellen chart is a wall chart hung at a distance of 20 feet from the patient (Fig. 3-13, A) although some charts have been configured for use at 10 feet. The chart consists of 11 lines of letters of decreasing size. The letter size indicates the degree of visual acuity when read from a distance of 20 feet. The patient is tested one eye at a time. Beside each line of letters is the corresponding acuity rating that should be recorded (e.g., 20/40, 20/100). The top number of the recording indicates the distance between the patient and the chart, and the bottom number indicates the distance at which a person with normal vision should be able to read that line of the chart. Ask the patient to name the colors of the horizontal lines as a screening for color perception. The top line is green, and the bottom line is red. Also ask the patient which line is longer as a screening for field perception measurement. The green line is longer.

is considered highly accurate in the measurement of oxygen saturation over the range of 70% to 100%.

Scale

Measurement of body height and weight is accomplished using a scale. A standing platform scale is used for older children and adults (Fig. 3-12, A). The scale should be calibrated to 0 (zero) before measuring a patient's weight. The weight can be recorded in increments as small as 0.25 lb or 0.1 kg. Height is measured using the height attachment. This should be pulled up before the patient stands on the platform and then lowered until it is in firm contact with the top of the patient's head. Height is usually recorded in inches for infants and in feet and inches for children, adolescents, and adults. Measurement of height and weight using a platform scale is discussed further in Chapter 4.

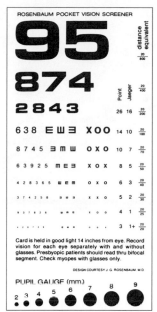

FIG. 3-14 Rosenbaum near-vision chart. (From Seidel et al., 2006.)

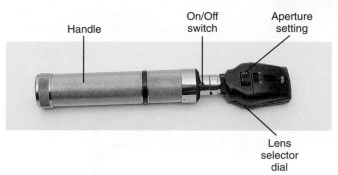

FIG. 3-15 Ophthalmoscope.

For young children or non–English-speaking individuals, the "E" chart may be used (Fig. 3-13, *B*). The nurse describes the "E" as a table with legs and asks the patient to point in the direction that the legs of the table point. The scoring of the "E" chart is the same as that of the Snellen chart. See Chapter 10 for further information regarding assessment of visual acuity.

Rosenbaum and Jaeger Charts

Two charts, the Rosenbaum and the Jaeger, are commonly used to evaluate near vision. The Rosenbaum chart consists of a series of numbers, *E*'s, *X*'s, and *O*'s in graduated sizes (Fig. 3-14). The patient should hold the chart 14 inches from the face. Each eye should be evaluated individually for visual acuity. Visual acuity is measured in the same distance equivalents as the far-vision acuity charts such as 20/20. The Jaeger equivalent is also shown on the Rosenbaum card. Alternatively near vision can be evaluated by asking the patient to read newspaper print that is held 14 inches from the face.

Ophthalmoscope

The ophthalmoscope is an instrument that consists of a series of lenses, mirrors, and light apertures permitting inspection of the internal structures of the eye (Fig. 3-15). This instrument consists of a head and a handle; the handle is a power source that contains batteries or connects to a wall-mounted electrical source. The head and handle fit together by a turn-and-lock system.

The head of the ophthalmoscope consists of two movable parts: the lens selector dial and the aperture setting. The lens selector dial allows the nurse to adjust a set of lenses that control focus. The unit of strength for each lens is referred to as a *diopter*. When the lens selector dial is turned clockwise, the positive, or black number–sphere, lenses are brought into place. The black numbers on the lens selector dial indicate increasingly positive diopter; these help the nurse focus on near objects within the patient's eye. Likewise, when the lens selector disk is turned counterclockwise, the negative, or red number–sphere, lenses are brought into place. The red numbers indicate increasingly negative diopter and help the nurse focus on objects that are further away within the patient's eye. The positive and negative lenses compensate for myopia or hyperopia in both the nurse's and patient's eyes and also permit focusing at different places within the patient's eye.

The aperture has several settings that permit light variations during the examination. The large light may be used for the internal eye examination if the patient's pupils have been dilated. The small light may be used if the patient's pupils are very small or if the pupils have not been dilated. The red-free filter actually shines a green beam of light. This filter facilitates the identification of pallor of the disc and permits the recognition of retinal hemorrhages by making the blood appear black. The slit light permits easy examination of the anterior of the eye and determination of elevation or depression of a lesion. The grid light facilitates an estimation of size, location, and pattern of a fundal lesion. Eye examination using an ophthalmoscope is discussed further in Chapter 10.

Otoscope

Inspection of the external auditory canal and tympanic membrane is performed with an otoscope. The traditional otoscope consists of two primary components: the head and the handle. Some otoscopes also have a pneumatic attachment (Fig. 3-16, *A*). The head of the otoscope consists of a magnification lens, a light source, and a speculum that is inserted into the auditory canal. On newer models of otoscopes such as the MacroView, an adjustable focus allows greater magnification and field of view compared to traditional otoscopes (Fig. 3-16, *B*). Specula come in various sizes. Choose the largest-size speculum that fits into the patient's ear canal. The handle of the otoscope is the power source; it either contains batteries or connects to a wall-mounted electrical source.

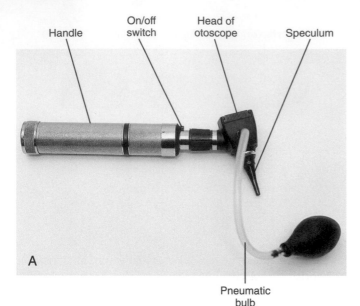

Handle   On/off switch   Head of otoscope   Speculum

A

Pneumatic bulb attachment

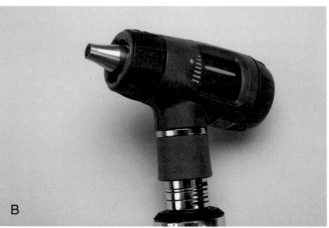

B

FIG. 3-16 A, Traditional otoscope with pneumatic bulb. **B,** MacroView otoscope.

The pneumatic attachment is used to evaluate the fluctuation of the tympanic membrane in children. This attachment consists of a small rubber tube with a bulb attached to the head of the otoscope. When the bulb is squeezed, it produces small puffs of air against the tympanic membrane, causing the membrane to move. No fluctuation of the membrane may indicate pressure from behind the membrane. See Chapter 10 for further discussion regarding use of the otoscope.

Penlight

The penlight provides a focused light source to facilitate inspection; thus it has many uses during a physical assessment (Fig. 3-17). It may be used to illuminate the inside of the mouth or nose, highlight a lesion, or evaluate pupillary constriction. To be effective the penlight must have a bright light source. The nurse can use the light transmitted from the otoscope if a penlight is not available.

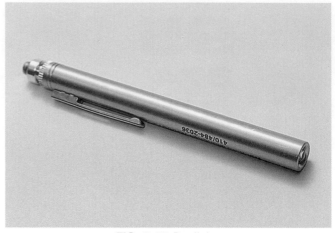

FIG. 3-17 Penlight.

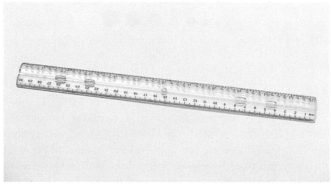

FIG. 3-18 Centimeter ruler.

Ruler and Tape Measure

Obtaining an accurate measurement of size is accomplished with a ruler or tape measure. A small transparent metric ruler that has both millimeter and centimeter markings is useful for measuring lesions or other marks on the skin (Fig. 3-18). A disposable paper tape measure is useful in various situations such as measuring the length of an infant or the circumference of an extremity. A tape measure that has inches on one side and centimeters on the reverse side is ideal. Nurses can estimate size using their hands or fingers if they know landmark measurements (e.g., the fingertip to the distal interphalangeal joint).

Nasal Speculum

A nasal speculum is used to spread the opening of the nares so the internal surfaces can be inspected. Two instruments can be used as a nasal speculum. The simple nasal speculum is used in conjunction with a penlight to visualize the lower and middle turbinates of the nose (Fig. 3-19). The instrument is used by gently squeezing the handle of the speculum, causing the blades of the speculum to open and spread the nares, which permits inspection of the internal nose. The second type of nasal speculum is a broad-tipped, cone-shaped device that is placed on the end of an otoscope. The nasal

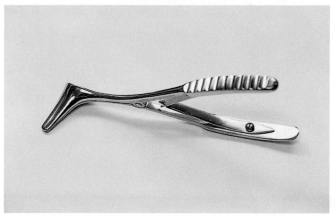

FIG. 3-19 Nasal speculum.

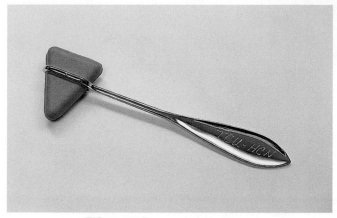

FIG. 3-21 Percussion hammer.

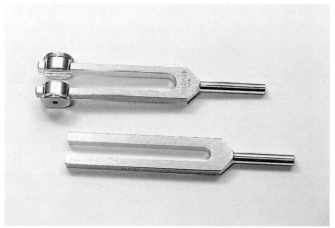

FIG. 3-20 Tuning forks for vibratory sensation *(top)* and auditory screening *(bottom)*.

cavity may be inspected by using the light source and viewing lens of the otoscope.

Tuning Fork

The tuning fork has two purposes in physical assessment: auditory screening and assessment of vibratory sensation. For auditory evaluation a high-pitched tuning fork with a frequency of 500 to 1000 Hz should be used (Fig. 3-20). A fork that vibrates in this frequency range can estimate hearing loss in the range of normal speech (300 to 3000 Hz). Hold the tuning fork at the base with one hand and squeeze the prongs together or tap them against your hand to engage. Vigorously striking the prongs results in a loud high pitch and could lead to inaccurate results. If a lower-frequency fork were used, overestimation of hearing ability could result. See Chapter 10 for further discussion of using a tuning fork to assess hearing with the Rinne and Weber tests.

For assessment of vibratory sensation, use a tuning fork with a pitch between 100 and 400 Hz. To engage, hold the tuning fork at the base and sharply strike the prongs on the heel of the hand. Place the vibrating tuning fork over a bone such as the malleus (ankle bone) and ask the patient if the vibration is felt. Patients who are unable to feel the vibration have reduced peripheral sensation. See Chapter 15 for further information on assessment using a vibratory sensation.

Percussion, or Reflex, Hammer

Deep tendon reflexes are tested with a percussion (reflex) hammer. This device consists of a triangular rubber component on the end of a metal handle (Fig. 3-21). The hammer is configured so either flat or pointed surfaces can be used to elicit the reflex response. The flat surface is more commonly used when striking the tendon directly and observing the patient response. The pointed surface may be used either to strike the tendon directly or to strike the nurse's finger, which is placed on a small tendon such as the patient's biceps tendon. A neurologic hammer can also be used to test deep tendon reflexes. It is similar to a percussion hammer, but the rubber striking end is rounded on both sides. The technique to assess deep tendon reflexes is found in Chapter 15.

Doppler

A Doppler is a device that amplifies sounds difficult to hear with an acoustic stethoscope. Ultrasonic waves are used to detect difficult-to-hear vascular sounds such as fetal heart tones or peripheral pulses (Fig. 3-22). To use the device, the nurse applies coupling gel to the patient's skin and slides the transducer over the skin surface until the blood flow source is heard in the nurse's earpieces. As blood in the vessels ebbs and flows, the probe on the distal end of the Doppler amplifies the subtle changes in pitch. The resulting sound heard is a swishing, pulsating sound. A volume control helps amplify the sound further.

Goniometer

The goniometer is a two-piece ruler that is jointed in the middle with a protractor-type measuring device used to determine the degree of flexion or extension of a joint (Fig. 3-23). The goniometer is placed over a joint; as the patient extends or flexes the joint, the nurse measures the degree of flexion and extension on the protractor. Goniometer use is discussed further in Chapter 14.

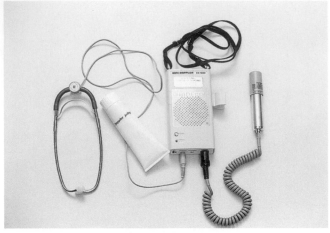

FIG. 3-22 Doppler.

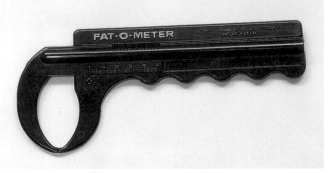

FIG. 3-24 Skinfold calipers.

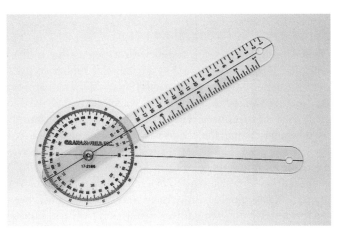

FIG. 3-23 Goniometer.

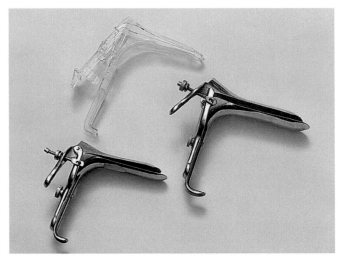

FIG. 3-25 Vaginal specula.

Calipers for Skinfold Thickness

Nurses estimate body fat by measuring the thickness of subcutaneous tissue with a skinfold caliper. Different models of calipers (e.g., Lang or Herpendem) may be used to measure the thickness of subcutaneous tissue at different points on the body (Fig. 3-24). The most frequent location for thickness evaluation is the posterior aspect of the triceps. Use of calipers to measure skinfold thickness is discussed further in Chapter 8.

Vaginal Speculum

A vaginal speculum is used to spread the walls of the vaginal canal as part of the pelvic examination. This allows the nurse to inspect the vaginal walls and cervix and collect samples for diagnostic testing. There are three types of vaginal specula: the Graves', the Pederson, and the pediatric or virginal. All of the specula are composed of two blades and a handle and are available as either reusable metal or disposable plastic models (Fig. 3-25). The Graves' speculum is available in a variety of sizes, with blades ranging from 3.5 to 5 inches in length and 0.75 to 1.25 inch in width. The bottom blade is slightly longer than the top blade. This configuration conforms to the longer posterior vaginal wall and aids with visualization. The Pederson speculum has blades that are as long as the Graves' speculum but much narrower and flatter. The pediatric or virginal speculum is smaller in all dimensions of width and length.

Plastic and metal specula differ slightly in ease of use and positioning. The metal speculum has two positioning devices. The top blade is hinged and has a thumb lever attached. When the thumb lever is pressed down, the distal end of the top blade rises and opens the speculum. The blade may be locked open at that point by tightening the screw on the thumb lever. The proximal end of the speculum may also be opened wider if necessary by loosening and then tightening another thumbscrew on the handle.

The bottom blade of the disposable plastic speculum is fixed to a posterior handle, and the upper blade is fixed to the anterior lever handle. When the lever is pressed, the distal end of the top blade opens; at the same time the base of the

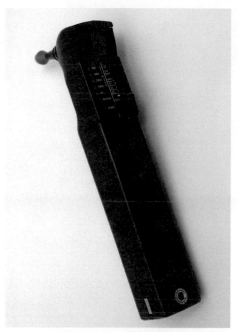

FIG. 3-26 Audioscope.

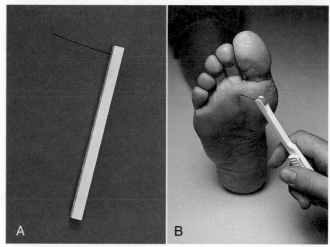

FIG. 3-27 A, Monofilament. **B,** Assessing peripheral sensation. (From Seidel et al., 2011.)

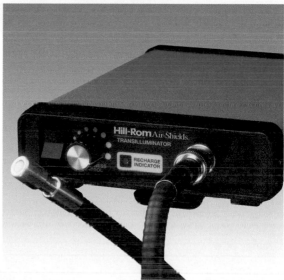

FIG. 3-28 Transilluminator. (Courtesy Draeger Medical, Inc., Telford, Pa.)

speculum widens. As the speculum opens, it goes through a series of clicking sounds until it snaps into the desired position. The patient should be forewarned about the clicking and snapping sounds. In addition, some of the plastic models have a port where a light source may be inserted directly into the speculum. See Chapter 17 for further discussion on use of the speculum.

Audioscope

An audioscope is used to perform basic screening for hearing acuity. The handheld, battery-operated audioscope is inserted into the patient's external ear (Fig. 3-26) and provides a fast, simple test to detect hearing problems. It systematically and automatically creates tones at the different frequencies: 1000, 2000, 4000, and 5000 Hz. A light appears when the specific tone at a given frequency is sounded. The patient is instructed to raise an index finger when the tone is heard, which should correspond to the light seen on the audiometer. Hearing assessment is discussed further in Chapter 10.

Monofilament

The monofilament is a small, flexible, wirelike device attached to a handle (Fig. 3-27, *A*) used to test for sensation on the lower extremities. The wire is placed on the skin surface and then bent (the wire bends at 10 g of liner pressure) (Fig. 3-27, *B*). The patient should indicate when and where the monofilament is felt. Patients who are unable to feel the monofilament when it is bent have reduced peripheral sensation. Typically the monofilament is used to assess sensation to the foot in several locations, including the plantar aspect of the foot, great toe, heel, and ball of the foot. It is used only over areas with intact skin. Examination of peripheral

sensation with a monofilament is discussed further in Chapter 15.

Transilluminator

A transilluminator is used to differentiate the characteristics of tissue, fluid, and air within a specific body cavity. It consists of a strong light source with a narrow beam at the distal section of the light (Fig. 3-28). When the examination room is darkened and the light is placed directly against the skin over a body cavity such as a sinus area, the transilluminator disseminates its light source under the surface of the skin. On the basis of the character of the glowing light tones, the nurse can determine if the area under the surface is filled with air, fluid, or tissue.

Wood's Lamp

The Wood's lamp produces a black-light effect and is used to detect fungal infections of the skin or corneal abrasions. The examination room should be darkened to enhance the determination of the lesion color. Skin lesions caused by a fungal infection exhibit a fluorescent yellow-green or blue-green color when examined with a Wood's lamp (Fig. 3-29). When fluorescein dye is placed in the eye, the Wood's lamp can also detect scratches or abrasions of the cornea.

Magnification Device

Many nurses use a small handheld magnification device to assist with inspection. Some of these devices come with a battery-powered light source. Magnification and lighting facilitate the inspection of wounds, skin lesions, and parasites.

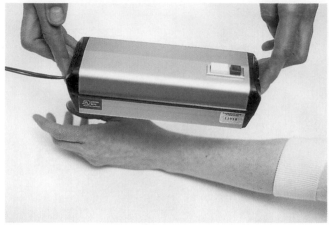

FIG. 3-29 Wood's lamp. The purple color on the skin indicates that no fungal infection is present.

CLINICAL APPLICATION AND CLINICAL REASONING

See Appendix D for answers to exercises in this section.

REVIEW QUESTIONS

1. The nurse is caring for a patient with a femur fracture. An external fixator is used to maintain alignment of the femur. The nurse palpates the top of the foot to make which determination?
   1. Amount of drainage from the wound
   2. Adequacy of blood perfusion to the foot
   3. Presence of air in the underlying tissue
   4. Range of motion to the foot

2. Auscultation is a component of which examination technique?
   1. Blood pressure measurement
   2. Visual acuity
   3. Examination of the ears
   4. Measurement of oxygen saturation

3. Which infection control intervention is used most frequently?
   1. Wearing gloves
   2. Using masks
   3. Wearing eye protection
   4. Hand hygiene

4. Which assessment data are determined by the application of a goniometer?
   1. Auscultation of fetal heart tones
   2. Inspection of the cervix
   3. Measurement of joint flexion
   4. Assessment of hearing

5. While examining a patient with an infected abdominal incision, the nurse notices that it is very malodorous. Which technique does this represent?
   1. Inspection
   2. Palpation
   3. Auscultation
   4. Percussion

General Inspection and Measurement of Vital Signs

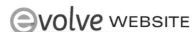

http://evolve.elsevier.com/Wilson/assessment

Initial data are collected from the patient before specific body systems are examined. These initial or baseline data are often referred to as *general inspection* and typically include the nurse's initial observations. Other terms include *general survey, general observations,* and *initial observations.* In addition to a general inspection, other baseline data collected include vital signs, height, and weight.

GENERAL INSPECTION

Begin the general inspection the moment you meet the patient. This involves observation of his or her physical appearance and hygiene, body structure, body movement, emotional and mental status, and behavior (Fig. 4-1). General inspection requires attention to detail and provides clues regarding possible problems the patient may be experiencing. Initial impressions gained from these preliminary observations direct the nurse to further examination in areas that do not initially appear normal.

Physical Appearance and Hygiene

The physical appearance includes a variety of general observations about patients, including general appearance, age, skin, and hygiene. Consider the patient's general appearance. Do you notice any obvious findings immediately (such as tremors or facial drooping)? Does the patient appear close to his or her stated age? Some patients appear older or younger than their stated age as a result of a number of factors such as drug and alcohol use, excessive sun exposure, chronic disease, and endocrine disorders (altered growth patterns or sexual development). Notice the color and condition of the patient's skin. Are there any variations in color or is there an

obvious presence of lesions? What is the patient's general hygiene? Is the patient clean and well groomed? Does the patient have a disheveled appearance? Are any odors detected? When unpleasant odors are detected, you must try to suppress reactions that may be communicated through facial expressions.

Body Structure and Position

Observations involving body structure include inspecting stature, general impression of nutritional status (i.e., well nourished, cachectic, or obese), and body symmetry (i.e., right and left sides of the body appear similar in size). Also note the patient's position or posture. Does he or she sit and stand up straight? For example, a patient with spinal deformities or back pain may have a slumped posture when standing or sitting. A patient who is having difficulty breathing may sit slightly forward, bracing the arms on his or her knees in what is referred to as a *tripod position.* A patient who is in pain may exhibit guarding or assume a *fetal position* while lying down.

Body Movement

Note how the patient moves. Does he or she walk with ease? Is the gait balanced and smooth with symmetric movement of all extremities? Note the use of assistive devices for ambulation such as a cane or walker. Note the ease of movement from standing to sitting and from sitting to lying. Does the patient move all extremities? Are there any limitations in range of motion of any of the extremities? Does the patient seem to guard extremities or show evidence of pain with movement? Also observe for the presence of involuntary movements such as a tremor or tic.

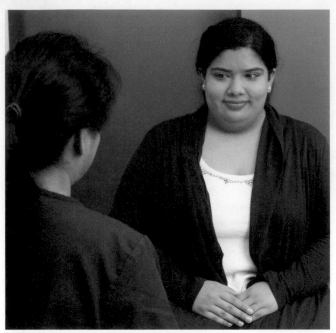

FIG. 4-1 General inspection begins immediately on meeting the patient. Note physical appearance, hygiene, body structure, movement, posture, emotional status, and behavior.

Emotional and Mental Status and Behavior

Emotional and mental status are evaluated by noting alertness, facial expressions, tone of voice, and affect. Does the patient maintain eye contact? Does he or she converse appropriately? Are the facial expressions and body language appropriate for the conversation? Is the clothing appropriate for the weather? Is the behavior appropriate?

MEASUREMENT OF VITAL SIGNS, HEIGHT, AND WEIGHT

Baseline indicators of a patient's health status include the measurement of vital signs (temperature, heart rate, respiratory rate, blood pressure, and oxygen saturation), height, and weight. Assessing the presence of pain is also considered standard baseline data to be collected on all patients and is often included with assessment of vital signs. Vital signs, pain assessment, height, and weight are usually assessed at the onset of the physical examination; however, they may also be integrated into the examination. Chapter 6 describes pain assessment.

Temperature

Body temperature is regulated by the hypothalamus. Heat is gained through the processes of metabolism and exercise and lost through radiation, convection, conduction, and evaporation. The expected temperature ranges from 96.4° to 99.1° F (35.8° to 37.3° C), with an average of 98.6° F (37° C). This is the stable core temperature at which cellular metabolism is most efficient.

Temperature changes occur as a result of normal variations and activities. Diurnal variations of 1° to 1.5° F (0.6° to 0.9° C) occur, with the lowest temperature early in the morning and the highest in the late afternoon and early evening. During the menstrual cycle a woman's temperature increases 0.5° to 1° F (0.3° to 0.6° C) at ovulation and remains elevated until menses ceases. This elevation is caused by progesterone secretion. Moderate-to-vigorous exercise increases temperature.

Temperature is measured by several routes, including oral, tympanic, temporal, axillary, and rectal. Thermometers measure body temperature in Fahrenheit and Celsius.

Oral Temperature

Temperature measurement by the oral route is safe and relatively accurate. Smoking or the ingestion of hot or cold liquids or food impacts the accuracy of measurement[1]; thus delay taking oral temperature readings for at least 10 minutes in such situations.

Cover the probe with a disposable sheath. Place the probe under the patient's tongue in the right or left posterior sublingual pocket. This location receives its blood supply from the carotid artery; thus it indirectly reflects inner core temperature. Ask the patient to keep the mouth closed while temperature is being measured. An electronic oral thermometer remains in place for 15 to 30 seconds until the audible signal occurs and the temperature registers on the display screen. Because the plastic sheath does not break, assessment of oral temperature with an electronic thermometer is safe for use with school-age children.

Another device is the pacifier thermometer. Pacifier thermometers have gained popularity in recent years because they are less invasive and well tolerated by children. They have also been shown to be comparable in accuracy to adjusted rectal core temperature.[2]

Temporal Artery Temperature

A temporal artery thermometer provides a temperature measurement of the temporal artery using infrared technology. Heat emitted from the skin surface of the forehead is detected while scanning the temporal artery to record the temperature.

To take the temperature, first place a disposable cover on the probe. Place the probe on the center of the patient's forehead, depress the scan button, and maintain contact with the skin while sliding the probe across the forehead into the hairline and behind the ear; then release the button and read the temperature measurement (Fig. 4-2). Movement of the probe to behind the ear before reading the thermometer accounts for evaporative cooling effect with diaphoresis. This device has shown a high level of accuracy among children and adults in a critical care settings.[3-4]

Tympanic Membrane Temperature

Tympanic thermometers measure temperature from the tympanic membrane. The probe is covered with a protective sheath and placed inside the external ear canal with firm but gentle pressure (Fig. 4-3). An ear tug in an upward direction on the helix for adults (and downward direction on the earlobe

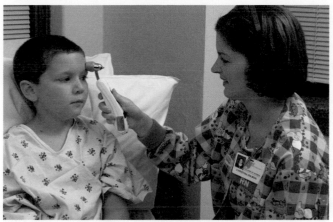

FIG. 4-2 Taking a temporal artery temperature. (From Potter et al., 2013.)

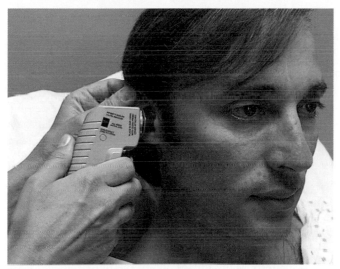

FIG. 4-3 Taking a tympanic membrane temperature. (From Harkreader, Hogan, and Thobaben, 2007.)

in infants and children) should be used to help straighten the external auditory canal to ensure measurement accuracy; the presence of impacted cerumen results in an inaccurate temperature measurement.[1] The probe must come in contact with all sides of the ear canal. (NOTE: The probe does not extend all the way to the tympanic membrane.) The thermometer is removed after the audible signal occurs (about 2 to 3 seconds) and the temperature reading is displayed.

Axillary Temperature

The axilla is a common site for temperature measurement on infants and children; however, it is an infrequently used site for adult temperature measurement. Results from research raise questions regarding the accuracy in measurement. Because it is not close to any major blood vessels and because it is placed between skin surfaces, the axillary site is thought to poorly reflect core body temperature. Multiple studies have shown that temperature measurements at the axillary site are less accurate than alternative sites.[5-6] To take an axillary temperature, place the probe of an electronic thermometer in the middle of the axilla with the arm held against the body until the audible signal occurs and the temperature appears on the screen. Normal temperature readings from the axilla are about 1° below the normal oral temperature.

Rectal Temperature

Rectal temperatures are taken less frequently than tympanic or oral measurements. Although rectal temperature measurement is considered safe and accurate for adults, it is less comfortable, requires more time, and has an increased risk of infection transmission compared to other routes.

To take a rectal temperature, place the patient in a Sims' position with the upper leg flexed. Appropriate privacy should be provided. Insert a disposable sheath over the thermometer probe and apply a water-soluble lubricant. Wearing gloves, insert the lubricated thermometer probe in the rectum 1 to 1.5 inches (2.5 to 3.8 cm) and hold in place until the audible signal occurs and the temperature is displayed on the screen. Rectal temperature readings are about 1° higher than oral readings.

Heart Rate

Heart rate is commonly assessed indirectly by palpating the pulse. The pulse *rate* is the number of pulsations felt in 1 minute. The *rhythm* refers to the regularity of the pulsations (i.e., the time between each beat). Further discussion of heart rates and rhythms is found in Chapter 12.

To take a pulse, place your fingers over the artery and feel for the pulsations and the rhythm. Pulses are palpated using the finger pads of the index and middle fingers. Firm pressure is applied over the pulse but not so hard that the pulsation is occluded. If the pulse is difficult to locate, vary the amount of pressure and palpate the location where you expect to find it. If the rhythm is regular (time between each beat is consistent), count the number of pulsations palpated for 30 seconds and multiply by 2 or count for 15 seconds and multiply by 4. If the pulse rhythm feels irregular (time between each beat varies), note whether there is a regularity to the rhythm (e.g., a skip every fourth pulsation), which is documented as a "regular irregularity"; or if the rhythm lacks regularity, which is documented as an "irregular irregularity." When rhythm irregularities are found, count the number of pulsations for 1 minute. Document an irregular pulse when recording vital signs. Expected heart rates for various age-groups are listed in Table 4-1.

Although a pulse can be taken in many areas, the radial artery is most frequently used to measure heart rate because it is accessible and easily palpated. The radial pulse is found at the radial side of the forearm at the wrist (Fig. 4-4). The brachial and carotid arteries are common alternative sites to assess pulse rate. The brachial pulse is located in the groove between the biceps and triceps muscles just medial to the biceps tendon at the antecubital fossa (in the bend of the elbow) (Fig. 4-5). The carotid pulse is found by palpating along the medial edge of the sternocleidomastoid muscle in the lower third of the neck (Fig. 4-6). The heart rate can also be assessed by auscultating the heart (known as the apical

TABLE 4-1	AVERAGE VITAL SIGNS THROUGHOUT THE LIFE SPAN				
VITAL SIGN	**NEWBORN**	**TODDLER**	**SCHOOL-AGE CHILD**	**ADOLESCENT**	**ADULT**
Heart rate (beats/min)					
• Range	120-160	90-140	75-100	60-90	60-100
• Average	140	110	85	70	70
Respiratory rate (breaths/min)	30-60	24-40	18-30	12-16	12-20
Blood pressure (mm Hg)					
• Systolic range	60-90	80-112	84-120	94-139	110-139
• Diastolic range	20-60	50-80	54-80	62-88	60-79

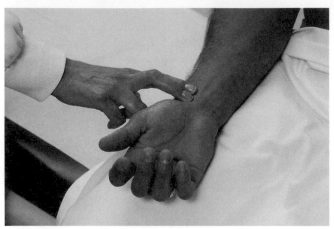

FIG. 4-4 Radial pulse.

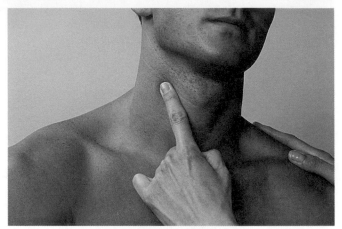

FIG. 4-6 Carotid pulse.

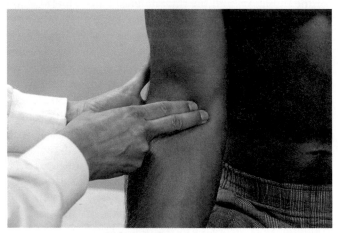

FIG. 4-5 Brachial pulse.

pulse) and counting the heart sounds for 1 minute. To auscultate the heart, place the bell or diaphragm of the stethoscope over the fifth intercostal space at the left midclavicular line over the mitral area. Auscultation of the heart is discussed further in Chapter 12.

Respiratory Rate

Assessment of the respiratory rate involves counting the number of times patients complete a ventilatory cycle (inhalation and exhalation) each minute. Men usually breathe diaphragmatically, which increases the movement of the abdomen; whereas women tend to be thoracic breathers,

which is noted with movement of the chest. Count the respiratory rate when patients are unaware that you are doing so; this prevents them from becoming self-conscious of the assessment and perhaps changing the breathing rate or pattern. Many nurses obtain the pulse rate and leave their fingers on the pulse site while they count the respirations so patients are unaware of when counting the pulse rate ends and counting the respiratory rate begins. Respiratory rates vary with age (see Table 4-1). Other factors that increase respiratory rate are fever, anxiety, exercise, and increased altitude. Respiratory changes associated with altitude are generally noticed beginning at about 8000 feet for those not acclimated; the higher the altitude, the greater the effects.[7]

In addition to assessing the rate, note the rhythm, depth, and effort of breathing. Rhythm is the pattern or regularity of breathing and is described as regular or irregular. Depth is assessed by observing the excursion or movement of the chest wall. It is described as deep (full lung expansion with full exhalation), normal, or shallow. Shallow breathing (small volume of air movement in and out of lungs) may be difficult to observe. The effort that goes into breathing is also observed. Normally breathing should be even, quiet, and effortless when patients are sitting or lying down.

Blood Pressure

Blood pressure is the force of blood against the arterial walls and reflects the relationship between cardiac output and peripheral resistance. Cardiac output is the volume of blood ejected from the heart each minute. Peripheral resistance is the force that opposes the flow of blood through vessels. For example, when the arteries are narrow, the peripheral resistance to blood flow is high, which is reflected in an elevated blood pressure. Blood pressure depends on the velocity of the blood, intravascular blood volume, and elasticity of the vessel walls.

Blood pressure is measured in millimeters of mercury (mm Hg). *Systolic blood pressure* is the maximum pressure exerted on arteries when the ventricles contract or eject blood from the heart. By contrast, *diastolic blood pressure* represents the minimum amount of pressure exerted on the vessels; this occurs when the ventricles of the heart relax and fill with blood. Blood pressure is recorded with the systolic pressure written on top of the diastolic pressure (e.g., 130/76), but it is not a fraction. The difference between the systolic and diastolic pressure is called the *pulse pressure,* which normally ranges from 30 to 40 mm Hg. Expected blood pressure ranges are shown in Table 4-1. A series of blood pressure measurements may also be taken when the patient is in a lying, sitting, and standing position to assess for *orthostatic hypotension.* (A 20– to 30–mm Hg drop in blood pressure when the patient goes from a lying or sitting position to standing indicates orthostatic hypotension.)

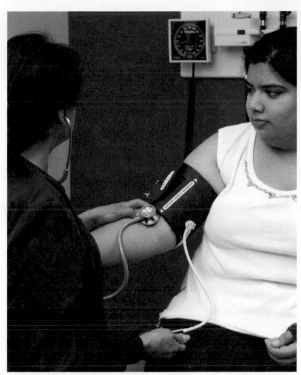

FIG. 4-7 Auscultating Korotkoff sounds to measure blood pressure.

Blood Pressure Measurement: Methods and Sites

Blood pressure can be measured directly or indirectly. Direct measurement is accomplished by inserting a small catheter into an artery that provides continuous blood pressure measurements and arterial waveforms. This direct measurement is done in the critical care setting when continuous monitoring is required. In all other settings blood pressure is measured indirectly either by auscultation (also known as *manual blood pressure measurement*) using a sphygmomanometer and a stethoscope (Fig. 4-7) or an automated blood pressure device—also known as *oscillometric blood pressure measurement* (see Chapter 3).

Indirect blood pressure typically is measured using the upper arm. Measuring blood pressure on a bare arm has been the gold standard for years, although findings reported from multiple studies show no significant differences in findings when measuring blood pressure over a thin layer of clothing.[8-9] Alternative sites to measurement include the thigh, calf, and ankle. A study comparing accuracy among sites recommended the ankle site in preference to the calf as an alternative site for blood pressure measurement if the upper arm is unavailable.[10] Approaches to measuring blood pressure using wrist and finger sites have been developed, but these lack acceptable accuracy and cost efficiency to be recommended for clinical practice.[11]

Measurement of Blood Pressure—Auscultation Method.
The procedure for measuring blood pressure by auscultation is described in detail in Box 4-1.

The auscultation method requires careful listening for *Korotkoff* sounds (named for the Russian physician who first described them). Blood flows freely through the artery until the inflated cuff occludes the artery enough to interrupt blood flow and silence any sounds. As the cuff pressure is slowly released, the nurse listens for the sounds of the blood pulsating through the artery again. The initial sound is called the *first Korotkoff sound* and is characterized by a clear, rhythmic thumping corresponding to the pulse rate that gradually increases in intensity (Fig. 4-8). The pressure reading at which this sound is first heard indicates the systolic pressure. A swishing sound heard as the cuff continues to deflate is the *second Korotkoff sound.* The *third Korotkoff sound* is a softer thump than the first; the *fourth Korotkoff sound* is muffled and low pitched as the cuff is further deflated. The *fifth Korotkoff sound* actually marks the cessation of sound and indicates that the artery is completely open. The manometer pressure noted at the fifth Korotkoff sound is the diastolic pressure. A great deal of practice is required to differentiate all five sounds, but this differentiation ordinarily is not necessary; in most cases only the first (systolic) and fifth (diastolic) Korotkoff sounds are recorded.

To take a thigh blood pressure reading, wrap a large cuff 7 to 7.9 inches (18 to 20 cm) around the lower third of the thigh, centering the bladder of the cuff over the popliteal artery. Follow the same procedure for taking a blood pressure measurement in the arm (see Box 4-1). Normally the systolic blood pressure is 10 to 40 mm Hg higher in the leg than in the arm. The diastolic pressures of arms and legs are similar.

BOX 4-1 PROCEDURE FOR MEASURING BLOOD PRESSURE (AUSCULTATION METHOD)

- With the patient sitting or lying down, position his or her upper arm slightly flexed at heart level with the palm turned up. The arm should be free of clothing.
- Palpate the brachial pulse in the antecubital space. Apply an appropriate-size blood pressure cuff (see Chapter 3) 1 inch (2.5 cm) above the site of brachial pulsation. The bladder of the cuff should be centered over the artery. The cuff should fit evenly and snugly around the arm.
- Position the sphygmomanometer at eye level no more than 3 feet (1 meter) away. Close the valve on the pressure bulb clockwise until it is tight but easily releasable with one hand.
- Palpate the brachial or radial pulse with the fingertips of one hand while inflating the cuff rapidly; note the point at which you no longer feel the pulse and continue to inflate 20 to 30 mm Hg above this point. Slowly release the valve to deflate the cuff and note the point at which the pulse reappears; this is the palpated systolic pressure. Immediately deflate the cuff completely.
- After waiting for 30 seconds, place the stethoscope over the brachial pulse and inflate the cuff to 30 mm Hg above the palpated systolic pressure. Release the valve and allow the cuff to deflate slowly at a rate of 2 to 3 mm Hg per second.
- Note the pressure reading on the sphygmomanometer when the first Korotkoff sound is heard: this is the systolic pressure. Continue to deflate the cuff slowly and note the point at which the sounds disappear: this is the diastolic pressure.
- Deflate the cuff completely and remove it from the patient's arm. Record the measurement.
- This procedure may be repeated on the other arm for comparison purposes.

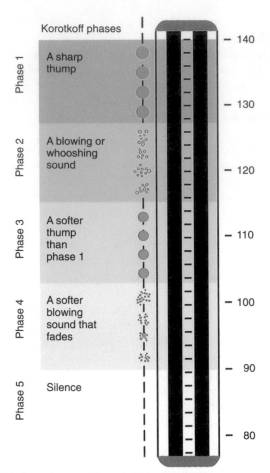

FIG. 4-8 Sounds auscultated during blood pressure measurement can be differentiated into five Korotkoff phases. In this example the blood pressure is 140/90. (From Potter et al., 2013.)

Measurement of Blood Pressure—Automated Blood Pressure Monitor. The procedure for measuring blood pressure with an automated blood pressure monitor differs somewhat from the procedure presented in Box 4-1. Because the automated monitor is an electronic device, Korotkoff sounds are not auscultated. The monitor senses circulating blood flow vibrations through a sensor in the blood pressure cuff, converts the vibrations into electric impulses, and translates the impulses into a digital readout indicating systolic and diastolic pressures.

One of the concerns raised with automated blood pressure devices relates to accuracy of blood pressure obtained. Familiarity with the equipment and following manufacturer guidelines are needed to optimize accurate results. For the automated blood pressure monitor to be accurate, the cuff must fit properly and be placed correctly on the arm so the sensor is directly over the brachial artery. Even when used correctly, the accuracy of automated blood pressure devices

has come into question. First, because of variability in calibration among devices, the potential for inconsistent readings occurs when multiple devices are used. Several studies comparing automated and manual approaches confirm acceptable accuracy and consistency for systolic readings; however, diastolic accuracy is less clear.[12-14] For this reason it is recommended that, if the blood pressure measurement using an automated device is very high or if there is any doubt about the blood pressure measurement obtained with an automated device, the blood pressure should be rechecked by auscultation as described in Box 4-1.

Physiologic Factors That Affect Blood Pressure Measurements

A number of patient-related factors affect blood pressure and should be considered when interpreting blood pressure measurements.

- *Age:* From childhood to adulthood there is a gradual rise.
- *Gender:* After puberty females usually have a lower blood pressure than males; however, after menopause, women's blood pressure may be higher than men's.

- *Race:* The incidence of hypertension is twice as high in African Americans as in Caucasians.
- *Diurnal variations:* Blood pressure is lower in the early morning and peaks in later afternoon or early evening.
- *Emotions:* Feeling anxious, angry, or stressed may increase the blood pressure.
- *Pain:* Experiencing acute pain can increase blood pressure.
- *Personal habits:* Ingesting caffeine or smoking a cigarette within 30 minutes before measurement may increase blood pressure.
- *Weight:* Obese patients tend to have higher blood pressures than nonobese patients.

Common Errors Associated with Blood Pressure Measurement

The accuracy of blood pressure measurement is significantly affected by technique. Research has found that many nurses demonstrated incorrect technique or lack of knowledge associated with blood pressure measurement.[11,14,15,16] In a study assessing improvements in accuracy among nurses, researchers[17] found that the technique among a sample of nurses was poor before an education program but improved significantly following remedial education.[17] This finding supports the recommendation from the Subcommittee of Professional and Public Education of the American Heart Association to retrain all health professionals on a regular basis.[14]

Incorrect technique can result in false-low or false-high measurements, potentially leading to inaccurate diagnosis or unnecessary medical care. Box 4-2 presents common errors in blood pressure measurement.

Oxygen Saturation

In many settings measurement of oxygen saturation is included routinely with vital signs. As discussed in Chapter 3, oxygen saturation is measured by a pulse oximeter—a device that estimates the oxygen saturation of hemoglobin in the blood. The probe is usually either clipped or taped to the patient's fingertip; the toe, earlobe, and nose are alternative sites. The oxygen saturation appears as a digital readout within 10 to 15 seconds after the oximeter is placed. Oxygen saturation levels lower than 90% are considered abnormal and require further evaluation. Although this is considered an easy procedure, deficiencies in nurses' knowledge of pulse oximetry measurement and interpretation of results have been reported.[18]

Pain

Routine assessment of a patient's pain or comfort level is standard practice in all health care settings and is often assessed with vital sign measurement. An in-depth discussion of pain assessment is presented in Chapter 6.

Weight

Body weight or mass is influenced by a number of factors, including genetics, dietary intake, exercise, and fluid volume. Genetics influence height and body size, including bone structure, muscle mass, and gender. Body weight is important for nutritional assessment to determine changes in weight over time (if previous body-weight measurements are available) and in some situations to calculate medication dosage. An unintentional change in weight can be a significant finding. For example, an increase in weight may be the first sign of fluid retention. For every liter of fluid retained

---

BOX 4-2 ERRORS IN BLOOD PRESSURE MEASUREMENT

Errors Resulting in False-High Blood Pressure Measurement
- Patient's legs are crossed during measurement
- Positioning the patient's arm below the level of the heart
- Using a cuff that is too narrow for the extremity
- Wrapping the cuff too loosely or unevenly
- Deflating the cuff too slowly (slower than 2 to 3 mm Hg per second)
- Reinflating the cuff without completely deflating it
- Failing to wait 1 to 2 minutes before obtaining a repeat measurement

Errors Resulting in False-Low Blood Pressure Measurement
- Positioning the patient's arm above the level of the heart
- Using a cuff that is too wide
- Not inflating the cuff enough
- Deflating the cuff too rapidly (faster than 2 to 3 mm Hg per second)
- Pressing the diaphragm too firmly on the brachial artery

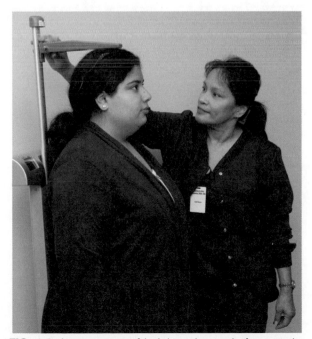

FIG. 4-9 Assessment of height using a platform scale.

(1000 mL, or about 1 quart), weight increases 2.2 lbs (1 kg). In addition, unexplained weight loss may be one indication of a disease process. Nutritional assessment is discussed further in Chapter 8.

Measure weight using a balance scale by asking the patient to stand in the middle of the scale platform while the large and small weights are balanced. The scale uses a counterbalance system of adding or subtracting weights in increments as small as 0.25 lb (0.1 kg) to achieve a level horizontal balance beam on the scale. Move the larger weight to the 50-lb (22.7-kg) increment less than the patient's weight. Adjust the smaller weight to balance the scale. Read the weight to the nearest 0.25 lb (0.1 kg).

Height

Height is also influenced by genetics and dietary intake. It is measured on a platform scale with a height attachment. The height attachment is pulled up, and the horizontal headpiece extended before the patient steps on the scale to avoid poking him or her as the headpiece is extended. Ask the patient to stand on the scale (without shoes); lower the attachment until the horizontal headpiece touches the top of the patient's head (Fig. 4-9). The vertical measuring scale can measure in inches or centimeters. Adult height is attained between ages 18 and 20.

AGE-RELATED VARIATIONS

This chapter discusses conducting a general inspection and measurement of vital signs with adult patients. These data are important to assess for individuals of all ages, but the approach and techniques used to collect the information may vary, depending on the patient's age.

INFANTS AND CHILDREN

The measurement of height (recumbent length), weight, head, and chest circumference is an important indicator of growth. These data are plotted on growth charts to assess growth patterns of infants and children and to compare growth to infants and children of the same age and gender. Although the same general process for general inspection and vital signs measurement among infants and children is followed as previously described, nurses use specific age-appropriate approaches and techniques as presented in Chapter 19.

OLDER ADULTS

The measurement of height, weight, and vital signs in the older adult is described previously.

CLINICAL APPLICATION AND CLINICAL REASONING

See Appendix D for answers to exercises in this section.

REVIEW QUESTIONS

1. The nurse obtains vital signs on a 42-year-old man having his annual physical examination. He has no medical conditions and states that his health is excellent. His blood pressure appears as 62/40 using an automated blood pressure device. Which action by the nurse is most appropriate?
   1. Obtain a different cuff and take the blood pressure again.
   2. Take the blood pressure again using the auscultation method.
   3. Place the patient in a supine position and take the pressure on the leg.
   4. Record the blood pressure and continue with the examination.

2. Which set of vital signs should the nurse recognize as out of the expected range?
   1. 42-year-old man: BP, 114/82; pulse, 74 beats/min; respiration, 16 breaths/min; temperature, 36.8° C
   2. 11-year-old girl: pulse, 88 beats/min; respiration, 22 breaths/min; temperature, 36.7° C
   3. 3-year-old boy: pulse, 130 beats/min; respiration, 44 breaths/min; temperature, 36.7° C
   4. 1-month-old girl: pulse, 120 beats/min; respiration, 42 breaths/min; temperature, 36.7° C

3. The nurse records the following general inspection findings on a patient: "41-year-old Hispanic male in no distress; very thin, skin tone slightly jaundiced, disheveled appearance, and appears older than stated age. Patient with flat affect and makes minimal eye contact." What additional information should be added to this general inspection?
   1. Body movement
   2. Family history
   3. Estimated size of his liver
   4. Palpation of pulses

4. A patient is brought to the emergency department with severe respiratory distress. Which method of temperature measurement would be most appropriate?
   1. Oral temperature with an electric thermometer
   2. Axillary with an electronic thermometer
   3. Temporal artery
   4. Rectal temperature

5. A 62-year-old patient tells the nurse that he has recently had frequent fainting spells. After palpating the radial pulse, 13 pulsations are counted in 15 seconds. The nurse determines that the patient has a pulse rate of 52, with a regularly irregular rhythm. What is the most appropriate action for the nurse to take at this time?
   1. Reassess the pulse rate after he walks around the room for several minutes.
   2. Reassess the pulse rate for 15 seconds using the carotid artery.
   3. Take an apical pulse for 5 full minutes, counting the number of skipped beats.
   4. Palpate the pulse for a full minute and note whether there is a pattern to the irregularity.

Ethnic, Cultural, and Spiritual Considerations

evolve WEBSITE

http://evolve.elsevier.com/Wilson/assessment

All people are influenced by their unique cultural and spiritual beliefs and practices. Culturally and spiritually competent care is delivered when nurses value health-illness experiences through the patient's eyes while helping them achieve their highest level of health. Nurses working together from diverse cultures may practice in different ways. Native American nurses report that their nursing practice may be different from practices of other nurses because they perceive life through a view that is different and that guides them in making their own sense of health care matters. For example, these nurses emphasize spirituality in their nursing practice, believing that the art of touching someone has spiritual power. Honor is a characteristic that includes the components of appreciation and respect. They feel honored to be present at a birth and at a death.[1]

ETHNIC, CULTURAL, AND SPIRITUAL AWARENESS

The United States has been called a *melting pot* because people from so many different cultures and religions live here. At one end of the continuum are people who moved to the United States from other countries and have not changed many of their behaviors or beliefs. They live in small communities inhabited by people with common cultural heritages. At the other end of the continuum are people who moved to the United States from other countries and adapted from the "old country" beliefs and behaviors to those of the American culture. Between the two ends of this continuum are people with varying cultural and spiritual behaviors and beliefs that represent a blending of foreign and American influences. Belief systems act as lenses through which people filter everything they view. As people interact with new individuals and new environments, their culture may change.

Although cultural diversity enriches America, it also creates challenges. About 20% of people in the United States speak a language other than English at home.[2] Diversity refers to differences in gender, age, culture, race, ethnicity, religion, sexual orientation, physical or mental disabilities, and social and economic status. As a nurse you have a responsibility to work with and care for individuals who may not have the same skin color, language, health practices, beliefs, religious practices, and values as your own. When this occurs, the goal is not to force patients and their families to comply with your beliefs, values, and practices but instead to meet patients where they are and to work with their belief and value systems. The challenge occurs not when patients are of the same heritage and speak the same language as the nurse but when the cultures, languages, and religions are different. Consider the following scenario:

You are caring for a 72-year-old Hispanic woman, Rosa Martinez, who speaks Spanish as her primary language. Conversing in broken English, she tells you that she has injured her lower back and now has continuing aches and stiffness. She was unsure about seeking care but came at the urging of her daughter. She says that she hasn't seen a physician in years because Maria, her curandera, takes good care of her. When you inquire whether she has seen Maria for her back, she replies yes and tells you that Maria had given her an herbal formula to take by mouth and had made herbal poultices to apply to her back at home. The patient tells you that she believes that these remedies are working and she is not sure if treatment from the clinic will help her.

The nurse caring for Mrs. Martinez is potentially challenged by three issues: (1) the language barrier; (2) an alternative health care provider, Maria the *cuerandera,* in whom Mrs. Martinez has much confidence; and (3) the use of alternative folk remedies (i.e., the herbal formulas and poultices). How the nurse interacts with this patient and her family depends partly on the nurse's own heritage and culture and partly on the nurse's knowledge of and attitude toward other cultures and other health beliefs and practices.

Understanding the meanings of *culture, ethnicity, race, spirituality, and religion* is necessary to improve cultural and spiritual awareness. There are many definitions of culture and they all overlap with ethnicity and religion. The Office of Minority Health defines culture as "the thoughts, communications, actions, customs, beliefs, values, and institutions of racial, ethnic, religious, or social groups."[3 p. 131] Thus *culture* includes all socially transmitted behavioral patterns, arts, beliefs, knowledge, values, morals, customs, life ways, and characteristics of a population that influence perception, behavior, and evaluation of the world. *Ethnicity* refers to characteristics that a group may share in some combination such as common geographic origin; race; language and dialect; religious beliefs; shared tradition and symbols; literature, folklore, and music; food preferences; settlement and employment patterns; and an internal sense of distinctiveness[4] (Fig. 5-1). Consider the following scenario:

A nurse is trying to obtain a history from a Navajo woman. After each question there is a long silence. The patient often stares at the floor. The nurse thinks that the patient is shy or does not understand the questions. However, the patient is indicating that she is paying close attention to the nurse using a culturally appropriate behavior. As a Navajo she values silence. A person who interrupts while someone is speaking is perceived as immature.[5]

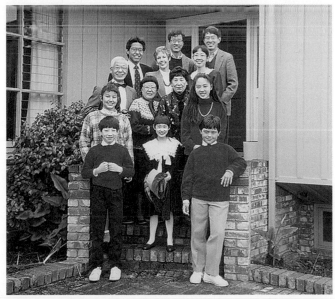

FIG. 5-1 Ethnicity indicates a common race, language, and dialect, and shared tradition.

The previous example illustrates how behaviors can be interpreted differently between two individuals from different cultural backgrounds.

Race is genetic in origin and includes physical characteristics such as skin color, bone structure, eye color, and hair color. The Human Genome Project provides evidence that all human beings share a genetic code that is more than 99% identical. Although less than a 1% difference exists in genetic code, the differences are evident when performing health assessments. People from a given racial group do not necessarily share a common culture.[6]

Spirituality has many definitions. A review of spirituality definitions in health care literature provides several themes: relationship to God, a spiritual being, a higher being, or reality greater than the self; existential, not of the material world; meaning and purpose in life; and life force or integrating aspect of the person.[7] Religion may or may not be part of one's spirituality. Religion refers to an organized system of beliefs, rituals, and practices in which an individual participates; whereas spirituality is broader. Spirituality practices may include prayer, meditation, walking in the woods, listening to music, painting, journaling, intentional appreciation of beauty, or being present in the world with others.[8] Spiritual and religious beliefs can influence interpersonal behaviors and expectations. This is illustrated in the following situation:

A Buddhist monk from Cambodia is in same-day surgery for a procedure. He is accompanied by his mother and cousin. When the nurse enters the room to greet him, she puts her hand on his shoulder to direct him to a chair across the room. The patient suddenly jumps in horror. The mother and cousin began shouting at the nurse in Cambodian. After an interpreter talks with the cousin, he explains to the nurse that the patient is a monk and cannot be touched by a woman. Should touch be necessary, the monk is not to look at the woman or move or respond in any way. Because of this incident the monk would have to do great penance.[5]

To emphasize the importance of culturally and linguistically appropriate services in health care, the U.S. Department of Health and Human Services, Office of Minority Health (OMH) issued national standards to ensure that all people entering the health care system receive equitable and effective treatment (Fig. 5-2). These 14 standards provide for culturally and linguistically appropriate services (CLAS) to help eliminate racial and ethnic health disparities and improve the health of all people who live in the United States of America. Although the CLAS standards are primarily directed at health care organizations, they guide health care providers, including nurses, to use the standards to make their practices more culturally and linguistically accessible. The standards are organized around three themes: culturally competent care, language access services, and organizational supports for cultural competence. Health care team members are affected by the first standard, which states that "healthcare organizations should ensure that patients/consumers receive from all staff members effective, understandable, and respectful care that is provided in a manner compatible with the cultural health

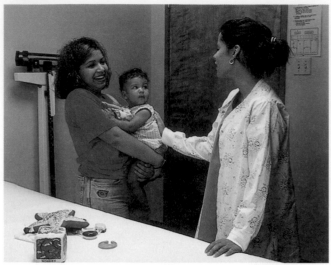

FIG. 5-2 Patients receive effective, understandable, and respectful care.

©The Joint Commission. Accessed at http://www.jointcommission.org/standards_information/jcfaqdetails.aspx?StandardsFaqId=290&ProgramId=1 on September 2, 2011.

BOX 5-1   SPIRITUAL ASSESSMENT

Examples of questions that could be asked in a spiritual assessment but are not required.

- Who or what provides you with strength and hope?
- Do you use prayer in your life?
- How do you express your spirituality?
- How do you describe your philosophy of life?
- What type of spiritual/religious support do you desire?
- What is the name of your clergy, ministers, chaplains, pastor, rabbi?
- What does suffering mean to you?
- What does dying mean to you?
- What are your spiritual goals?
- Is there a church/synagogue role in your life?
- How does your faith help you cope with illness?
- How do you keep going day after day?
- What helps you get through this health care experience?
- How has illness affected you and your family?

BOX 5-2   BARRIERS TO ASSESSING SPIRITUAL NEEDS

Personal and Individual Barriers

- Nurses view assessing patients' spiritual needs as private or family matters or pastoral responsibilities, not their responsibility.
- Nurses may experience personal embarrassment, discomfort, or uncertainty with their own spirituality.
- Nurses may be uncomfortable dealing with conditions and situations that frequently result in spiritual distress (e.g., suffering, grief).

Knowledge Barriers

- Nurses lack knowledge about spirituality and the religious beliefs of others.
- Nurses have minimal, if any, education related to spiritual assessment.
- Nurses mistake spiritual needs for psychosocial needs.

Adapted from McEwen M: Spiritual nursing care: State of the art, *Holistic Nurs Pract* 19:161-168, 2005.

---

beliefs and practices and preferred language."[3] The following scenario exemplifies the need to consider organizational environment and its impact for some individuals:

> A 70-year old Cambodian woman is admitted to a Catholic hospital following a motor vehicle accident. Instead of responding to the nurse during the shift assessment, the patient stares at the wall across from the bed. The nurse assumes that the response is caused by the shock of the accident. Later the patient's daughter asks the nurse to remove the crucifix from the wall because it is bothering her mother. The patient is a Buddhist and later explains that the crucifix makes her feel that she is being influenced to worship a God that she does not recognize.[5]

Using interpreters as communicators between patients and health care team members may improve communication, but words in one language may not translate to another language. For example, some languages have no equivalent word for "pain," whereas others have several words to describe it. A patient might describe severe pain as feeling like "electric shocks." If an interpreter translates "electric shocks" as "twinges," the nurse may interpret the pain as mild rather than severe.[2]

The Joint Commission (TJC) requires that a spiritual history be taken and documented on every patient admitted to a hospital, nursing home, or home health agency. TJC expects health care organizations to define the content and scope of spiritual assessment and the qualifications of the person(s) performing the assessment.[9] Box 5-1 has questions that TJC suggests that nurses consider when assessing spiritual needs of patients or their families. Box 5-2 describes barriers to assessing spiritual needs. The following situation illustrates the importance of asking about spiritual needs:

> A man enjoying a cruise to Alaska becomes ill on the cruise ship and is transported to a local hospital. During the admission history the nurse asks the man if the hospital could help

him with any spiritual needs. He replies, "Yes, I'm Muslim and will be praying five times a day. Which way do I face to pray to Mecca?" The nurse responds that she does not know the answer to his question but would find out for both of them. Later the nurse reports to the patient that Muslims in Alaska face north to pray to Mecca.

Improving cultural awareness and meeting Standard 1 of CLAS require that nurses take several steps: (1) become culturally competent through sensitivity to differences between their own culture and that of the patient; (2) avoid stereotyping and assuming the meaning of others' behavior; and

(3) develop a template that may be used for cultural and spiritual assessment of patients and the families.

DEVELOP CULTURAL COMPETENCE

Nurses who are culturally competent have the ability to respect patients as unique persons; to assess their beliefs, values, preferences and needs; and to determine the meaning of their illnesses. These nurses are aware of their biases and either have knowledge of other cultures or know the questions to ask to learn about the unique cultures of patients.[10]

Five interrelated attributes of the concept of cultural competence include knowledge, consideration, understanding, respect, and tailoring. *Knowledge* refers to gaining information about cultural differences and values that can be acquired through training and education and by talking with people from different cultures about their beliefs and practices. Although knowledge of and respect for cultural beliefs and practices for different cultures are valued, familiarity with *all* cultural perspectives that a nurse might encounter is impractical. *Consideration* is implemented after knowledge is acquired when nurses use knowledge of patients' and others' languages, practices, and customs in providing care. *Understanding* involves thoughtful consideration of the effects and importance of another's values and experiences. *Respect* is communicated when nurses show appreciation and regard for patient's cultural differences and for other nurses with whom they work. The final attribute of cultural sensitivity is *tailoring*, which is adapting interactions based on cultural practices and beliefs of others.[10] Box 5-3 describes ways to achieve cultural competence.

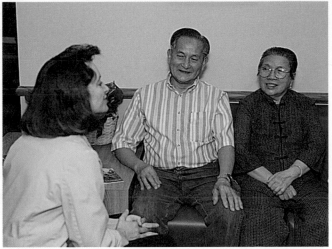

FIG. 5-3 When interviewing patients, recognize that cultural diversity exists.

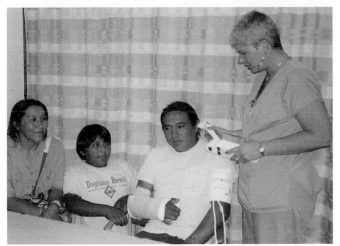

FIG. 5-4 Developing sensitivity to the differences between your culture and that of patients from another culture is important in providing patient-centered care.

Of the IOM Core Competencies, providing patient-centered care and working in interdisciplinary teams apply to cultural and spiritual assessment.[11] Table 5-1 presents knowledge, skills, and attitudes to use when demonstrating patient-centered care or working with interdisciplinary team members to assess cultural and spiritual needs.

AVOID STEREOTYPING

Regardless of a person's skin color, physical features, cultural heritage, social group, or spirituality, the nurse must acknowledge that individual's uniqueness. Cultural heritage plays an important part in helping to identify the individual's "roots" and perhaps helps to explain attitudes, beliefs, and health practices. However, each major cultural group is composed of unique individuals and families who may have values and attitudes that differ from the cultural norm. Nurses must not

---

BOX 5-3   WAYS TO DEVELOP CULTURAL COMPETENCE

- Acknowledge that cultural diversity exists (Fig. 5-3).
- Recognize the uniqueness of and demonstrate respect for individuals and families of cultures other than your own (Fig. 5-4). Each person's cultural values are ingrained and are a part of who that person is.
- Demonstrate knowledge and understanding of the patient's culture, health-related needs, and meanings of health and illness. When the patient's culture is unfamiliar, ask the patient about his or her culture using the template for assessment. Recognize that some cultural groups have definitions of health and illness that may differ from yours and thus use health and healing practices that may be different from yours.
- Respect the unfamiliar and learn more about it so it is no longer unfamiliar. Be open to cultural encounters. Identify and explore your own cultural beliefs as you learn about those of others.
- Be willing to modify health care delivery to be more congruent with the patient's cultural background.

Modified from Seidel HM et al: *Mosby's guide to physical examination*, ed 7, St Louis, 2011, Mosby; Purnell L, Paulanka B: *Guide to culturally competent care*, Philadelphia, 2005, FA Davis.

TABLE 5-1	QUALITY IMPROVEMENT COMPETENCIES FOR NURSES: CULTURAL AND SPIRITUAL ASSESSMENT	
KNOWLEDGE	**SKILLS**	**ATTITUDES**
Patient-Centered Care		
Describe how diverse ethnic, cultural, spiritual, and social backgrounds function as sources of patient, family, and community values.	Elicit patient values, preferences, and expressed needs as part of clinical interview. Communicate patient values, preferences, and expressed needs to other members of the health care team. Provide patient-centered care with sensitivity and respect for the diversity of human experiences.	Value seeing health care situations through patients' eyes. Respect and encourage individual expression of patient values, preferences, and expressed needs. Value the patient's expertise with own health and symptoms. Recognize personally held attitudes about working with patients from different ethnic, cultural, spiritual, and social backgrounds. Willingly support patient-centered care for individuals and groups whose values differ from own.
Interdisciplinary Teamwork		
Recognize contributions of chaplains, ministers, rabbis, priests, or other spiritual leaders in helping patients and families express and meet their spiritual needs.	Act with integrity, consistency, and respect for differing views. Integrate the contributions of chaplains, ministers, rabbis, priests, or other spiritual leaders in helping patients and families express and meet their spiritual needs.	Respect the centrality of the patient and family as core members of any health care team. Respect the unique attributes that chaplains, ministers, rabbis, priests, or other spiritual leaders bring to the team, including variations in professional orientation and accountabilities.

Adapted from www.qsen.org.

assume that because individuals or families are Asian or Pacific Islander they all share culturally similar beliefs. Within the Asian or Pacific Islander people are Chinese, Filipino, Japanese, Asian Indian, Korean, Vietnamese, Cambodian, Thai, Bangladeshi, Burmese, Indonesian, Malayan, Laotian, Kampuchean, Pakistani, Sri Lankan, Hawaiian, Samoan, Tongon, Tahitian, Palauan, Fijian, and Northern Mariana Islanders; and each of these groups has a unique heritage and set of beliefs. Thus nurses should avoid making assumptions based on racial or ethnic backgrounds. The following scenario illustrates this point:

A 52-year-old Hispanic man seeks health care after injuring his hand in an agricultural accident. When the nurse enters the room, the patient is talking in Spanish to another man who has accompanied him. Because of the number of migrant workers in the area, the nurse assumes that he is a poor illegal migrant worker who speaks no English. She decides that the best course of action is to ask another nurse in the clinic who speaks Spanish to see the patient. She excuses herself without talking with either man and finds another nurse who agrees to see the patient. After a brief introduction the Spanish-speaking nurse determines that the patient is fluent in both Spanish and English. The nurse also learns that the patient is actually the owner of the large ranch and oversees multiple agricultural operations and that he has a master of science in agricultural economics.

Likewise individuals who identify with one religion do not necessarily have the same beliefs or practices. For example, people can claim to be Methodists but not practice their religion in the same way or accept all of the beliefs of the faith.

This variation applies to those of all faiths. Thus assessing each person's faith beliefs is necessary to gain an accurate understanding of that individual.

Personal beliefs and knowledge about other cultures in the United States have been influenced by stereotyped images and misinformation presented through the media, educational and political institutions, and family beliefs. Understanding how your beliefs were formed increases your receptiveness to different beliefs. Some common misbeliefs and stereotyped images include the following:

- All African Americans have large families.
- All welfare recipients are minorities.
- All Asians excel in mathematics and science.
- All Native Americans live on reservations.
- All Hispanics speak Spanish.

If you learn nothing else from this text, learn that all individuals are unique, deserving of a personalized assessment of their beliefs, values, and traditions. Even people who share the same culture and background are not necessarily the same. In addition, they may act one way in one role but differently in another role.

DEVELOP A TEMPLATE FOR ASSESSMENT

When assessing the patient and family, nurses ask about health beliefs and practices that may reflect their cultural heritage. They also ask patients about spiritual beliefs and practices important to them. Because there is so much diversity, nurses are *not* responsible for knowing about the health beliefs, practices, religions, and values of all cultural and racial groups. However, they are responsible for asking patients about their health beliefs, practices, religious beliefs, attitudes, and values because this information is essential for providing patient-centered, holistic care for people. A person may be from one of the major racial and cultural groups (e.g., Native American; African American; Asian; white, nonhispanic; or Hispanic) or one of the often unrecognized cultural groups (e.g., the homeless, migrant workers, gay men, or lesbians).

To improve cultural awareness and sensitivity, nurses notice patients' behaviors during the initial interview for clues about preferred communication practices. For example, if patients do not make eye contact, they may be demonstrating that this is a preferred way of communicating in their culture. If patients back up as nurses approach them, they may prefer more personal space. Nurses ask questions to gather information about the unique beliefs, value systems, and spiritual practices of individuals of other cultures and backgrounds. They ask one question at a time, allow ample time for a response, use active voice, and avoid medical jargon. This assessment forms part of the personal and psychosocial history described in Chapter 2.

Personal and Psychosocial History
Introductory Questions
- Where were you born?
- With what particular cultural group (or groups) do you identify?
- Which cultural practices are important to you?

Primary Language and Method of Communication
- Which language is usually spoken in your home?
- How well do you speak, read, and write English?
- In which language do you think?
- Do you have to translate in your mind when communicating in English?
- Will you need the services of a translator during the time you are in this health care facility?
- Are there special rituals of communication in your family? (For example, is there someone special to whom questions should be directed?) Tell me about these.
- Are there unique customs in your culture that influence nonverbal or verbal communication? Tell me about them.
- What are some ways of indicating respect for others?
- What are appropriate ways to enter and leave situations?

Personal Beliefs About Health and Illness
- Do you believe that you have control over your health? If not, what or whom do you believe controls it?
- Which are some practices or rituals that you believe will improve your health?
- Do you use or have you used any alternative healing methods such as acupuncture, acupressure, *ayurveda*, healing touch, or herbal products? If so, how effective was the treatment?

- Whom do you consult when you are ill?
- Which specific practices or rituals do you believe should be used to treat your health problem?
- Who makes the health decisions in your family?
- Which health topics make you feel uncomfortable?
- Which examination procedures do you consider to be immodest?
- What can the members of the health care team do to help you stay healthy (or become healthy again)?

Beliefs About a Current Health Problem (Sickness)[12,13]
- What do you call this sickness?
- What do you think caused the sickness?
- Why do you think it started when it did?
- What do you think the sickness does? How does it work?
- How severe is your sickness?
- What kind of treatment do you think you should receive?
- What are the most important results you hope to receive from this treatment?
- What do you fear most about this sickness?

Religious or Spiritual Influences
- If time or situation only permits asking one question, ask, "Do you have any spiritual needs or concerns related to your health?"[14]
- Do you belong to a specific religious or faith community?
- What role does your spirituality play in your daily life?
- Do particular rituals or religious practices help you deal with daily life and its obstacles? If so, describe them.
- How do your beliefs affect your health practices?
- Box 5-4 contains a spiritual assessment tool using the acronym *FICA*.

Roles in the Family
- Who makes the decisions in your family?
- What is the composition of your family? How many generations of family members live in your household?
- What is the role of and attitude toward children in the family?

BOX 5-4 SPIRITUAL ASSESSMENT TOOL

The five questions immediately below are remembered using the acronym FICA, which represents the topics: *Faith, Importance, Community, Apply, Address.*
- What is your *faith* tradition?
- How *important* is your faith to you?
- What is your *church or community* of faith?
- How do your religious and spiritual beliefs *apply* to your health?
- How might we *address* your spiritual needs?

From Puchalski CH, Romer AL: Taking a spiritual history allows clinicians to understand patients, *Journal of Palliative Medicine* 3:129-137, 2000.

- Do you or the members of your family have special beliefs and practices surrounding conception, pregnancy, childbirth, lactation, and childrearing?

Special Dietary Practices

- What is the main type of diet eaten in your home?
- Are there special types of foods that are forbidden by your culture or foods that are a cultural requirement in observance of a rite or ceremony? If so, what are they?
- Who in your family is responsible for food preparation?
- How is the food in your culture prepared?
- Are there specific beliefs or preferences concerning food such as those believed to cause or cure illness?

Notice the Patient's Surroundings

- While asking the patient questions, look around the immediate area for religious symbols.
- Notice religious books such as the Koran, Bible, or Torah, a cross, or rosary beads. If you notice any, you may be able to gather more data by commenting on it, saying something like: "I notice you have your rosary beads." In response the patient may comment on its meaning to him or her.
- Notice if the patient is wearing an amulet, which is an object with magical powers such as a charm worn on a string or chain the around neck, wrist, waist to protect the patient from physical and psychological illness, harm, or misfortune.[4] If you notice an amulet, you may be able to gather additional data by commenting on it. For example, you might say, "I notice that you have something on a chain around your neck. Tell me more about it."

REMEMBER...

The most important behaviors in cultural assessment are to be sensitive; to ask questions; to gather information specific to the individual patient; to avoid stereotyping; and to not assume that, just because you took care of a similar patient last week, you know exactly how this patient feels and what he or she believes.

Regardless of the patient's race or cultural heritage, each individual is unique. Before you become involved in the detailed task of a physical assessment, first take the time to get to know the patient and his or her family.

CLINICAL APPLICATION AND CLINICAL REASONING

See Appendix D for answers to exercises in this section.

REVIEW QUESTIONS

1. A school nurse notices a boy with a bandage on his arm and black fluid under the edge of the bandage. She asks the teen what happened to his arm. He replies that his mother applied axle grease to a boil. What is the nurse's most appropriate response to this boy?
   1. Tell the teen to remove the bandage and wash his arm.
   2. Ask the teen what the boil looks like, what it feels like, and if the axle grease is helping it get better.
   3. Advise the teen to tell his mother to use antibiotic cream rather than axle grease.
   4. Suggest that the teen see a health care provider because the axle grease will infect the boil.

2. The nurse is caring for a woman who has just been pronounced dead. Her adult children are in the room. Which statement by the nurse indicates culturally competent care?
   1. "Which funeral home would you like notified of your mother's death?"
   2. "We will be moving her to the morgue in about 30 minutes."
   3. "Would you like time alone with your mother for any specific ceremonies?"
   4. "Here are some of her personal belongings that were in the drawer."

3. A nurse is assessing a woman whose religious beliefs do not allow blood transfusions. She has severe anemia, is very weak, and has altered mental status. What behavior by the nurse is needed to provide effective care to this woman?
   1. Examine his or her own feelings about the importance of religious beliefs in making decisions about life.
   2. Recognize that he or she cannot provide care to patients whose religious beliefs endanger their lives.
   3. Try to convince the patient to have a blood transfusion to save her own life.
   4. Determine whether the patient is competent to make her own decisions about health care.

4. A nurse is teaching a family from Guatemala about the importance of exercise to reduce body weight. The husband asks, "What exercise do we do?" Considering the time orientation of this family, which response by the nurse is most effective?
   1. "In the past research has shown that walking 30 minutes most days of the week is best."
   2. "Is there an exercise that you can do today for 30 minutes and make it part of your daily routine?"
   3. "If you exercise 30 minutes most days of the week, you can lose weight by your next visit."
   4. "I have always found that resistance weight training each day for 30 minutes is effective."

5. An older man who is near death has been admitted to the hospital, and family members are at his bedside. During the admission assessment the nurse uses which question or statement to appropriately address spiritual needs?
   1. What is your religion? I'll make the appropriate spiritual arrangements?
   2. Tell me what death means to people from your culture.
   3. Are there any special needs or rituals that you and your family request at this time?
   4. I'll call the hospital priest so he can administer last rites.

CHAPTER

6

Pain Assessment

evolve WEBSITE

http://evolve.elsevier.com/Wilson/assessment

Working with people to relieve their pain is a primary responsibility of all health care providers. The ethical principles of beneficence (the duty to benefit another) and nonmaleficence (the duty to do no harm) compel health care professionals to provide pain management and comfort.[1] The first step in managing pain is assessing the patient. Because pain is an important component of patient well-being, it is often referred to as one of the vital signs after temperature, blood pressure, pulse, and respirations.

A widely accepted definition of pain is the one adopted by the International Association for the Study of Pain (IASP), which states that pain is an unpleasant sensory and emotional experience associated with actual or potential tissue damage.[2] A practical definition of pain is that of Margo McCaffery, who believes that "Pain is whatever the experiencing person says it is, existing wherever he says it is."[3] This definition represents the belief that one person cannot judge the perception or meaning of pain experienced by another person.

Although pain occurs when tissues are damaged, there is no correlation between the amount of tissue damage and the degree or intensity of pain experienced. For example, patients with extensive traumatic injuries may not report the intensity of pain expected, whereas patients with chronic cancer pain may experience intense pain for which no tissue damage can be found.

CONCEPT OVERVIEW

The feature concept for this chapter is *Pain*. This concept represents an unpleasant sensory and emotional experience associated with actual or potential tissue damage, or pain processing.

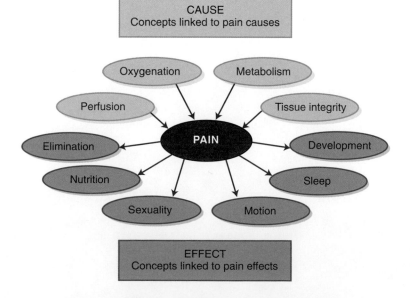

Pain (regardless of the cause) links to several other concepts presented in this book; this relationship is presented in the Pain Cause and Effect Model.

This model shows the potential effects of pain on an individual. Any cause of reduced perfusion interrupts oxygen supplied to tissues and can lead to impaired tissue integrity if not corrected. Pain can reduce mobility, impair sleep, and contribute to a loss of appetite. An individual taking narcotic medications to relieve pain may experience a change in elimination patterns (constipation). Having an understanding of the interrelationship of these concepts helps the nurse recognize risk factors and thus increases awareness when conducting a health assessment.

The following case provides a clinical example featuring several of these interrelated concepts.

Haim is a 41-year-old man who has peripheral arterial disease that prevents blood from carrying oxygen to his legs, causing pain and potentially impairing tissue integrity. This pain prevents him from walking long distances (reduced motion). At times it interrupts his sleep.

COGNITIVE AND CULTURAL INFLUENCES ON PAIN PERCEPTION

A person's pain perception and responses are influenced by cognitive factors, cultural influences, and previous experiences with pain. Cognitive factors include the attention people give to their pain, their expectation/anticipation of pain, and their appraisal or explanation of the pain. When people direct attention to specific stimuli, they shift attention away from or are distracted from other stimuli. Thus people who direct their full attention to their pain report more pain than those who direct attention elsewhere. This principle helps to explain how distraction is an effective pain-relieving strategy. People with persistent (chronic) pain having similar diagnoses and pain histories may report their pain differently based on their beliefs about the meaning of pain and their ability to function. Individuals who consider their pain to be an unexplainable mystery and doubt their abilities to control or decrease the pain are less likely to rate their coping strategies as effective. When a new pain is felt, people try to make sense of it or make an appraisal. For example, a woman wakes up one morning with pain in her upper back. In one appraisal she attributes this backache to muscular strain from gardening the previous day. In comparison, a different appraisal may be that the backache indicates a herniated disk requiring surgery and convalescence, which could lead to a different response. Thus, although the physiologic response may be equivalent, the person's cognitive appraisal or interpretation contributes to different behavioral responses. If the interpretation is that pain came from gardening, there is little emotional response, and treatment is sought with over-the-counter drugs, a hot shower, and rest. However, if fears of a herniated disk arise, the response is more emotional and prompts a visit to a health care provider. Over time every person develops cognitive patterns for attending to, anticipating, and appraising pain. These patterns, uniquely defined by one's cultural and environmental factors, are constantly changing as new and repeated pain perception is experienced.[4]

Individuals' cultures and their personal experiences with pain affect how they communicate, respond to, treat, and explain its meaning.[5] Several questions in the problem-based history are asked to determine the patient's cultural influence on the pain experience.

TYPES OF PAIN

Pain is categorized in several ways, but a clear distinction among types of pain may not always be possible. Types of pain include acute, persistent (also called chronic), nociceptive, and neuropathetic.[6] *Acute pain* has a recent onset (less than 6 months) and results from tissue damage, is usually self-limiting, and ends when the tissue heals. It is a stressor that initiates a generalized stress response and may cause physiologic signs associated with pain. By contrast, *persistent pain* may be intermittent or continuous, lasting more than 6 months. Clinical manifestations of persistent pain are not those of physiologic stress because people adapt to the pain, resulting in symptoms of irritability, depression, withdrawal, and insomnia.[7]

Another way to categorize pain is by the inferred pathology (i.e., nociceptive and neuropathic pain). *Nociceptive pain* arises from stimulation of somatic structures such as bone, joint, muscle, skin, and connective tissue or from stimulation of visceral organs such as the gastrointestinal tract or pancreas. This type of pain results from activation of essentially normal neural systems. In contrast, *neuropathic pain* occurs from abnormal processing of sensory input by the central or peripheral nervous systems.[6] Nociceptive pain and neuropathic pain are explained in Fig. 6-1.

Referred pain is pain felt in a location away from the area of tissue injury or disease. This type of pain often occurs during visceral pain because many abdominal organs have no pain receptors. As a result, when sensory nerves carrying pain impulses from abdominal organs enter the spinal cord, they stimulate sensory nerves from unaffected organs found in the same spinal cord segment as the nerves in areas where tissue injury or disease is located. For example, gallbladder disease may cause referred pain to the right shoulder, and myocardial infarction may cause referred pain to the left shoulder, arm, or jaw.

Phantom pain is pain that a person feels in an amputated extremity after the residual limb has healed. This type of pain commonly occurs in a person who experienced pain in that limb before amputation. If the nerve pathway from the amputated extremity is stimulated anywhere along the pathway, nerve impulses ascend to the cerebral cortex so the person perceives pain even though the limb has been removed. Phantom pain also is influenced by emotions and sympathetic stimulation.[7]

CLASSIFICATION OF PAIN BY INFERRED PATHOPHYSIOLOGY

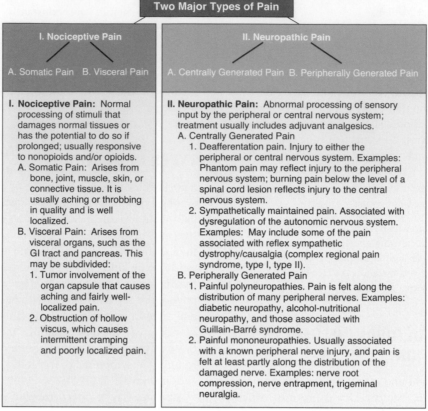

FIG. 6-1 A method of classifying pain is by the pathophysiology involved. *I*, Nociceptive pain (stimuli from somatic and visceral structures). *II*, Neuropathic pain (stimuli abnormally processed by nervous system). (From Pasero and McCaffery, 2011.)

STANDARDS FOR PAIN ASSESSMENT

Among criteria for accreditation for hospitals, The Joint Commission (TJC) set a standard that patients have the right to appropriate assessment and management of pain. This standard includes: (1) initial assessment and regular reassessment of pain, taking into account personal, cultural, spiritual, and ethnic beliefs; (2) education of all relevant health care personnel in pain assessment and management; and (3) education of patients and families regarding their roles in managing pain and the potential limitations and adverse effects of pain treatments. Another standard of TJC states that pain is assessed in all patients. Expectations for nurses implementing this standard include assessing pain intensity, location, quality, duration, and alleviating and aggravating factors and determining the effects of pain on the patient's life (e.g., daily function) and pain goal.[8]

A common reason for inadequate pain management in hospitals in the United States is the failure of nurses to assess pain and the ineffectiveness of pain-relief interventions.[9] When patients' expressions or reactions to pain do not conform to the nurses' beliefs or expectations, nurses may consider the patient's behavior inappropriate. However, the patient's response to pain is not right or wrong; it is different from that of the nurse. A survey of 2949 nurses across the United States found that most of them understand principles of pain management. Interestingly, the results reveal that pain assessment is one area in which nurses need more education. Some nurses remain misinformed about certain key issues related to pain assessment. One issue is not believing the patient's self-report. Although most nurses know that the patient's self-report of pain is the most reliable indicator of pain, many remarks contradict this understanding. For example, some nurses comment about trying to determine the "real" status of pain in patients who are labeled *drug seeking, frequent flyers,* or *clock watchers.* Patients who are thought to be clock watchers often are undertreated and should be labeled *relief seekers* rather than *drug seekers.* Another issue is relying on increases in vital signs as indicators of pain. Although increases in heart and respiratory rates and blood pressures may occur briefly during acute pain, these parameters may increase for many other reasons. Patients with persistent pain usually do not experience changes in vital signs because they have adapted to the pain. Vital sign changes are not indicators of pain.[10] Box 6-1 contains self-assessment questions to help nurses determine their cultural norms concerning pain assessment.[11]

The competency of patient-centered care described by the Institute of Medicine (IOM) is demonstrated by providing pain assessment for patients. Specific knowledge, skills, and attitudes related to pain assessment are found in Table 6-1.

BOX 6-1   SELF-ASSESSMENT QUESTIONS TO HELP NURSES DETERMINE THEIR CULTURAL NORMS CONCERNING PAIN

When you were a child, how did those who cared for you react when you were in pain?
- How did they expect you to behave when you had a minor injury?
- How did they encourage you to cope when you had severe pain?
- How did they encourage you to behave during an injection or procedure?

When those who cared for you as a child were in pain, how did they react?
- Which words did they use to describe the pain?
- How did they cope with their pain?
- Do you tend to follow their example?

Consider a painful experience that you've had as an adult (e.g., childbirth, a fracture, a procedure).
- How did you express (or not express) your pain?
- Did the pain cause you fear? What did you fear?
- How did you cope with the pain?
- How did you want others to react while you were in pain?

Have you ever felt "uncomfortable" with the way a patient was reacting (or not reacting) to pain?
- What did the patient do that concerned you?
- Why did you feel that way?

Do you have "feelings" (make value judgments) about patients in pain who:
- Behave more stoically or expressively than you would in a similar situation?
- Ask for pain medicine frequently or not often enough?
- Choose treatments that you don't believe to be effective or with which you are unfamiliar?
- Belong to a cultural group (ethnic, linguistic, religious, socioeconomic) different from your own?

Do you tend to think that certain reactions to pain are "right" or "wrong?" Why? What about these reactions makes them seem right or wrong?
- Are some expressions or verbalizations of pain "right" or "wrong?"
- Some descriptions of pain?
- Some treatments for pain?

From Narayan M: Culture's effects on pain assessment and management, *AJN* 110:40, 2010.

TABLE 6-1   QUALITY IMPROVEMENT COMPETENCIES FOR NURSES: PAIN ASSESSMENT

KNOWLEDGE	SKILLS	ATTITUDES
Demonstrate comprehensive understanding of the concepts of pain and suffering, including physiologic models of pain and comfort.	Assess presence and extent of pain and suffering. Assess levels of physical and emotional comfort. Elicit expectations of patient and family for relief of pain.	Recognize personally held values and beliefs about the management of pain and suffering.
Discuss principles of effective communication.	Assess own level of communication skill in encounters with patients and families.	Value continuous improvement of own communication skills.

www.qsen.org. Accessed March 26, 2011.

ANATOMY AND PHYSIOLOGY

PAIN PROCESS

The physiology of pain involves a journey from the site of stimulation of peripheral receptors to the spinal cord, up the spinal cord to the cerebral cortex, and back down the spinal cord.

The pain process begins with a response of nociceptors to noxious stimuli that cause tissue damage. These nociceptors are primary sensory nerves located in tendons, muscles, subcutaneous tissue, epidermis, dermis, and skeletal muscles.

As nociceptors are stimulated, they initiate the second step in the journey, which is to stimulate sensory peripheral nerves. These sensory nerve fibers that carry pain impulses include the large A-delta and the small C fibers shown in Fig. 6-2. The A-delta fibers are associated with sharp, pricking, acute, well-localized pain of short duration. The C fibers are associated with a dull, aching, throbbing, or burning sensation that has a diffuse nature, slow onset, and relatively long duration. When these fibers are stimulated by nociceptors, they initiate an action potential that travels along peripheral nerves to the dorsal horn of the spinal cord. Located in the dorsal horn is the substantia gelatinosa, called the *gate,* which controls the stimulation of sensory tracts within the spinal cord. According to the gate theory of pain, when the gate is opened, pain impulses enter the spinal cord and ascend in the spinothalamic tract to the thalamus, resulting in the perception of pain.[12]

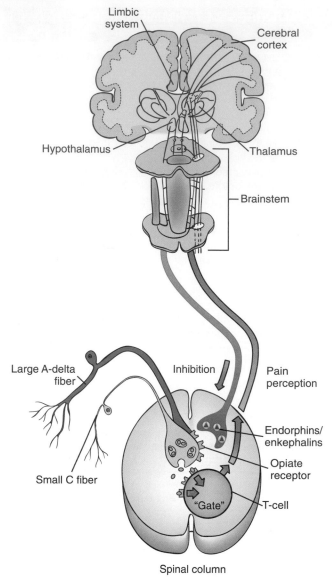

FIG. 6-2 The journey of the pain process. (1) Nociceptors stimulate the free nerve endings; (2) nociceptor stimulation initiates action potentials along large A-delta or small C fibers to open the gate in the substantia gelatinosa and ascend to the brain in the spinothalamic tract through the thalamus; (3) impulses move from the thalamus to the parietal lobe and limbic system; and (4) the body produces endorphins and enkephalins to occupy the opiate receptor sites to close the gate to slow or stop pain experience.

The third step in the journey occurs when the thalamus receives impulses from the spinothalamic tract and sends these impulses to the parietal lobe in the cerebral cortex and to the limbic system. When impulses reach the parietal lobe, the patient feels the pain. Although the journey of the pain stimulus takes a fraction of a second to reach the brain, people do not perceive their pain until the parietal lobe is stimulated. Stimulation of the limbic system generates the emotional response to the pain such as crying or anger.

The pain journey ends when the body produces substances to reduce pain perception. As sensory nerve fibers travel through the brainstem, they stimulate descending nerves that inhibit nociceptor stimuli. These nerves are descending fibers because they start in the brainstem and travel down to the dorsal horn of the spinal cord, where they release substances such as endogenous opioids (e.g., endorphins and enkephalins) that inhibit the transmission of noxious stimuli and produce analgesia.[6] For example, endorphins and enkephalins occupy the opioid receptor sites throughout the brain and spinal cord that prevent A and C nerve fibers from opening the gate (see Fig. 6-2).

Pain Threshold and Pain Tolerance

Both pain threshold and pain tolerance affect a person's pain experience. *Pain threshold* is the point at which a stimulus is perceived as pain. This threshold does not vary significantly over time. By contrast, *pain tolerance* is the duration or intensity of pain that a person endures or tolerates before responding outwardly. A person's culture, pain experience, expectations, role behaviors, and physical and emotional health influence pain tolerance. Pain tolerance decreases with repeated exposure to pain, fatigue, anger, boredom, apprehension, and sleep deprivation. The tolerance increases after alcohol consumption, medications, hypnosis, warmth, and distracting activities and as a result of strong faith beliefs.[7]

HEALTH HISTORY

GENERAL HEALTH HISTORY

Nurses interview patients to collect subjective data about their present health and their experiences with pain. In addition to present health status, nurses ask patients about how they usually manage their pain.

Present Health Status

Do you have any chronic illnesses? If so, do they cause you pain? Describe.

Some chronic illnesses such as osteoarthritis or the neuropathic pain experienced by patients with diabetes mellitus cause pain. The patient may have both persistent and acute pain from a current disorder.

Do you take any medications? If so, what do you take and how often? How well do they relieve your pain? Are you allergic to any medications? If yes, what kind of allergic reaction do you have from these medications?

Both prescription and over-the-counter medications should be noted. Ineffective medications should be reevaluated by the health care provider. Allergies are always noted so the patient will not be given a medication that would cause an allergic reaction. Patients are asked to describe the reaction because sometimes what they report as allergic is actually an adverse effect of the drug.

PROBLEM-BASED HISTORY

Unlike other chapters in this book that contain several problems, this chapter deals with only one problem: pain. Nurses rely on patients' self-reports as the most reliable parameter for pain assessment. When obtaining a patient's health history related to pain, the nurse is sensitive to the influences of culture on communication and responses to pain because pain has psychological, social, spiritual, and physical dimensions. Because pain is a complex, multidimensional, subjective experience, nurses collect data from patients using a symptom analysis applying the mnemonic OLD CARTS, which includes the *o*nset, *l*ocation, *d*uration, *c*haracteristics, *a*ggravating factors, *r*elated symptoms, *t*reatment by the patient, and *s*everity (see Box 2-3).

What are your beliefs about discussing your pain with others? How do you usually communicate your pain to others?

For accurate data collection, nurses need to know the patient's preferred method for communicating pain (i.e., verbally or nonverbally). Culture influences how people communicate their pain. In some cultures people may express their pain overtly, whereas those in other cultures may be stoic, remain silent, or even smile. Some people believe that using nonverbal communication such as wincing or groaning is sufficient for communicating pain. People holding this belief may not think that verbally expressing their pain is necessary. Communication of pain may not be acceptable in some cultures in which people believe that asking for pain medication is a sign of their weakness or a lack of respect for the health care provider.[13]

Onset

When does the pain occur? During activity? Before or after eating?

The answer may help determine the source of the pain. Physical activity may aggravate joint pain. Eating may increase peptic ulcer pain.

Does the pain occur suddenly or gradually?

The answer may help determine the causes of the pain. Acute pain has a sudden onset. Ischemic pain gradually increases in intensity.

What do you think is causing your pain? Why do you think the pain started when it did?

Knowing patients' insights into the cause of their pain is a patient-centered approach and may help determine its occurrence and assist in pain management.

Location

Where do you feel the pain? Can you point to the location(s)?

Location may provide information about the cause of pain and its type (e.g., somatic versus visceral) (see Fig. 6-1). The patient may describe pain location away from the site of pathology when it is referred.

Duration

How long does the pain last? Is it constant or intermittent? If it is intermittent, how often does it occur, and how long does it last?

The answer to these questions may suggest a cause of the pain. For example, patients with mild peripheral artery disease experience intermittent leg pain when walking as a result of ischemia. When they stop walking, their pain is relieved. As the disease progresses, the pain with walking become constant and is not relieved by rest.

Characteristics

Can you describe what the pain feels like?

The McGill Pain Questionnaire in Fig. 6-3 is a multidimensional tool that provides information about the patient's characteristics and effect on the patient's daily life.[14] Somatic pain is usually well localized and described as aching or throbbing in quality.

Visceral pain caused by a tumor is aching and well localized; but, if caused by obstruction, the pain may be poorly localized and described as intermittent cramping.[7]

Aggravating Factors

What makes the pain worse?

The answer may help to determine the cause of the pain or understand the impact that pain may have on the patient. For example, patients with a penetrating gastric peptic ulcer report that their pain increases when they eat. Patients who have pneumonia may complain of a sharp pain when taking a deep breath (termed *pleuretic chest pain*).

Related Symptoms

Do you have other symptoms during the pain such as palpitations; shortness of breath; sweating; rapid, irregular breathing; nausea; or vomiting?

During low-to-moderate acute pain intensity the sympathetic nervous system may cause palpitations, diaphoresis, or increasing respiratory rate; whereas during severe or deep pain the parasympathetic nervous system may cause pallor; rapid, irregular breathing; nausea; and vomiting.

Treatment by the Patient

How have you tried to relieve this pain? How effective have these measures been?

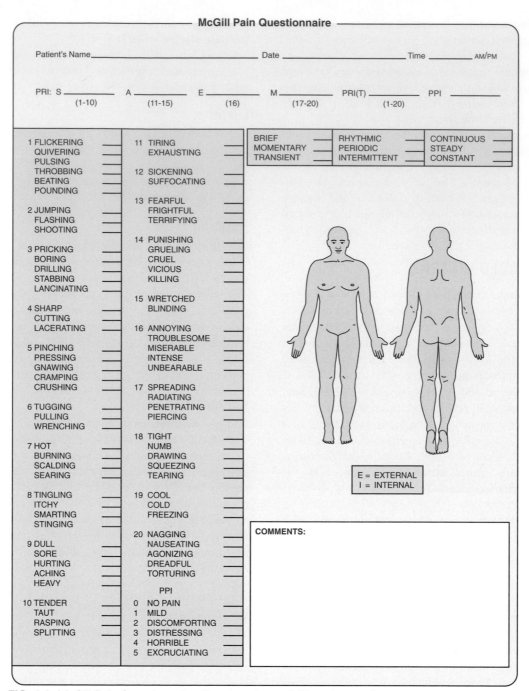

FIG. 6-3 McGill Pain Questionnaire. The descriptors fall into four major groups: sensory, 1 to 10; affective, 11 to 15; evaluative, 16; and miscellaneous, 17 to 20. The rank value of each descriptor is based on its position in the word set. The sum of the rank values is the pain rating index *(PRI)*. The present pain intensity *(PPI)* is based on a scale of 0 to 5. (From Melzack and Katz, 1994.)

A broad, open-ended question is purposefully asked first to encourage patients to report all forms of therapy (i.e., medications and alternative therapies). The response to this question helps the nurse know which therapies to continue and which to ignore in providing pain relief. All forms of pain relief should be noted: prescription and over-the-counter medications and alternative treatments. Inquiring about the amount of drug taken is important to detect possible toxic effects such as drugs that contain acetaminophen, which can be toxic to the liver. Asking about the effectiveness of pain relief is important because the patient may not volunteer this information and ineffective medications should be reevaluated by the health care provider. The question reminds patients that pain can often be relieved with alternative treatments such as movement-based therapies, nutritional and herbal remedies, mind-body medicine, energy healing, massage, and lifestyle changes.[15]

How much pain relief are you expecting?
Cultural beliefs may affect the extent of pain relief expected. When caring for patients who have a low expectation for pain relief, the nurse asks about their beliefs regarding pain and satisfaction with current pain level. Nurses do not assume that patients have the same expectation of pain relief as they would have in a similar situation. The patient's satisfaction with pain relief is assessed, and both alternative treatments and pharmacologic interventions are offered to achieve the patient's desired pain expectation.

Severity

How would you describe the intensity, strength, or severity of the pain on a scale of 0 to 10, with 0 being no pain and 10 being the most intense pain possible?
These data provide further description of how "bad" the patient's pain feels. Pain assessment tools allow the patient to communicate how severe the pain feels (pain quantity) and are appropriate for cultural groups that read horizontally from left to right. However in cultures such as Chinese or Japanese that read vertically, they may be confusing or yield inaccurate data. People from different cultures use various communication styles to express their pain. For example, when asked to rate pain using a numeric scale from 0 to 10, some Native American patients may select a favorite or sacred number instead of the number that accurately indicates their pain level.[11]

Frequently used pain rating scales are the numeric rating scale (NRS) and the FACES rating scale. These scales, shown in Fig. 6-4, give patients a choice of rating their pain either on a scale showing a horizontal line with markings from 0 to 10 or a face that represents their pain. Pasero and McCaffery[16] recommend using both the NRS and FACES in clinical practice with cognitively intact adolescents, adults, and older adults. The NRS scale in this format has been used successfully and translated into many languages, including Chinese, French, German, Greek, Hawaiian, Hebrew, the Philippine language, Italian, Japanese, Korean, Pakistan, Polish, Russian, Samoan, Spanish, Tagalog, Tingan, and Vietnamese.[16]

At which point on this scale of 0 to 10 do you usually take medication for your pain?
This question seeks knowledge about the patient's pain tolerance, which is influenced by culture, pain experience, expectations of pain, and its ability to be relieved.

Response to Pain

How do you react to your pain? How do you express it (e.g., anger, frustration, crying, or no expression at all)? What do you fear most about your pain? What problems does it cause?
Pain can affect people physically, psychologically, socially, and spiritually. Patients' responses to pain may be influenced by culture and previous experience with it. Pain can evoke a variety of emotional responses such as anxiety, fear, depression, and anger. Conversely anxiety and fear can exacerbate a pain experience.[5] The nurse acknowledges these feelings as the patient's personal response to pain without trying to change them.

Does this pain have any particular meaning for you? If so, what is it?
The meaning of pain is unique for each person. For some people it is based on a particular action they took that contributed to the pain (e.g., "I should not have tried to steal home base"). To others the meaning is spiritual or psychologic. For example, they may believe that they are being punished or that they have had impure thoughts. In some cultures people grow up not expecting a great deal of pain relief because they believe that having pain is a part of the healing process. Knowing the meaning of the pain helps the nurse understand the patient's subjective experience of it. The nurse's role is to encourage the patient to describe the meaning of pain without judging the patient's response.

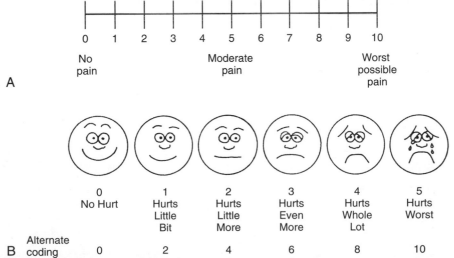

FIG. 6-4 A, Numeric rating scale (NRS). **B,** Wong-Baker FACES pain rating scale. (**B** from Hockenberry MJ, Wilson D: *Wong's essentials of pediatric nursing,* ed 8, St Louis, 2009, Mosby. Used with permission. Copyright © Mosby.)

What has been your past experience with pain and pain relief?

These questions address the cognitive response to pain. Patients use their past experiences to respond to pain. When nurses know what these experiences are, they can help patients relieve their pain more therapeutically and better understand patients whose expectations for pain relief are high (greater than 6 on a scale of 0 to 10).

Do you have any concerns about taking medications for pain relief?

Some patients do not ask for pain relief medication because they fear that it will cause an addiction. This misconception can be remedied by appropriate patient education.

How has the pain affected your quality of life? How has it altered your life (e.g., does it interfere with sleep, mood, walking ability, work, relationships with others)?

Pain can alter a patient's usual daily activity. Those who have compensated for or adjusted to persistent, chronic pain may perceive a higher quality of life than those who have not adjusted to the pain. However, persistent pain is often associated with a sense of hopelessness and helplessness. Patients with persistent pain may report depression, difficulty sleeping and eating, and preoccupation with the pain.[7]

Pain Reassessment

After taking the pain medication and/or using other pain-relieving strategies, how would you rate your pain on a scale of 0 to 10?

The Agency for Health Care Policy and Research (AHCPR) Clinical Practice Guidelines (CPG) state that pain should be reassessed within 30 minutes after parenteral analgesic drug administration and within 1 hour of oral analgesic drug administration.[17]

ASSESSING PAIN OF PATIENTS WHO CANNOT COMMUNICATE

Nurses acknowledge that pain cannot be assessed accurately without adequate communication with the patient. When patients are unable to communicate, how do nurses complete a pain assessment? Herr[1] suggests a hierarchy of five pain-assessment approaches when patients cannot communicate. First, attempt a self-report from the patient or explain why self-report cannot be used. The second approach is used when self-reports are not possible, such as for infant and toddlers, older adults with dementia, or adults with a decreased level of consciousness. In these cases the nurse searches for potential causes of pain, including pathologic conditions and common problems or procedures known to cause pain such as surgery, rehabilitation, wound care, positioning, blood draws, heel sticks, and a history of persistent pain. The third approach recommended is to list the patient's behaviors that may indicate pain. Fourth, the nurse identifies behaviors that caregivers and others knowledgeable about the patient think may indicate pain. Finally the nurse attempts an analgesic trial by giving an analgesic appropriate to the estimated intensity of pain based on the patient's pathology and analgesic history, even when the patient cannot communicate pain. Notice changes in behaviors when the analgesic becomes effective.[1]

EXAMINATION

PROCEDURE AND TECHNIQUES WITH EXPECTED FINDINGS	ABNORMAL FINDINGS

ROUTINE TECHNIQUES: PAIN

CLEAN hands.

OBSERVE patient for posture, facial expressions, and behavior to relieve pain.

Posture should be erect, and no movement to relieve pain should be evident. Facial muscles appear relaxed.

Guarding of a painful body part, rubbing or pressing the painful area, distorted posture, or fixed or continuous movement may indicate acute pain. Patients may lie very still to avoid movement or may be restless. Head rocking, pacing, or inability to keep hands still, a wrinkled forehead, tightly closed eyes, lackluster eyes, grimace, clenched teeth, or lip biting may be other signs of acute pain. Facial grimacing may indicate pain. Behaviors associated with pain may include agitation, restlessness, irritability, confusion, and combativeness.[1]

PROCEDURE AND TECHNIQUES WITH EXPECTED FINDINGS	ABNORMAL FINDINGS
LISTEN for sounds the patient makes. Sounds other than those of conversation are not expected.	Moaning, grunting, screaming, crying, or gasping may indicate acute pain; but some patients make no verbal sounds when they are in pain. Pain may be expressed during movement of an affected extremity during examination.
MEASURE blood pressure and pulse. Blood pressure and pulse should be within expected limits for age.	Systolic blood pressure and heart rate may be increased by the sympathetic stimulation during acute pain.
ASSESS respiratory rate and pattern. Respirations should be even, quiet, and unlabored. Respiratory rate should be within expected limits for age.	Respiratory rate and pattern may vary from slow and deep to rapid and shallow, depending on which provides more comfort to the patient. Some patients may use slow, deep breathing to relax as a pain-relieving strategy.
INSPECT site of pain for appearance. Skin should be intact without edema. Skin color should be consistent over the body area inspected.	The area of pain may appear inflamed (red, edematous) and have an incision or visible injury.
PALPATE site of pain for tenderness. The patient may report feeling the pressure of the nurse's palpation but should not report tenderness or pain. If the site of pain is an open wound, the nurse wears gloves during palpation.	Tissue damage or an incision may result in pain on palpation.

AGE-RELATED VARIATIONS

This chapter discusses variables influencing a nurse's assessment of pain in adults. Nurses adapt their approach to pain assessment and find different responses to pain depending on the age of the patient.

INFANTS AND CHILDREN

This chapter discusses variables influencing a nurse's assessment of pain in adults. Nurses adapt their approach to pain assessment and find different responses to pain depending on the age of the patient. Neonates respond to pain in a global response, as evidenced by increased heart rate, hypertension, decreased oxygenation saturation, pallor, and sweating.[18] Infants and young children are unable to communicate their pain and have difficulty distinguishing between anxiety and pain intensity. Indicators of pain for infants may be crying and reflex withdrawal; whereas indicators for toddlers may be pursed lips, wide opening of eyes, rocking, rubbing, or defensive behavior (e.g., biting, hitting, kicking, running away).[9] Young children have difficulty understanding pain and the procedures that cause it; however, they have developed a basic ability to describe pain and its location. School-age children are better able to understand pain and to describe its location. Chapter 19 presents further information regarding pain assessment for this age-group.

For children the FACES rating has been developed. The Wong-Baker FACES has been translated into various languages, including Chinese, French, Italian, Japanese, Portuguese, Romanian, Spanish, and Vietnamese and has been used with children as young as 3 years old.[16]

OLDER ADULTS

Although transmission and perception of pain may be slowed in the older person, their pain perception is no different from that of any other adult. Older adults may underreport their pain because of fear, cultural factors, or stoicism. Assessment of their pain may be hampered by vision or hearing impairment when they must look at an assessment tool such as the visual analog scale and follow verbal directions on how to use it.[9] Many older adults have a lifetime of experience in coping with pain, but pain is not an expected part of aging. Chapter 21 presents further information regarding pain assessment in this age-group.

CLINICAL APPLICATION AND CLINICAL REASONING

See Appendix D for answers to exercises in this section.

REVIEW QUESTIONS

1. What is the most reliable way to assess a patient's pain?
   1. Type and frequency of analgesic medications the patient takes
   2. Patient's most recent vital signs (e.g., blood pressure and pulse rate)
   3. Extent of tissue damage the patient has had
   4. Report from the patient describing the pain experienced

2. A patient had a knee replaced because of arthritis. He reports that he has not slept well in several nights. He states that he can't get comfortable. Today he is asking for pain medication more often. What might be a reason for this increase in pain?
   1. Arthritis pain is variable; it can be mild one day and severe the next.
   2. Pain tolerance decreases with sleep deprivation.
   3. The anesthesia from surgery is wearing off.
   4. The patient is using the pain medication to help him sleep during the day.

3. A patient complains of chest pain. Which question is pertinent to ask to gain additional information?
   1. "What were you doing when the pain first occurred?"
   2. "What does the pain feel like?"
   3. "Do you have shortness of breath with the chest pain?"
   4. "Has anyone in your family ever had similar pain?"

4. A patient complains of leg pain. Which question is pertinent to ask to gain additional information?
   1. "What were you doing when the pain first occurred?"
   2. "How do you feel about having this pain?"
   3. "Do you think the pain is caused by a cramp?"
   4. "Has anyone in your family ever had similar pain?"

5. A female has been admitted to the emergency department with severe abdominal pain. She is lying on a stretcher quietly, with very little movement. The nurse preparing to assess her abdomen should expect to see which behavior when it is time to palpate this patient's abdomen?
   1. Flushing of the face and neck
   2. Guarding over the abdomen
   3. Relaxation of abdominal muscles
   4. Decreased peristalsis

CASE STUDY

A patient comes to the emergency department with a chief complaint of severe right abdominal and flank pain.

Interview Data

The patient tells the nurse, "The pain came on rather suddenly about an hour ago. I was doing some work at my desk, and it suddenly started." He points to the right flank areas as the location of the pain, but it extends into the right lower abdominal area as well. The patient describes the pain as "severe," sharp pain. On a scale of 0 to 10, he states, "This is off your pain scale—at least a 12." He describes the pain as constant, with intensity being intermittent since it may lighten slightly and intensify again. The other symptom he describes is nausea.

Examination Data

- *General survey:* BP, 128/96 mm Hg; pulse, 108 beats/min; respirations, 24 breaths/min; temperature, 101.8° F (38.8°

C). Patient is curled up on a stretcher in the fetal position; appears uncomfortable, groaning.
- *Skin:* Pale, diaphoretic, and warm to touch.
- *Abdomen:* Flat, no scars observed; bowel sounds active in all quadrants; soft, nontender to abdominal palpation. Costovertebral angle (CVA) pain on percussion of kidneys.

Clinical Reasoning

1. Which data deviate from expected findings, suggesting a need for further investigation?
2. Which additional information should the nurse gather?
3. With which other health care team member could the nurse consult to help relieve this patient's pain?

Mental Health and Abusive Behavior Assessment

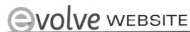 WEBSITE

http://evolve.elsevier.com/Wilson/assessment

Comprehensive assessment of individuals includes mental and emotional health in addition to physical health. Mental health is an integral and essential component of health. *Mental health* is defined as a state of well-being in which people realize their own abilities, can cope with normal stresses of life, can work productively, and are able to make contributions to their communities.[1] Changes in people's lives may affect their mental health, requiring periodic mental health and mental status assessment. *Mental status* is defined as the degree of competence that a person shows in intellectual, emotional, psychologic, and personality functioning. Abusive experiences may influence a person's mental health. Examples of abusive experiences include alcohol, drug, and personal abuse, called *interpersonal violence*. Interpersonal violence is not an illness; it is a crime (i.e., a human rights violation that can have negative impacts on patients' mental and physical health).[2] The purpose of this chapter is to describe ways to assess for an individual's mental health and identify any abnormal findings that may indicate the need for a referral to mental health professionals.

ANATOMY AND PHYSIOLOGY

Memory and basic emotions such as fear, anger, and sex drive are regulated by the limbic system, also called the *emotional brain*. The limbic system structures are shown in Fig. 7-1 and include the limbic lobe, cingulate gyrus, hippocampus, amygdala, thalamus, and portions of the hypothalamus. These structures enable communications between the limbic system and cerebral cortex. For example, when a person sees something that jogs a memory about a happy event, communication occurs among the occipital lobe for vision, prefrontal lobe for memory, and limbic system for the happy emotion and the memory.

Neurotransmitters have an essential function in the role of human emotion and behavior. They are chemical vehicles that provide synaptic transmission of messages from neuron to neuron or from neurons to muscle cells. These neurotransmitters are synthesized in neurons, released in the synaptic cleft, and bind to receptor sites on other neurons or effector cells as shown in Fig. 7-2. After release, any neurotransmitters not used during impulse transmission are stored through reuptake mechanisms, are degraded by enzymes, or diffuse into the nerve terminal.[3] Neurotransmitters affecting mental health include dopamine, norepinephrine, serotonin, histamine, acetylcholine, and gamma-aminobutyric acid (GABA). The neurotransmitters associated with mental illness are described in Table 7-1.

⊕ ETHNIC, CULTURAL, AND SPIRITUAL VARIATIONS

Culturally Relevant Phenomena in Mental Health Nursing

The concept of mental health is formed within a culture, and deviance from cultural expectations can be defined as *illness* by other members of the group. Mental health nursing is based on personality and development theories promoted by Europeans and Americans and grounded in western cultural ideals and values. Nurses are as influenced by their own professional and ethnic cultures as patients are by theirs and thus must guard against ethnocentric tendencies.

Continued

🌐 ETHNIC, CULTURAL, AND SPIRITUAL VARIATIONS

Culturally Relevant Phenomena in Mental Health Nursing—cont'd

Phenomena include the following:

- *Perception of reality*—Perception may be culturally pre-scribed, spiritually induced in a traditional healing system, or otherwise sanctioned by the cultural group. For example, a Native American patient may appear to a Cau-casian American to have lost touch with reality, but the Native American is practicing his or her spiritual healing ritual, which is important to attain or maintain health.
- *Needs, feelings, thoughts of others and self*—Patients need to attend to their needs, feelings, and thoughts of self and others, whether they are internal or external. Events considered as stressors vary from one culture to another. For example, Kenyans are taught not to discuss or show their feelings of sadness or pain. If a Kenyan were seen by an American health care provider for a suspected mental health disorder, he or she would not willingly share feelings, which is a large part of the health history for mental health nursing. This patient may be seen as uncooperative, when in fact he or she is comply-ing with the Kenyan culture.
- *Decision making*—The ability to make decisions may be culturally prescribed so families and cultures designate decision makers, which may include health care deci-sions. Inability to make decisions is a clinical manifesta-tion of depression and anxiety. For example, in traditional Vietnamese families the oldest male makes decisions about health care. As a result, a female patient may delay seeking health care until she consults with the oldest male in the family.

From Zoucha R, Narayan M: Cultural implications for psychiatric mental health nursing. In Varcarolis EM, Halter M: *Foundations of psychiatric mental health nursing: a clinical approach,* ed 6, Philadelphia, 2010, Saunders, pp 101-117.

TABLE 7-1 NEUROTRANSMITTERS ASSOCIATED WITH MENTAL ILLNESS

NEUROTRANSMITTER	ASSOCIATION WITH MENTAL ILLNESS
Dopamine (DA)	Decreased in depression Increased in schizophrenia and mania
Norepinephrine (NE)	Decreased in depression Increased in schizophrenia, mania, and anxiety states
Serotonin (5 HT)	Decreased in depression Increased in anxiety states
Histamine	Decreased in depression
Acetylcholine (Ach)	Increased in depression
Gamma aminobutyric acid (GABA)	Decreased in anxiety states and schizophrenia

Data from Varcarolis E, Halter M: *Foundations of psychiatric mental health nursing,* ed 6, Philadelphia, 2010, Saunders.

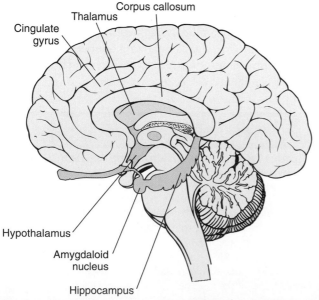

FIG. 7-1 The limbic system. (From McKenry and Salerno, 2003.)

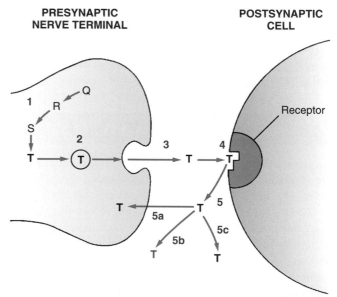

FIG. 7-2 Steps in synaptic transmission. Step 1, Synthesis of transmitter *(T)* from precursor molecules *(Q, R,* and *S).* Step 2, Storage of transmitter in vesicles. Step 3, Release of trans-mitter: In response to an action potential, vesicles fuse with the terminal membrane and discharge their contents in the synaptic gap. Step 4, Action at receptor: Transmitter binds (reversibly) to its receptor on the postsynaptic cell, causing a response in that cell. Step 5, Termination of transmission: Transmitter dissociates from its receptor and is then removed from the synaptic gap by (a) reuptake into the nerve terminal, (b) enzymatic degradation, or (c) diffusion away from the gap. (From Lehne, 2010.)

HEALTH HISTORY

Nurses interview patients to collect subjective data about their present health and any past medical experiences. In addition to present health status, past medical history, and family history, nurses ask patients about their self-concept; interpersonal relationships, including domestic violence; stressors; anger; and alcohol and drug use, which may affect their mental health.

GENERAL HEALTH HISTORY

Most data needed for a mental health assessment are collected by talking with patients. Thus most pertinent data are collected during history taking rather than during a physical examination. When nurses determine or suspect deviations from expected behavior, they ask additional questions (discussed later in this chapter). During the health history nurses notice and compare the patient's appearance, behavior, and cognitive functions with the characteristics of a healthy personality. Data collection begins when nurses first see the patients. Quality Improvement Competencies for Nurses include providing patient-centered care and interdisciplinary teamwork with the health care provider and community mental health professionals. Refer to Table 11-1 on p. 196 for specific competencies.

Notice:

- Is the patient dressed appropriately for the weather?
- Does his or her mood seem appropriate?
- Is the affect (emotional state) appropriate?
- What is the patient's body posture?
- Is the patient slumped over and looking at the ground with a sad facial expression or walking tall with a brisk step and a smiling face?
- What is the patient's tone of voice?
- Does he or she talk in a monotone or a happy, expressive tone?
- Does the patient's conversation flow in a logical or meaningful sequence?

Present Health Status

Are you having any medical problems?
Some medical problems (e.g., endocrine disorders such as hypothyroidism or adrenal insufficiency) may cause changes in mood or behavior.

What medications are you taking?
The nurse needs to document medications the patient is taking for mental health disorders. Adverse effects of these medications may cause changes in mood and behavior. In addition, medications taken for physical disorders may have adverse effects that may cause changes in mood and behavior. For example, some oral contraceptives, antihypertensives, or corticosteroids can cause depression as an adverse reaction.

Past Health History

In the past have you experienced any behaviors that could indicate a mental health problem? If yes, describe your experience. How have you coped in the past with this disorder? Are these coping strategies still working for you?
Identifying the person's previous problems with mental health provides a baseline for interviewing, knowing that this person has had experience with mental health disorders. If previous coping strategies are working, they should be used again. If they have not been successful, other strategies may be suggested.

Family History

Do you have any blood relatives who have behaviors that could indicate a mental health problem? If so, can you describe the behavior they experience?
Some mental illnesses such as anxiety, depression, and schizophrenia have genetic links. Having a family member with a mental illness may be associated with the patient's behavior.

Some people witnessed or experienced violence during their childhood. Did you have any experience with violence in the home while growing up?
Children raised in violent homes may be at increased risk for perpetrating or experiencing violence in adulthood. However, not all abusive partners or abused women or men were exposed to family violence while growing up.[4]

Personal and Psychosocial History
Self-Concept

How have you been feeling about yourself? Do you consider your present feelings to be a problem in your daily life? If so, do you think that the problem is temporary or curable?
These questions invite the patient to discuss feelings and may help to identify problems (e.g., depression, stress, anger). One's perception of an event determines his or her emotional reaction to that event. Each culture influences how events are perceived and acceptable ways to respond. Some cultures allow a verbal or physical response, whereas others refrain from any outward expression of emotion.

How would you describe yourself to others? What are your best characteristics? What do you like about yourself?
This determines how patients perceive themselves. Those with positive self-esteem regard themselves favorably and can name their positive attributes. Those with negative self-esteem tend to list primarily negative attributes and may be at risk for depression.

Interpersonal Relationships

How satisfied are you with your interpersonal relationships? Are there people to whom you can talk about feelings and problems?

Achieving satisfying interpersonal relationships is needed for mental health. Patients who have few or no interpersonal relationships may be depressed or out of touch with reality. Social support is important for healthy interpersonal relationships.

I am going to ask you a few routine questions that I ask all patients because abuse and violence have become more common. Have you been physically injured (hit, kicked, punched) by someone in your home in the last year? Are you fearful of an individual with whom you have previously had a relationship? Do you feel safe in your current relationship with your partner?[2]

These questions screen for interpersonal violence. They are introduced as questions asked of all patients so the nurses do not imply that they suspect abuse for this specific patient. If the answer is "yes" to any of these questions, the patient is further screened as described under Problem-Based History later in this chapter.

Stressors

Have there been any recent changes in your life? How have these changes affected your stress level?

Inquire about stressors such as money, intimate relationships, death or illness of a family member or friend, and employment problems. One way to inquire further about stress is to administer the Holmes Social Readjustment Rating Scale (Table 7-2).

What are the major stressors in your life now? How do you deal with stress? Are these methods of stress relief currently effective for you?

Coping with the stress of daily life is essential to maintain mental health. Answers to these questions help identify the patient's stressors and how well they are being managed. The nurse may take this opportunity to teach patients alternate ways to react to their stress. These may include relaxation techniques, physical exercise, or journaling. When patients describe difficulty dealing with stress, they can be referred to agencies for care and support.

Anger

Have you been feeling angry? How do you react when you are angry? Do you react verbally or physically or do you keep your anger inside? Can you talk about what has caused this anger?

Learning how patients react to anger gives the nurse insight into how healthy their responses to anger are and provides an opportunity to teach them alternate ways to express their feelings (e.g., hit a pillow instead of a person, verbally express anger in an empty room or elevator). Talking about the cause of the anger can be therapeutic and provides an opportunity for the nurse to make referrals for help.

We all have disagreements with people. What happens when you and your partner fight or disagree?

Nurses may not feel the need to ask this question. It is included with the topic of anger to further screen for interpersonal violence.[4]

Alcohol Use

How often do you drink alcohol, including beer, wine, or liquor?

Every adult and adolescent should be asked about alcohol consumption to determine if it is a health problem. Additional data are collected when a male patient reports drinking more than five standard drinks daily or 15 weekly, a female patient reports more than five standard drinks daily or eight drinks weekly, or adults age 65 and older report more than one standard drink daily or seven weekly. Refer to Problem-Based History, Alcohol Abuse, later in this chapter.

Recreational Drug Use

Some people use recreational drugs. Do you ever use them? If yes, tell me about your drug use.

Every adult and adolescent should be asked about recreational drug use to determine if it is a health problem. The opening statement encourages patients to be honest in reporting their use. When people report recreational drug use, nurses collect additional data as described in Problem-Based History, Drug Abuse, later in this chapter.

PROBLEM-BASED HISTORY

Commonly reported problems related to mental health include depression, anxiety, and altered mental status; whereas common problems of abusive behaviors include alcohol abuse, drug abuse, and interpersonal violence. When data from the Present Health Status suggest that further assessment is indicated, nurses ask additional questions to identify common problems. Although a symptom analysis is used when assessing physical manifestations, it is not as useful when asking questions about the patient's behavior and feelings.

Depression

Document the gender and age of the patient.

Women are at risk for depression 2:1 over men. About one in eight women develop depression at some point in life. Depression can occur at any age, but it is most common in women between the ages of 25 and 44 years. After puberty depression rates are higher in females than in males. This depression gender gap lasts until after menopause.[5]

Notice the facial expression, eye contact, body language, and tone of voice of the patient.

Patients who are depressed may have a sad facial expression or evidence of tearfulness. They may avoid eye contact, speak in a monotone, show little facial expression, and have a slumped posture.[6]

During the past month have you often felt down, depressed, or hopeless? During the past month have you often had little interest or pleasure in doing things?

These two questions are used to screen for major depression. An affirmative answer to either question warrants a follow-up clinical interview.[7]

TABLE 7-2   HOLMES SOCIAL READJUSTMENT RATING SCALE

EVENT	EVENT VALUE	EVENT	EVENT VALUE
1. Death of a spouse	100	22. Change in responsibilities at work	29
2. Divorce	73	23. Son or daughter leaving home	29
3. Marital separation	65	24. Trouble with in-laws	29
4. Jail term	63	25. Outstanding personal achievement	28
5. Death of a close family member	63	26. Spouse begins or stops work	26
6. Personal injury or illness	53	27. Beginning or ending school	26
7. Marriage	50	28. Change in living conditions	25
8. Fired at work	47	29. Revision of personal habits	24
9. Marital reconciliation	45	30. Trouble with boss	23
10. Retirement	45	31. Change in work hours or conditions	20
11. Change in health of family member	44	32. Change in residence	20
12. Pregnancy	40	33. Change in schools	20
13. Sex difficulties	39	34. Change in recreation	19
14. Gain of a new family member	39	35. Change in church activities	19
15. Business readjustment	39	36. Change in social activities	19
16. Change in financial state	38	37. Change in sleeping habits	16
17. Death of a close friend	37	38. Change in number of family get-togethers	15
18. Change to different line of work	36	39. Vacation	13
19. Change in number of arguments	35	40. Christmas	12
20. Mortgage or loan over $10,000	31	41. Minor violations of the law	11
21. Foreclosure of mortgage or loan	30	**Total Points**	—

Directions for completion: Add the point values for each of the events that you have experienced during the past 12 months.

Scoring

Below 150 points:
The amount of stress that you are experiencing as a result of changes in your life is normal and manageable. There is only a one in three chance that you might develop a serious illness over the next 2 years based on stress alone. Consider practicing a daily relaxation technique to reduce your chance of illness even more.

150 to 300 points:
The amount of stress that you are experiencing as a result of changes in your life is moderate. Based on stress alone, you have a 50/50 chance of developing a serious illness over the next 2 years. You can reduce these odds by practicing stress management and relaxation techniques on a daily basis.

Over 300 points:
The amount of stress that you are experiencing as a result of changes in your life is high. Based on stress alone, your chances of developing a serious illness during the next 2 years approaches 90%, unless you are already practicing good coping skills and regular relaxation techniques. You can reduce the chance of illness by practicing coping strategies and relaxation techniques daily.

Modified from Holmes TH, Rahe RJ: Social readjustment rating scale, *Journal of Psychosomatic Research* 11:213-218, 1967.

Are you able to fall asleep and stay asleep without difficulty? Have you noticed any marked changes in your eating habits? Have you recently gained or lost weight without trying? Have you noticed a lack of energy?

A depressed mood can interrupt sleep habits. Insomnia is reported frequently with variations, including difficulty falling asleep and staying asleep. Appetite may decrease or increase. Profound fatigue that is not relieved by rest is reported.

Describe your mood. Do you have crying spells? Do you have difficulty concentrating or making decisions? Have you noticed an increase in irritability? How often have you experienced these feelings, how long did the feelings last, and how many of them occurred together in a 2-week period?

These questions help identify possible symptoms of depression. Some patients can recognize symptoms but do not realize that the group of symptoms may indicate depression. Experiencing five or more of these symptoms in a 2-week period may indicate a need for a referral to a mental health professional.[3]

Do you have friends whom you can trust and who are available when you need them?
Friends can be a source of social support to listen to the patient's feelings and demonstrate their caring for the patient.

Have you had depressive feelings like this before? What did you do about them?
Depression may be a recurring disorder. Treatment that was successful in the past may be useful again.

Have there been times when you wanted to escape? Have you ever thought about escaping by hurting yourself or ending your life? If yes, do you feel like hurting yourself now? Do you have a plan for hurting yourself? If yes, what will you do to end your life? Where will this occur? Have you told anyone else about your plan? What would happen if you were dead?
These questions screen for suicidal thoughts. A patient who has a specific plan for suicide is at higher risk than one who has no plan. Steps must be taken to protect the person who has a plan to hurt himself or herself. Women attempt suicide three times as often as men, but men complete suicide at a rate four times that of women. The higher attempted suicide rate in women is attributed to their elevated rate of mood disorders such as major depression and seasonal affective disorder. Firearms are now the leading method of suicide in women and men. Suicide rates for men rise with age, most significantly after age 65. Suicide rates for women peak between ages 45 and 54 and again after 75 years.[8]

FREQUENTLY ASKED QUESTIONS

When patients say that they want to end their life, the nurse is supposed to ask if they have thought about hurting themselves or if they have a plan for hurting themselves. Doesn't that suggest to them that they should hurt themselves? Aren't you putting ideas in their head?

Asking patients about a plan to hurt themselves may seem like a suggestion, but it is not. The purpose for asking the question is to determine if they are depressed enough or serious enough to make a plan to end their life. If the nurse learns that patients have a plan, they need immediate referral to a mental health professional.

What has kept you from hurting yourself in the past?
Reminding the patient of factors that prevented suicide may be useful again. Ambivalence often keeps patients from ending their lives.

Anxiety

Have you had difficulty concentrating or making decisions? Have you been preoccupied or forgetful? Are you able to fall asleep and stay asleep without difficulty?
Sleep deprivation is a risk factor for anxiety.

Have you noticed a change in the amount of energy that you have (fatigue)? Have you been more irritable than usual? Do your muscles seem tense? Do you feel a tightening in your throat?
These are symptoms of anxiety. See the description of the four levels of anxiety under Common Problems and Conditions later in this chapter.

Have you felt nauseated? Do you feel your heart racing? Have you had to urinate more often than usual?
Nausea, urinary frequency, and palpitations may be physiologic responses to anxiety.

Have you noticed a change in your feelings? If yes, describe these feelings. What do you think initiated them? How did you handle or cope with them?
Feelings of anger, guilt, worthlessness, and anguish often accompany anxiety. The patient may report feeling that he or she is going to die or have a sense of impending doom.

Altered Mental Status

Changes in mental status may become evident when there is change in the patient's orientation to person, place or time, attention span, or memory. When nurses suspect that a patient's orientation has changed, they ask questions to collect additional data. Long-term memory can be assessed during the history by asking patients where they were born or about their previous surgeries.

Assess mental status by determining orientation, memory, calculation ability, communication skills, judgment, and abstraction.

Orientation

Ask the patient what year it is, where he or she is, and his or her name. Orientation to time is the first orientation to be lost; to place, the second orientation to be lost; and to person, the last orientation to be lost.

Memory

Ask patients to repeat three unrelated objects that are spoken slowly such as "dog," "cloud," and "apple."

Calculation Ability

The calculation ability can be tested by asking patients about making change. For example, the nurse asks a patient, "You buy fruit that costs $2.45 and you give the cashier $3.00. How much change would you expect to receive?"

Communication Skills (Naming, Repeating, Writing, and Copying)

Ask patients to *name* common objects such as a watch or pencil. *Repetition* is tested by asking patients to repeat a phrase such as, "No ifs, ands, or buts." *Reading* is tested by asking patients to read a phrase that is written on a piece of paper and to do what it says such as, "Lift your right hand." When patients complete this task, the nurse knows that they can read, comprehend what they read, and follow instructions. *Writing* is tested by asking patients to write a sentence. Do not tell them what to write. The sentence must have a subject and a verb to be sensible, but correct punctuation and grammar are not assessed. *Copying* is assessed by asking patients to copy a drawing of two geometric figures that overlap such as an intersecting pentagon about 1 inch on a side.

Judgment and Reasoning

Ask a question such as, "What would you do if a car were speeding toward you?"

Abstract Reasoning

Ask the meaning of a proverb such as, "A bird in the hand is worth two in the bush."[9]

Alcohol Abuse

Patients with an alcohol use disorder are likely to deny or minimize their drinking to avoid being judged by others. Thus the nurse uses a matter-of-fact and nonjudgmental approach when assessing these patients.[10]

Many people drink alcohol. Do you sometimes drink beer, wine, or other alcoholic beverages? If yes, how many times in the past year have you had more than five drinks in a day (for men) or four drinks in a day (for women)?

The National Institute on Alcohol Abuse and Alcoholism (NIAAA) recommends that all health care providers screen every patient for alcohol use disorders. Not all alcohol use is dangerous; however, alcohol causes or increases the risk of alcohol-related problems such as cirrhosis and injuries from falls and complicates management of other medical problems. Every adult and adolescent should be asked about alcohol consumption to determine if it is a health problem. For the general adult population, NIAAA recommends these limits:

- Men: fewer than five standard drinks daily or 15 weekly
- Women: fewer than four standard drinks daily or eight weekly
- Adults age 65 and older: no more than one standard drink daily or seven weekly
- Pregnant women: No level of alcohol consumption is safe[11]

The standard drinks are shown in Fig. 7-3.

In the past 2 months has your drinking repeatedly caused or contributed to:
- **Risk of bodily harm (e.g., drinking and driving, operating machinery, swimming)?**
- **Relationship trouble with family or friends?**
- **Role failure (e.g., interference with home, work, school obligations)?**
- **Run-ins with the law (e.g., arrests or other legal problems)?**

When patients answer "yes" to one or more of these questions, they are abusing alcohol and need to be screened for alcohol dependence.[12]

Accurate information about alcohol intake may be difficult to obtain because patients are unwilling to disclose their actual consumption. One tool used to screen for alcoholism is called the Alcohol Use Disorders Identification Test (AUDIT). It has 10 questions that ask about quantity and frequency of drinking, binging, and consequences of drinking (Table 7-3). Another screening tool is the CAGE questions, which is an acronym for Cut down, Annoyed, Guilty and Eye opener. This tool is available at www.addictionsandrecovery.org/addiction-self-test.htm.

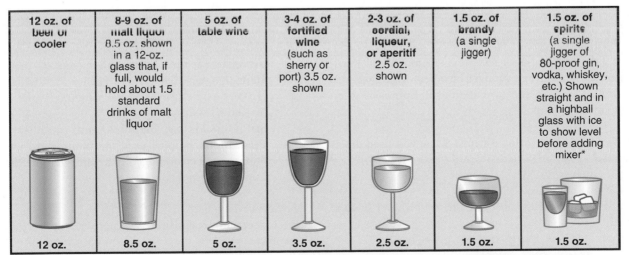

FIG. 7-3 U.S. standard drink equivalents. These are approximate, since different brands and types of beverages vary their actual alcohol content. A standard drink in the United States is any drink that contains about 14 g of pure alcohol (about 0.6 fluid ounces or 1.2 tablespoons). (From National Institute on Alcohol Abuse and Alcoholism (NIAAA): *Helping patients who drink too much: a clinician's guide, Patient Education Materials: What's a standard drink,* 2005, available at www.niaaa.nih.gov, accessed September 7, 2011.)

TABLE 7-3   AUDIT STRUCTURED INTERVIEW*

QUESTION	SCORE				
	0	1	2	3	4
How often do you have a drink containing alcohol?	Never	Monthly or less	2-4 times/ month	Monthly 2-3 times/week	4 or more times/week
How many drinks do you have on a typical day when you are drinking?	None	1 or 2	3 or 4	5 or 6	7-9†
How often do you have 6 or more drinks on one occasion?	Never	Less than monthly	Monthly	Weekly	Daily or almost daily
How often during the last year have you found that you were unable to stop drinking once you had started?	Never	Less than monthly	Monthly	Weekly	Daily or almost daily
How often last year have you failed to do what was normally expected from you because of drinking?	Never	Less than monthly	Monthly	Weekly	Daily or almost daily
How often during the last year have you needed a first drink in the morning to get yourself going after a heavy drinking session?	Never	Less than monthly	Monthly	Weekly	Daily or almost daily
How often during the last year have you had a feeling of guilt or remorse after drinking?	Never	Less than monthly	Monthly	Weekly	Daily or almost daily
How often during the last year have you been unable to remember what happened the night before because you had been drinking?	Never	Less than monthly	Monthly	Weekly	Daily or almost daily
Have you or someone else been injured as a result of your drinking?	Never	Yes, but not in last year (2 points)		Yes, during the last year (4 points)	
Has a relative, doctor, or other health worker been concerned about your drinking or suggested that you cut down?	Never	Yes, but not in last year (2 points)		Yes, during the last year (4 points)	

From Report of the U.S. Preventive Services Task Force: *Guide to clinical preventive services,* ed 2, U.S. Department of Health and Human Services, 1996, Washington, DC.
AUDIT, Alcohol Use Disorders Identification Test.
*Score of greater than 8 (out of 41) suggests problem drinking and indicates need for more in-depth assessment. Cut-off of 10 points is recommended by some to provide greater specificity.
†5 points if response is 10 or more drinks on a typical day.

Drug Abuse

Patients with drug use disorders are likely to deny or minimize their use to avoid being judged by others. Thus the nurse uses a matter-of fact and nonjudgmental approach when assessing these patients.[10]

Some people use recreational drugs. Have you used drugs in the past?
If the patient answers "yes," ask:

Which of the following substances have you used in your lifetime?
- **Cannabis (e.g., marijuana, pot, grass, hash)**
- **Cocaine (e.g., coke, crack)**
- **Prescription stimulants (e.g., methylphenidate [Ritalin, Concerta], dextroamphetamine [Dexedrine], Adderall, diet pills)**
- **Methamphetamine (e.g., speed, ice)**
- **Inhalants (e.g., nitrous, glue, gas, paint thinner)**

- **Sedatives or sleeping pills (e.g., diazepam [Valium], oxazepam [Serepax], alprazolam [Xanax])**
- **Hallucinogens (e.g., D-lysergic acid diethylamide [LSD], acid, mushrooms, phencyclidine [PCP], Special K, ecstasy)**
- **Street opioids (e.g., heroin, opium)**
- **Prescription opioids used for nonmedical use (e.g., fentanyl, oxycodone, hydrocodone, methadone, buprenorphine)**

Any other drug use?
If no lifetime drug use is reported, the screening is complete.

For each drug use reported, nurses ask the following questions:

In the past 3 months how often have you used each of the substances you mentioned?

How often have you had a strong desire or urge to use?

How often has your drug use led to health, social, legal or financial problems?

How often have you failed to do what was normally expected of you because of your use of this (these) drug(s)?

Has a friend, relative, or anyone else ever expressed concern about your use?

Have you ever tried and failed to control, cut down, or stop using this (these) drug(s)?

Have you ever used any drug by injection for nonmedical use?

Screening for drug abuse by asking these questions is an important first step in identifying patients who need to be referred for intervention procedures.[13]

Interpersonal Violence

If a patient answered "yes" to any of the screening questions about interpersonal violence, the nurse asks additional questions in private, with only the patient and nurse present. Be calm, matter-of-fact, and nonjudgmental. Listen carefully and let the patient define the problem. Gather descriptions of the behavior rather than why it happened and what it means. The nurse may preface comments by saying:

⊕ ETHNIC, CULTURAL, AND SPIRITUAL VARIATIONS

Legality of Drugs

Drugs that are considered illegal in one society may be considered legal and useful in another. For example, in the United States and parts of Western Europe, caffeine, alcohol, and nicotine are used widely and accepted. In the Middle East cannabis is considered a legal drug, whereas alcohol is forbidden. Some Native American tribes use peyote, a hallucinogen causing visual and auditory hallucinations, for religious services.

From McKenry L, Tessier E, Hogan M: *Mosby's pharmacology in nursing*, ed 22, St Louis, 2006, Mosby.

HEALTH PROMOTION FOR EVIDENCE-BASED PRACTICE

Mental Illness, Suicide Prevention, Interpersonal Violence, and Substance Abuse

Goals: *Healthy People 2020*

Healthy People 2020 outlines the national policy initiatives for health. Three topics associated with this area of assessment include Mental Health and Mental Disorders, Substance Abuse, and Injury and Violence Prevention. The specific goals for these topic areas are as follows:

- Improve mental health through prevention and by ensuring access to appropriate, quality mental health services
- Prevent unintentional injuries and violence and reduce their consequences
- Reduce substance abuse to protect the health, safety, and quality of life for all, especially children

Recommendations to Reduce Risk (Primary Prevention)
Substance Abuse: National Institute on Drug Abuse

Strategies for prevention of drug abuse focus on two primary principles:

1. *Enhance protective factors:* Protective factors include strong, positive bonds within the family; parental monitoring; clear rules of conduct consistently enforced within the family; parent involvement in the lives of children; success in school performance; strong bonds with institutions such as church and school; and adoption of conventional norms regarding drug use.
2. *Reduce risk factors:* Risk factors include a chaotic home environment (especially with parents who have substance abuse problems or mental illness); ineffective parenting; lack of mutual attachments; shy or aggressive behavior in the classroom; failure in school performance; poor social coping skills; association with deviant peer group; and adoption of attitude that approves of drug use.

Screening Recommendations (Secondary Prevention)
U.S. Preventive Services Task Force

Screening for depression:

- U.S. Preventive Services Task Force (USPSTF) recommends screening of adolescents (12-18 years of age) for major depressive disorder when systems are in place to ensure accurate diagnosis, psychotherapy (cognitive-behavioral or interpersonal), and follow-up.
- USPSTF recommends screening adults for depression when staff-assisted depression care supports are in place to ensure accurate diagnosis, effective treatment, and follow-up.

Screening for substance abuse:

- The USPSTF recommends screening and behavioral counseling interventions to reduce alcohol misuse by adults, including pregnant women, in primary care settings.
- Screen all adults for problem drinking through a history of alcohol use or use of standardized
- Use screening tools such as AUDIT.
- Current evidence is insufficient to assess the balance of benefit and harm of screening adolescents, adults, and pregnant women for illicit drug use.

Screening for violence:

- There is insufficient evidence to recommend for or against routine screening of parents or guardians for physical abuse or neglect of children, of women for intimate partner violence, or of older adults or their caregivers for elder abuse.

Data from US Department of Health and Human Services: US Preventive Services Task Force: *The guide to clinical preventive services, 2010-2011,* available at www.ahrq.gov; National Institute on Drug Abuse: Risk and protective factors in drug abuse prevention, *NIDA Notes 23*(4), 2011, available at *www.drugabuse.gov/NIDA_Notes*; US Department of Health and Human Services: *Healthy people 2020: understanding and improving health,* Washington, DC, 2011, US Government Printing Office, available at www.healthypeople.gov/2020/topicsobjectives2020/default.aspx.

- You are asked about violence because so many women are dealing with this problem in their home. Nobody deserves to be afraid in their home. If abuse is a problem for you, you may talk with me about it safely.[2]
- Are you in a relationship in which you have been physically hurt or threatened by your partner?
- Are you in a relationship in which you felt you were treated badly? In which ways?
- Has your partner ever destroyed things that you valued?
- Has your partner ever threatened or abused your children?
- Has your partner ever forced you to have sex when you weren't willing? Does he force you to engage in sex that makes you feel uncomfortable?

- What happens when you and your partner fight or disagree?
- Do you ever feel afraid of your partner?
- Has your partner ever prevented you from leaving home, seeing friends, getting a job, or continuing your education?
- You mentioned that your partner uses drugs/alcohol. How does he act when he is drinking or on drugs? Is he ever verbally or physically abusive?
- Do you have guns in your home? Has your partner ever threatened to use them when he was angry?[4]

EXAMINATION

ROUTINE TECHNIQUES

- OBSERVE the patient's posture and movement.
- OBSERVE for appropriate dress.
- NOTICE changes in voice tone, rate of speech, perspiration, and muscle tension or tremors.
- MEASURE blood pressure.
- PALPATE a pulse for rate.
- OBSERVE and COUNT respirations for rate and breathing pattern.
- OBSERVE eye movements and MEASURE pupil size.

Most data related to mental health and abusive behavior assessment are collected during interviews with patients. However, additional data can be obtained through observations and assessment of vital signs and the eyes.

PROCEDURES AND TECHNIQUES WITH EXPECTED FINDINGS	ABNORMAL FINDINGS

ROUTINE TECHNIQUES

CLEAN hands.

OBSERVE the patient's posture and movements.

The posture should be erect, and the body relaxed.

Tense muscles, fidgeting, or pacing may indicate anxiety; a slumped posture and slow movements may indicate depression.

OBSERVE dress and hygiene.

The clothing worn by the patient should be clean and appropriate for the weather or situation. The patient should show evidence of basic hygiene.

Outlandish dress and makeup may be worn by a patient in a manic phase of a bipolar disorder. Soiled clothing or lack of hygiene may indicate depression or organic brain syndrome.

NOTICE changes in voice tone, rate of speech, perspiration, and muscle tension or tremors.

Speech should be smooth, even, and without effort. The conversation should be clear, spontaneous, understandable, and appropriate to the context of the discussion. There should be no visible perspiration, and the patient should appear relaxed.

Physical signs of anxiety include changes in tone of voice and rate of speech, body tremors, increased muscle tension, perspiration, and sweaty palms.

PROCEDURES AND TECHNIQUES WITH EXPECTED FINDINGS	ABNORMAL FINDINGS

MEASURE the blood pressure.

Blood pressure varies with sex, body weight, and time of day; but the upper limits for adults are <120 mm Hg systolic and <80 mm Hg diastolic.

Anxiety, especially severe anxiety or panic, may cause elevated blood pressure as a result of sympathetic stimulation.

PALPATE a pulse for rate.

Rate: 60 to 100 beats/min
(See Chapter 12 for descriptions of pulses.)

Pulse rates for patients with anxiety may be elevated as a result of sympathetic stimulation from their anxious thoughts. Substance abuse may increase pulse rate.

OBSERVE and COUNT respirations for rate and breathing pattern.

Note the respiratory rate. Breathing should be smooth and even. In adults breathing should occur at a rate of 12 to 20 breaths/min. Evaluate the rhythm or pattern of breathing. The chest wall should symmetrically rise and expand and then relax. It should appear easy, without effort. (See Chapter 11 for descriptions of respirations.)

Respiratory rate may be increased during anxiety as a result of sympathetic stimulation. The patient may appear to be dyspneic. Respiratory rate may be decreased during depression, and the breathing pattern may include frequent, deep sighs.

OBSERVE eye movements and MEASURE pupil size.

When you suspect that the patient has drug intoxication, complete the rapid eye test in Box 7-1.

Table 7-4 on p. 78 describes clinical findings of acute drug intoxication. Table 7-5 describes common eye signs detected after abuse of selected drugs.

BOX 7-1   RAPID EYE TEST TO DETECT CURRENT DRUG INTOXICATION

General Observation
Look for redness of sclera, ptosis, retracted upper lid (white sclera visible above iris, causing blank stare), glazing, excessive tearing of eyes, and swelling of eyelids.

Pupil Size
Dilated (>6.5 mm) or constricted (<3 mm).

Pupil Reaction to Light
Slow, sluggish, or absent response.

Nystagmus
Hold finger in vertical position and have patient follow it as it moves to the side, in a circle, and up and down. Positive test is failure to hold gaze or jerkiness of eye movements.

Convergence
Inability to hold the cross-eyed position after an examining finger is moved 1 foot away from patient's nose and held there for 5 seconds.

Corneal Reflex
Decreased rate of blinking after touching cornea with cotton.

AGE-RELATED VARIATIONS

This chapter discusses assessment of the effects of alcohol and drug abuse in adults, which may affect neonates and infants. Assessing drug and alcohol use by children and adolescents is important. Nurses assess for depression and dementia in older adults.

INFANTS, CHILDREN, AND ADOLESCENTS

Variations for neonates and infants include asking about drug and alcohol use of the mother during the pregnancy. Children are asked about their experiences in school, how they like school, and if they get into trouble at school. They are also asked about their fears of any aspect of their life, including violence in their home. Adolescents are asked about school experience as well. In addition, they are asked about drug and alcohol use, and feelings of depression or anxiety. Assessing the self-esteem of this age-group is important. Chapter 19 presents further information regarding the mental health assessment of these age-groups.

OLDER ADULTS

Indications of depression in an older adult may be misinterpreted as expected manifestations of aging. For example, decrease in appetite or fatigue may be explained as a decrease in metabolism or a loss of taste buds that occur with aging. When older adults report problems concentrating or sleeping, it may be interpreted as an expected change with advanced age. Many older adults think that depression will go away without intervention, they are too old to get help, or reporting sadness may be a sign of weakness. Chapter 21 presents further information regarding the mental health assessment of this age-group.

COMMON PROBLEMS AND CONDITIONS

RISK FACTORS
Depression and Anxiety

Risk Factors for Depression
- *Gender:* Women at risk for depression 2:1 over men
- *Age:* Adolescents at risk for depression and anxiety because of peer pressure and desire to fit in and be independent of parents; In adults onset typically between 24 and 44 years of age
- *Genetics:* Children of parents who have depression likely to develop the disorder; risk doubles if both parents affected
- *Psychosocial environment:* People who have a history of trauma, sexual abuse, physical abuse, physical disability, alcoholism, or drug abuse or who have experienced death of a relative, divorce, changing jobs, or moving
- *Personal characteristics:* Low self-esteem; distorted perception of others' views; being pessimistic; inability to acknowledge personal accomplishment; having a serious illness, few friends or personal relationships; recently given birth (M)

Risk Factors for Anxiety
- *Gender:* Women more likely than men to be diagnosed with an anxiety disorder
- *Genetics:* A 20% risk for general anxiety disorder in blood relatives of people with the disorder and a 10% risk among relatives with depression
- *Physical health:* Stress from an illness, sleep deprivation (M)
- *Psychosocial environment:* Childhood trauma; illness; excessive stress (e.g., financial concerns, health, relationships, school or work problems); or alcohol or drug abuse (M)

Data from www.mayoclinic.com/health/depression/DS00175/DSECTION=risk-factors, updated Feb 11, 2010, accessed September 6, 2011; and www.mayoclinic.com/health/anxiety/DS01187/DSECTION=risk-factors, updated June 29, 2010, accessed September 6, 2011.
M, Modifiable risk factor.

MAJOR DEPRESSION

Major depression is an abnormal mood state in which a person characteristically has a sense of sadness, hopelessness, helplessness, worthlessness, and despair resulting from some personal loss or tragedy. A person may experience a single episode or have recurrent episodes of depression. Feeling depressed is not the same thing as the illness of depression. Major depression may interfere with the patient's ability to work, study, sleep, eat, and enjoy pleasurable activities. **Clinical Findings:** A person must have been in a depressed mood or have lost interest or pleasure for at least 2 weeks and have at least five of the classic clinical findings. These classic findings include persistent sad, anxious, or "empty" mood; feelings of hopelessness or pessimism; feelings of guilt, worthlessness, and helplessness; reduced appetite with weight loss or increased appetite with weight gain; insomnia; excessive fatigue; difficulty concentrating and making decisions; and suicidal thoughts.[3]

BIPOLAR DISORDER

Bipolar disorder is a type of depression characterized by episodes of mania, depression, or mixed moods. Sometimes the mood swings are dramatic and rapid, but most often they are gradual. **Clinical Findings:** Characteristics of the manic phase are excessive emotional displays, excitement, euphoria, hyperactivity accompanied by elation, boisterousness, impaired ability to concentrate, decreased need for sleep, and limitless energy, often accompanied by delusions of grandeur. In contrast, in the depressive phase there is marked apathy and feelings of profound sadness, loneliness, guilt, and lowered self-esteem.[6]

SCHIZOPHRENIA

Schizophrenia is group of mental disorders characterized by severe disturbance of thought and associative looseness, impaired reality testing (hallucinations, delusions), and limited socialization. **Clinical Findings:** Fundamental signs include changes in affect, associative looseness, autism, and ambivalence. Examples of affect are flat, blunted, inappropriate or bizarre emotions. Associative looseness includes disorganized thinking as manifested by jumbled and illogical speech and impaired reasoning. Autism is recognized by thinking that is not bound to reality but reflects the private perceptual world of the individual. Delusions and hallucinations are examples of autistic thinking. Ambivalence is holding two opposing emotions, attitudes, ideas, or wishes toward the same person, situation, or object.[6]

ANXIETY DISORDERS

Anxiety

Anxiety is a feeling of uneasiness or discomfort experienced in varying degrees, from mild anxiety to panic. Unlike fear, which is a response to an actual object or event, anxiety is a fearful response when no actual danger is present. Other characteristics of anxiety include emotional distress that interferes with everyday life and avoidance of situations that cause anxiety. The energy that anxiety provides may mobilize a person to take constructive action such as solving a major problem or filling an unmet need. When used destructively, it can immobilize a person.[3] **Clinical Findings:** Four levels of anxiety have been described: mild, moderate, severe, and panic. A mildly anxious person has a broad perceptual field because the anxiety heightens awareness to sensory stimuli. The person sees more, hears more, and thinks more logically. Learning occurs during mild anxiety. The moderately anxious person has a narrower field of perception and uses selective inattention to ignore stimuli in the environment to focus on a specific concern. The severely anxious person has reduced perception of stimuli and develops compulsive mechanisms to avoid the anxiety-provoking object or situation. During severe anxiety the person experiences impaired memory, attention, and concentration; has difficulty solving problems; and is unable to focus on events in the environment. The panic level of anxiety is characterized by complete disruption of the perceptual field. The person experiences intense terror and is unable to think logically or make decisions. Physical manifestations of anxiety represent sympathetic nervous system stimulation. The person experiences muscle tension, tachycardia, dyspnea, hypertension, increased respiration, and profuse perspiration.[6]

Obsessive-Compulsive Disorder

Obsessive-compulsive disorder is classified as an anxiety disorder because of the anxiety symptoms that develop when the patient tries to resist an obsession or compulsion. *Obsessions* are defined as unwanted, intrusive, persistent ideas, thoughts, impulses, or images that cause marked anxiety or distress. *Compulsions* are ritualistic behaviors that an individual feels driven to perform in an attempt to reduce anxiety. The person recognizes that the behaviors are excessive or unreasonable but continues them because of the relief from the discomfort of anxiety that they provide. **Clinical Findings:** Common obsessions include repeated thoughts about contamination, repeated doubts, a need to have everything in a particular order, and sexual imagery.[6]

SUBSTANCE ABUSE DISORDERS

Alcohol Withdrawal Syndrome

Ethyl alcohol, or ethanol, is a central nervous system depressant found in alcoholic beverages. The blood alcohol level is used to measure the amount of alcohol in blood. The legal intoxication level in most states is 100 mg/dL (0.10%), with some states using 0.08%.

There are two phases of alcohol withdrawal syndrome (AWS): alcohol withdrawal and alcohol withdrawal delirium, or delirium tremens (DT). **Clinical Findings:** When patients are dependent on alcohol, clinical findings of AWS may become evident within 6 to 24 hours after their last drink, peak in 24 to 36 hours, and end after 48 hours of abstinence. For most people manifestations subside within a few days. For patients with severe withdrawal, manifestations may continue for 2 or more weeks. With mild-to-moderate AWS clinical findings include fine tremors, nausea and vomiting, diaphoresis, increases in heart rate and blood pressure, anxiety, irritability, and insomnia. With severe AWS (also called *alcohol withdrawal delirium,* formerly called *delirium tremors*) patients experience delirium that may be accompanied by seizures. The patient's tremors become uncontrolled shaking, diaphoresis becomes diffuse, hypertension and tachycardia become worse, tachypnea develops, and hyperthermia may occur. The mental state may include extreme agitation, fluctuating disorientation, confusion, and hallucinations (visual, tactile, and occasionally auditory).[10]

Drug Intoxication

Clinical findings of intoxication from commonly abused drugs (cannabis, cocaine, opiates, barbiturates, amphetamines, and hallucinogenic agents) are presented in Tables 7-4 and 7-5.

DELIRIUM AND DEMENTIA

Delirium

Delirium is a cognitive disorder characterized by a disturbance of consciousness and a change in cognition that develops rapidly over a short period of time. Manifestations arise suddenly, last a short duration (i.e., 1 week, rarely more than 1 month), and are reversible with treatment. **Clinical Findings:** These findings include altered level of consciousness; impaired memory, judgment, and calculation; and a fluctuating attention span. The emotional state can change abruptly and range from fearful to aggressive with hallucinations and delusions. Activity may be increased or decreased and worsens at night (sundowning). The sleep cycle may be reversed. Speech may be rapid, inappropriate, and rambling.[6]

Dementia

Dementia is a cognitive disorder characterized by memory impairment and one of the following disorders: aphasia (language disturbance), apraxia (impaired ability to perform motor activities despite intact motor function), agnosia (failure to recognize familiar objects despite intact sensory function), and disturbance of executive functions. Dementia usually is not reversible—a characteristic that distinguishes it from delirium. **Clinical Findings:** Onset occurs slowly over months. Although level of consciousness is intact, memory, judgment, and calculation are impaired. The individual has a flat affect and may have delusions. Speech is slow and incoherent.[6]

TABLE 7-4 CLINICAL FINDINGS OF ACUTE DRUG INTOXICATION

DRUG(S) ABUSED	CLINICAL FINDINGS
Cannabis drugs	Tachycardia and postural hypotension, conjunctival vascular congestion, distortions of perception, dryness of mouth and throat, possible panic
Cocaine	Increased stimulation, euphoria, increased blood pressure and heart rate, anorexia, insomnia, agitation; in overdose, increased body temperature, hallucinations, seizures, death
Opiates	Depressed blood pressure and respiration; fixed, pinpoint pupils; depressed sensorium; coma; pulmonary edema
Barbiturates and other general CNS depressants	Depressed blood pressure and respirations; ataxia, slurred speech, confusion, depressed tendon reflexes, coma, shock
Amphetamines	Elevated blood pressure, tachycardia, other cardiac dysrhythmias, hyperactive tendon reflexes, pupils dilated and reactive to light, hyperpyrexia, perspiration, shallow respirations, circulatory collapse, clear or confused sensorium, possible hallucinations, paranoid feelings
Hallucinogenic agents	Elevated blood pressure, hyperactive tendon reflexes, piloerection, perspiration, pupils dilated and reactive to light, anxiety, distortion of body image and perception, delusions, hallucinations

From McKenry L, Tessier E, Hogan M: *Mosby's pharmacology in nursing*, ed 22, St Louis, 2006, Mosby.
CNS, Central nervous system.

TABLE 7-5 COMMON EYE SIGNS DETECTED AFTER ABUSE OF SELECTED DRUGS

	MARIJUANA	HEROIN	ALCOHOL	COCAINE	PCP
Pupil size	Normal	Constricted	Normal	Dilated	Normal
Slow or no reaction of pupil to light	Yes		Yes	Yes	Yes
Nonconvergence	Yes				
Redness of sclera	Yes		Yes		
Glazing of cornea	Yes	Yes	Yes		
Nystagmus	Yes		Yes		Yes
Swollen eyelids	Yes	Yes			Yes
Watering eyes	Yes				
Ptosis		Yes			
Decreased corneal reflex		Yes		Yes	Yes

Data from Tennant F: Is your patient abusing? *Postgrad Med* 84:108-114, 1988.
PCP, Phencyclidine.

CLINICAL APPLICATION AND CLINICAL REASONING

See Appendix D for answers to exercises in this section.

REVIEW QUESTIONS

1. Which question is appropriate for a nurse to ask at the beginning of a mental health history?
   1. "Have you been feeling anxious or sad?"
   2. "How have you been feeling about yourself?"
   3. "Are you alone a lot, or do you have friends with whom you socialize?"
   4. "How are you dealing with the stressors in your life?"

2. During a history the patient says that she is so uncomfortable with her life that she wishes that it were over. Which is an appropriate follow-up question from the nurse?
   1. "Have you thought of hurting yourself?"
   2. "Oh, I've felt that way many times."
   3. "That feeling will go away; just give it some time."
   4. "In which ways has your life been uncomfortable?"

3. During a health history a patient says, "Stressors? Oh, yeah, I have stressors. I got a promotion at work; and, with the extra income I'm going to move into a new house, but that has been delayed because my mother is in the hospital and my son is going off to college. To get through this time I just keep using my support systems, exercising, and meditating." How does a nurse interpret these comments by this patient?
   1. Flight of ideas
   2. Moderate anxiety
   3. Positive coping strategies
   4. Rationalization and denial

4. Difficulty sleeping, financial concerns, problems with personal or work relationships, difficulty making decisions, tense muscles, and fatigue are indicators of which disorder?
   1. Depression
   2. Anxiety
   3. Delirium
   4. Alcohol withdrawal syndrome

5. A patient reports nausea and vomiting; and the nurse observes hand tremors, agitation, and sweating. In view of these findings, which additional data would the nurse need to collect?
   1. Which fears or stressors the patient has been experiencing
   2. When the patient last took illegal drugs and which one was taken
   3. Which kinds of obsessions or compulsions the patient has been experiencing
   4. When the patient last drank alcohol and how much was consumed

CASE STUDY

Sarah Ubina comes to the student health clinic with complaints of fatigue. The following data are collected by the nurse from interview and examination.

Interview Data

Ms. Ubina tells the nurse that she has constantly felt tired and all she wants to do is sleep. She says that she doesn't have time to be tired because final examinations are approaching and she is very concerned about her grades. She begins to cry. "I'm so afraid that I won't pass my classes. If I don't pass, my parents won't help me with school anymore." When asked to describe herself, Sarah replies, "Friendly, but not very smart." Ms. Ubina tells the nurse that she has a boyfriend but only sees him occasionally because he lives in another state. When asked about other friends, Ms. Ubina replies, "I know all of the people in my class."

Examination Data

- *General survey:* Well-nourished, overweight young woman appearing unkempt, with slightly swollen red eyes from crying. Makes infrequent eye contact.

- *Vital signs:* BP, 128/84 mm Hg; pulse, 96 beats/min; respirations, 22 breaths/min; temperature, 98.6° F (36.7° C); height: 5 ft 3 in (160 cm); weight: 148 lbs (67 kg).
- *Mental status:* Oriented to person, place, and time. Slow speech pattern with flat affect.
- All body system findings are within expected limits.

Clinical Reasoning

1. Which data deviate from normal findings, suggesting to the nurse that Ms. Ubina may have a mental health issue?
2. For what additional information should the nurse ask or assess?
3. Based on the data, which risk factors for depression does this patient have?
4. With which other health care team members could you collaborate to help this patient?

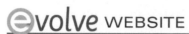 WEBSITE

http://evolve.elsevier.com/Wilson/assessment

Because food and fluid are basic biologic needs, a nutritional assessment of the patient is an integral part of the total health assessment. Nutritional assessment is not typically done in isolation: collecting data specifically related to nutritional status and identifying risk factors for nutritional problems are usually part of a general examination. In addition to collecting a general health history, nurses explore questions detailing dietary intake and perceived nutrition-related problems. The nutritional examination includes anthropometric measurements, biochemical tests, and nutrition-focused assessment with select body systems. Although data collection varies with age-groups and various stages in the life cycle (such as pregnancy), the general approach is consistent for patients of all ages.

ANATOMY AND PHYSIOLOGY

Nutrients are necessary to provide the body calories for energy, build and maintain body tissues, and regulate body processes. The base energy requirement is called the *basal metabolic rate* (BMR), which is influenced by several factors. Activity levels, illness, injury, infection, ingestion of food, and starvation can all affect the BMR. When caloric intake meets energy needs, no weight change occurs. When energy needs exceed caloric intake, weight loss occurs. When caloric intake exceeds energy needs, weight gain occurs. Nutrients are classified into one of three groups: macronutrients, micronutrients, and water.

MACRONUTRIENTS

Carbohydrates, proteins, and fats are considered *macronutrients,* meaning nutrients needed in large amounts.

Carbohydrate is the main source of energy and fiber in the diet. Each gram of carbohydrate produces 4 kcal of energy. Fiber passes through the digestive tract partially undigested, providing bulk that stimulates peristalsis. The two main sources of carbohydrates are plant foods (fruits, vegetables, and grains) and lactose (from milk). Although a small amount of carbohydrates are stored in the liver and muscle in the form of glycogen (to serve as energy reserves between meals), moderate amounts of carbohydrates must be ingested at regular intervals to meet the energy demands. If more carbohydrates are ingested than needed, the excess is stored as adipose tissue. The recommended daily allowance (RDA) for carbohydrate intake is 130 g/day for children and adults but increases to 175 g/day during pregnancy and 210 g/day for lactating women.[1] Carbohydrates should account for 55% to 60% of total calories. Many carbohydrate sources are classified as high energy, nonnutrient dense. Examples include sugar-sweetened beverages, desserts, and candy. Sedentary people should decrease consumption of energy-dense carbohydrates to maintain ideal body weight.[2]

Protein plays an essential role in facilitating growth and repair of body tissues. It can also be a source of energy. The simplest form of protein is an amino acid. There are 20 different amino acids, and these combine in a number of different ways to form proteins. Ten of the amino acids are considered essential in the diet because they are not synthesized by the body. A complete-protein food contains all of the essential amino acids; complete proteins are also referred to as high–biologic value proteins. Foods containing the highest-quality proteins (complete proteins) come from animal sources (meat, fish, poultry, milk, and eggs). Foods that contain incomplete proteins include cereals, legumes, and some vegetables. Combinations of incomplete-protein foods can provide all the essential amino acids. If more protein is ingested than needed, the extra is used to supply energy or is

BOX 8-1 CALCULATING GRAMS OF A MACRONUTRIENT

To calculate the recommended number of grams of carbohydrates, proteins, and fats based on the number of calories in a diet, multiply the total calories by the recommended percent and then divide by the number of kilocalories per gram.

(total kcal × recommended %) / kcal/g

Example: Grams of carbohydrate, protein, and fat in a 1500-kcal diet

Carbohydrates	1500 kcal × 55% carbohydrate = 825 calories/4 kcal = 206 g
Protein	1500 kcal × 20% protein = 300 calories/4 kcal = 75 g
Fat	1500 kcal × 25% fat = 375/9 kcal = 42 g

BOX 8-2 CALCULATING THE PERCENT OF CALORIES FROM MACRONUTRIENTS

To calculate the percent of calories from carbohydrate, protein, and fat in a given food source, multiple the total grams by the kilocalories per gram and divide by the total number of calories.

(g × kcal/g) / total kcal

Example: Percent of kilocalories from carbohydrate, protein, and fat in 8 oz of 2% milk. According to the label, 8 oz of milk has 125 kcal comprised of 12 g of carbohydrate, 8 g of protein, and 5 g of fat.

Carbohydrates	12 g of carbohydrates × 4 kcal/g = 48 kcal/125 kcal = 0.38 or 38% carbohydrates
Protein	8 g of protein × 4 kcal/g = 32 kcal/125 kcal = 0.26 or 26% protein
Fat	5 g of fat × 9 kcal/g = 45 kcal/125 kcal = 0.36 or 36% fat

stored as fat. Each gram of protein provides 4 kcal of energy. The RDA for protein intake in the adult diet is 0.8 g/kg of body weight, or an average of 56 g/day for adult males, 46 g/day for adult females, and 71 g/day for pregnant or lactating females.[1] Ideally protein should account for 12% to 20% of total kilocalories. These requirements are based on ideal body weight.[2]

Fat is the main source of fatty acids, which are essential for normal growth and development. Other functions of fat include synthesis and regulation of certain hormones, tissue structure, nerve impulse transmission, energy, insulation, and protection of vital organs. There are two essential fatty acids for metabolic processes: linoleic (or omega 3) and linolenic (or omega 6) acids. Fat is the major form of stored energy of the body. One gram of fat yields 9 kcal of energy. If energy needs exceed carbohydrate intake, fat can be converted to glucose by a process known as gluconeogenesis. If more fat is ingested than needed, it is stored in adipose tissue. Current recommendations are to limit saturated fatty acid intake to less than 7% of total calories and dietary cholesterol to less than 300 mg/day.[2] Basic macronutrient calculations are shown in Box 8-1 and Box 8-2.

MICRONUTRIENTS

Micronutrients are nutrients required in small quantities. The two groups of micronutrients, vitamins and minerals, are essential for growth, development, and metabolic processes that occur continuously throughout the body.

Vitamins are classified as water soluble or fat soluble (Table 8-1). Water-soluble vitamins cannot be stored in the body; thus they must be ingested in the diet daily. Fat-soluble vitamins can be stored in the body, and vitamin toxicity can result if they are taken in large quantities. Deficiencies or toxicities in micronutrients result in nutritionally based diseases; when these deficiencies are observed, they are usually a late sign of depletion.

Minerals are grouped into two categories: major minerals and trace minerals (Table 8-2). Major minerals are present in the body in large amounts with a required intake of over 100 mg/day. Trace minerals are present in the body in smaller

TABLE 8-1 VITAMINS

FAT-SOLUBLE VITAMINS	WATER-SOLUBLE VITAMINS
Vitamin A	Vitamin C
Vitamin D	B vitamins
Vitamin E	Thiamin
Vitamin K	Riboflavin
	Niacin
	Pyridoxine (B_6)
	Pantothenic acid
	Biotin
	Folate
	Cobalamin (B_{12})

TABLE 8-2 MINERALS

	TRACE MINERALS	
MAJOR MINERALS	**ESSENTIAL**	**UNCLEAR ROLE**
Calcium	Iron	Silicon
Phosphorus	Iodine	Vanadium
Magnesium	Zinc	Nickel
Sodium	Copper	Tin
Potassium	Manganese	Cadmium
Chloride	Chromium	Arsenic
Sulfur	Cobalt	Aluminum
	Selenium	Boron
	Molybdenum	
	Fluoride	

amounts; 10 of these are considered essential and have a required intake of under 100 mg/day.

WATER

Water composes 60% to 70% of total body weight, making it a critical component of the body. Cellular function depends on a well-hydrated environment. Because water is continually lost from the body, replacement is required on an ongoing basis. Without water an individual can survive only a few days. The average adult metabolizes 2.5 to 3 L of water every day in the form of both foods and fluids. Fluid needs are increased in certain situations, especially fever, infection, gastrointestinal (GI) losses, and respiratory illness.

HEALTH HISTORY

A nutritional history is a component of the health history discussed in Chapter 2. The nurse asks questions to elicit information about present health status, past medical history, family history, personal and psychosocial history, and risk factors. Specific questions are asked to assess the patient's actual or potential nutritional needs and to assess for nutrition-related problems. Data gained from the history are used to evaluate the adequacy of the diet and identify areas needed for patient education to make necessary dietary modifications. Quality Improvement Competencies for Nurses include providing patient-centered care and interdisciplinary teamwork with a health care provider and a dietitian. Refer to Table 11-1 on p. 196 for specific competencies.

GENERAL HEALTH HISTORY

Present Health Status

Do you have any chronic illnesses? If so, describe.
Many chronic illnesses are associated with nutritional problems or require special dietary measures and referral to a registered dietitian (e.g., diabetes mellitus, cystic fibrosis, phenylketonuria, celiac disease, heart failure, renal failure, and cancer). Individuals with GI disease are at greater risk for malnutrition.[3]

Which medications do you take? How often do you take them? Can you recall the dose?
Many medications can affect nutritional status. Some medications affect appetite; others may cause GI discomfort such as nausea, fullness, constipation, or diarrhea. Some medications are affected by foods ingested; thus food restrictions may be necessary.

Do you take vitamins or dietary supplements? If so, what do you take, how often, and for what reason?
Many individuals use vitamins and/or nutritional supplements as health promotion measures or to manage nutritional deficiencies. Iron deficiency occurs among many adolescents and women of childbearing years[3]; many older women take calcium and vitamin D supplementation to treat or prevent osteoporosis. Overuse of fat-soluble vitamins (A, E, D, and K) can lead to toxicity. Dietary supplements and vitamins are not intended to serve as a substitute food intake but are useful sources for one or two nutrients.[4]

Have you noticed any unexplained changes in your weight in the last 6 months? If so, describe.
Weight should remain fairly stable over time. Significant or rapid changes in weight require further evaluation.

Past Health History and Family History
What concerns have you had in the past regarding your weight or problems eating? Which measures did you take to try to correct the problems (e.g., diet modification, exercise, medications, surgery)? How effective were these measures?
A personal history of excessive weight gain (such as during a pregnancy) or weight loss with an illness is important to note. Most individuals who have experienced weight gain try to lose weight. Determine which measures they have used or attempted in the past and if they were effective.

Have you or has anyone in your family ever had nutrition-related problems such as obesity or diabetes mellitus?
Obesity in one or both parents makes an individual at higher risk for excessive weight, which is partly genetic and partly from learned patterns of behavior regarding eating. Obesity is the prime risk factor for type 2 diabetes mellitus. Individuals with a family history of diabetes are at risk of developing the disease.

Have you or has anyone in your family suffered from an eating disorder such as compulsive eating disorders, bulimia, or anorexia nervosa?
Eating disorders most commonly occur during adolescence and may cause lingering deficiency-related or psychologic-related problems in adulthood. Eating disorders tend to run in families and are thought to have a genetic basis.[5]

Personal and Psychosocial History
Describe your activity level and exercise pattern.
Physically active people have a reduced risk of becoming overweight or obese. Specifically, sedentary lifestyle is a known risk factor for weight gain and obesity. Children and adults should avoid inactivity and are encouraged to meet the 2010 Physical Activity Guidelines.[2]

Do you follow any specific diet or have any known dietary restrictions? Do you have any food intolerances of allergies? If so, describe.
Individuals may be following a prescribed dietary plan to manage a health condition, for weight management, or for religious or cultural reasons. Many people have intolerance to foods such as lactose or are allergic to foods such as nuts or shellfish. This information is important when assessing dietary intake.

Do you have any problems obtaining, preparing, or eating foods? If so describe.

ETHNIC, CULTURAL, AND SPIRITUAL VARIATIONS

Lactose Intolerance

Lactose intolerance affects a large percentage of people. Worldwide an estimated 75% of the population has some degree of lactose intolerance—the most common races include Asian, South American, and African descent. In the United States approximately 25% of Caucasian Americans have lactose intolerance compared to 75% to 90% of Native, Asian, and African Americans.

Data from Roy et al: *Lactose intolerance*, 2011, Medscape, available at http://emedicine.medscape.com/article/187249-overview.

 ETHNIC, CULTURAL, AND SPIRITUAL VARIATIONS

Jewish Dietary Laws

Some people of the Jewish culture adhere to kosher standards. Laws that dictate which foods are permissible under religious law are found in Leviticus and Deuteronomy. The term *kosher* means "fit to eat"; it is not a method of food preparation. Because life is sacred and animal cruelty is forbidden, the kosher slaughter of animals is performed so the animals die instantaneously. All blood is drained from the animal before eating it.

Milk and meat may not be mixed together in cooking, serving, or eating. To avoid mixing foods, utensils used to prepare food and plates used to serve them are separated. Jewish people who follow these dietary laws have one set of dishes, pots, and utensils for milk products and one set for meat products. Because glass is nonabsorbent, it can be used for either meat or milk products.

From Purnell LD, Paulanka BJ: *Transcultural health care: a culturally competent approach*, ed 2, Philadelphia, 2003, FA Davis.

Obtaining adequate nutrition may be a problem for low-income groups, the elderly, or those with disabilities. Many individuals with physical deficits or illness may have difficulty with food procurement and preparation. If this is an issue, assess support systems (someone willing to purchase and prepare food) or assess for community resources (e.g., meals on wheels).

Do you use street drugs or drink alcohol? If so, describe.
The use of drugs or alcohol can contribute to nutritional deficiencies. Alcohol is a source of "empty" calories (i.e., calories that supply no nutrients), which in turn suppresses the appetite. Alcohol also impairs the absorption of nutrients. In addition, money spent on drugs and alcohol may replace money available for the purchase of food. Alcohol consumption and drug use are often underreported by patients with a history of substance abuse.

PROBLEM-BASED HISTORY

The most commonly reported problems related to nutrition include weight loss, weight gain, difficulty chewing and swallowing, and loss of appetite or nausea. As with symptoms in all areas of health assessment, the nurse completes a symptom analysis using the mnemonic OLD CARTS from Box 2-3, which includes *O*nset, *L*ocation, *D*uration, *C*haracteristics, *A*ggravating and *A*lleviating, *R*elated symptoms, *T*reatment by the patient, and *S*everity.

Weight Loss

When did the weight loss start? What is your normal weight? What is your weight now? How many pounds have you lost in the last 6 months?
Determining onset and extent of weight loss and if weight loss has been sudden or gradual are important.

To what do you attribute the weight loss? Was it desired or undesired? If desired, which measures did you take to lose the weight? If undesired, what do you think is causing you to lose weight?
Desired weight loss may be the result of a change in eating habits or an increase in exercise. Strict calorie intake, fasting, bulimia, laxative abuse, and excessive exercise are indications of a preoccupation with body weight or a possible eating disorder. Undesired weight loss may be caused by loss of appetite, vomiting, illness, stress, or medications. Individuals are usually able to explain what they think is causing the weight loss. Advanced age is a known risk factor for undernutrition.

Have you had any symptoms associated with the loss of weight such as fatigue, headaches, bruising, constipation, hair loss, or cracks in corners of the mouth?
Excessive weight loss may cause a number of symptoms because of inadequate energy and protein and deficiency in vitamins and minerals.

Weight Gain

When did you start gaining weight? What do you consider your normal weight? What is your weight now? How many pounds have you gained in the last 6 months?
Establish the total weight gained and the time frame over which it occurred, whether sudden or gradual.

To what do you attribute your weight gain? Has it been intentional? Unintentional?
Desired weight gain usually occurs from an intentional increase in caloric intake or use of dietary supplements (or both). Undesired weight gain may result from a decrease in activity levels, change in eating habits, increased appetite, or smoking cessation. It may also be associated with fluid retention as a result of certain medical conditions (e.g., heart failure) or as a side effect of certain medications (e.g., corticosteroids).

Difficulty Chewing or Swallowing

Tell me about the problems that you are experiencing with chewing or swallowing (or both). When did they start?
Ask the patient about the nature of the problem. Determine the time frame over which the chewing or swallowing

difficulties have occurred. Choking and coughing are common symptoms associated with impaired swallowing.

Eating which type of food causes you the most problems?
Thin liquids and foods requiring forceful chewing (such as meat) may not be tolerated well.

Which types of foods are you able to consume without difficulty?
Foods that are soft and highly viscous are chewed and swallowed most easily.

Has your weight changed since this problem developed?
Weight loss, particularly if undesired, may be an indication that food intake is hampered by chewing or swallowing difficulties.

Loss of Appetite or Nausea

Tell me about the problems you are experiencing with appetite or nausea (or both). When did you first notice them? Are they constant or do they come and go?
Establish the onset of the problem—this may provide clues to the cause and potential nutritional deficiencies. Appetite may fluctuate from time to time. A reduction in appetite over an extended period of time may result in nutritional deficiencies.

To what do you attribute the loss of appetite or nausea (e.g., medications, illness, pregnancy, depression)?
The patient often has an idea of what is causing a change in appetite or nausea. Medications, pregnancy, certain chronic illnesses, and depression can all contribute to changes in appetite or nausea.

Which types of foods are the most offensive or intolerable? Which types of foods are you able to consume without difficulty?
In some cases an individual may avoid an entire food group and eat from another. Determining which nutrients the patient is consuming and identifying possible deficiencies in the diet are important.

Have you had a change of weight since these problems developed?
A significant change in weight indicates a problem and may suggest nutritional deficiencies as well.

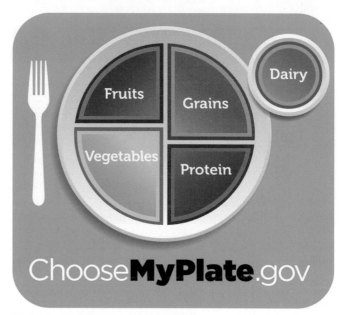

FIG. 8-1 MyPlate. (From the US Department of Agriculture, http://www.choosemyplate.gov/.)

TABLE 8-3	TECHNIQUES TO ASSESS DIETARY INTAKE	
TECHNIQUE	**DESCRIPTION**	**COMMENTS**
24-hour recall	Patient recalls what he or she has eaten in the last 24 hours.	Very easy to use; does not need a trained interviewer Useful as a quick screening tool May not be reflective of typical daily intake
Typical food intake	Patient describes which types of food that he or she typically eats at specified times—breakfast, lunch, dinner, snacks.	Does not require trained interviewer Can be directed at specific nutrients (e.g., protein or fats) May not be accurate reflection of actual intake
Food diary	Patient is asked to record all food eaten for a specified length of time (e.g., 3 days or 1 week).	Provides detailed information Not convenient—requires follow-up visit May not accurately reflect actual intake over time Analysis of data gained is time consuming
Food frequency questionnaires	Patient indicates frequency of intake of certain foods over a period of time (e.g., number of servings and types of fruit eaten in a typical week).	Easy to use Patient recalls types of foods typically eaten as opposed to actual foods eaten Does not assess intakes of all available foods—foods listed are usually those that are considered major contributors to the nutrients under study
Comprehensive diet history	An in-depth interview provides detailed information regarding food intake.	May provide more accurate reflection of nutrient intake Is time consuming to acquire Requires a trained/skilled dietary interviewer

ASSESSMENT OF DIETARY INTAKE

To complete an individual nutritional assessment, information regarding the patient's dietary intake is collected. Obtaining accurate information about total dietary intake is a challenge because of the high incidence of underreporting, the wide variation in the day-to-day intake, and variations in serving portions. Thus a "snapshot" of nutrient intake over 1 day or even over a course of several days may not be an accurate reflection of intake over a long period of time. Nutrient intakes are estimated using a variety of instruments and techniques (Table 8-3). In addition to determining nutrient intakes, ask patients about their appetite, food preferences, food dislikes, and food intolerances. Also specifically ask patients about special diets they may be following and the use of dietary supplements or herbs. Diets may be followed for weight loss, weight gain, or disease control (e.g., low-salt diet) or as part of cultural/religious practice.

Once the patient's dietary intake is obtained, the nurse can use several methods to determine its adequacy. Comparing diet intake to the United States Department of Agriculture *MyPlate* guide is the simplest approach to dietary assessment.[6] Determine the portion of food on a typical plate for a rough comparison to the recommended intake (Fig. 8-1). An Internet-based interactive program and additional information for consumers and health care professionals are easily located on the Internet at http://www.choosemyplate.gov/.

HEALTH PROMOTION FOR EVIDENCE-BASED PRACTICE

Nutrition and Weight Status

Nutrition and weight status is one of the topics identified by *Healthy People 2020*. Obesity is one of the most serious health care problems in the United States, not only because of the significant incidence found in all age-groups but also because obesity contributes to many other diseases, including hypertension, hyperlipidemia, type 2 diabetes mellitus, cardiovascular disease, gallbladder disease, sleep disturbances, respiratory disease, degenerative joint disease, and certain types of cancer. According to the 2007-2008 National Health and Nutrition Examination Survey, an estimated 16.9% of children ages 2 to 19 years and 33.8% of adults ages 20 and over are obese.

Goal: *Healthy People 2020*
The *Healthy People 2020* goal for nutrition and weight status is to promote health and reduce chronic disease risk through the consumption of healthful diets and achievement and maintenance of healthy body weights.

Clinical Recommendations
U.S. Preventive Services Task Force
- Provide behavioral counseling in primary care to promote a healthy diet.
- Provide screening for obesity among all adults, adolescents, and children ages 6 years and older.
- Offer or refer obese patients for intensive counseling and behavioral interventions to promote weight loss.

From US Department of Health and Human Services: *Healthy People 2020*, available at http://www.healthypeople.gov/2020/; US Preventive Services Task Force: *Behavioral counseling in primary care to promote a healthy diet; Screening for obesity in children and adolescents; Screening for obesity in adults; Counseling for a healthy diet;* and *Screening and interventions to prevent obesity in adults*, available at http://www.uspreventiveservicestaskforce.org/index.html. National Center for Health Statistics: *National health and nutrition examination survey 2007-2008*, available at http://www.cdc.gov/nchs/nhanes.htm.

EXAMINATION

Many nutritional deficiencies may become apparent through routine examination. Several basic examination techniques provide important information regarding nutritional status. However, sometimes assessment findings associated with nutritional deficiencies may be caused by nonnutritionally related problems. For example, multiple bruises could be associated with nutritional deficiency, be related to tissue trauma, or be caused by low platelets. For this reason findings must be considered in association with a detailed history. Table 8-4 summarizes common findings associated with nutritional deficiencies.

Before beginning the examination, wash your hands.

ROUTINE TECHNIQUES

- MEASURE height and weight.
- ASSESS general appearance and level of orientation.
- INSPECT skin.
- INSPECT hair and nails.
- INSPECT eyes.
- INSPECT oral cavity.
- INSPECT and PALPATE extremities.

SPECIAL CIRCUMSTANCES OR ADVANCED PRACTICE

- CALCULATE desirable body weight.
- CALCULATE percent change in weight.
- CALCULATE the waist-to-hip ratio.
- ESTIMATE body fat by measuring triceps skinfold. ★
- ASSESS nutritional status by reviewing laboratory tests (if available).

EQUIPMENT NEEDED

Weight and height scale • Calculator • Tape measure • Skinfold calipers • Tongue blade • Pen light

★ Advanced practice.

TABLE 8-4 CLINICAL MANIFESTATIONS OF VARIOUS NUTRIENT DEFICIENCIES

AREA OF EXAMINATION	CLINICAL MANIFESTATION	POTENTIAL NUTRIENT DEFICIENCY
Hair	Alopecia	Zinc, essential fatty acids
	Easy pluckability	Protein, essential fatty acids
	Lackluster	Protein, zinc
	"Corkscrew" hair	Vitamin C, vitamin A
	Decreased pigmentation	Protein, copper
Eyes	Xerosis of conjunctiva	Vitamin A
	Corneal vascularization	Riboflavin
	Keratomalacia	Vitamin A
	Bitot's spots	Vitamin A
Gastrointestinal tract	Nausea, vomiting	Pyridoxine
	Diarrhea	Zinc, niacin
	Stomatitis	Pyridoxine, riboflavin, iron
	Cheilosis	Pyridoxine, iron
	Glossitis	Pyridoxine, zinc, niacin, folate, vitamin B_{12}
	Magenta tongue	Riboflavin
	Swollen, bleeding gums	Vitamin C
	Fissured tongue	Niacin
	Hepatomegaly	Protein
Skin	Dry and scaling	Vitamin A, essential fatty acids, zinc
	Petechiae/ecchymoses	Vitamin C, vitamin K
	Follicular hyperkeratosis	Vitamin A, essential fatty acids
	Nasolabial seborrhea	Niacin, pyridoxine, riboflavin
	Bilateral dermatitis	Niacin, zinc
Extremities	Subcutaneous fat loss	Kilocalories
	Muscle wastage	Kilocalories, protein
	Edema	Protein
	Osteomalacia, bone pain, rickets	Vitamin D
	Arthralgia	Vitamin C
Neurologic	Disorientation	Niacin, thiamin
	Confabulation	Thiamin
	Neuropathy	Thiamin, pyridoxine, chromium
	Paresthesia	Thiamin, pyridoxine, vitamin B_{12}
Cardiovascular	Congestive heart failure, cardiomegaly, tachycardia	Thiamin
	Cardiomyopathy	Selenium

From Ross Products Division, Abbott Laboratories. In Seidel HM et al: *Mosby's guide to physical examination,* ed 7, St Louis, 2011, Mosby.

PROCEDURES AND TECHNIQUES WITH EXPECTED FINDINGS

ROUTINE TECHNIQUES: NUTRITION

CLEAN hands.

MEASURE height and weight for body mass index (BMI).

BMI is a weight-to-height ratio that is significantly correlated with total body fat. It is an alternative to the traditional height-weight tables for assessing nutritional status. BMI can be estimated using a BMI table (Table 8-5), or it can be specifically calculated using the formula in Box 8-3.

The normal range for BMI is 18.5 to 24.9.

ABNORMAL FINDINGS

Patients increase their risk of developing nutrition-related problems the farther their weight varies from the normal range.
- BMI <18.5: underweight
- BMI 25-29.9: overweight
- BMI 30-34.9: obesity class I
- BMI 35-39.9: obesity class II
- BMI >40: obesity class III (extreme obesity)

TABLE 8-5 BODY MASS INDEX CHART*

BMI	19	20	21	22	23	24	25	26	27	28	29	30	31	32	33	34	35
HEIGHT (INCHES)	BODY WEIGHT (POUNDS)																
58	91	96	100	105	110	115	119	124	129	134	138	143	148	153	158	162	167
59	94	99	104	109	114	119	124	128	133	138	143	148	153	158	163	168	173
60	97	102	107	112	118	123	128	133	138	143	148	153	158	163	168	174	179
61	100	106	111	116	122	127	132	137	143	148	153	158	164	169	174	180	185
62	104	109	115	120	126	131	136	142	147	153	158	164	169	175	180	186	191
63	107	113	118	124	130	135	141	146	152	158	163	169	175	180	186	191	197
64	110	116	122	128	134	140	145	151	157	163	169	174	180	186	192	197	204
65	114	120	126	132	138	144	150	156	162	168	174	180	186	192	198	204	210
66	118	124	130	136	142	148	155	161	167	173	179	186	192	198	204	210	216
67	121	127	134	140	146	153	159	166	172	178	185	191	198	204	211	217	223
68	125	131	138	144	151	158	164	171	177	184	190	197	203	210	216	223	230
69	128	135	142	149	155	162	169	176	182	189	196	203	209	216	223	230	236
70	132	139	146	153	160	167	174	181	188	195	202	209	216	222	229	236	243
71	136	143	150	157	165	172	179	186	193	200	208	215	222	229	236	243	250
72	140	147	154	162	169	177	184	191	199	206	213	221	228	235	242	250	258
73	144	151	159	166	174	182	189	197	204	212	219	227	235	242	250	257	265
74	148	155	163	171	179	186	194	202	210	218	225	233	241	249	256	264	272
75	152	160	168	176	184	192	200	208	216	224	232	240	248	256	264	272	279
76	156	164	172	180	189	197	205	213	221	230	238	246	254	263	271	279	287

From National Institutes of Health/National Heart, Lung, and Blood Institute: *Clinical guidelines on the identification, evaluation, and treatment of overweight and obesity in adults: the evidence report,* June 1998. NIH Publication 98-4093. Accessed from http://www.nhlbi.nih.gov/guidelines/obesity/ob_gdlns.pdf.

*To use the table, find the appropriate height in the left-hand column. Move across to a given weight. The number at the top of the column is the BMI at that height and weight. Pounds have been rounded off.

BOX 8-3 CALCULATION OF BODY MASS INDEX (BMI)

Calculation Using Kilograms and Meters

$$BMI = \frac{Weight\ (kg)}{Height\ M^2}$$

Calculation Using Pounds and Inches

$$BMI = \frac{Weight\ (lb) \times 705}{Height\ (in^2)}$$

Example: A woman is 65 inches tall and weighs 156 pounds.

$$156 \times \frac{705}{65^2} = \frac{109980}{4225} = BMI\ 26.03$$

FREQUENTLY ASKED QUESTIONS

Why is body mass index (BMI) now used as opposed to the height and weight tables?

BMI still takes into account height and weight, but the difference is that a mathematic formula is applied to these data so the same range is used for all individuals. A person with a BMI between 18.5 and 25 is within the normal range, regardless of whether he or she is 5 feet 2 inches or 6 feet 7 inches tall.

ETHNIC, SPIRITUAL, AND CULTURAL VARIATIONS

Obesity

Prevalence of self-reported obesity (BMI >30) differs among various racial groups.

- The highest prevalence of obesity is among African Americans (36.8%), followed by Hispanics (30.7%); the prevalence of obesity among Caucasians is 25.2%.
- Among women African Americans have the highest prevalence of obesity (41.9%), followed by Hispanics (30.8%). The prevalence of obesity among Caucasian women is 23.3%.
- Among men the prevalence of obesity based on racial group is less significant. Hispanics, 30.6%; African Americans, 30.9%; Caucasians, 27.1.

From Centers for Disease Control and Prevention: Vital signs: State-specific obesity prevalence among adults—United States, 2009, *MMWR* 59:1-5, August 3, 2010.
BMI, Body mass index.

| PROCEDURES AND TECHNIQUES WITH EXPECTED FINDINGS | ABNORMAL FINDINGS |

ASSESS general appearance and level of orientation.

A well-nourished individual is alert and has a body that is well proportioned and within an acceptable weight range.

Poor nutritional status may be recognized from general observation. Excessive obesity or generalized edema is an obvious indicator of poor nutritional status. Prominent cheek and clavicle bones or wasted-appearing limbs (cachexia) suggest malnutrition. A patient with insufficient caloric intake may be irritable or have a flat affect. Disorientation can be caused by niacin deficiency.

INSPECT the skin for surface characteristics, hydration, and lesions.

The skin should be smooth; elastic; and without lesions, cracks, or bruising (Fig. 8-2).

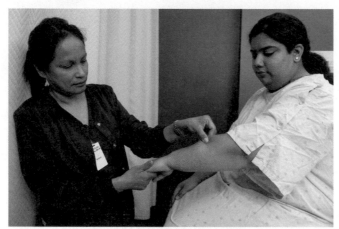

FIG. 8-2 Inspection of the skin.

Many nutritional deficiencies and fluid imbalances can be recognized by changes in the skin. The presence of edema indicates fluid retention (which may reflect protein depletion), whereas dry skin and decreased skin turgor may reflect dehydration. Multiple bruises are associated with vitamin C and K deficiencies; essential fatty acid deficiencies lead to dry flaking skin and eczema. Follicular hyperkeratosis is associated with vitamin A deficiency (Fig. 8-3).

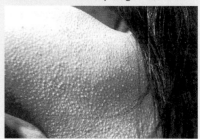

FIG. 8-3 Follicular hyperkeratosis. (From McLaren, 1992.)

INSPECT the hair and nails for appearance and texture.

In well-nourished individuals hair appears shiny, smooth, and firm. Nails should be pink, smooth, intact, and firm (Fig. 8-4).

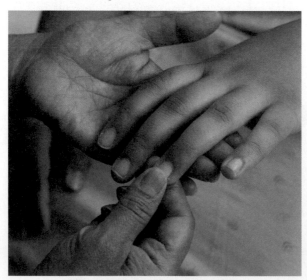

FIG. 8-4 Inspection of the nails.

Hair that is dull and falls out easily or observable hair loss indicates protein and fatty acid deficiencies. Spoon-shaped nails may be associated with iron deficiency (Fig. 8-5).

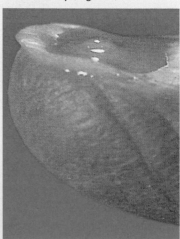

FIG. 8-5 Severe spooning with thinning of the nail.

PROCEDURES AND TECHNIQUES WITH EXPECTED FINDINGS

ABNORMAL FINDINGS

INSPECT the eyes for surface characteristics.

Mucous membranes (conjunctivae) around the eyes should be pink, moist, and free of lesions or drainage. The corneas should be clear and shiny (Fig. 8-6).

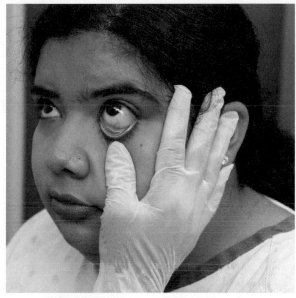

FIG. 8-6 Inspection of the conjunctiva.

Conjunctivae that are pale may be a sign of anemia. Excessively red conjunctivae may indicate riboflavin deficiency. Foamy-looking areas on the eyes (known as Bitot's spots) or excessively dry eyes are caused by vitamin A deficiency; with further deficiency the cornea becomes dry and hard, a condition known as xerophthalmia (Fig. 8-7).

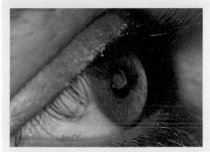

FIG. 8-7 Xerophthalmia. (Courtesy Lemmi and Lemmi, 2013.)

INSPECT the oral cavity for dentition and intact mucous membranes.

A penlight and tongue blade are used to improve visualization of the oral cavity. The teeth should be present, clean, and intact; dentures, if present, should be assessed for fit. The mucous membranes and gums should be moist, pink, and free of lesions. The tongue and lips should be pinkish red, smooth, and without lesions (Fig. 8-8).

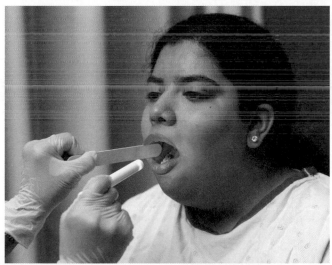

FIG. 8-8 Inspection of the oral cavity with penlight and tongue depressor.

Poor dentition and painful oral lesions can negatively affect food intake. Dry mucous membranes may indicate dehydration. Bleeding gums may be a sign of vitamin C or vitamin K deficiency; vitamin B complex deficiency can cause cracks in the corners of the mouth or on the lips or an excessively red tongue. A reddish purple tongue can be caused by riboflavin deficiency.

PROCEDURES AND TECHNIQUES WITH EXPECTED FINDINGS

ABNORMAL FINDINGS

INSPECT and PALPATE the extremities for shape, size, coordinated movement, and sensation.

Well-developed muscles should be observed, and these should be bilaterally equal. The patient should have muscle strength and coordinated muscle movement and full sensation to the extremities (Fig. 8-9).

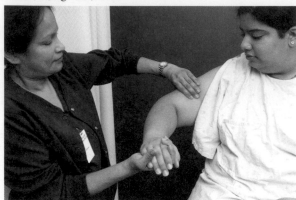

FIG. 8-9 Inspection of the extremities for muscle mass as an indication of nutritional status.

Muscle weakness and muscle wasting may be signs of inadequate protein intake or excessive protein wasting. Uncoordinated muscle movements may interfere with the ability to feed self. Vitamin D deficiency can cause skeletal malformation. Thiamin deficiency can cause peripheral neuropathy and paresthesia.

SPECIAL CIRCUMSTANCES OR ADVANCED PRACTICE: NUTRITION

CALCULATE desirable body weight (DBW).

Calculate the patient's DBW and compare this to the actual body weight. These calculations allow you to express the current weight as a percentage of the DBW. The calculated weight can be increased or decreased by 10% to account for bone structure and amount of muscle or fat tissue. DBW is calculated using the formula in Box 8-4. Ideally the patient falls between 90% and 110% of DBW.

Patients increase their risk of developing nutrition-related problems the further their weight varies from desired body weight.
- Severely underweight: 70% or less of DBW
- Moderately underweight: 70% to 80% or less of DBW
- Mild obesity: 20% to 40% above DBW
- Moderate obesity: 40% to 100% above DBW
- Morbid obesity: over 100% above DBW or over 45 kg higher than DBW

BOX 8-4	CALCULATION OF DESIRABLE BODY WEIGHT (DBW)

Females: 100 lb (45.5 kg) for the first 5 feet (60 in); 5 lb (2.27 kg) for each inch greater than 5 feet; ±10%
Males: 106 lb (48 kg) for the first 5 feet (60 in); 6 lb (2.7 kg) for each inch greater than 5 feet; = ±10%
Express the weight as a percentage of DBW by dividing the current weight by the DBW and multiplying by 100.

$$\text{Current weight} / \text{DBW} \times 100 = \% \text{ DBW}$$

Example:
    Current weight 150 lb/DBW 160 lb = 0.9375 × 100 = 93.8% of DBW

CALCULATE percent change in weight.

Document the amount of weight loss over a period of time to determine the severity of weight loss. To determine the rate of weight loss, calculate the percentage change of weight by dividing current body weight by the usual body weight (UBW) and multiplying by 100.

$$\text{Current body weight}/\text{UBW} \times 100 = \% \text{ UBW}$$

- Moderate weight loss: 1% to 2% weight change over 1 week
- Severe weight loss: >2% weight change over 1 week
- Moderate weight loss: 5% weight loss over 1 month
- Severe weight loss: >5% weight loss over 1 month, >7.5% weight loss over 3 months, or >10% weight loss over 6 months[7]

| PROCEDURES AND TECHNIQUES WITH EXPECTED FINDINGS | ABNORMAL FINDINGS |

CALCULATE the waist-to-hip ratio.

Waist-to-hip ratio is an indication of the risk of unhealthy fat distribution. To obtain the waist-to-hip ratio, measure the waist at the narrowest point and measure the hips at the widest point. Calculate the waist-to-hip ratio using the following formula:

$$\text{Waist (inches [cm]) / Hips (inches [cm])}$$

For example, if a man has a 44-inch (112 cm) waist and 40-inch (101 cm) hips, the calculation would be as follows:

$$112 \text{ cm} / 101 \text{ cm} = 1.1 \text{ waist-to-hip ratio}$$

The desired waist-to-hip ratio for women is 0.8 or less and for men is 1 or less.

A ratio that exceeds the desired ratio indicates upper body obesity. This increases the risk of developing health problems related to obesity (e.g., diabetes, hypertension, coronary artery disease, gallbladder disease, osteoarthritis, and sleep apnea). Women typically collect fat in their hips, giving their bodies a pear (gynecoid) shape. However, men build up fat around their waists, giving them an apple (android) shape (Fig. 8-10).

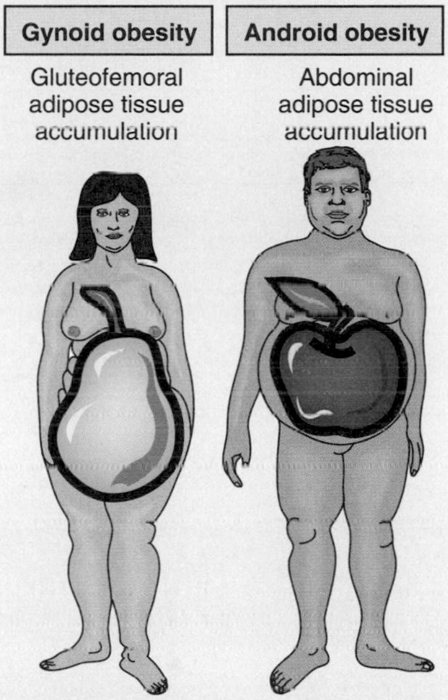

Gynoid obesity — Gluteofemoral adipose tissue accumulation

Android obesity — Abdominal adipose tissue accumulation

FIG. 8-10 Distribution of body fat. *Left,* Pear shape. *Right,* Apple shape. (From Lewis et al., 2011.)

★ ESTIMATE body fat by measuring triceps skinfold.

Skinfold measurements provide an estimate of total body fat (Fig. 8-11). Triceps skinfold measurements are made with skinfold calipers. The nurse uses the thumb and index finger to grasp and lift a fold of skin and fat about ½ inch (1.27 cm) on the posterior aspect of the patient's arm halfway between the olecranon process (tip of the elbow) and acromial process on the lateral aspect of the scapula. Opened caliper jaws are placed horizontally to the raised skinfold; the nurse releases the lever of the calipers to make the measurement to the nearest millimeter.

Two or three measurements at the same site should be taken, and the numbers averaged. Normal ranges for triceps skinfold fat measurements for men and women are included in Table 8-6. The desired skinfold measurement falls at or near the 50th percentile. Accuracy of this measurement is related to the skill of the nurse using the calipers. In addition, these measurements are not useful in patients who are acutely ill because of shifts in fluid.

Values significantly higher than normal can indicate increased fat mass. Values significantly lower than normal can indicate decreased fat mass secondary to either an increase in lean mass or depleted fat stores.

ASSESS nutritional status by reviewing laboratory tests.

Many laboratory tests are helpful in assessment of nutritional status. Not all of these tests are indicated for all situations. These tests include serum albumin, prealbumin, hemoglobin and hematocrit, blood glucose, lipid profile, BUN/creatinine ratio, and urine specific gravity.

Table 8-7 summarizes the normal ranges of laboratory tests, their purposes, and significances of abnormal findings for adults.

★ Advanced practice.

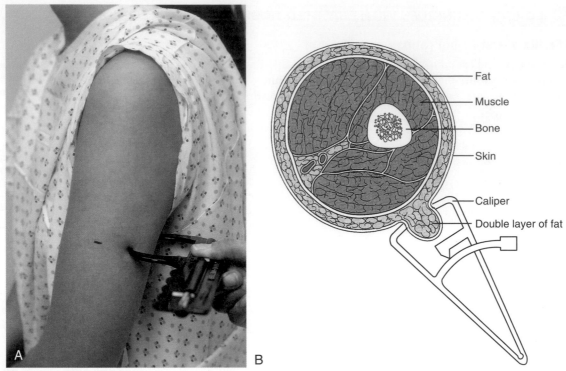

FIG. 8-11 A, Placement of calipers for triceps skinfold thickness measurement. **B**, Cross-section of arm with triceps skinfold measurement. (**B** From Barkauskus et al., 2002.)

TABLE 8-6	PERCENTILES FOR TRICEPS SKINFOLD MEASUREMENTS (ADULTS)		
	TRICEPS SKINFOLD		
GENDER	**5TH**	**50TH**	**95TH**
Males			
18-19	4	9	24
19-25	4	10	22
25-34	5	12	24
35-45	5	12	23
45-54	6	12	25
55-64	5	11	22
65-74	4	11	22
Females			
18-19	10	18	30
19-25	10	18	34
25-34	10	21	37
35-45	12	23	38
45-54	12	25	40
55-64	12	25	38
65-74	12	24	36

From Frisancho AR: New norms of upper limb fat and muscle areas for assessment of nutritional status, *Am J Clin Nutr* 34:2540-2545, 1981.

FREQUENTLY ASKED QUESTIONS

What is the difference between serum albumin and prealbumin?
Serum albumin simply measures circulating protein. Albumin can be affected by a number of factors, including fluid status, blood loss, liver function, and stress. Fluctuation of albumin levels occurs over 3 to 4 weeks. Prealbumin is a reflection of protein and calorie intake over the previous 2 to 3 days.

TABLE 8-7 LABORATORY TESTS USED FOR NUTRITIONAL ASSESSMENT

TEST AND NORMAL VALUE*	PURPOSE	SIGNIFICANCE OF ABNORMAL FINDINGS
Serum Albumin 3.5-5 g/dL or 35-50 g/L (SI units)	Serum albumin measures circulating protein; levels can be affected by fluid status, blood loss, liver function, trauma, and surgery. Fluctuations in albumin levels occur over a 3- to 4-week period.	Low albumin levels suggest protein-calorie malnutrition. Levels between 2.8 and 3.5 g/dL are consistent with moderate protein deficiency; levels below 2.5 g/dL represent severe protein depletion. Rapid changes in albumin are most likely caused by factors other than nutrition.
Prealbumin 15-36 mg/dL or 150-360 mg/L (SI units)	Prealbumin is a reflection of protein and calorie intake for the previous 2 to 3 days.	A deficiency of either calories or protein can cause prealbumin to decline. A malnourished individual undergoing refeeding therapy can produce rises in prealbumin levels.
Hemoglobin (Hgb) and Hematocrit (Hct) Male: Hgb 14-18 g/dL or 8.7-11.2 mmol/L (SI units); Hct 42%-52% or 0.42-0.52 volume fraction (SI units) Female: Hgb 12-16 g/dL or 7.4-9.9 mmol/L (SI units); Hct 37%-47% or 0.37-0.47 volume fraction (SI units) Pregnancy: Hgb >11 g/dL; Hct >33%	Hgb and Hct provide information regarding erythrocytes. These are clinically useful to screen for anemia caused by dietary deficiency such as iron, folate, and vitamin B_{12}. Hematocrit is also useful in evaluation of hydration.	Low Hgb and Hct levels suggest anemia. Causes of anemia are numerous; but dietary deficiencies of iron, vitamin B_{12}, or folate are a few possible causes. Elevated Hgb and Hct levels may occur in dehydration, chronic anoxia, and polycythemia. Elevated hematocrit levels suggest dehydration.
Blood Glucose 70-105 mg/dL or 3.9-5.8 mmol/L (SI units)	Blood glucose reflects carbohydrate metabolism. A fasting glucose level is used to screen for the presence of diabetes mellitus or glucose intolerance.	Hypoglycemia (blood glucose level less than 70 mg/dL) may indicate inadequate caloric intake. Hyperglycemia (blood glucose level over 126 mg/dL) may be an indication of diabetes mellitus.
Lipid Profile *Serum Cholesterol* <200 mg/dL or 5.2 mmol/L (SI units) *Serum Triglyceride* Male: 40-160 mg/dL or 0.45-1.81 mmol/L Female: 35-135 mg/dL or 0.40-1.52 mmol/L *High-Density Lipoproteins (HDLs)* Male: >45 mg/dL or >0.75 mmol/L Female: >55 mg/dL or >0.91 mmol/L *Low-Density Lipoproteins (LDLs)* Male and female: <130 mg/dL or <3.37 mmol/L *Cholesterol to HDLs* Male: 5.0 Female: 4.4	Lipid profile includes several tests that are indicators of lipid metabolism and important determinants of risk factors for cardiovascular disease. A lipid profile includes total cholesterol and triglyceride levels, HDL level, LDL level, and cholesterol/HDL ratio. The cholesterol-to-HDL ratio is calculated by dividing the total cholesterol value by the HDL value.	Values ≥200 mg/dL for total cholesterol and triglyceride levels indicate that the patient is at increased risk for vascular disease. Elevations of LDL are associated with increased risk for developing coronary heart disease; elevated HDL levels reduce the risk.
BUN/Creatinine Ratio Up to 20:1	Blood test is used as an indication of hydration.	Levels 21:1-24:1 are associated with impending dehydration; levels >25:1 indicate dehydration.
Urine Specific Gravity	Urine test is used as an indication of hydration.	Levels >1.029 are associated with dehydration.

Data from Pagana DK, Pagana TJ: *Mosby's diagnostic and laboratory test reference*, ed 10, St Louis, 2011, Mosby.
BUN, Blood urea nitrogen.
*Values for adults only; refer to a laboratory reference for other age-groups.

AGE-RELATED VARIATIONS

INFANTS AND CHILDREN

The pediatric nutritional assessment includes many of the same components described for the adult, although some specific differences exist, including assessing feeding patterns; assessing body weight; plotting weight, length, and head circumference on a growth chart; observing for the presence of rooting reflex and effective suck effort and swallowing in infants; and observing for presence of tooth decay in children. Childhood obesity is one of the most significant of all nutritional concerns. Chapter 19 presents further information regarding the nutritional assessment from this age-group.

OLDER ADULTS

The nutritional assessment for an older adult essentially is the same as previously described for adults with a few exceptions, including ability to acquire and prepare food, social interactions, and general functional assessment. Chapter 21 presents further information regarding the nutritional assessment of older adults.

COMMON PROBLEMS AND CONDITIONS

RISK FACTORS

Nutrition

Obesity	Protein-Calorie Malnutrition	Eating Disorders
• Sedentary lifestyle (M)	• Age	• Preoccupation with weight (M)
• High-fat diet (M)	• Acute or chronic illness	• Perfectionist (M)
• Genetics	• Side effects from medications or treatments	• Poor self-esteem (M)
• Ethnicity/race	• Hospitalization for acute illness	• Self-image disturbances (M)
• Female	• Resident of long-term care facility (M)	• Peer pressure (M)
• Low socioeconomic status (M)	• Low socioeconomic status (M)	• Athlete—drive to excel (M)
		• Compulsive or binge eating (M)
		• First-generation relative with eating disorder or alcoholism

M, Modifiable risk factor.

OBESITY

Obesity occurs when there is greater energy intake than energy expenditure. This condition is caused by genetics, overeating, and inactivity. The number of children, adolescents, and adults who are overweight or obese has become an epidemic and contributes to significant morbidity and mortality. In the United States 66% of individuals are classified as overweight or obese; 5.7% of the adult population is extremely obese.[8] **Clinical Findings:** Obesity is characterized by excessive adipose tissue to the face and neck, trunk, and extremities (Fig. 8-12). Overweight, obesity, and extreme obesity are clinically defined as a body mass index greater than 25, 30, and 40 respectively.

HYPERLIPIDEMIA

Hyperlipidemia is a condition associated with elevated serum lipids that can include cholesterol, triglycerides, and phospholipids. Causes include excessive dietary fat and genetics. Over 100 million American adults have total blood cholesterol values of 200 mg/dL and higher; 40 million American adults have levels of 240 mg/dL or above.[9] **Clinical Findings:**

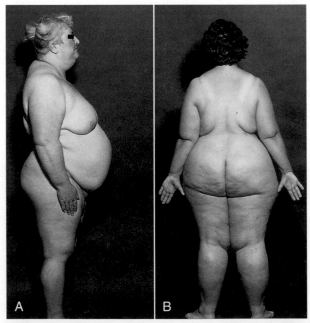

FIG. 8-12 Obesity. (From Forbes and Jackson, 2003.)

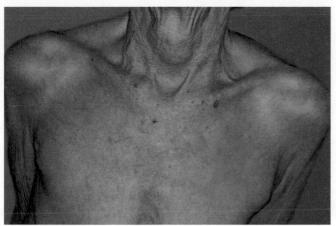

FIG. 8-13 Loss of subcutaneous fat and muscle wasting. (Courtesy Lemmi and Lemmi, 2013.)

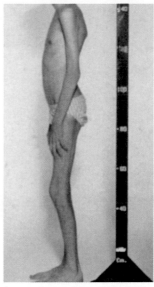

FIG. 8-14 Anorexia nervosa. (From Taylor, 1995.)

Hyperlipidemia is not associated with any clinical symptoms until a significant cardiovascular event occurs. Biochemical indications include elevations in serum lipids. In adults total cholesterol levels from 200 to 239 mg/dL are considered borderline high; levels of 240 mg/dL or higher are considered high.

PROTEIN-CALORIE MALNUTRITION

Protein-calorie malnutrition (PCM) refers to the state of inadequate protein and calorie intake. PCM is the most common form of undernutrition and can result from poor or limited food intake, wasting disease (such as cancer), malabsorption syndromes, endocrine imbalances, and poor living conditions. Among hospitalized elderly, up to 55% are undernourished; up to 85% of elderly who live in an institutional setting are undernourished.[10] **Clinical Findings:** The malnourished individual often appears thin with muscle wasting and a loss of subcutaneous fat (Fig. 8-13) and other protein deficiency findings presented in Table 8-4. One is considered underweight with a body mass index of less than 18.5 or if more than 10% below desired body weight. Biochemical indications such as low serum levels of albumin or protein may exist.

EATING DISORDERS

Eating disorders refer to a group of psychiatric conditions resulting in altered food consumption. Three prevalent eating disorders are anorexia nervosa, bulimia nervosa, and binge-eating disorder. An estimated 9% of women and 3% of men experience anorexia nervosa during their lifetime; the lifetime bulimia nervosa prevalence is 5% of women and 1% of men. Binge eating disorders affect an estimated 2% of men and women.[11] **Clinical Findings:** Clinical findings depend on the type of eating disorder. *Anorexia nervosa:* refusing to eat, extreme thinness, along with other symptoms of PCM (Fig. 8-14). *Bulimia nervosa:* recurrent binge-and-purge eating cycles, electrolyte imbalances, chronic irritation or erosion of the pharynx, esophagus, and teeth (from exposure to hydrochloric acid). *Binge eating disorder:* consumption of large quantities of food until uncomfortably full. Frequently the individual experiences feelings of being out of control during the binge episodes.

CLINICAL APPLICATION AND CLINICAL REASONING

See Appendix D for answers to exercises in this section.

REVIEW QUESTIONS

1. The nurse is teaching a patient how to evaluate the percentage of fat in a serving of food. She explains that the label on a package of a toaster pastry states that there are 6 g of fat and 210 calories per serving, What is the percentage of fat per serving?

1. 26%.
2. 35%.
3. 54%.
4. 72%.

2. A man weighs 265 pounds and is 6 feet 4 inches tall. Based on these data, how does the nurse classify his weight?
   1. Overweight
   2. Class I obesity
   3. Class II obesity
   4. Class III obesity

3. An older woman is 5 feet 2 inches tall and weighs 100 pounds. To best understand her dietary intake, which question is most appropriate?
   1. "Who prepares your meals?"
   2. "What are your favorite foods?"
   3. "How do you get to the grocery store?"
   4. "Could you describe what you eat on a typical day?"

4. Why does the nurse ask a patient which medications he takes as part of a nutritional assessment?
   1. Medications must be taken with food to avoid irritation to the gastrointestinal system.
   2. Many drugs affect nutritional intake requirements; thus adjustments to the diet must be made.
   3. The absorption and bioavailability of some medications are affected by food.
   4. Some medications taste bad and may interfere with the appetite.

5. A patient states that he has experienced "a lot" of unintentional weight loss over the past 4 months. The nurse measures his height and weight (5 feet 11 inches, 170 pounds) and determines that his body mass index is 22.7. Which of the following is the most appropriate action to better evaluate his recent weight loss?
   1. Calculate his desirable body weight.
   2. Ask, "What is your usual body weight?"
   3. Record what he ate in the last 24 hours.
   4. Determine his hip-to-waist ratio.

CASE STUDY

Marian Parker is a 45-year-old woman who is brought to the hospital after an episode of fainting.

Interview Data

Ms. Parker states that she has been very tired lately and gets short of breath and fatigues very easily. She also complains of cracks in the corners of her mouth that won't heal. When asked about her diet, she tells the nurse that she is a "new vegetarian." She states that she started a vegetarian diet about 4 months ago "to prevent diseases and because animals are unclean." She acknowledges weight loss since starting the diet but states, "I am healthy because of what I eat and because I am thin." She refuses foods that contain meat or animal products. Her diet is described as "healthy"; she typically eats beans, rice, breads, and salad. She is not specific about portions, stating, "I eat until I'm full." Her fluid intake consists of coffee, tea, and water. She does not use drugs or alcohol. She also tells the nurse that her financial resources are very limited.

Examination Data

- *Vital signs and other measurements:* BP, 118/76 mm Hg; pulse, 92 beats/min; respirations, 20 breaths/min; temperature, 98.2° F (36.8° C); height, 5 ft 4 in (162 cm); weight, 110 lb (50 kg)
- *General observation:* Very thin, protruding bony prominence to cheeks and clavicles
- *Skin:* Warm, very dry with scaling—especially on arms and legs
- *Hair:* Brown, thin, dull, easily plucked
- *Oral cavity:* Pink, moist mucous membranes without lesions; teeth present, in good repair; cracks noted in corners of mouth
- *Eyes:* Conjunctivae pale; no drainage or lesions
- *Extremities:* Bilaterally equal; extremities thin; small amount of muscle mass noted; muscle strength 4/5

Clinical Reasoning

1. Which data deviate from normal findings, suggesting a need for further investigation?
2. For which additional information should the nurse ask or assess?
3. Which risk factors for nutritional problems can be identified?
4. With which additional health care professionals should you consider collaborating to meet her health care needs?

Skin, Hair, and Nails

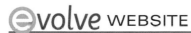

evolve WEBSITE

http://evolve.elsevier.com/Wilson/assessment

CONCEPT OVERVIEW

The feature concept for this chapter is *Tissue Integrity.* This concept represents the structural intactness and physiologic function of tissues and conditions that affect integrity. In this chapter the tissues are referred to as skin, hair, and nails. Several concepts are interrelated to *tissue integrity* and include perfusion, oxygenation, motion, tactile sensory perception, elimination, nutrition, and pain. These are shown in the illustration to the right.

The maintenance of tissue integrity requires adequate perfusion to carry oxygenated blood and nutrients to tissues; interference with perfusion results in tissue injury or necrosis. Adequate nutrition is also required to maintain tissues. Sustained pressure over tissue may occur if an individual has limited mobility and/or limited tactile sensory perception. Urinary or bowel incontinence can also contribute to impairment of tissue integrity. Finally a loss of tissue integrity often results in pain. Understanding the interrelationships among these concepts helps the nurse recognize risk factors and thus increases awareness when conducting a health assessment.

The following case provides a clinical example featuring several of these interrelated concepts.

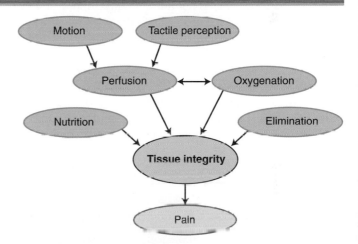

Roberta is a 24-year-old female who has been confined to a wheelchair for the last 2 years as a result of a spinal cord disease that has left her partially paralyzed. She has been very depressed; as a result she has a poor appetite, which has resulted in weight loss. She has developed skin breakdown over her sacrum as a result of sustained pressure that impaired perfusion (caused by reduced motion and tactile sensation); the condition is exacerbated by her poor nutritional status.

ANATOMY AND PHYSIOLOGY

The skin and the accessory structures (i.e., hair, nails, sweat glands, and sebaceous glands) form what is referred to as the *integumentary system.* The skin is an elastic, self-regenerating cover for the entire body. Because they are composed of several tissues that perform specialized tasks, the skin and related structures are considered a body organ. The skin has several important functions. The primary functions are to protect the

body from microbial and foreign-substance invasion and to protect internal body structures from minor physical trauma. The skin also helps retain body fluids and electrolytes; without skin an individual would suffer tremendous water loss. The skin provides the body with its primary contact with the outside world, providing sensory input about the environment. Its sensitive surface detects and reports comfort factors such as temperature and surface textures, enabling the body to adapt through either temperature regulation or position changes. This regulation of body temperature is accomplished continuously through radiation, conduction, convection, and evaporation. Other functions of the skin include production of vitamin D; excretion of sweat, urea, and lactic acid; expression of emotion (e.g., blushing); and even repair of its own surface wounds through the normal process of cell replacement. The skin and appendages often mirror systemic disease and thus may provide valuable clues to an internal disorder such as jaundice resulting from liver disease.

SKIN

The skin is composed of three layers that are functionally related: the epidermis; the dermis; and the subcutaneous layer, also known as the *hypodermis*. The main components of each of these layers and their functional and spatial relationships are shown in Fig. 9-1.

Epidermis

The epidermis is the thin, outermost layer of the skin and is composed of stratified squamous epithelium. This layer of skin is *avascular,* meaning that it has no direct blood supply. The deepest aspect of the epidermis is the stratum germinativum. This layer lies adjacent to the dermis, which provides a rich supply of blood. Within this deepest layer of epidermis, active cell generation takes place. As cells are produced, they push up the older cells toward the skin surface. As the cells move toward the surface, they begin to die (because they move away from their nutritional source); and they undergo a process known as *keratinization,* in which keratin (a protein)

is deposited, causing the cells to become flat, hard, and waterproof. The outermost aspect of the epidermis, the stratum corneum, is composed of 30 layers of these dead, flattened, keratinized cells. This exposed layer serves as the protective barrier and regulates water loss. The dead cells are continuously sloughed off and replaced by new cells moving up from the underlying epidermal layers. The entire process takes about 30 days.

Melanocytes, located in the basal cell layer of the epidermis, secrete melanin, which provides pigment for the skin and hair and serves as a shield against ultraviolet radiation.

Dermis

The dermis is made up of highly vascular connective tissue. The blood vessels dilate and constrict in response to external heat and cold and internal stimuli such as anxiety or hemorrhage, resulting in the regulation of body temperature and blood pressure. The dermal blood nourishes the epidermis, and the dermal connective tissue provides support for the outer layer. The dermis also contains sensory nerve fibers that react to touch, pain, and temperature. The arrangement of connective tissue enables the dermis to stretch and contract with body movement. Dermal thickness varies from 1 to 4 mm in different parts of the body.

Subcutaneous Layer

The subcutaneous tissue (hypodermis) is not actually skin tissue but a support structure for the dermis and epidermis—literally acting as an anchor for these upper layers. This layer is composed primarily of loose connective tissue interspersed with subcutaneous fat. These fatty cells help to retain heat, provide a protective cushion, and provide calories.

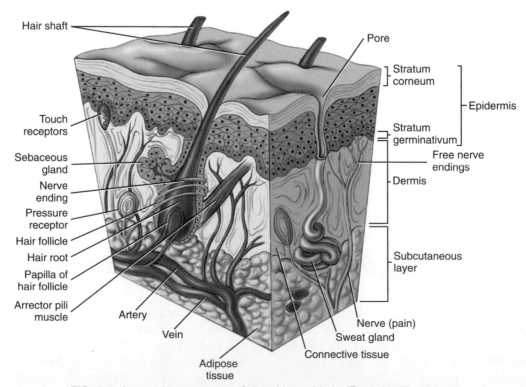

FIG. 9-1 Anatomic structures of the skin and hair. (From Herlihy, 2011.)

APPENDAGES

Hair, nails, and glands (the eccrine sweat glands, the apocrine sweat glands, and the sebaceous glands) are considered appendages. These structures are formed at the junction of the epidermis and the dermis.

Hair

Epidermal cells in the dermis form hair. Each hair consists of a root, a shaft, and a follicle (the root and its covering). At the base of the follicle is the papilla, a capillary loop that supplies nourishment for growth. Melanocytes within the hair shaft provide color. Variations in hair color, density, and pattern of distribution vary considerably as a result of age, gender, race, and hereditary factors. Structures of the hair follicle are shown in Fig. 9-1.

Nails

Nails are really epidermal cells converted to hard plates of keratin. The nails assist in grasping small objects and protect the fingertips from trauma. The nail is composed of a free edge, the nail plate, and the nail root (i.e., the site of nail growth). The white, crescent-shaped area at the base, the lunula, represents new nail growth (Fig. 9-2). Skin tissue adjacent to the nail is referred to as *paronychium;* the cuticle is epidermal tissue (stratum corneum) that grows on the nail plate at the nail base. Tissue directly under the nail plate is highly vascular, providing clues to oxygenation status and blood perfusion.

Eccrine Sweat Glands

Eccrine sweat glands regulate body temperature by water secretion through the surface of the skin. They are the most numerous and widespread sweat glands on the body. They

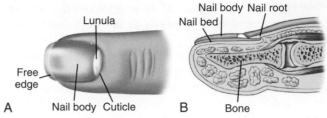

FIG. 9-2 Structures of the nail. (From Herlihy, 2011.)

are distributed almost everywhere throughout the surface of the skin, found in greatest numbers on the palms of the hands, the soles of the feet, and the forehead. Sweat glands are controlled primarily by the nervous system.

Apocrine Sweat Glands

These structures are much larger and deeper than the eccrine glands; they are found only in the axillae, nipples, areolae, anogenital area, eyelids, and external ears. They begin secretion at puberty and are strongly influenced by hormones. In response to emotional stimuli, the glands secrete an odorless fluid containing protein, carbohydrates, and other substances. Decomposition of apocrine sweat produces what we associate with body odor.

Sebaceous Glands

These glands secrete a lipid-rich substance called *sebum,* which keeps the skin and hair lubricated. The greatest distribution of sebaceous glands is found on the face and scalp, although they are found in all areas of the body with the exception of the palms and soles. Sebum secretion, stimulated by sex hormone activity, accelerates during puberty and varies throughout the life span.

HEALTH HISTORY

Nurses interview patients to collect subjective data about their present health and any past experiences. In addition to present health status, past medical history, family history, and personal and psychosocial history, nurses ask patients about their home environment, occupational environment, and travel, which may affect the health condition of their skin, hair, and nails. Quality Improvement Competencies for Nurses include providing patient-centered care and interdisciplinary teamwork with the health care provider, dietitian, and wound care nurse. See Table 11-1 on p. 196 for examples of competencies.

GENERAL HEALTH HISTORY

Present Health Status

Do you have any chronic illnesses? If so, describe.
Some chronic illnesses (e.g., liver failure, renal failure, venous insufficiency, and autoimmune disease) cause changes to the skin such as pruritus, excessive dryness, discoloration, and skin lesions.

Do you take any medications? If so, what do you take and how often? What are the medications for?
Medications can cause a number of side effects that are manifested in the skin, including allergic reactions in the form of hives or rashes, lesions associated with photosensitivity, or other systemic effects such as acne, thinning of the skin, and stretch marks. The nurse should document medications that are used to treat skin problems.

Have you noticed any changes in the way your skin, hair, or nails look or feel? Any changes in the sensation of your skin? If so, where? Describe.
Ask patients if they have noticed changes as opposed to asking them if they have any problems. The development of lesions or other changes such as how the skin feels indicate a skin condition or an underlying systemic disease. Patients do not always perceive skin or hair changes as a "problem"; for this reason it is important to specifically ask.[1]

What type of work do you do? To your knowledge are you exposed to chemicals at home or in the workplace? If so, describe.

Dangerous chemicals are found in the home and in the workplace. According to the Centers for Disease Control and Prevention, it is estimated that more than 13 million workers in the United States are potentially exposed to chemicals that can be absorbed through the skin. Occupations with highest incidence of chemical exposures to the skin include food service, cosmetology, health care, agriculture, cleaning, painting, mechanics, printing/lithography, and construction.[2]

Past Medical History and Family History

Have you ever had problems with your skin such as skin disease, infections involving the skin or nails, or trauma involving the skin? If so, describe.

Past skin injuries and conditions may provide clues to current skin lesions or findings.

Has anyone in your family ever had skin-related problems such as skin cancer or autoimmune-related disorders such as systemic lupus erythematosus?

A family history helps determine predisposition to certain skin disorders. Some skin disorders have familial or genetic links. Autoimmune disorders tend to be familial and may manifest in a number of ways, including rash and alopecia.

Personal and Psychosocial History

What do you do to keep your skin healthy (e.g., hygiene measures, use of lotions, protection from sun exposure, use of sunscreen)?

Health care practices may provide clues for underlying skin problems and areas for education. Specifically determine products and frequency used. Excessive exposure to sun and ultraviolet light is a known risk factor for skin cancer.[3]

PROBLEM-BASED HISTORY

The most commonly reported symptom of skin disease is pruritis.[4] Other common problems related to the skin include rashes; pain/discomfort; lesions; wounds; and changes in skin color or texture, hair, or nails. As with symptoms in all areas of health assessment, the nurse completes a symptom analysis using the mnemonic OLD CARTS, which stands for the *Onset, Location, Duration, Characteristics, Aggravating factors, Related symptoms, Treatment by the patient, and Severity* (see Box 2-3).

Skin
Pruritus

When did the itching first start? Did it start suddenly or gradually? Where did it start? Has it spread?

Understanding the onset and location of the itching may provide clues to the cause.

Does anything make the itching worse? Is there anything that relieves it? What have you done to treat yourself?

Document characteristics and aggravating and alleviating factors of the itching; these data may provide clues to the cause. For example, if taking an antihistamine relieves the itch, the cause may be an allergy.

What were the circumstances when you first noticed the itching? Taking medications? Contact with possible allergens such as animals, foods, drugs, plants?

Pruritus may be caused by several factors. Common factors include an allergic response (hives); exposure to chemicals; or infestation of scabies, lice, or insect bites. Systemic diseases such as biliary cirrhosis and some types of cancer such as lymphoma may also cause pruritus.[4]

Do you have dry or sensitive skin?

Dry or sensitive skin may make an individual more prone to itching.

Rash

When did the rash start? Where did you first notice the rash? Describe the appearance of the rash initially: Flat? Raised? How long has the rash been present?

Determining onset, location, and duration of the rash may provide clues to the cause.

Does the rash itch or burn? What makes it better? Worse? What have you done to treat it? Have you noticed any other symptoms associated with this rash such as joint pains, fatigue, or fever?

Document aggravating factors, related symptoms, and measures of self-treatment to better understand the cause.

Do you have any known allergies to foods, plants, skin/hair products, laundry detergent, chemicals, or animals? Does anyone else in your family have a similar rash? Have you been exposed to others with a similar rash?

A rash is not generally a disease in itself but rather a symptom of an allergic response, skin disorder, or systemic illness. Some of these questions help differentiate the cause of the rash.

Pain/Discomfort of Skin

Describe the pain or discomfort that you are experiencing. When did the pain start? Describe its location. Does the pain or discomfort spread anywhere? Does the pain stay on the skin surface, or does it go deep inside?

There are multiple causes of pain; onset and location are important factors in determining the cause.

Describe the pain or discomfort (e.g., sharp, dull, achy, burning, itching). How bad is your pain on a scale of 0 to 10? Is it constant, or does it come and go? If constant, does the pain vary? If pain comes and goes, how long does it last?

Document characteristics of the pain or discomfort to better understand the cause.

What triggers the pain? Are there things that make it worse? Better?

Document aggravating factors and measures of self-treatment for the discomfort.

Lesion or Changes in Mole

Describe the lesion with which you are concerned. Where is the lesion? When did you first notice it? Do you have any symptoms associated with the lesion such as pain, discomfort, pruritus, or drainage? If so, describe.

Lesions may result from acne, trauma, infections, exposure to chemicals or other irritants, tumors, or other systemic disease.

Describe the changes you have noticed in the mole (i.e., color, shape, texture, tenderness, bleeding, or itching).

A changing or irregular mole may be a sign of a malignant lesion.

Change in Skin Color

Has there been any generalized change in your skin color such as a yellowish tone or paleness?

Changes in overall skin color may have a number of causes, including medications, anemia, or an internal systemic disease such as liver disease causing jaundice.

Have there been any localized changes in your skin color such as redness, discoloration of one or both feet, or areas of bruises or patches? What do you think caused the change in skin color?

Localized changes may be associated with changes in tissue perfusion, causing a discoloration to the affected area, cyanosis, bruising (may be a sign of a hematologic condition, abuse, frequent falls), or vitiligo (i.e., a loss of pigmentation in the skin). Notice the answer the patient gives to the cause of the discoloration. Does the explanation fit the discoloration? Should you suspect interpersonal violence?

Skin Texture

In what way has the texture of your skin changed (e.g., skin thinning, fragile, excessive dryness)?

Changes in the skin texture may be expected (e.g., associated with aging) or may indicate a metabolic or nutritional problem.

Do you have excessively dry (xerosis) or oily (seborrhea) skin? If so, is it seasonal, intermittent, or continuous? What do you do to treat it?

A history of dry skin may provide information about an existing system disease (e.g., thyroid disease), or it may be related to an environmental condition such as low humidity. Dry skin may also be associated with poor skin lubrication.

Wounds

Where is your wound located? What caused it? How long have you had it? Do you have any associated symptoms such as pain or drainage? If so, describe.

The location of a wound and how long it has been there are important to document. These may provide clues as to the cause of the wound. For example, chronic wounds on the lower legs suggest problems with peripheral perfusion. Leg ulcers associated with venous insufficiency tend to recur after healing.[5] If the explanation for the cause of the wound does not seem to fit, suspect interpersonal violence.

What have you done to treat the wound?

Self-treatment of a wound may provide insight to the its appearance, particularly if the patient reports problems associated with wound healing.

Do you typically have problems with wound healing?

A history of problems associated with wound healing can point to nutritional or metabolic problems, infection, or poor circulation.

Hair

What changes or problems with your hair are you experiencing? When did you notice the changes? Did they occur suddenly or gradually?

Establish the type of problem, the onset, and the nature of the changes with the hair. Common problems associated with hair include excessive dryness, brittleness, hair loss, and pain/dryness to the scalp.

Can you think of any contributory factors associated with the problems or changes? Have you recently experienced stress? Fever? Other illness? Itching? What kinds of hair products have been used on your hair recently?

Reports of changes in the hair such as excessive dryness or brittle hair may indicate stress or systemic disease. Exposure to hair care products may account for changes in texture or condition of hair.

Has there been a change in your diet in the last few months?

Nutritional deficiencies may be observed by changes in hair appearance or texture. For example, dullness and hair that is easily plucked could be caused by a protein deficiency.

Have you noticed any changes in the distribution of hair growth on your arms or legs?

A decrease in hair growth on an extremity, particularly the lower extremity, may indicate problems with arterial circulation. Increases in hair growth may be caused by an ovarian or adrenal tumor.

Nails

What type of problem or changes are you experiencing with your nails? When did you first notice the changes?

The appearance and consistency of the fingernails and toenails may be an important sign about the patient's general health. Establish onset of the changes or problem.

Have you been exposed to or do you handle any chemicals at home or work?

Exposure to chemicals can cause the nails to change in appearance or consistency.

Are your nails brittle? Have you noticed a pitting type of pattern to your nail?

Pitting, brittle nails, crumbling, and changes in color can be caused by nutritional deficiencies, systemic diseases, or localized fungal infections.

Do you chew your nails? Do you now have, or have you ever had, an infection of the nail or around the nail bed? If so, describe.

Patients who have a habit of nail biting may use the biting as an unconscious way to handle stress. The nails may show signs of local infection such as fungal infection.

Do you have difficulty keeping your nails clean? Do they appear dirty?

Hyperthyroidism may cause the nail to separate from the nail bed and make the nail appear "dirty."

BOX 9-1   EARLY SIGNS OF MELANOMA

To help you remember the early signs of melanoma, use the mnemonic ABCDEF:

A—Asymmetry (not round or oval)
B—Border (poorly defined or irregular border)
C—Color (uneven, variegated)
D—Diameter (usually greater than 6 mm)
E—Elevation (recent change from flat to raised lesion)
F—Feeling (sensation of itching, tingling, or stinging within the lesion)

HEALTH PROMOTION FOR EVIDENCE-BASED PRACTICE

Skin Cancer

Skin cancer is the most common cancer, accounting for almost half of all cancers. The number of nonmelanoma (basal and squamous cell) skin cancers is difficult to estimate because reporting these types of cancers is not required. However, estimates are that over 3 million cases are diagnosed per year. Melanoma accounts for 76,250 new cases of skin cancer per year. The estimated number of skin cancer–related deaths in 2012 was 12,190, of which 9180 were related to melanoma. In the elderly, melanoma tends to be diagnosed at a later stage and is more likely to be lethal. According to the American Cancer Society (ACS), the International Agency for Research on Cancer upgraded its classification of indoor tanning devices from "probably" to "definitively" carcinogenic to humans. Despite this evidence, about 15% of adolescents and adults report intentional exposure to artificial source ultraviolet light for tanning purposes. Also of concern is that only 9.3% of adolescents follow protective measures for sun exposure compared to 73% of adults.

Goals and Objectives—Healthy People 2020

The overall *Healthy People 2020* goal related to cancer is to reduce the number of new cancer cases and reduce illness, disability, and death caused by cancer. Two specific objectives relate to skin cancer:

- Reduce the rate of melanoma cancer deaths.
- Increase the proportion of persons who participate in behaviors that reduce their exposure to harmful ultraviolet irradiation and avoid sunburn.

Recommendations to Reduce Risk (Primary Prevention)
American Cancer Society

- Skin should be protected from sun exposure by:
  - Covering with tightly woven clothing and a wide-brimmed hat.
  - Applying sunscreen that has sun protection factor (SPF) of 15 or higher to exposed skin (even on cloudy or hazy days).
  - Wearing sunglasses to protect the skin around the eyes.
- Seeking shade (especially at midday) whenever possible.
- Avoiding sunbathing and indoor tanning.

Screening Recommendations (Secondary Prevention)
American Cancer Society

- Adults should examine their skin periodically; new or unusual lesions should be evaluated promptly by a health care provider.
- Use the ABCDEF mnemonic for evaluating lesions (see Box 9-1).

From American Cancer Society: *Cancer facts & figures 2012*, Atlanta, American Cancer Society; 2012; US Department of Health and Human Services: *Healthy People 2020*, available at http://www.healthypeople.gov/2020/.

EXAMINATION

ROUTINE TECHNIQUES

- INSPECT the skin.
- PALPATE the skin.
- INSPECT and PALPATE the scalp and hair.
- INSPECT facial and body hair.
- INSPECT and PALPATE the nails.

SPECIAL CIRCUMSTANCES OR ADVANCED PRACTICE

- INSPECT and PALPATE skin lesions.
- INSPECT lesions using a Wood's lamp. ★

EQUIPMENT NEEDED

Light source (e.g., overhead light, penlight) • Centimeter ruler • Magnifying lens if needed • Gloves (if open lesions present) • Wood's lamp

★ Advanced practice.

| PROCEDURES AND TECHNIQUES WITH EXPECTED FINDINGS | ABNORMAL FINDINGS |

ROUTINE TECHNIQUES

Start with a general survey, noticing the color of the skin, general pigmentation, vascularity or bruising, and lesions or discoloration. Note any unusual odors. Next inspect and palpate the skin more closely, moving systematically from the head and neck to the trunk, arms, legs, and back. In a head-to-toe assessment you can examine the skin in conjunction with other body systems. Before you begin, be sure to have adequate lighting so subtle changes are not missed. Be alert for cuts, bruises, scratches, and welts that may indicate interpersonal violence, especially when the explanation for their cause does not seem to fit the lesions observed.

CLEAN hands.

INSPECT the skin for general color.

Inspect the skin for general color and uniformity of color. The skin color should be consistent over the body surface, with the exception of vascular areas such as the cheeks, upper chest, and genitalia, which may appear pink or have a reddish-purple tone. The normal range of skin color varies from whitish pink, to olive tones, to deep brown. Table 9-1 compares clinical findings of patients with light and dark skin. Sun-exposed areas may show evidence of slightly darker pigmentation.

Abnormal skin color may be evidence of local or systemic disease. Common abnormal findings of particular importance include *cyanosis, pallor,* and *jaundice* (see Table 9-1). Less common findings include:

- *Hypopigmentation,* also known as *albinism* (a complete absence of pigmentation; pale white skin tone is noted over the entire body surface).

- *Hyperpigmentation* (increased melanin deposition) may be an indication of an endocrine disorder (e.g., Addison's disease) or liver disease.

TABLE 9-1	COMPARISON OF SKIN-RELATED FINDINGS IN LIGHT- AND DARK-SKINNED PATIENTS	
CLINICAL SIGN	**LIGHT SKIN**	**DARK SKIN**
Cyanosis	Grayish-blue tone, especially in nail beds, earlobes, lips, mucous membranes, palms, and soles of feet	Ashen-gray color most easily seen in the conjunctiva of the eye, oral mucous membranes, and nail beds
Ecchymosis (bruise)	Dark red, purple, yellow, or green color, depending on age of bruise	Deeper bluish or black tone; difficult to see unless it occurs in an area of light pigmentation
Erythema	Reddish tone with evidence of increased skin temperature secondary to inflammation	Deeper brown or purple skin tone with evidence of increased skin temperature secondary to inflammation
Jaundice	Yellowish color of skin, sclera of eyes, fingernails, palms of hands, and oral mucosa	Yellowish-green color most obviously seen in sclera of eye (do not confuse with yellow eye pigmentation, which may be evident in dark-skinned patients), palms of hands, and soles of feet
Pallor	Pale skin color that may appear white	Skin tone appears lighter than normal; light-skinned African Americans may have yellowish-brown skin; dark-skinned African Americans may appear ashen; specifically evident is a loss of the underlying healthy red tones of the skin
Petechiae	Lesions appear as small, reddish-purple pinpoints	Difficult to see; may be evident in the buccal mucosa of the mouth or sclera of the eye
Rash	May be visualized and felt with light palpation	Not easily visualized but may be felt with light palpation
Scar	Narrow scar line	Frequently has keloid development, resulting in a thickened, raised scar

| PROCEDURES AND TECHNIQUES WITH EXPECTED FINDINGS | ABNORMAL FINDINGS |

INSPECT the skin for localized variations in skin color.

Almost all healthy individuals have natural variations in skin pigmentation. A common intentional localized variation in skin color is a tattoo. If a tattoo is present, its location and the characteristics of the surrounding areas should be examined and documented. Normal localized variations of the skin pigmentation include the following:

- *Pigmented nevi (moles):* Moles are considered an expected finding; most adults have between 10 and 40 moles scattered over the body. They are most commonly located above the waist on sun-exposed body surfaces (chest, back, arms, legs, and face). They tend to be uniformly tan to dark brown, are typically less than 5 mm in size, and may be raised or flat. The expected shape of a mole is round or oval with a clearly defined border (see Table 9-2 later in this chapter).
- *Freckles:* Freckles are small, flat, hyperpigmented macules that may appear anywhere on the body, particularly on sun-exposed areas of the skin. The most common locations are on the face, arms, and back.
- *Patch:* A patch is an area of darker skin pigmentation that is usually brown or tan and typically is present at birth (birthmarks). Some of these patches fade, but many do not change over time.
- *Striae:* Striae are silver or pink "stretch marks" secondary to weight gain or pregnancy (see Table 9-3 later in this chapter).

Melanoma: The nurse should be familiar with abnormal characteristics of pigmented moles that might point to melanoma (Box 9-1 on p. 102). Moles located below the waist or on the scalp or breast are rarely "normal" moles.

Vitiligo is an acquired condition associated with the development of unpigmented patch or patches; it is more common in dark-skinned races and thought to be an autoimmune disorder (see Table 9-2 later in this chapter).

Localized areas of hyperpigmentation may be associated with endocrine disorders (pituitary, adrenal) and autoimmune disorders (systemic lupus erythematosus).

⊕ ETHNIC, CULTURAL, AND SPIRITUAL VARIATIONS
Coining and Cupping

- Coining is a treatment practiced by Cambodians and Vietnamese. The body is rubbed vigorously with a coin while exerting pressure until red marks appear over the bony prominence of the rib cage on the back and chest. Marks created by this treatment frequently have been mistaken as signs of abuse or mistreatment.
- Cupping is an alternative medicine therapy for arthritis, stomach aches, bruises, and paralysis. Glass cups with negative pressure are applied to the skin; the negative pressure may be achieved by heating the air in the cups before application. As a result of the heat, the cup adheres to the skin and may leave a reddened area or mark. This is practiced by Latin American and Russian cultures.[6]

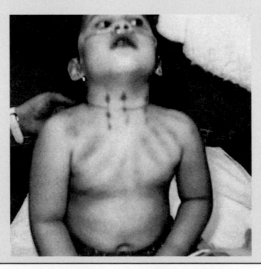

PROCEDURES AND TECHNIQUES WITH EXPECTED FINDINGS	**ABNORMAL FINDINGS**

PALPATE the skin for texture, temperature, moisture, mobility, turgor, and thickness.

Texture

The skin should be smooth, soft, and intact, with an even surface. Expected variations include calluses over the hands, feet, elbows, and knees.

Excessive dryness, flaking, cracking, or scaling of the skin may occur secondary to environmental conditions or may be signs of systemic disease or nutritional deficiency. Look for areas of maceration, discoloration, or rashes under skinfolds (Fig. 9-3).

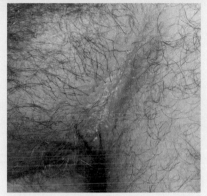

FIG. 9-3 Maceration in a skinfold. (From Habif, 2010.)

Temperature

The skin temperature is best evaluated using the dorsal aspect of your hands. The skin should be warm. The skin temperature should be consistent for the entire body with the exception of the hands and feet, which may be cooler, particularly in a cool environment.

Cool Skin: Generalized cool or cold skin is an abnormal finding and may be associated with shock or hypothermia. Localization of cold skin, particularly in the extremities, may be an indication of poor peripheral perfusion.

Hot Skin: Generalized hot skin is a reflection of hyperthermia. This may be associated with a fever, increased metabolic rate (e.g., hyperthyroidism), or exercise. Localized areas of skin that are hot may reflect an inflammation, infection, traumatic injury, or thermal injury such as sunburn.

Moisture

The skin is normally dry. There should be minimal perspiration or oiliness, although increased perspiration may be an expected finding associated with increased environmental temperatures, strenuous activity, or anxiety.

Diaphoresis (excessive sweating) is an abnormal finding in the absence of strenuous activity. This may be a reflection of hyperthermia, extreme anxiety, pain, or shock. Excessively moist skin may often be seen with metabolic conditions such as hyperthyroidism.[7]

PROCEDURES AND TECHNIQUES WITH EXPECTED FINDINGS

Mobility and Turgor

Skin mobility and turgor are assessed by picking up and slightly pinching the skin on the forearm or under the clavicle. The skin should be elastic (i.e., move easily when lifted) and return to place immediately when released. The technique and expected findings for skin turgor are shown in Fig. 9-4.

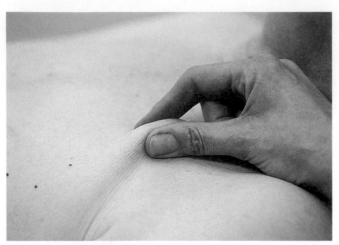

FIG. 9-4 Elastic skin turgor.

Thickness

Skin thickness varies based on age and area of the body. Typically skin thickens until adulthood and decreases in thickness after age 20. The skin is thickest over the palms of hands and soles of feet and thinnest over the eyelids. A callus is an area of excessive thickening of skin that is an expected variation associated with friction or pressure over a particular surface area. A callus is commonly found on the hands or feet (Fig. 9-6).

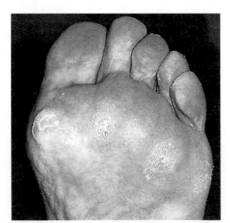

FIG. 9-6 Callus. (From White and Cox, 2000.)

ABNORMAL FINDINGS

Edema, excessive scarring to the skin, or some connective tissue disorders (such as scleroderma) reduce skin mobility. Poor skin turgor is noted if "tenting" is observed or the skin slowly recedes back into place. Decreased turgor may result from dehydration or may be a finding in an individual who has experienced significant weight loss (Fig. 9-5).

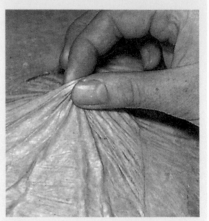

FIG. 9-5 Poor skin turgor. (From Kamal and Brocklehurst, 1991.)

An increase in skin thickness is seen in patients with diabetes mellitus and is thought to be caused by abnormal collagen resulting from hyperglycemia.[8] Excessively thin skin may take on a shiny or transparent appearance and is seen in hyperthyroidism, arterial insufficiency, and aging.

PROCEDURES AND TECHNIQUES WITH EXPECTED FINDINGS

INSPECT and PALPATE the scalp and hair for surface characteristics, hair distribution, texture, quantity, and color.

The scalp should be smooth to palpation and show no evidence of flaking, scaling, redness, or open lesions. The hair should be shiny and soft. The texture of the hair may be fine or coarse. Note the quantity and distribution of the hair for balding patterns and isolated areas of hair loss. If there are areas of isolated hair loss, note whether the hair shaft is broken off or absent completely. Men may show a gradual, symmetric hair loss on the scalp caused by genetic disposition and elevated androgen levels.

INSPECT facial and body hair for distribution, quantity, and texture.

Examine the quantity and distribution of facial and body hair. Men generally have noticeable hair present on the lower face, neck, nares, ears, chest, axilla, back, shoulders, arms, legs, and pubic region. The noticeable hair distribution in women is most commonly limited to the arms, legs, axillae, pubic region, and around the nipples. Women may also have fine or light-colored hair on the back, face, and shoulders. The women in some cultural groups may also have facial or chin hair. Fine vellus hair covers the body; whereas coarser hair is found on the eyebrows and lashes, pubic region, axillary area, male beards, and to some extent the arms and legs. The male pubic hair configuration is an upright triangle, with the hair commonly extending midline to the umbilicus. The female pubic hair configuration forms an inverse triangle; the hair may also extend midline to the umbilicus.

INSPECT and PALPATE the nails for shape, contour, consistency, color, thickness, and cleanliness.

Inspect the edges of the nails to determine if they are smooth and rounded. The nail surface should be flat in the center and slightly curved downward at the edges. The skin adjacent to the nail should be intact, the same color as adjacent skin and without edema.

ABNORMAL FINDINGS

Dull, coarse, and brittle hair is seen with nutritional deficiencies, hypothyroidism, and exposure to chemicals in some hair products and bleach. Hyperthyroidism makes the hair texture fine.[7] *Parasitic infection* with lice is characterized by the presence of nits (eggs) found on the scalp at the base of the hair shaft. *Alopecia* (hair loss) often occurs as a manifestation of many systemic diseases, including autoimmune disorders, anemic conditions, and nutritional deficiencies, or treatment with radiation or antineoplastic agents.

Hair loss on the legs may indicate poor peripheral perfusion. Thinning of the eyebrows is a prominent finding in hypothyroidism.[9] *Hirsutism* (hair growth in women with an increase of hair on the face, body, and pubic area) may be a sign of an underlying endocrine disorder. Pubic hair distribution that deviates from typical gender patterns may indicate a hormonal imbalance.

Inflammation characterized by edema and erythema of the folds of the finger tissue may indicate infection.

Koilonychia (spoon nail) presents as a thin, depressed nail with the lateral edges turned upward (Fig. 9-7). This is associated with anemia or may be congenital.[10]

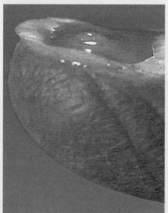

FIG. 9-7 Severe spooning with thinning of the nail. (From Beaven and Brooks, 1994.)

PROCEDURES AND TECHNIQUES WITH EXPECTED FINDINGS

In light-skinned individuals nails are pink and blanch with pressure. Individuals with darker-pigmented skin typically have nails that are yellow or brown, and vertical banded lines may appear (Fig. 9-8).

ABNORMAL FINDINGS

Leukonychia appears as white spots on the nail plate (Fig. 9-9). This is usually caused by minor trauma or manipulation of the cuticle.

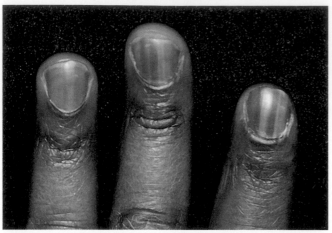

FIG. 9-8 Nail bed color of a dark-skinned person (pigmented bands occur as a normal finding in over 90% of African Americans). (From Habif, 2010.)

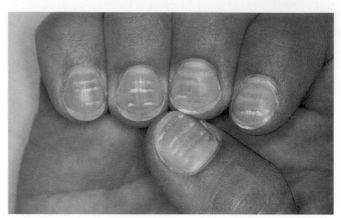

FIG. 9-9 Leukonychia punctata. Transverse white bands result from repeated minor trauma to the nail matrix. (From Baran, Dawber, and Levene, 1991.)

Inspect the nail base angle (i.e., the angle of the proximal nail fold and the nail plate). The expected angle of the nail base is 160 degrees.

Clubbing is present when the angle of the nail base exceeds 180 degrees (Fig. 9-10). It is caused by proliferation of the connective tissue, resulting in an enlargement of the distal fingers. Clubbing is most commonly associated with chronic respiratory or cardiovascular disease.

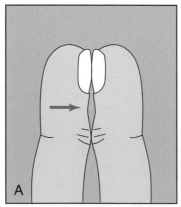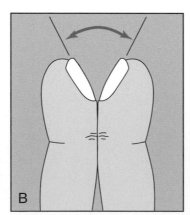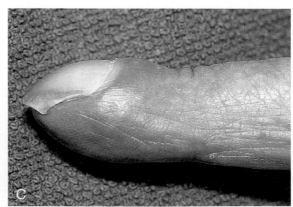

FIG. 9-10 Assessment of finger clubbing. **A,** Normally when opposing fingers are placed together, a small space is visible between the place where the fingers and the nail beds meet. **B,** With finger clubbing no space is observed between the fingers, and the nail beds angle away from one another. **C,** With finger clubbing the base of the nail is enlarged and curved. (**A** and **B,** From Seidel et al., 2011; **C** From White and Cox, 2000.)

PROCEDURES AND TECHNIQUES WITH EXPECTED FINDINGS

Inspect the nail surface itself to determine its smoothness. Note grooves, depressions, pitting, and ridges.

Examine the thickness of the nail itself. The nail should have a uniform thickness. Finally palpate the nail to ensure that the nail base feels firm and adheres to the nail bed.

ABNORMAL FINDINGS

Beau's lines manifest as a groove or transverse depression running across the nail (Fig. 9-11). They result from a stressor such as trauma that temporarily impairs nail formation. The groove first appears at the base of the nail by the cuticle and moves forward as the nail grows out.

Pitting of the nail is commonly associated with psoriasis. Minor pitting may also be seen in persons with no health care problems (Fig. 9-12).

Thinning or brittleness of the nail may be secondary to poor peripheral circulation or inadequate nutrition.

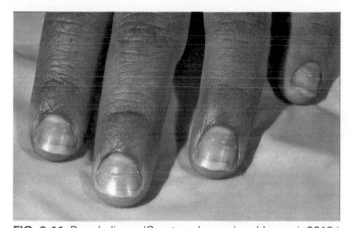

FIG. 9-11 Beau's lines. (Courtesy Lemmi and Lemmi, 2013.)

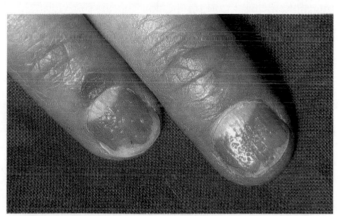

FIG. 9-12 Nail pitting. (From White and Cox, 2000.)

PROCEDURES AND TECHNIQUES WITH EXPECTED FINDINGS	**ABNORMAL FINDINGS**

SPECIAL CIRCUMSTANCES OR ADVANCED PRACTICE

INSPECT and PALPATE the skin for lesions.

An in-depth examination of lesions is not performed routinely during every health assessment. However, when the patient has a new lesion or when a lesion has changed (i.e., it has changed in appearance or become painful), it should be examined. A strong light source to determine the exact color, elevation, and borders and a centimeter ruler to measure the size of lesions are helpful. The lesion is documented based on its characteristics, including location, distribution, color, pattern, edges, depth, and size (Fig. 9-13 and Box 9-2). Lesions are classified as primary, secondary, or vascular.

Primary Lesions

Many primary lesions are considered expected variations of the skin and include moles, freckles, patches, and comedones (acne) among adolescents and young adults. These have been discussed in previous sections (Table 9-2).

Many primary lesions are considered abnormal findings and are associated with a specific disease process or injury (see Table 9-2).

★ Use a Wood's lamp to identify fluorescing lesions, indicating fungal infection. Darken the room and shine the light on the area to be examined. If there is no fungal infection, the light tone on the skin appears soft violet.

A yellow-green or blue-green fluorescence indicates the presence of fungal infection.

★ Advanced practice.

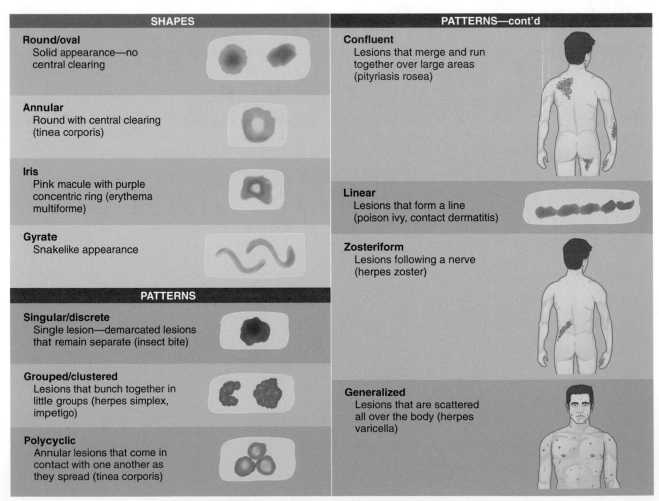

FIG. 9-13 Shapes and patterns of lesions.

SHAPES

Round/oval
Solid appearance—no central clearing

Annular
Round with central clearing (tinea corporis)

Iris
Pink macule with purple concentric ring (erythema multiforme)

Gyrate
Snakelike appearance

PATTERNS

Singular/discrete
Single lesion—demarcated lesions that remain separate (insect bite)

Grouped/clustered
Lesions that bunch together in little groups (herpes simplex, impetigo)

Polycyclic
Annular lesions that come in contact with one another as they spread (tinea corporis)

PATTERNS—cont'd

Confluent
Lesions that merge and run together over large areas (pityriasis rosea)

Linear
Lesions that form a line (poison ivy, contact dermatitis)

Zosteriform
Lesions following a nerve (herpes zoster)

Generalized
Lesions that are scattered all over the body (herpes varicella)

BOX 9-2 LESION CHARACTERISTICS TO BE NOTED DURING EXAMINATION

- Note the **location** and **distribution** of the lesion. Is the lesion generalized over the entire body or section of the body; or is it localized to a specific area such as around the waist, under a piece of jewelry, or in the hair?
- Describe the **color** of the lesion and how this lesion may be different in color from other lesions noted on the body (e.g., a mole or freckle). Has the patient noticed a change in the color of the lesion?
- What is the **pattern** of the lesion? Are the lesions clustered? Are they in a line? How does the patient describe the development of the pattern of the lesion? (See Fig. 9-13.)

- What are the **edges** of the lesion like? Is the edge of the lesion regular or irregular? Has the patient noticed a change in the shape of the lesion?
- Is the lesion flat, raised, or sunken?
- What is the current **size** of the lesion? Measure using a centimeter ruler. Has the patient noticed a change in the size?
- What are the **characteristics** of the lesion? Is it hard, soft, or fluid filled? If there is an exudate, what is the color of the drainage fluid? Does the exudate have an odor? Note both the color and odor if present. Has the patient noticed a change in either the characteristics or drainage of the lesion? If so, how and when?

TABLE 9-2 PRIMARY SKIN LESIONS

SKIN LESIONS	EXAMPLES		
Macule Flat, circumscribed area that is a change in the color of the skin; less than 1 cm in diameter	Freckles, flat moles (nevi), petechiae, measles, scarlet fever	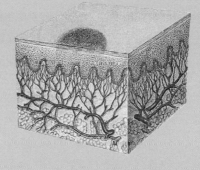	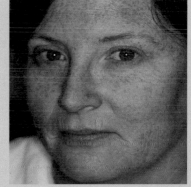 Freckles are a very common macule (Courtesy Lemmi and Lemmi, 2013.)
Papule Elevated, firm, circumscribed area less than 1 cm in diameter	Wart (verruca), elevated moles, lichen planus, cherry angioma, neurofibroma, skin tag	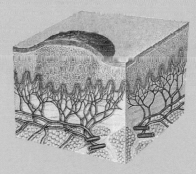	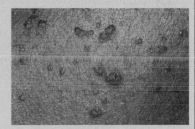 Moles. (Courtesy Lemmi and Lemmi, 2013.)
Patch A flat, nonpalpable, irregular-shaped macule more than 1 cm in diameter	Vitiligo, port wine stains, mongolian spots, café-au-lait spots	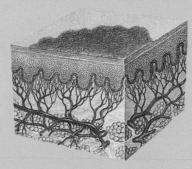	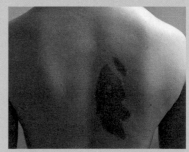 Café-au-lait patch. (Courtesy Lemmi and Lemmi, 2013.)

Continued

TABLE 9-2   PRIMARY SKIN LESIONS—cont'd

SKIN LESIONS	EXAMPLES		
Plaque Elevated, firm, and rough lesion with flat top surface greater than 1 cm in diameter	Psoriasis, seborrheic and actinic keratoses, eczema	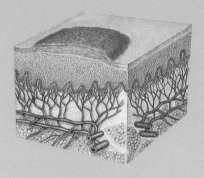	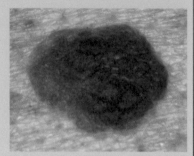Seborrheic keratosis. (Courtesy Lemmi and Lemmi, 2013.)
Wheal Elevated irregular-shaped area of cutaneous edema; solid, transient; variable diameter	Insect bites, urticaria, allergic reaction, lupus erythematosus	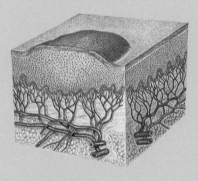	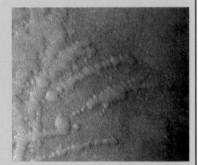Urticaria. (Courtesy Lemmi and Lemmi, 2013.)
Nodule Elevated, firm, circumscribed lesion; deeper in dermis than a papule; 1 to 2 cm in diameter	Dermatofibroma erythema nodosum, lipomas, melanoma, hemangioma, neurofibroma	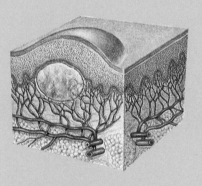	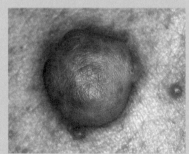Neurofibroma. (Courtesy Lemmi and Lemmi, 2013.)
Tumor Elevated and solid lesion; may or may not be clearly demarcated; deeper in dermis; greater than 2 cm in diameter	Neoplasms, lipoma, hemangioma	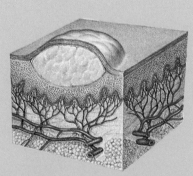	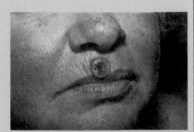Tumor of upper lip. (From Goldstein and Goldstein, 1997.)

TABLE 9-2   PRIMARY SKIN LESIONS—cont'd

SKIN LESIONS	EXAMPLES		
Vesicle Elevated, circumscribed, superficial, not into dermis; filled with serous fluid; less than 1 cm in diameter	Varicella (chickenpox), herpes zoster (shingles), impetigo, acute eczema	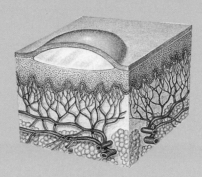	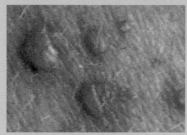 Vesicles. (From Farrar et al., 1992.)
Bulla Vesicle greater than 1 cm in diameter	Blister, pemphigus vulgaris, lupus erythematosus, impetigo, drug reaction	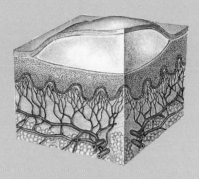	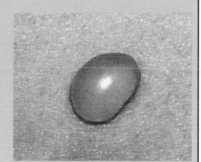 Blister. (From White, 1994.)
Pustule Elevated, superficial lesion; similar to a vesicle but filled with purulent fluid	Impetigo, acne, folliculitis, herpes simplex	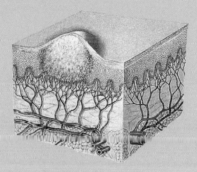	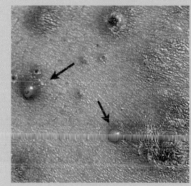 Acne. (From Weston, Lane, and Morelli, 2002.)
Cyst Elevated, circumscribed, encapsulated lesion; in dermis or subcutaneous layer; filled with liquid or semisolid material	Sebaceous cyst, cystic acne	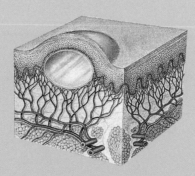	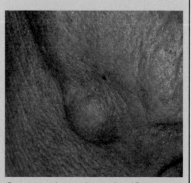 Cyst on lateral neck. (Courtesy Lemmi and Lemmi, 2013.)

PROCEDURES AND TECHNIQUES WITH EXPECTED FINDINGS

Secondary Lesions

Some secondary lesions are considered expected variations. For example, a scar is a common variation seen on the skin, caused by injury to the skin. A multitude of skin injuries can cause a scar; thus in many cases scars lack significance.

ABNORMAL FINDINGS

Abnormal secondary lesions result from changes from or trauma to a primary lesion (Table 9-3). Although scars can be an expected finding, they also may be an indication of past physical abuse. Examples may include excessive scars or those that appear on skin surfaces typically protected. Scarring caused by needle-track marks generally indicates intravenous drug use.

TABLE 9-3 SECONDARY SKIN LESIONS

SKIN LESIONS	EXAMPLES		
Scale Heaped-up keratinized cells; flaky skin; irregular; thick or thin; dry or oily; variation in size	Flaking of skin with seborrheic dermatitis following scarlet fever or flaking of skin following a drug reaction; dry skin, pityriasis rosea, eczema, xerosis	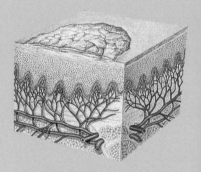	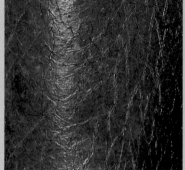 Scaling. (From White, 2004.)
Lichenification Rough, thickened epidermis secondary to persistent rubbing, itching, or skin irritation; often involves flexor surface of extremity	Chronic dermatitis, psoriasis	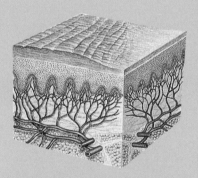	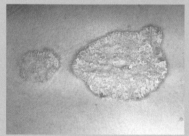 Psoriasis on the leg. (Courtesy Lemmi and Lemmi, 2013.)
Keloid Irregular-shaped, elevated, progressively enlarging scar; grows beyond the boundaries of the wound	Keloid formation following surgery	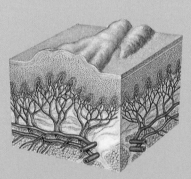	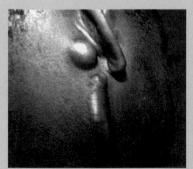 Keloid. (From Weston, Lane, and Morelli, 2002.)

TABLE 9-3 SECONDARY SKIN LESIONS—cont'd

SKIN LESIONS	EXAMPLES		
Scar Thin-to-thick fibrous tissue that replaces normal skin following injury or laceration to the dermis	Healed wound or surgical incision	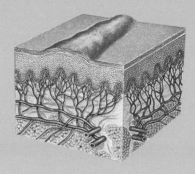	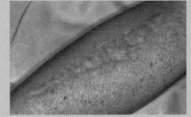Scar on forearm from an open reduction following a fracture. (Courtesy Lemmi and Lemmi, 2013.)
Excoriation Loss of the epidermis; linear hollowed-out crusted area	Abrasion or scratch, scabies	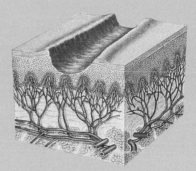	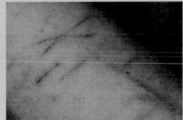Excoriation. (From Lemmi and Lemmi, 2000.)
Fissure Linear crack or break from the epidermis to the dermis; may be moist or dry	Athlete's foot, cracks at the corner of the mouth, chapped hands, eczema, intertrigo labialis	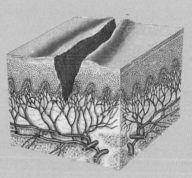	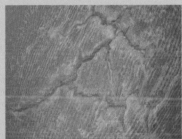Fissure. (Courtesy Lommi and Lemmi, 2013.)
Crust Dried drainage or blood; slightly elevated; variable size; colors variable—red, black, tan, or mixed	Scab on abrasion, eczema	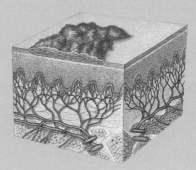	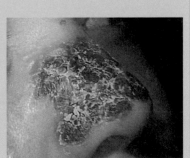Scab. (From Seidel et al., 2011.)

Continued

TABLE 9-3 SECONDARY SKIN LESIONS—cont'd

SKIN LESIONS	EXAMPLES		
Erosion Loss of part of the epidermis; depressed, moist, glistening; follows rupture of a vesicle or bulla	Varicella, variola after rupture, candidiasis, herpes simplex	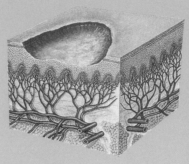	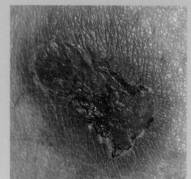Erosion resulting from rupture of a bulla. (Courtesy Lemmi and Lemmi, 2013.)
Ulcer Loss of epidermis and dermis; concave; varies in size	Pressure ulcer, stasis ulcers, syphilis chancre	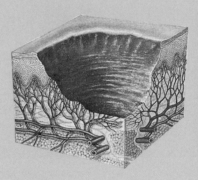	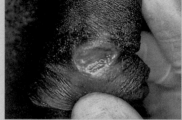Ulcer caused by syphilis. (From Goldstein and Goldstein, 1997.)
Atrophy Thinning of the skin surface and loss of skin markings; skin appears translucent and paperlike	Aged skin, striae, discoid lupus erythematosus	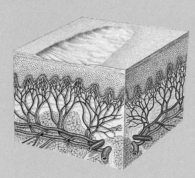	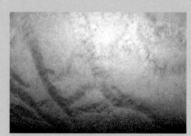Striae. (Courtesy Antoinette Hood, MD, Dept. of Dermatology, University of Indiana, Dept. of Medicine, Indianapolis. From Seidel et al., 2011.)

PROCEDURES AND TECHNIQUES WITH EXPECTED FINDINGS

Vascular Lesions

Many vascular lesions are considered common variations (Table 9-4). Ecchymosis (bruising) on a bony prominence is generally considered a common finding secondary to the activities of daily living. Other vascular lesions include the following:

- *Telangiectasia:* A fine, irregular, red line caused by permanent dilation of a group of superficial blood vessels.
- *Cherry angioma:* A small, slightly raised, bright red area that typically appears on the face, neck, and trunk of the body. These increase in size and number with advanced age (Fig. 9-14).

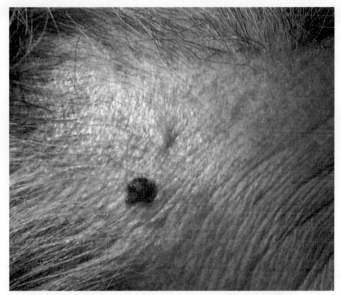

FIG. 9-14 Cherry angioma. (From Baran, Dawber, and Levene, 1991.)

ABNORMAL FINDINGS

Abnormal vascular lesions are presented in Table 9-4. A *hematoma* forms when there is a leakage of blood in a confined space caused by a break in a blood vessel. Bruising over soft tissue areas of the body in the absence of injury or the presence of multiple bruises on the body in various stages of healing is considered an abnormal finding warranting further investigation. Possible causes include physical abuse or a bleeding disorder.

TABLE 9-4	VASCULAR SKIN LESIONS		
SKIN LESIONS	**CAUSE/EXAMPLES**		
Petechiae			
Tiny, flat, reddish-purple, nonblanchable spots in the skin less than 0.5 cm in diameter; appear as tiny red spots pinpoint to pinhead in size	Cause: tiny hemorrhages within the dermal or submucosa—caused by intravascular defects and infection	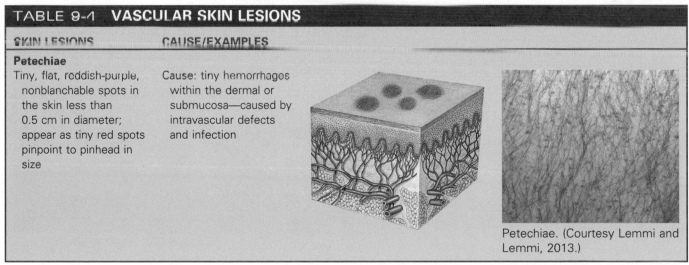	Petechiae. (Courtesy Lemmi and Lemmi, 2013.)

Continued

TABLE 9-4 VASCULAR SKIN LESIONS—cont'd

SKIN LESIONS	CAUSE/EXAMPLES		
Purpura Flat, reddish-purple, nonblanchable discoloration in the skin greater than 0.5 cm in diameter	Cause: infection or bleeding disorders resulting in hemorrhage of blood into the skin Examples: senile, actinic purpura, progressive pigmented purpura, vasculitis purpura, thrombocytopenic purpura	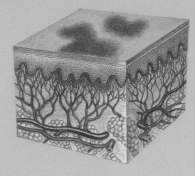	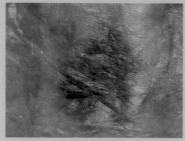 Senile purpura. (Courtesy Lemmi and Lemmi, 2013.)
Ecchymosis (Bruise) Reddish-purple, nonblanchable spot of variable size	Cause: trauma to the blood vessel resulting in bleeding under the tissue	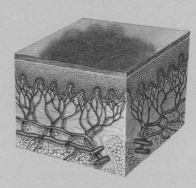	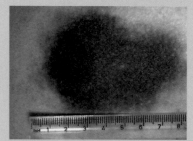 Ecchymosis. (From Lemmi and Lemmi, 2000.)
Angioma Benign tumor consisting of a mass of small blood vessels; can vary in size from very small to large	Examples: cherry angioma, hemangioma, cavernous hemangioma, strawberry hemangioma	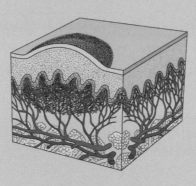	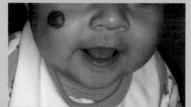 Strawberry hemangioma. (From Rakel and Bope, 2004. Courtesy Richard P. Usatine.)
Capillary Hemangioma (Nevus Flammeus) Type of angioma that involves the capillaries within the skin producing an irregular macular patch that can vary from light red to dark red to purple in color	Cause: congenital vascular malformation of capillaries Example: port wine stain, stork bite	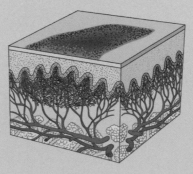	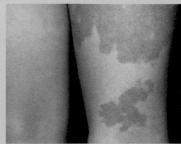 Port wine stain. (From McCance and Huether, 2002.)

TABLE 9-4   VASCULAR SKIN LESIONS—cont'd

SKIN LESIONS	CAUSE/EXAMPLES		
Telangiectasia Permanent dilation of preexisting small blood vessels (capillaries, arterioles, or venules) resulting in superficial, fine, irregular red lines within the skin	Causes: rosacea, collagen vascular disease; actinic damage, increased estrogen levels Examples: essential telangiectasia, hereditary hemorrhagic telangiectasia, spider telangiectasia	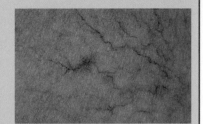	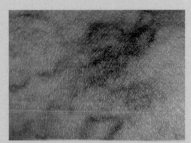 Telangiectasia. (Courtesy Lemmi and Lemmi, 2000.)
Vascular Spider (Spider Angioma) Type of telangiectasia characterized by a small central red area with radiating spiderlike legs; this lesion blanches with pressure	Causes: may occur in absence of disease, with pregnancy, in liver disease, or with vitamin B deficiency	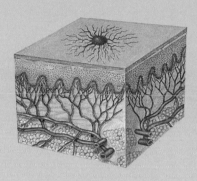	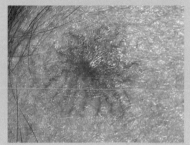 Spider angioma. (Courtesy Lemmi and Lemmi, 2013.)
Venous Star Type of telangiectasia characterized by a nonpalpable bluish, star-shaped lesion that may be linear or irregularly shaped	Cause: increased pressure in the superficial veins	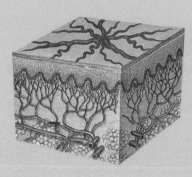	 Venous star. (From Lemmi and Lemmi, 2000.)

FREQUENTLY ASKED QUESTIONS

What is the best way to memorize all the different types of skin lesions?

As a student it is much more important that you learn to accurately describe a lesion than memorize the types of lesions themselves. As you become more proficient with descriptions, you will also begin to remember the names. When you describe a lesion, be sure to include the following information:

- Location, size, and color of the lesion
- Shape (oval, round, irregular) and borders (regular or irregular)
- Elevation (flat, raised, or sunken)
- Characteristics (e.g., hard, soft, fluid filled)
- Pattern (if more than one lesion)

DOCUMENTING EXPECTED FINDINGS

The skin is the expected color for race: it is smooth, soft, warm, dry, and intact with an even surface and elastic turgor. Freckles are noted on the face, back, arms, and legs. Hair on the scalp is red, shiny, soft, and fine. Facial and body hair are consistent with female distribution. Nails are clean, pink, smooth, and unpolished and blanch with pressure.

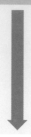 **CLINICAL REASONING: THINKING LIKE A NURSE**

Skin, Hair, and Nails

A 74-year-old man with type 2 diabetes mellitus and peripheral vascular disease arrives at a medical clinic complaining of a painful area on his right lower leg near the ankle.

Interpreting

Early in the encounter, the nurse considers two possible causes of this patient's leg pain: potential deep vein thrombosis or infection; the patient is at high risk for both. To determine whether either has any probability of being correct, the nurse gathers additional data. *Has there been a recent injury to the area, creating a mechanism for bacterial entrance into the skin?* The only injury the patient can recall is scratching his leg in that area the previous week while cutting weeds. The experienced nurse not only recognizes inflammation and infection by the signs (erythema, heat, and edema) and symptoms (pain) but also interprets this information in the context of an injury to an extremity of an individual with type 2 diabetes mellitus and peripheral artery disease. The nurse verifies medication allergies in anticipation of the need of antibiotics.

Nurse's Background, Experience, Perspective

The experienced nurse immediately has a perceptual grasp of the situation at hand. Extensive practical knowledge about what to expect with this age-group and diagnoses allows the nurse to recognize risk factors given his situation: age, diabetes mellitus, and peripheral vascular disease impact perfusion and immunity.

Noticing

This background knowledge sets up the possibility of noticing signs of a prevalent complication in an individual presenting with these data. The man indicates that the pain started several days ago and has become progressively worse. The nurse observes a large area of redness and swelling over the medial aspect of the lower left leg; the area is extremely painful to the touch and hot.

Responding

The nurse initiates appropriate initial interventions to reduce the inflammation and treat the infection, determine which type of health care provider may best assist the patient, and ensure that the patient receives appropriate immediate and follow-up care, including instruction about how to prevent infections.

Reflecting

The nurse evaluates the presentation and outcomes of interventions (reflection-in-action); this experience contributes and deepens the expertise on which he or she will draw (reflection-on-action) when encountering a similar situation.

AGE-RELATED VARIATIONS

The discussion thus far has featured the assessment of skin, hair, and nails for the adult patient. This assessment is performed for individuals across the life span. In general, the approach is the same, but there are variations in findings.

INFANTS AND CHILDREN

The assessment of skin among infants and children follows the same general principles as previously described for the adult. Skin lesions common to infants and children include milia, erythema toxicum, diaper rash, and rashes associated with allergens. Chapter 19 presents further information regarding the assessment of skin, hair, and nails for these age-groups.

ADOLESCENTS

The most common skin lesions of concern among adolescents are acne because of the increase in sebaceous gland activity. Not only are these lesions painful, but also they are of concern to the patient because of personal appearances. Chapter 19 presents further information.

OLDER ADULTS

The skin and hair undergo significant changes with aging. Lesions are commonly found on older adults. Although many lesions are considered expected variations associated with the aging process, the incidence of skin cancer increases with age. Further information related to changes of the skin and lesions commonly found among older adults is presented in Chapter 21.

SITUATIONAL VARIATIONS

PATIENTS WITH LIMITED MOBILITY (HEMIPLEGIA, PARAPLEGIA, QUADRIPLEGIA)

Patients with limited mobility are at risk for skin breakdown secondary to pressure and body fluid pooling because of an inability to feel pressure or a decreased ability to independently change position to relieve pressure. A pressure ulcer, as defined by the National Pressure Ulcer Advisory Panel, is a localized injury to the skin and/or underlying tissue usually over a bony prominence as a result of pressure or pressure in combination with shear and/or friction.[11] The nurse should examine the patient's skin, especially over bony prominences. The nurse may need assistance to turn the patient so a complete skin assessment may be performed. In addition, patients who operate their own wheelchairs are at high risk for developing hand calluses. Therefore special care should be taken to examine the patient's hands.

Assessing for pressure ulcers gained additional importance in 2006 when the Centers for Medicaid and Medicare Services (CMS) eliminated payment to hospitals for conditions deemed "reasonably preventable," also referred to as *never events.* Because hospital-acquired pressure ulcers are included as never events, all patients admitted are carefully assessed for pressure ulcers.[12] When found, these patients' ulcers are photographed to document their presence at the time of admission as opposed to being hospital acquired. In addition, to prevent pressure ulcers from developing, nurses assess patients at risk for them (e.g., those who are immobile, are incontinent of urine or stool, or have nutritional deficiencies). They then implement preventive interventions such as keeping the skin clean, dry, and free of prolonged pressure. Further, nurses collaborate with dietitians to plan a diet to maintain skin integrity (e.g., a diet including protein, vitamin C, and zinc). If nurses assess a pressure ulcer after admission to the hospital, they collaborate with a wound care nurse for prompt, early interventions to prevent further skin damage and regain skin integrity.

Expected and Abnormal Findings (Skin)

Assess all contact and skin pressure points for patients who have limited mobility (Fig. 9-15). When a red area of skin is noted, blanch the skin by applying gentle pressure over the red areas. If the skin becomes white (blanches) when pressure is applied and reddens again after pressure is relieved, the circulation to that area is sufficient, and the redness will disappear. If the skin does not blanch when pressure is applied, a stage I pressure ulcer has developed. Pressure ulcers are staged as follows: stage I, prolonged redness with unbroken skin; stage II, partial-thickness skin loss that appears as a shallow, open ulcer with pink wound bed and without slough; stage III, full-thickness skin loss with damage to the subcutaneous tissue with no bone, tendon, or muscle exposed; and stage IV, full-thickness tissue loss with exposed bone, muscle, or tendon. Eschar or slough may be present in some parts of the wound bed. If the entire wound bed is covered by slough or eschar, the stage cannot be determined; thus it is considered unstagable[11] (Table 9-5).

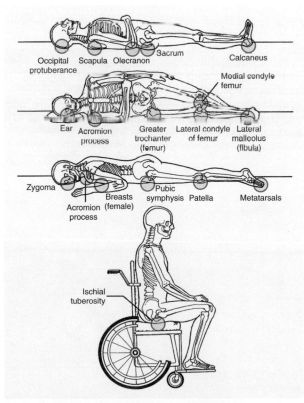

FIG. 9-15 Bony prominences vulnerable to pressure.

TABLE 9-5 STAGING OF PRESSURE ULCERS

DESCRIPTION	DIAGRAM	CLINICAL PRESENTATION

Suspected Deep Tissue Injury
Localized area of discolored (purple or maroon) intact skin or blood-filled blister caused by underlying soft tissue damage resulting from pressure or shear. May be difficult to detect among individuals with dark skin tone. May include a blister over a dark wound bed; wound may become covered with eschar.

Stage I
Intact skin with nonblanchable redness, usually over a bony prominence. The area may be painful, firm, soft, warmer, or cooler compared to adjacent tissue. May be difficult to detect among individuals with dark skin tones.

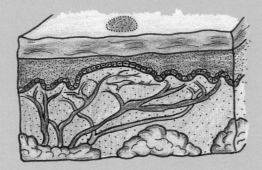

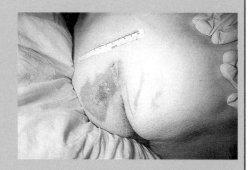

Stage II
Partial-thickness loss of dermis. Presents as a shiny or dry shallow open ulcer with pink wound bed without slough or bruising. May also present as an intact or open/ruptured serum-filled blister.

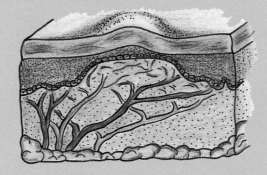

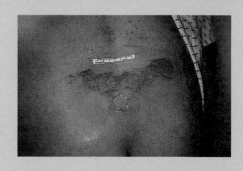

Stage III
Full-thickness skin loss involving damage to or necrosis of subcutaneous tissue. Subcutaneous fat may be visible; but bone, tendon, or muscles are not exposed. Slough may be present; wound may include undermining and tunneling. Depth of a stage III ulcer varies by anatomic location because of variation in presence and depth of subcutaneous tissue.

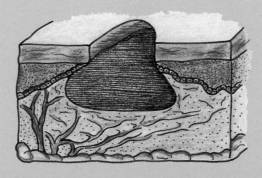

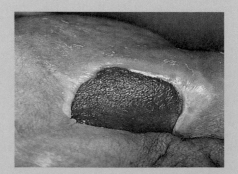

TABLE 9-5 STAGING OF PRESSURE ULCERS—cont'd

DESCRIPTION	DIAGRAM	CLINICAL PRESENTATION

Stage IV

Full-thickness tissue loss with exposed bone, tendon, or muscle. Slough or eschar may be present within the wound bed. Undermining and tunneling often present. Depth of a stage IV ulcer varies by anatomic location because of variation in presence and depth of subcutaneous tissue.

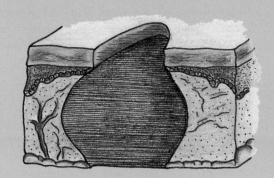

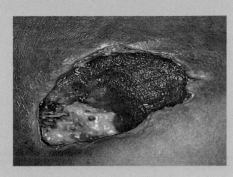

Unstageable Ulcer

Full-thickness tissue loss in which base of ulcer is covered by slough (yellow, tan, gray-green, or brown) and/or eschar (tan, brown, or black). True depth of the wound cannot be determined until the slough and/or eschar is/are removed to expose the base of the wound.

From National Pressure Ulcer Advisory Panel: *Updated staging system*. 2007, available at www.npuap.org. Images from Lewis, Heitkemper, and Dirksen, 2007, 2011.

COMMON PROBLEMS AND CONDITIONS

RISK FACTORS

Skin, Hair, and Nails

- Systemic disease (e.g., liver, kidney, collagen, endocrine, or autoimmune disease)
- Infection (viral, bacterial, or fungal)
- Family history of skin cancer or autoimmune disease
- Immobility
- Excessive sun exposure (M)
- Exposure to chemicals or allergens (M)
- Medications (allergic outbreaks, photosensitive response) (M)

M, Modifiable risk factor.

SKIN

Hyperkeratosis
Clavus (Corn)

A corn is a lesion that develops secondary to chronic pressure from a shoe over a bony prominence. **Clinical Findings:** The corn is a flat or slightly raised, painful lesion that generally has a smooth, hard surface (Fig. 9-16). A "soft" corn is a whitish thickening commonly found between the fourth and fifth toes. A "hard" corn is clearly demarcated and has a conical appearance.

Dermatitis

The term *dermatitis* is used to describe a variety of superficial inflammatory conditions of the skin that can be acute or chronic.

Atopic Dermatitis

Atopic dermatitis is a chronic superficial inflammation of the skin with an unknown cause; however, it is commonly associated with hay fever and asthma and is thought to be familial. It is seen in all age-groups, although it is more common in infancy and childhood. **Clinical Findings:** During infancy and early childhood red, weeping, crusted lesions appear on the face, scalp, extremities, and diaper area (Fig. 9-17). In older children and adults, lesion characteristics include erythema, scaling, and lichenification. The lesions are usually localized to the hands, feet, arms, and legs (particularly at the antecubital fossa and popliteal space) and are associated with intense pruritus.

Contact Dermatitis

Contact dermatitis is an inflammatory reaction of the skin in response to irritants or allergens such as metals, plants, chemicals, or detergent. This condition affects people of all ages and ethnic groups. **Clinical Findings:** Contact dermatitis developed in an area exposed to the causative irritant or allergen and appears as localized erythema that may also include edema, wheals, scales, or vesicles that may weep, ooze, and become crusted. Pruritus is a common associated symptom of contact dermatitis (Fig. 9-18). The inflammatory response is highly individualized; it can vary from no-to-extreme reaction.

Seborrheic Dermatitis

Seborrheic dermatitis is a chronic inflammation of the skin of unknown cause affecting individuals throughout their life, often with periods of remission and exacerbation. (In infants this condition is known as cradle cap.) **Clinical Findings:** The lesions appear as scaly, white, or yellowish plaques involving skin on the scalp, eyebrows, eyelids, nasolabial folds, ears, axillae, chest, and back. Lesions typically cause mild pruritus; lesions on the scalp cause dandruff (Fig. 9-19).

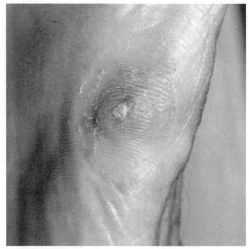

FIG. 9-16 Corn (clavus). (From White, 1994.)

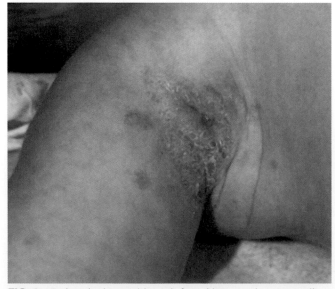

FIG. 9-17 Atopic dermatitis on infant. Note erythema, scaling, and lichenification. (Courtesy Lemmi and Lemmi, 2013.)

Stasis Dermatitis

Stasis dermatitis is an inflammation of the skin on the lower legs most commonly seen in older adults. It is thought to be caused by venous stasis, chronic edema, and poor peripheral circulation. **Clinical Findings:** Initially this condition is characterized by an area or areas of erythema and pruritus followed by scaling, petechiae, and brown pigmentation (Fig. 9-20). Stasis dermatitis progresses to ulcerated lesions (known as stasis ulcers) if untreated.

Psoriasis

This is a common chronic skin disorder that can occur at any age but usually develops by age 20. Inflammatory cytokines from activated helper T-cells cause lesions of psoriasis, and the disease can range from mild to severe. **Clinical Findings:** The lesions appear as well-circumscribed, slightly raised, erythematous plaques with silvery scales on the surface. They appear most frequently on the elbows, knees, buttocks, lower back, and scalp. A specific characteristic of this condition is the observance of small bleeding points if the lesion is scratched. Associated symptoms include pruritus, burning, and bleeding of the lesions and pitting of the fingernails (Fig. 9-21, *A* and *B*).

Pityriasis Rosea

Pityriasis rosea is a common, acute, self-limiting inflammatory disease that usually occurs in young adults during the

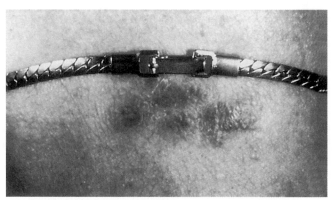

FIG. 9-18 Contact dermatitis caused by an allergic reaction to nickel. (From Cohen, 1993.)

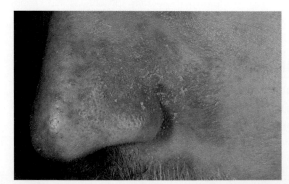

FIG. 9-19 Seborrheic dermatitis. (From McCance and Huether, 2010. Courtesy Department of Dermatology, School of Medicine, University of Utah.)

winter months. The cause is unknown but might be associated with a virus. **Clinical Findings:** The initial manifestation is a lesion referred to as a *herald patch* (i.e., a single lesion, usually located on the trunk, resembling tinea corporis) (Fig. 9-22, *A*). At 1 to 3 weeks following the initial lesion, a generalized eruption of pale, erythematous, and macular lesions occurs on the trunk and extremities (Fig. 9-22, *B*); occasionally they appear as vesicular lesions. The patient generally feels well but may complain of mild itching.

Lesions Caused by Viral Infection
Warts (Verruca)

A wart is a small benign lesion caused by human papillomavirus (HPV) and transmitted by contact. Because there are more than 60 different types of HPV, many different types of warts occur in many locations and in many sizes. They may appear at any age. **Clinical Findings:** Common warts (verrucae vulgaris) are round or irregular-shaped papular lesions that are light gray, yellow, or brownish black. They commonly appear on hands, fingers, elbows, and knees (Fig. 9-23). Plantar warts are found on the sole of the foot and are typically tender to pressure.

Herpes Simplex

The term *herpes simplex* represents a group of eight deoxyribonucleic acid (DNA) viruses. Herpes simplex virus (HSV) is a chronic, noncurable condition transmitted by contact; between outbreaks the virus is dormant. Outbreaks are triggered by a number of factors, including sun exposure, stress, and fever. **Clinical Findings:** Before the onset of lesions, many patients report a sensation of slight stinging and increased sensitivity. The classic manifestation of HSV is the development of grouped vesicles on an erythematous base. The lesions are very painful and highly contagious after direct contact with skin. Lesions caused by herpes simplex virus type 1 (HSV-1) often appear on the upper lip (often referred to as a *cold sore*), nose, around the mouth, or on the tongue (Fig. 9-24). HSV type 2 (HSV-2) lesions usually appear on the genitalia. As the lesions erupt, they move through maturational stages of vesicles, pustules, and finally crusting. They typically last for approximately 2 weeks. (See Chapter 17 for further discussion of HSV-2.)

Herpes Varicella (Chickenpox)

This is a highly communicable viral infection that spreads by droplets. It commonly occurs in children but can also infect

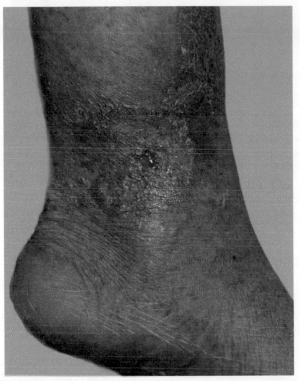

FIG. 9-20 Stasis dermatitis on lower leg with ulceration. (Courtesy Lemmi and Lemmi, 2013.)

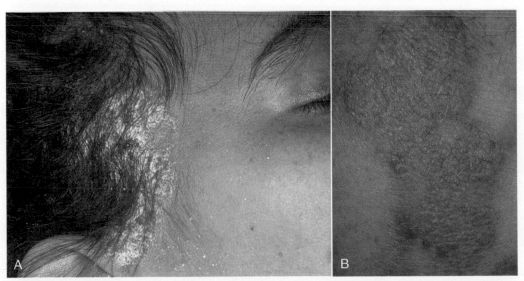

FIG. 9-21 Psoriasis. **A,** On the scalp. **B,** On the leg. (Courtesy Lemmi and Lemmi, 2013.)

adults who did not have the infection as children. **Clinical Findings:** The lesions first appear on the trunk and then spread to the extremities and the face. Initially the lesions are macules; they progress to papules and then vesicles, and finally the old vesicles become crusts. The lesions erupt in crops over a period of several days. For this reason lesions in various stages are seen concurrently. The period of infectivity is from a few days before lesions appear until the final lesions have crusted, usually about 6 days after the first lesions erupt (Fig. 9-25, *A* and *B*).

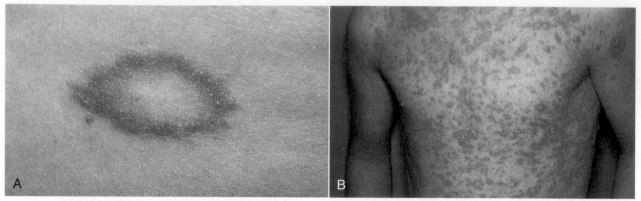

FIG. 9-22 Pityriasis rosea. **A,** Large herald patch on the chest. **B,** Many oval lesions on the chest. (**A** from Cohen, 1993; **B** Courtesy Lemmi and Lemmi, 2013.)

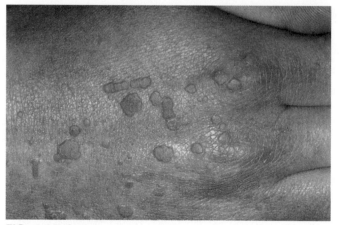

FIG. 9-23 Common warts on hand and fingers. (Courtesy Lemmi and Lemmi, 2013.)

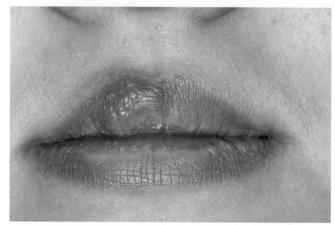

FIG. 9-24 Herpes simplex. Typical manifestation with vesicles appearing on the lips and extending onto the skin. (From Lemmi and Lemmi, 2000.)

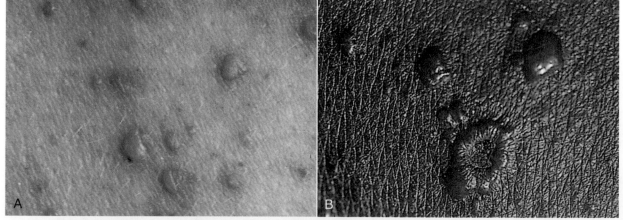

FIG. 9-25 Herpes varicella (chickenpox). Lesions in various stages of development, including red papules, vesicles, umbilicated vesicles, and crusts. **A,** Light-skinned person. **B,** Dark-skinned person. (From Farrar et al., 1992.)

Herpes Zoster (Shingles)

A dormant herpes varicella virus causes herpes zoster, which is an acute inflammation by reactivation of the virus. Herpes zoster follows years after the initial varicella infection in some individuals. **Clinical Findings:** Linearly grouped vesicles appear along a cutaneous sensory nerve line (dermatome) (Fig. 9-26). As the disease progresses, the vesicles turn into pustules followed by crusts. This painful condition is generally unilateral and commonly appears on the trunk and face. Pain may precede lesion eruption by several days.

Lesions Caused by Fungal Infections
Tinea Infections

Tinea infections are caused by a number of dermophyte fungal infections involving the skin, hair, and nails that affect children and adults. **Clinical Findings:** *Tinea corporis* (ringworm) involves generalized skin areas (excluding scalp, face, hands, feet, and groin) and appears as circular, well-demarcated lesions that tend to have a clear center (Fig. 9-27, *A*). They are hyperpigmented in light-colored skin and hypopigmented in dark-skinned persons. *Tinea cruris* ("jock itch") affects the groin area and is characterized by small erythematous and scaling vesicular patches with a well-defined border spreading over the inner and upper surfaces of the thighs (Fig. 9-27, *B*). *Tinea capitis* involves the scalp, causing scaling and pruritus with balding areas resulting from hair that breaks easily (Fig. 9-27, *C*). *Tinea pedis* is a chronic infection involving the foot ("athlete's foot"). It initially appears as small weeping vesicles and painful macerated areas between the toes and sometimes on the sole of the foot. As the lesions develop, they may become scaly and hard and cause discomfort and itching (Fig. 9-27, *D*).

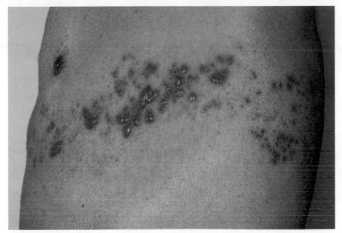

FIG. 9-26 Herpes zoster (shingles). (Courtesy Lemmi and Lemmi, 2013.)

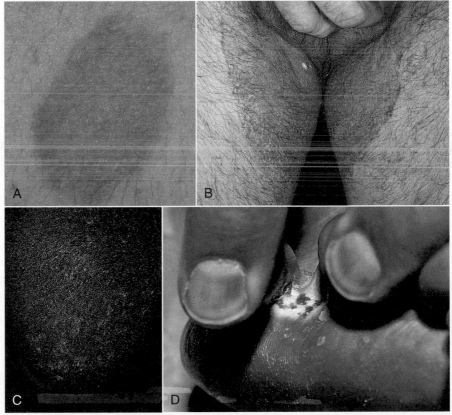

FIG. 9-27 Fungal infections. **A,** Tinea corporis on chest—pink, oval-shaped with scaling. **B,** Tinea cruris. **C,** Tinea capitis. **D,** Tinea pedis. (**A** and **B** courtesy Lemmi and Lemmi, 2013; **C** and **D** from White, 2004.)

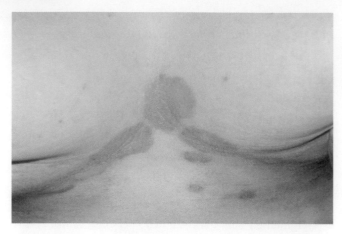

FIG. 9-28 Candidiasis. (From Lemmi and Lemmi, 2000.)

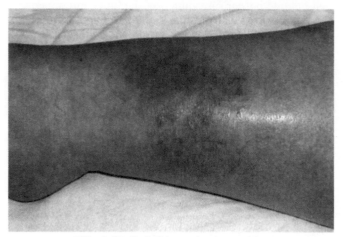

FIG. 9-29 Cellulitis to the lower leg.

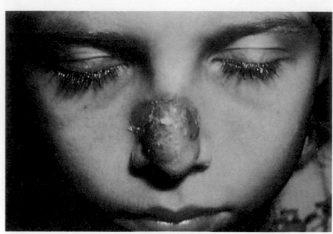

FIG. 9-30 Impetigo. (From Goldstein and Goldstein, 1997. Courtesy Department of Dermatology, University of North Carolina at Chapel Hill.)

Candidiasis

This fungal infection is caused by *Candida albicans* and is normally found on the skin, mucous membranes, gastrointestinal tract, and vagina. However, candidiasis can develop under certain conditions such as a favorable environment (warm, moist, or tissue maceration); disease states (diabetes mellitus, Cushing's syndrome, debilitated states, immunosuppression); and systemic antibiotic administration. **Clinical Findings:** A *Candida* infection affects the superficial layers of skin and mucous membranes. It appears as a scaling red rash with sharply demarcated borders. The area is generally a large patch but may have some loose scales. Common areas for candidiasis involving the skin include the genitalia, the inguinal areas, and along gluteal folds (Fig. 9-28).

Lesions Caused by Bacterial Infections
Cellulitis

Cellulitis is an acute streptococcal or staphylococcal infection of the skin and subcutaneous tissue. Cellulitis can occur at any age and can involve any skin area on the body. **Clinical Findings:** The skin is red, warm to the touch and tender, and appears to be indurated. There may be regional lymphangitic streaks and lymphadenopathy (Fig. 9-29).

Impetigo

This is a common and highly contagious bacterial infection caused by group A streptococcus and transmitted by contact.[13] It can occur in any age- group; however, it is most prevalent in children, especially among individuals living in crowded conditions with poor sanitation. Impetigo occurs most commonly in mid-to-late summer, with the highest incidence in hot, humid climates. **Clinical Findings:** This infection appears as an erythematous macule that becomes a vesicle or bulla and finally a honey-colored crust after the vesicles or bullae rupture (Fig. 9-30). The lesions commonly occur on the face around the nose and mouth, although other skin areas can be involved.

Folliculitis

This is an inflammation of hair follicles. **Clinical Findings:** An acute lesion appears as an area of erythema with a pustule surrounding the hair follicle (Fig. 9-31), most commonly on the scalp and extremities. A chronic condition occurs when deep hair follicles are infected (usually seen in bearded areas).

Furuncle or Abscess

A furuncle, also known as a *boil,* is a localized bacterial lesion caused by a staphylococcal pathogen. Furuncles often develop from folliculitis. **Clinical Findings:** Initially a furuncle is a nodule surrounded by erythema and edema. As it progresses it becomes a pustule; the center (or core) fills with a sanguineous purulent exudate. The skin around a furuncle is red, hot, and extremely tender (Fig. 9-32).

Lesions Associated with Arthropods
Scabies

Scabies is a highly contagious infestation associated with the mite *Sarcoptes scabiei.* The female mite burrows into the superficial layer of skin and lays eggs. Transmission usually occurs with direct skin-to-skin contact. **Clinical Findings:** Severe pruritus is the hallmark of scabies caused by a hypersensitivity to the mite and its feces. The lesions are small

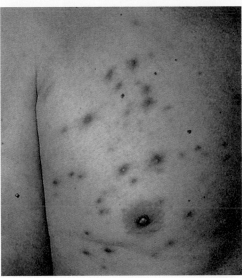

FIG. 9-31 Folliculitis. (From Goldstein and Goldstein, 1997. Courtesy Beverly Sanders, MD.)

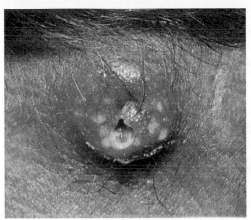

FIG. 9-32 Furuncle. (From Thompson et al., 2002. Courtesy JA Tschen, MD, Baylor College of Medicine, Department of Dermatology, Houston, Tex.)

papules, vesicles, and burrows that result from the mite entering the skin to lay eggs. The burrows appear as short, irregular marks that look as if they were made by the end of a pencil. Areas most commonly affected include the hands, wrists, axillae, genitalia, and inner aspects of the thigh.

Lyme Disease

Lyme disease occurs after a bite from a tick infected with *Borrelia burgdorferi* and is the most commonly reported vectorborne illness in the United States. The large majority of Lyme disease cases in the United States occur in the northeast states.[14] **Clinical Findings:** The classic manifestation of Lyme disease is the development of an expanding erythemic rash with central clearing at the site of the tick bite (Fig. 9-33). This rash typically exceeds 5 cm and persists for several weeks. Most individuals also have flulike symptoms (e.g., fever, headache, muscle aches).

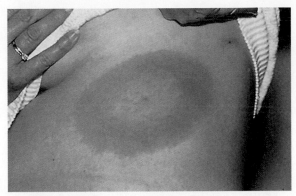

FIG. 9-33 Lyme disease. Note expanding erythematous lesion with central clearing on trunk. (From Goldstein and Goldstein, 1997. Courtesy John Cook, MD.)

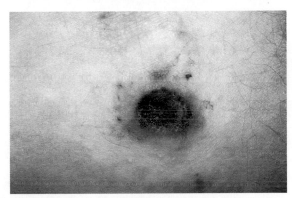

FIG. 9-34 Brown recluse spider bite. Note necrotic ulcer and erythema. (From Goldstein and Goldstein, 1997. Courtesy Marshall Guill, MD.)

Spider Bites

Most bites that are of concern to humans are caused by two spiders—the black widow and the brown recluse spider. Black widow spiders are found throughout the United States; brown recluse spiders are found predominantly in the central and south central United States. **Clinical Findings:** The bite of the black widow and brown recluse spiders tends to cause minimal symptoms at the time of the bite. The initial lesion of a black widow spider bite appears as an area of erythema with two red puncta at the bite site. Within a few hours symptoms of severe abdominal pain and fever typically develop. The bite of a brown recluse spider initially appears as a lesion with erythema and edema that evolves into a necrotic ulcer with erythema and purpura (Fig. 9-34). Other symptoms include fever, nausea, and vomiting.

Malignant Neoplasia
Basal Cell Carcinoma

Basal cell carcinoma is the most common form of skin cancer. It predominantly afflicts light-skinned individuals between ages 40 and 80. This malignancy is locally invasive and rarely metastasizes. The incidence increases with age and is more common in males than females.[3] **Clinical Findings:** The lesion has different forms but usually appears as a nodular

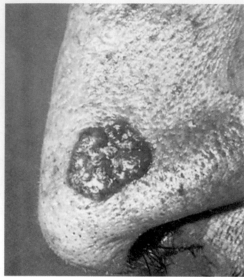

FIG. 9-35 Basal cell carcinoma. (From Thompson et al., 1993. Courtesy Gary Monheit, MD, University of Alabama at Birmingham School of Medicine.)

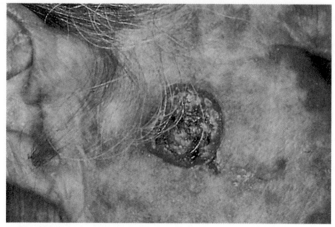

FIG. 9-36 Squamous cell carcinoma. (From Goldstein and Goldstein, 1997. Courtesy Department of Dermatology, Medical College of Georgia.)

pigmented lesion with depressed centers and rolled borders. In some cases the center is ulcerated. It is usually found in areas that have had repeated exposure to the sun or ultraviolet light such as the face (Fig. 9-35).

Squamous Cell Carcinoma

Squamous cell carcinoma is the second-most frequent form of skin cancer. It is an invasive skin cancer that typically appears on the head and neck and occurs as a result of excessive sun or ultraviolet light exposure. Those most commonly affected are individuals over age 50 who have blue eyes and childhood freckling (light pigmentation). Men are more commonly affected than women.[3] **Clinical Findings:** Initially this cancer appears as a red, scaly patch that has a sharply demarcated border (Fig. 9-36). As the lesion develops further, it is soft, mobile, and slightly elevated. As the tumor matures, a central ulcer may form with surrounding redness.

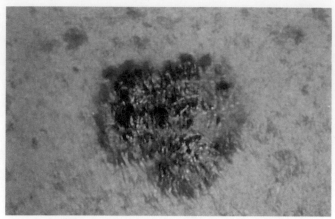

FIG. 9-37 Malignant melanoma. (From Hill, 1994.)

Melanoma

Melanoma is the most serious form of skin cancer, responsible for a large majority of skin cancer-related deaths.[3] It is a malignant proliferation of pigmented cells (melanocytes). These lesions typically arise from already present nevi. **Clinical Findings:** The mnemonic ABCDEF (see Box 9-1) is used to remember the classic manifestations of melanoma: *A*symmetry, *B*order irregularity, *C*olor variation, *D*iameter greater than 6 mm, *E*levation (recent change from a flat to raised lesion), and *F*eeling (a reported sensation of itching, tingling, or stinging within the lesion). The lesion may have a flaking or scaly texture; its color may vary from brown to pink to purple, or it may have mixed pigmentation (Fig. 9-37).

Kaposi's Sarcoma

Kaposi's sarcoma is a malignant neoplasm that develops in connective tissues such as cartilage, bone, fat, muscle, blood vessels, or fibrous tissues. It affects those with acquired immunodeficiency syndrome (AIDS) and those who have drug-induced immunosuppression. **Clinical Findings:** The initial lesions appear on the lower extremities and are characterized by dark blue–purple macules, papules, nodules, and plaques (Fig. 9-38, *A* and *B*). The lesions eventually spread all over the body, particularly the trunk, arms, neck, face, and oral mucosa. Associated symptoms are pain and pruritus to the lesions.

Skin Lesions Caused by Abuse

Injuries to the skin are among the most easily recognized signs of physical abuse. When abuse is suspected, compare the type of injury or injuries to the history and the developmental level (if it involves an infant or child). Injuries to the skin are generally recognized in three forms: bruises, bites, and burns.

Bruise (Ecchymosis)

A bruise is a discoloration of the skin or mucous membrane caused by blood seeping into the tissues as a result of a trauma to the area. It can indicate superficial or deep injury such as injury to muscle or abdominal organs. Consider the location,

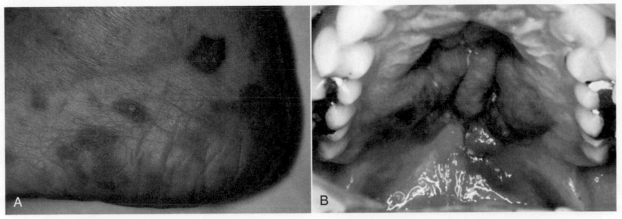

FIG. 9-38 **A,** Kaposi's sarcoma of the heel and lateral foot. **B,** Oral Kaposi's sarcoma. (**A** from Grimes, 1991. **B** Courtesy Sol Silverman, Jr., DDS, University of California, San Francisco.)

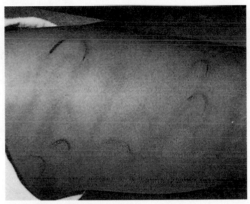

FIG. 9-39 Loop mark pattern of bruising caused by whipping with an electrical cord. (From Monteleone, 1996.)

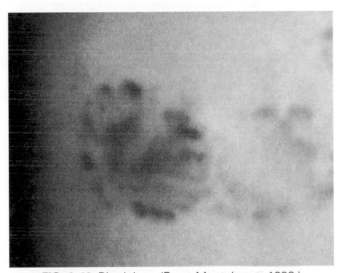

FIG. 9-40 Bite injury. (From Monteleone, 1996.)

appearance, and pattern of bruises and the type of mark made. **Clinical Findings:** A recent bruise (1 to 3 days old) is purple to deep black in appearance. A bruise that is 3 to 6 days old is green to brown in color, whereas an older bruise (6 to 15 days old) changes from green to tan to yellow and then fades. Look for a pattern in the bruise markings. Bruises associated with abuse may be caused by objects that leave distinctive patterns such as a loop pattern from being hit with a cord[15] (Fig. 9-39).

Bites

Bites are always intentional and are a common injury associated with abuse (Fig. 9-40). Bite marks are ovoid with tooth imprints that may or may not break the skin. They may have a suck mark (bruising) in the middle. The size of the bite mark is important to note to determine the age of the person who may have left the mark (i.e., child versus adult). Bite marks on infants and children are frequently located on the genitals or buttocks.[15]

Burns

Burns are frequently associated with abuse. The most common type is an immersion burn. This is easily recognizable by a

"glove" or "stocking" burn pattern (a line of demarcation) in which the child is immersed into scalding hot water. Look for this pattern on hands and arms, feet and legs, and buttocks (Fig. 9-41). Another common type of burn associated with abuse is a *contact burn* (i.e., a burn caused by intentionally placing a hot object such as a cigarette, light bulb, lighter, or hot iron on the skin) (Fig. 9-42). Intentional contact burns are easily recognizable because they literally leave a "branded pattern" on the skin. An accidental burn with an object typically leaves a glancing burn pattern with a nonuniform pattern.[16]

HAIR

Pediculosis (Lice)

Lice are parasites that invade the scalp, body, or pubic hair regions. Lice on the body are called *pediculosis corporis*, and pubic lice are called *pediculosis pubis*. Lice infestations are spread most commonly by close person-to-person contact.[17] **Clinical Findings:** The eggs (nits) are visible as small, white

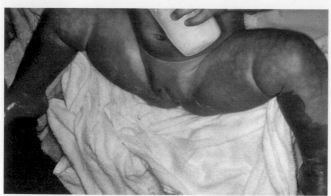

FIG. 9-41 Stocking burn patterns to perineum, thighs, legs, and feet. (From Zitelli, McIntire, and Nowalk, 2012. Courtesy Thomas Layton, MD.)

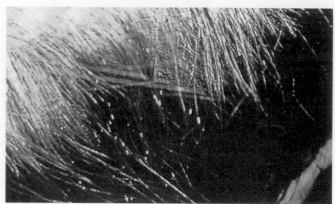

FIG. 9-43 Pediculosis (lice). The eggs, or nits, are visible, attached to hair shafts. (From Farrar et al., 1992. Courtesy Dr. E. Sahn.)

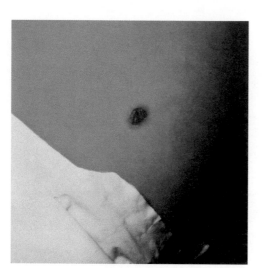

FIG. 9-42 Cigarette burn to a child's abdomen. (From Zitelli, McIntire, and Nowalk, 2012.)

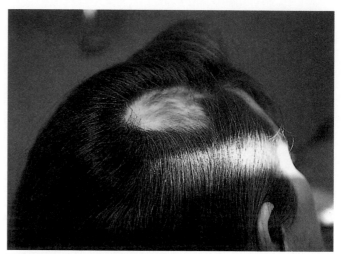

FIG. 9-44 Alopecia areata. Note areas of regrowth (fine, light-colored hairs). (From Goldstein and Goldstein, 1997.)

particles at the base of the hair shaft (Fig. 9-43). The skin underlying the infested area may appear red and excoriated.

Alopecia Areata

Alopecia areata is a chronic inflammatory disease of the hair follicles resulting in hair loss on the scalp. The cause is unknown but is associated with autoimmune disorders, metabolic disease, and stressful events. **Clinical Findings:** Hair loss is observed in multiple round patch areas of the scalp (Fig. 9-44). The affected areas are either completely smooth or have short shafts of hair. The poorly developed and fragile hair shafts break and generally grow back within 3 to 4 months, although some individuals suffer total scalp hair loss.

Hirsutism

This is a condition associated with an increase in the growth of facial, body, or pubic hair in women. Hirsutism has familial tendency and can be associated with endocrine disorders; polycystic ovarian disease; menopause; and side effects of medications, especially corticosteroid or androgenic steroid therapy.[18] **Clinical Findings:** An increase of body or facial

hair is seen; the amount of hair varies (Fig. 9-45). This condition is more pronounced among individuals with darkly pigmented hair. Increased hair growth may or may not be associated with other signs of virilization when secondary male sexual characteristics are acquired by females.

NAILS

Onychomycosis

This is a fungal infection of the nail plate caused by tinea unguium. Although the prevalence varies, it occurs in up to 18% of the population in given areas.[19] **Clinical Findings:** The nail plate turns yellow or white as hyperkeratotic debris accumulates. As the problem progresses, the nail separates from the nail bed, and the nail plate crumbles (Fig. 9-46).

Paronychia

Paronychia involves an acute or chronic infection of the cuticle. The infection is usually caused by staphylococci and streptococci, although *Candida* may also be the causative organism. **Clinical Findings:** Acute infection involves the

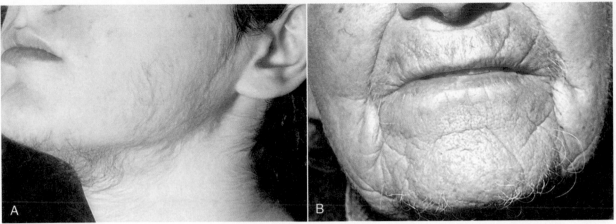

FIG. 9-45 Facial hirsutism. **A,** Hair growth on the jaw line and neck of a young woman. **B,** Hair growth on the chin of a postmenopausal woman. (From Baran, Dawber, and Levene, 1991.)

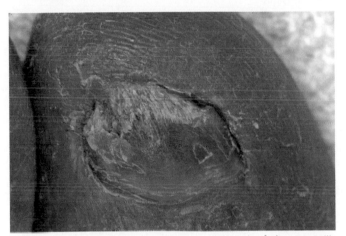

FIG. 9-46 Onychomycosis (fungal infection) of the toenail). (Courtesy Lemmi and Lemmi, 2013.)

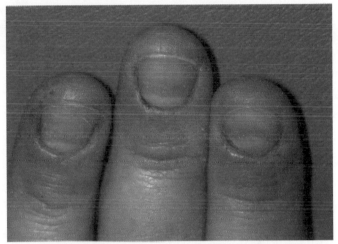

FIG. 9-47 Chronic paronychia with swollen posterior nail folds and nail dystrophy. (Courtesy Lemmi and Lemmi, 2013.)

rapid onset of very painful inflammation at the base of the nail, often after minor trauma to the area. In some cases an abscess may form. With chronic paronychia the inflammation develops slowly, usually starting at the base of the nail within the cuticle and working up along the sides of the nails (lateral nail folds). Frequent exposure of the hands to moisture is a risk factor for chronic paronychia (Fig. 9-47).

Ingrown Toenail

An ingrown toenail is a relatively common problem that occurs when the nail grows through the lateral nail and into the skin. This condition usually involves the great toe and is usually caused by cutting the nail too far down the sides, wearing shoes that fit too tightly, or injury.[20] **Clinical Findings:** The individual experiences pain, redness, and edema. An acute infection may occur, resulting in purulent drainage (Fig. 9-48). Common risk factors for an ingrown toenail include trauma, poorly fitting shoes, and excessive trimming of the lateral nail plate.

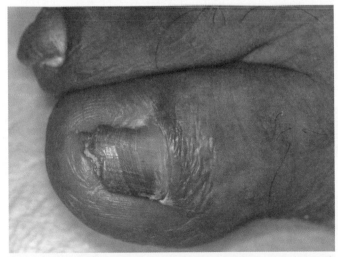

FIG. 9-48 Ingrown toenail. (Courtesy Lemmi and Lemmi, 2013.)

CLINICAL APPLICATION AND CLINICAL REASONING

See Appendix D for answers to exercises in this section.

REVIEW QUESTIONS

1. A patient has edema and redness of the skin surrounding the nail on his right index finger. Which data elicited from his history best explains this condition?
    1. He has a family history of liver disease.
    2. There has been a scabies outbreak among his family members.
    3. He has a new full-time position as a dishwasher at a local restaurant.
    4. He had several warts removed from his hands 2 years ago.

2. When examining a 16-year-old male patient, the nurse notes multiple pustules and comedones on the face. The nurse recognizes that increased activity of which cells or glands produce these manifestations?
    1. Epidermal cells.
    2. Eccrine glands.
    3. Apocrine glands.
    4. Sebaceous glands.

3. A patient with darkly pigmented skin has been admitted to the hospital with hepatitis. What is the best way for the nurse to assess for jaundice in this patient?
    1. Jaundice is best seen in the sclera.
    2. In dark-skinned persons, jaundice results in a darkening of genitalia.
    3. Jaundice is best determined by blanching the fingernails.
    4. Jaundice cannot be assessed in patients with darkly pigmented skin.

4. A patient has multiple solid, red, raised lesions on her legs and groin that she describes as "itchy insect bites." How does the nurse document these lesions?
    1. Wheals.
    2. Bullae.
    3. Tumors.
    4. Plaques.

5. The nurse observes multiple red circular lesions with central clearing that are scattered all over the abdomen and thorax. How does the nurse document the shape and pattern of these lesions?
    1. Gyrate and linear.
    2. Annular and generalized.
    3. Iris and discrete.
    4. Oval and clustered.

6. Which disorder is an example of a vascular lesion?
    1. Dermatofibroma
    2. Vitiligo
    3. Sebaceous cyst
    4. Port wine stain

7. A 60-year-old male patient states that he has a sore above his lip that has not healed and is getting bigger. The nurse observes a red scaly patch with an ulcerated center and sharp margins. These findings are commonly associated with which malignancy?
    1. Kaposi's sarcoma.
    2. Malignant melanoma.
    3. Basal cell carcinoma.
    4. Squamous cell carcinoma.

8. A 48-year-old woman asks the nurse how to best protect herself from excessive sun exposure while at the beach. Which response would be most appropriate?
    1. "Limit your time in the sun to 5 minutes every hour."
    2. "Wear a wet suit that covers your arms and legs."
    3. "Apply a waterproof sunscreen (SPF 15 or higher) to exposed skin surfaces; reapply at least every 2 hours."
    4. "Apply sunscreen with a minimum SPF 50 to all skin surfaces before leaving for the beach; this will provide all-day coverage."

CASE STUDY

Don Hillerman is a 38-year-old male paraplegic admitted to the hospital for unexplained weakness and depression. The following data are collected by the nurse during an interview and assessment.

Interview Data

Don states that he became a paraplegic 2 years ago after a motorcycle accident. He claims that he is fully independent and needs no assistance. However, for about the past month he has felt weak and has had a loss of appetite. Normally he is able to transfer himself in and out of a wheelchair but admits that he has engaged in very little activity during the last few weeks. His mother and father keep telling him that he is depressed, and this makes him feel very angry. He has no other medical problems and no allergies to medications.

Examination Data

- *General survey:* Alert, very thin male with flat affect lying in a supine position. Height, 6 ft 2 in (188 cm); weight, 153 lb (69.5 kg). Slight foul-smelling odor noted.
- *Skin:* Skin color is pale. No evidence of bruising, no skin discoloration. Presence of stage 2 skin breakdown involving the epidermis over the left greater trochanter and sacrum.
- *Hair:* Full hair distribution on head with soft texture.
- *Abdomen:* Active bowel sounds. Abdomen soft, nondistended, nontender.
- *Musculoskeletal:* Paralysis, atrophy to both lower extremities; upper extremities fully functional.

Clinical Reasoning

1. Which data deviate from normal findings, suggesting a need for further investigation?
2. For which additional information should the nurse ask or assess?
3. Which risk factors for pressure ulcers does this patient have?
4. With which interdisciplinary team members can the nurse collaborate to help meet this patient's needs?

Head, Eyes, Ears, Nose, and Throat

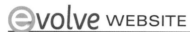 WEBSITE

http://evolve.elsevier.com/Wilson/assessment

CONCEPT OVERVIEW

The feature concept for this chapter is *Sensory Perception.* The concept of sensory perception refers to the ability to understand and interact with the environment through senses (sight, hearing, smell, taste, and touch) and conditions that negatively affect these perceptions. Sensory perception occurs through a variety of body systems and a complex interaction between sensory structures and neurologic function shown in the model below.

This model shows the interrelationship of concepts that are impacted by sensory perception and the relationship that sensory perception has to neurologic function. As an example, a child with chronic ear infections may be impacted by pain, interrupted sleep, and developmental delay. An individual with a visual disturbance may experience changes in mobility. Having an understanding of the interrelationships of these

concepts helps the nurse recognize potential risk factors and thus increases awareness when conducting a health assessment. This is an important step associated with clinical judgment. The following case provides a clinical example featuring several of these interrelated concepts.

Mr. Rodriquez is a 79-year-old man who lives alone. He has a long history of diabetes mellitus and hypertension. Over the past 8 years he has experienced progressive loss of vision as a result of retinopathy (a complication from diabetes). The loss in vision has resulted in frequent falls; and, because he no longer cooks for himself, he has lost weight. He also has hearing loss and tinnitus (ringing in the ears), which interferes with his sleep. Mr. Rodriquez has become progressively withdrawn to the point at which his grown children are exploring alternative living arrangements for him.

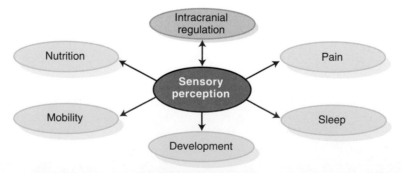

ANATOMY AND PHYSIOLOGY

The head and neck regions contain multiple structures that make examination of these areas complex. The skull encloses the brain; facial structures include the eyes, ears, nose, and mouth. Structures of the neck include the upper portion of

the spine, the esophagus, the trachea, the thyroid gland, arteries, veins, and lymph nodes. Because of the regional relationship, all of these structures are presented in this chapter.

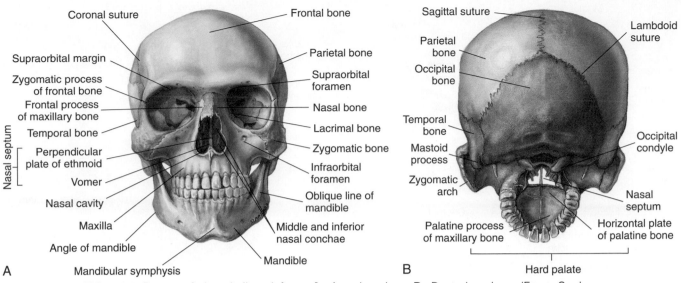

FIG. 10-1 Bones of the skull and face. **A,** Anterior view. **B,** Posterior view. (From Seeley, Stephens, and Tate, 1995. The McGraw Hill Companies, Inc.)

THE HEAD

The skull is a bony structure that protects the brain and upper spinal cord (Fig. 10-1). The special senses of vision, hearing, smell, and taste are also contained within the brain. Six bones form the skull (one frontal bone, two parietal bones, two temporal bones, and one occipital bone) and are fused together at sutures. The skull is covered by scalp tissue, which is typically covered with hair.

The face consists of 14 bones that protect facial structures, including the eyes, ears, nose, and mouth; these structures are generally symmetric. Like the skull, these bones are immobile and are fused at sutures, with the exception of the mandible. The mandible articulates with the temporal bone of the skull at the temporomandibular joint, allowing for movement of the jaw up, down, in, out, and from side to side. The facial muscles are innervated by cranial nerves V (trigeminal) and VII (facial).

THE EYES

External Ocular Structures

The external eye is composed of the eyebrows, upper and lower eyelids, eyelashes, conjunctivae, and lacrimal glands (Fig. 10-2). The opening between the eyelids is termed the *palpebral fissure.* The eyelashes curve outward from the lid margins, filtering out dirt. Two thin, transparent mucous membranes termed *conjunctivae* lie between the eyelids and the eyeball. The bulbar conjunctiva covers the scleral surface of the eyeballs. The palpebral conjunctiva lines the eyelids and contains blood vessels, nerves, hair follicles, and sebaceous glands. One of the sebaceous glands, the meibomian gland, secretes an oily substance that lubricates the lids, prevents excessive evaporation of tears, and provides an airtight seal when the lids are closed. Tears, formed by the lacrimal glands, combine with sebaceous secretions to maintain a constant film over the

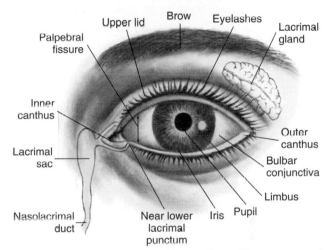

FIG. 10-2 External ocular structures. (From Thompson et al., 2002.)

cornea. In the inner (or medial) canthus small openings termed the *lacrimal puncta* drain tears from the eyeball surface through the lacrimal sac into the nasolacrimal ducts.

Ocular Structures

The globe of the eye, also known as the "eyeball," is surrounded by three separate layers: the sclera, uvea, and retina (Fig. 10-3). The *sclera* is a tough, fibrous outer layer commonly referred to as the *white* of the eye. The sclera merges with the cornea in front of the globe at a junction termed the *limbus.* The cornea covers the iris and the pupil. It is transparent, avascular, and richly innervated with sensory nerves via the ophthalmic branch of the trigeminal nerve (cranial nerve V). The constant wash of tears provides the cornea with its oxygen supply and protects its surface from drying. An important corneal function is to allow light transmission through the lens to the retina.

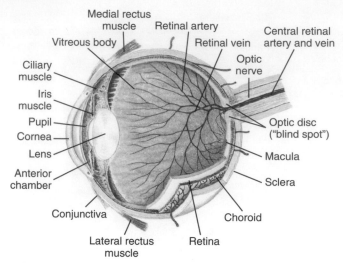

FIG. 10-3 Anatomy of the human eye. (From Seidel et al., 2011.)

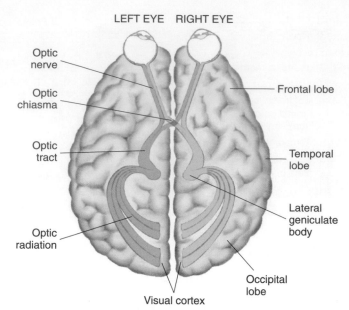

FIG. 10-4 Visual pathway. (From Thompson et al., 2002.)

The middle layer, termed the *uvea,* consists of the choroid posteriorly and the ciliary body and iris anteriorly. The choroid layer is highly vascular and supplies the retina with blood. The iris is a circular, muscular membrane that regulates pupil dilation and constriction via the oculomotor nerve (cranial nerve III). The central opening of the iris, the pupil, allows light transmission to the retina through the transparent lens. The ciliary body is a thickened region of the choroid that has two functions: it adjusts the shape of the lens to accommodate vision at varying distances, and it produces transparent aqueous humor—a fluid that helps maintain the intraocular pressure and metabolism of the lens and posterior cornea. Aqueous humor fills the anterior chamber between the cornea and lens and flows between the lens and the iris.

The inner layer of the eye, the *retina,* is an extension of the central nervous system. This transparent layer has photoreceptor cells, termed *rods* and *cones,* scattered throughout its surface. As the term *photoreceptor* suggests, these cells perceive images and colors in response to varying light stimuli. Rods respond to low levels of light, and cones to higher levels of light. Although these rods and cones are scattered throughout the retina, they are not evenly distributed. The macula lutea, a pigmented area about 4.5 mm in diameter, is densely packed peripherally with rods. The fovea centralis, a small depression in the center of the macula lutea on the posterior wall of the retina, is concentrated with cones but contains no rods.

Perforating the retina is the optic disc, which is the head of the optic nerve (cranial nerve II). It contains no rods or cones, causing a small blind spot located about 15 degrees laterally from the center of vision. The central retinal artery and central vein bifurcate at the optic disc and feed into smaller branches throughout the retinal surface as shown in Fig. 10-3. (Also see Fig. 10-28.)

Ocular Function

Vision, the primary function of the eyes, occurs when rods and cones in the retina perceive images and colors in response

to varying light stimuli. The lenses are constantly adjusting to stimuli at different distances through accommodation. When the lenses bring an image into focus, nerve impulses transmit the information from the retina along the optic nerve and optic tract, reaching the visual cortex (located in the occipital lobe of each cerebral hemisphere) for cognitive interpretation (Fig. 10-4).

Six extraocular muscles and three cranial nerves allow for eye movement in six directions. The medial, inferior, and superior rectus muscles and the inferior oblique muscles, guided by the oculomotor nerve (cranial nerve III), control upward outer, lower outer, upward inner, and medial eye movements. The superior oblique muscle controls lower medial movement, innervated by the trochlear nerve (cranial nerve IV). The lateral rectus muscle controls lateral eye movement, innervated by the abducens nerve (cranial nerve VI).

THE EAR

External Ear

The external ear is composed of the auricle (pinna) and the external auditory ear canal. The auricle is composed of cartilage and skin. The helix is the prominent outer rim; the concha is the deep cavity in front of the external auditory meatus (Fig. 10-5). The bottom portion of the ear is referred to as the *lobule.* The auricle is attached to the head by skin, extension cartilage to the external auditory canal cartilage, ligaments, and muscles (the anterior, superior, and posterior auricular muscles). The auricle serves three main functions: collection and focus of sound waves, location of sound (by turning the head until the sound is loudest), and protection of the external ear canal from water and dirt.

The adult's external ear canal is an S-shaped pathway leading from the outer ear to the tympanic membrane (TM), commonly known as the *eardrum* (Fig. 10-6). The lateral one third of the ear canal has a cartilaginous framework; the medial two thirds of the canal is surrounded by bone. The skin covering the cartilaginous portion of the auditory canal has hair follicles surrounded by sebaceous glands that secrete cerumen (earwax). The hair follicles and cerumen protect the middle and inner ear from particles and infection.

Middle Ear

The middle ear is an air-filled cavity separated from the external ear canal by the TM. The TM, composed of layers of skin, fibrous tissue, and mucous membrane, is shiny and pearl gray. It is translucent, permitting limited visualization of the

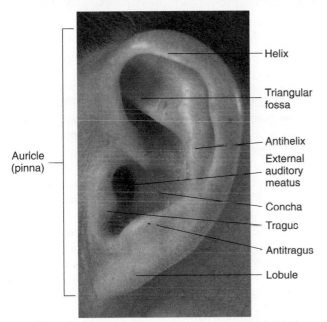

FIG. 10-5 Anatomic structure of the auricle (pinna).

middle ear cavity. The middle ear contains three tiny bones—the malleus, incus, and stapes—that are collectively known as ossicles (see Fig. 10-6). Lying between the nasopharynx and the middle ear is the eustachian tube. It opens briefly during yawning, swallowing, or sneezing to equalize the pressure of the middle ear to the atmosphere.

The function of the middle ear is amplification of sound. Sound waves cause the TM to vibrate; this vibration is transmitted through the ossicles to the inner ear. The amplification results from the ossicles and from the size (area) difference between the TM and the oval window, an oval-shaped aperture in the wall of the middle ear leading to the inner ear.

Inner Ear

The inner ear is encased in a bony labyrinth that contains three primary structures: the vestibule, the semicircular canals, and the cochlea (see Fig. 10-6). The vestibule and the semicircular canals contain receptors responsible for balance and equilibrium. The coiled snail-shaped cochlea contains the organ of Corti, the structure that is responsible for hearing. Specialized hair cells on the organ of Corti act as sound receptors. Sound waves that reach the cochlea cause movement of the hair cells, which in turn transmit the impulses along the cochlear nerve branch of the acoustic nerve (cranial nerve VIII) to the temporal lobe of the brain, where interpretation of sound occurs.

THE NOSE

The nose serves as a passageway for inspired and expired air. It humidifies, filters, and warms air before it enters the lungs and conserves heat and moisture during exhalation. Other functions of the nose include identifying odors and giving resonance to laryngeal sounds.

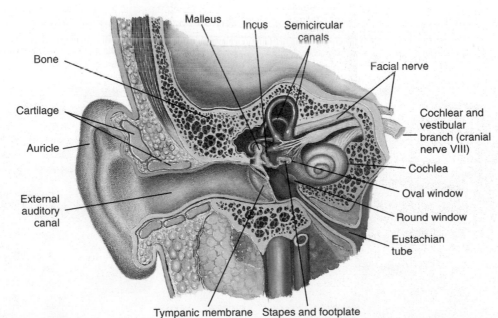

FIG. 10-6 Anatomy of the ear showing outer ear, external auditory canal, tympanic membrane, and structures of the middle and inner ear. (From Seidel et al., 2011.)

The upper third of the nose is encased in bone, and the lower two thirds are composed of cartilage. The floor of the nasal cavity is the hard palate. The septal cartilage maintains the shape of the nose and separates the nares (nostrils), which maintain an open passage for air. The nasal cavity is lined with highly vascular mucous membranes containing cilia (nasal hairs) that trap airborne particles and prevent them from reaching the lungs. Three turbinates (inferior, middle, and superior) line the lateral walls of the nasal cavity, providing a large surface area of nasal mucosa for heat and water exchange as air passes through the nose. The space between the inferior and middle turbinates is the middle meatus, which is an outlet for drainage from the frontal, maxillary, and anterior ethmoid sinuses. The nasolacrimal duct drains into the inferior meatus, and the posterior ethmoid sinus drains into the middle and superior meatus (Fig. 10-7).

Paranasal sinuses extend out of the nasal cavities through narrow openings into the skull bones to form four paired,

air-filled cavities (i.e., sphenoid, frontal, ethmoid, and maxillary) that make the skull lighter (Fig. 10-8, A and B). They are lined with mucous membranes and cilia that move secretions along excretory pathways.

THE MOUTH AND OROPHARYNX

Within the mouth are several structures, including the lips, tongue, teeth, gums, and salivary glands (Fig. 10-9, A and B). The roof of the mouth consists of the hard palate, near the front portion of the oral cavity, and the soft palate, toward the back of the pharynx. The tongue has hundreds of taste buds (papillae) on its dorsal surface. The taste buds distinguish sweet, sour, bitter, and salty tastes. The ventral (bottom) surface of the tongue is smooth and highly vascular.

Humans have two sets of teeth: deciduous teeth (baby teeth) and permanent teeth. There are 32 permanent teeth: 12 incisors, 8 premolars, and 12 molars. Teeth are tightly encased in mucous membrane–covered, fibrous gum tissue and rooted in the alveolar ridges of the maxilla and mandible.

Three pairs of salivary glands—the parotid, submandibular, and sublingual—release saliva through small openings (ducts) in response to the presence of food (see Fig. 10-9). The parotid glands lie anterior to the ears, immediately above the mandibular angle, and drain into the oral cavity through Stensen's ducts (parotid gland openings). These are visible adjacent to the upper second molars. The submandibular glands are tucked under the mandible and lie approximately midway between the chin and the posterior mandibular angle. Wharton's ducts, the openings for the submandibular glands, are visible on either side of the lingual frenulum under the tongue. The sublingual glands, the smallest salivary glands, lie on the floor of the mouth and drain through 10 to 12 tiny ducts that cannot be seen with the naked eye.

Oropharynx

The oropharynx includes the structures at the back of the mouth that are visible on examination: the uvula, the anterior

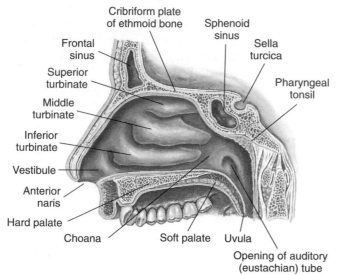

FIG. 10-7 Cross-sectional view of structures of the nose and nasopharynx. (From Seidel et al., 2011.)

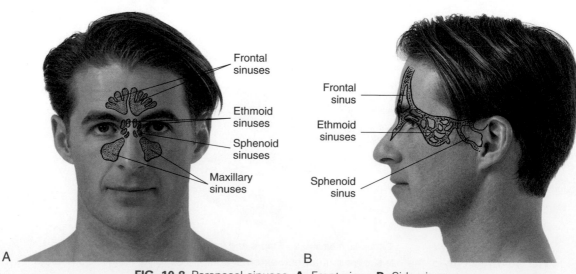

FIG. 10-8 Paranasal sinuses. **A,** Front view. **B,** Side view.

and posterior pillars, the tonsils, and the posterior pharyngeal wall (see Fig. 10-9). The uvula is suspended midline from the soft palate, which extends out to either side to form the anterior pillar. The tonsils are masses of lymphoid tissue that are tucked between the anterior and posterior pillars. These may be atrophied in adults to the point of being barely visible. The posterior pharyngeal wall is visible when the tongue is extended and depressed. This wall is highly vascular and may show color variations of red and pink because of the presence of small vessels and lymphoid tissue. The epiglottis, a cartilaginous structure that protects the laryngeal opening, sometimes projects into the pharyngeal area and is visible as the tongue is depressed.

NECK

Structures within the neck include the cervical spine, sternocleidomastoid muscle, hyoid bone, larynx, trachea, esophagus, thyroid gland, lymph nodes, carotid arteries, and jugular veins (Fig. 10-10). The neck is formed by the bones within the upper spine (cervical vertebrae), which are supported by ligaments and the sternocleidomastoid and trapezius muscles. These structures allow for the extensive movement within the neck. The relationship of neck muscles to one another and to adjacent bones creates anatomic landmarks called *triangles* (Fig. 10-11). The medial borders of sternocleidomastoid muscles and the mandible form the anterior triangle. Inside this triangle lie the hyoid bone, thyroid and cricoid cartilage, larynx, trachea, esophagus, and anterior cervical lymph nodes. The hyoid bone is a U-shaped bone at the base of the mandible that anchors the tongue. It is the only bone in the

body that does not articulate with another bone. The posterior triangle is formed by the trapezius and sternocleidomastoid muscles and the clavicle; it contains the posterior cervical lymph nodes.

Larynx

The larynx (also known as the *voice box)* lies just below the pharynx and just above the trachea. The larynx acts as a passageway for air (into the trachea) and allows for vocalization with the vocal cords. The largest component of the larynx is the thyroid cartilage (also known as the *Adam's apple*), located in the anterior portion of the neck (see Fig. 10-10). The thyroid cartilage is a tough, shield-shaped structure with a notch in the center of its upper border that protrudes in the front of the neck, protecting the other structures within the larynx (epiglottis, vocal cords, and upper aspect of the trachea).

Thyroid Gland

The thyroid gland, the largest endocrine gland in the body, produces two hormones, thyroxine (T_4) and triiodothyronine (T_3), which regulate cellular metabolism. Mental and physical growth and development depend on thyroid hormones. The thyroid gland is positioned in the anterior portion of the neck, just below the larynx, situated on the front and sides of the trachea (see Fig. 10-10). The right and left lobes of the thyroid gland are butterfly shaped, joined in the middle by the isthmus. The isthmus lies across the trachea under the cricoid cartilage (the uppermost ring of the tracheal cartilages) and tucks behind the sternocleidomastoid muscle.

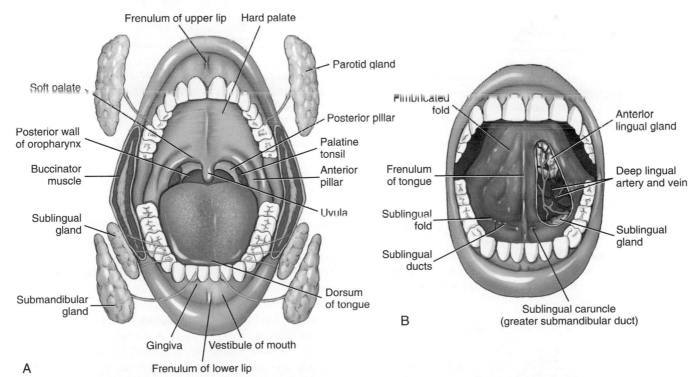

FIG. 10-9 Structures of the mouth. **A,** View of dorsal tongue surface. **B,** View of ventral tongue surface.

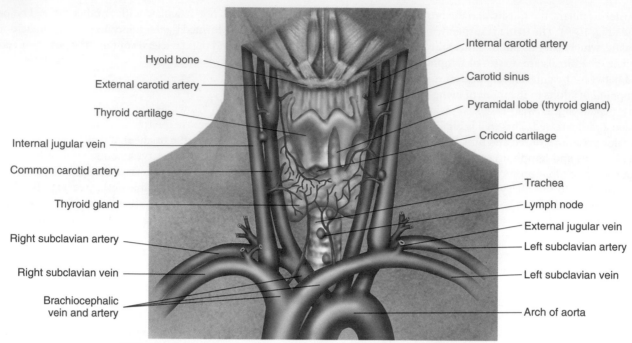

FIG. 10-10 Underlying structures of the neck. (From Seidel et al., 2011.)

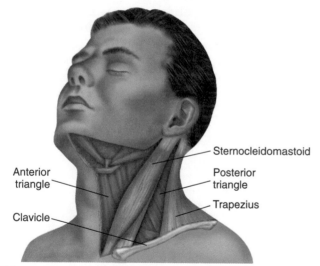

FIG. 10-11 Anterior and posterior triangles of the neck. (From Seidel et al., 2011.)

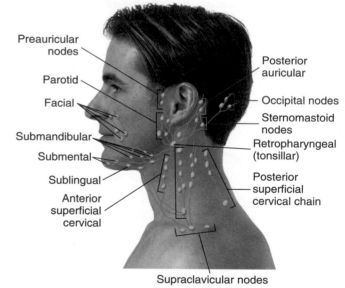

FIG. 10-12 Lymph nodes of the head and neck. (Modified from Seidel et al., 2011.)

Cardiovascular Structures

The carotid arteries and internal jugular veins lie deep and parallel to the anterior aspect of the sternocleidomastoid muscle (see Fig. 10-10). The carotid pulses are palpated along the medial edge of the sternocleidomastoid muscle in the lower third of the neck. See Chapter 12 for further information about these vessels.

LYMPH NODES

Lymph nodes are tiny oval clumps of lymphatic tissue, usually located in groups along blood vessels. Nodes located in subcutaneous connective tissue are called *superficial nodes;* those beneath the fascia of muscles or within various body cavities

are called *deep nodes.* Deep nodes are not accessible to inspection or palpation. However, superficial nodes are accessible and can become enlarged and tender, providing early signs of inflammation.

In the head, lymph nodes are categorized as preauricular, postauricular, occipital, parotid, retropharyngeal (tonsillar), submandibular, submental, and sublingual. In the neck, lymph nodes are found in chains and are named according to their relation to the sternocleidomastoid muscle and the anterior and posterior triangles of neck. Lymph nodes in the neck include the anterior and posterior cervical chains, sternomastoid nodes, and the supraclavicular nodes (Fig. 10-12).

HEALTH HISTORY

Nurses interview patients to collect subjective data about their present health status, past medical history, family history, and personal and psychosocial history, which may affect the health condition of their head, eyes, ears, mouth, and neck. Quality Improvement Competencies for Nurses include providing patient-centered care. See Table 11-1 on p. 196 for examples of competencies.

GENERAL HEALTH HISTORY

Present Health Status

Have you noticed any changes in your overall health or changes to your head, eyes, ears, nose, or mouth?
The patient may have noticed a change but may not consider it a "problem." This question allows you to potentially identify problems.

Do you have any chronic conditions that affect your eyes, ears, nose, mouth, head, or neck regions (e.g., cataracts, glaucoma, migraine headaches, hearing loss, oral cancer, hypothyroidism)? Do you have other chronic conditions (e.g., hypertension, human immunodeficiency virus [HIV] infection, diabetes mellitus, autoimmune disorders)?
Chronic diseases can impact clinical findings. For example, cataracts may impact visual acuity and may be visible on examination. Other chronic illnesses such as hypertension and diabetes mellitus can lead to visual changes; HIV infection and immunodeficiency disorders can lead to mouth lesions. Hypertension is a risk factor for macular degeneration, and autoimmune disorders increase risk for hearing loss.[1]

Do you take any medications? If so, what do you take and how often?
Adverse effects of medications can cause symptoms associated with the head and neck regions. Taking ototoxic medications such as aminoglycosides increases one's risk for hearing loss.[2] Long-term corticosteroid use is a known risk factor for glaucoma and cataracts. Headaches, dizziness, changes in vision, ringing in the ears, and dry mouth are all examples of medication adverse effects.

Past Health History

Have you ever had an injury to your head, eyes, ears, mouth, or neck? If so, describe when and what happened. Do you continue to have any problems related to the injury?
Injuries, either recent or past, may provide information relevant to a patient's clinical findings. Although not common, some individuals have lost an eye as a result of disease or injury and have an eye prosthesis.

Have you had surgery involving your eyes, nose, ears, mouth, or neck? If so, what was the purpose of the surgery?
Knowledge of past surgeries may provide information that may be applied to clinical findings. Teeth extraction and removal of tonsils are common surgical procedures that affect findings within the mouth. Common surgical procedures on the eyes include cataract and surgery for corrective vision. Myringotomy is a common surgical procedure of the ears among children.

In the past have you had a chronic infection affecting your eyes, ears, sinuses, or throat? If so, did it occur during childhood? Adulthood? How was the problem treated?
Establish baseline information for people with a history of chronic infections, even if they don't currently have problems. These data may shed light on other findings.

Family History

Is there a history of cancer in your family? If so, which family member(s)? Which kind of cancer was diagnosed?
The patient could have a genetic predisposition to cancer.

Does anyone in your family have conditions impacting hearing, vision, or thyroid?
Cataracts, glaucoma, presbycusis, Meniere's disease, and hyperthyroidism are examples of conditions that have familial tendencies and may increase a patient's risk.

Personal and Psychosocial History

When were your last routine examinations (dental, vision, hearing)? Do you use any corrective devices (e.g., contact lenses, glasses, hearing aids, dentures)?
These questions help to understand a patient's health promotion practices. Routine dental examinations and examination of the eyes and ears are recommended. The frequency of examinations depends on the patient's age, underlying medical conditions, and use of corrective devices.

Describe some of your daily practices to maintain the health of your eyes, ears, and mouth (e.g., brushing and flossing teeth, cleaning contact lenses, wearing sunglasses).
These questions help understand a patient's health promotion practices and potential risks.

Do you know of any occupational or recreational risks for injury to your eyes, ears, or mouth?
Assessment of environmental risk factors that can contribute to vision or hearing loss is an important component of a health history. Patients should be encouraged to take protective action to minimize injury such as avoiding loud sounds, wearing ear plugs, wearing goggles, and wearing eye and/or mouth protection when engaging in contact sports. Regulatory agencies such as the Occupational Safety and Health Administration[3] have guidelines and regulations to reduce injuries in the work environment.

Do you use nicotine products or drink alcohol? If so, how much and how often?
These questions help understand a patient's potential risks for problems involving the head, eyes, ears, and mouth. Chronic alcohol intake and smoking are risk factors for many

problems, including cataracts, glaucoma, and cancers of the oropharynx.

PROBLEM-BASED HISTORY

The most commonly reported problems related to the head and related structures (eyes, ears, nose, throat, and neck) include headache, dizziness, difficulty with vision, hearing loss, ringing in the ears, earache, nasal discharge, sore throat, and mouth lesions. As with symptoms in all areas of health assessment, a symptom analysis is completed using the mnemonic OLD CARTS, which includes the *Onset, Location, Duration, Characteristics, Aggravating* factors, *Related* symptoms, *Treatment,* and *Severity* (see Box 2-3).

Headache

How long have you been having headaches? How often do you have a headache? How long does it last? Does it follow a pattern?

Many times a headache may be a sign of stress. At other times it may be a sign of chemical imbalance in the body or even of a more serious pathologic condition. Identification of headache patterns may help determine aggravating factors and causes. Cluster headaches occur more than once a day and last for less than an hour to about 2 hours. They may follow this pattern for a couple of months and then disappear for months or years. Migraine headaches may occur at periodic intervals and may last from a few hours to 1 to 3 days.

What is the location of the headaches? Is the pain in one area, or is it generalized? What does it feel like? How severe is it on a scale of 0 to 10?

Sinus headaches may cause tenderness over frontal or maxillary sinuses. Tension headaches tend to be located in the front or back of the head, and migraine and cluster headaches are usually unilateral. Cluster headaches produce pain over the eye, temple, forehead, and cheek. Tension headaches are described as viselike, migraine headaches produce throbbing pain, and cluster headaches cause a burning or stabbing feeling behind one eye.

What other symptoms do you experience with the headaches?

Migraines may be accompanied by visual disturbances, nausea, and vomiting. Cluster headaches may occur with nasal stuffiness or discharge, red teary eyes, or drooping eyelids.

Can you think of any factors that trigger headaches? If so, describe.

Possible triggers include stress, fatigue, exercise, food, and alcohol. Box 10-1 lists foods that trigger headaches for some individuals. Conditions that can precipitate headaches include hypertension, hypothyroidism, and vasculitis. Migraines are frequently associated with menstrual periods.

What do you usually do to treat the headache? If medication, what kind? Is the medication effective in relieving the pain? How often do you take the medication?

BOX 10-1 HEADACHE-TRIGGERING FOODS

- Alcohol: sulfites
- Avocado
- Bacon: nitrites
- Bananas
- Canned figs
- Chicken livers
- Chocolate
- Citrus fruits: lemon, lime, orange, grapefruit
- Herring
- Hot dogs
- Meats, processed: bologna, salami, pepperoni
- Monosodium glutamate (Chinese food)
- Nuts
- Onions
- Sunflower seeds
- Tea and coffee (caffeinated or decaffeinated)
- Yogurt

From Smith L, Schumann L: Differential diagnosis of headache, *J Am Acad Nurse Pract* 10(11):519, 1998.

Knowing what brings relief may help in determining the cause of the headache. Rest can help relieve migraine headaches, whereas movement helps relieve cluster headaches.

Dizziness and Vertigo

Describe the sensation of dizziness that you are experiencing. When did it first begin? How often does it occur? How long does it last?

Ask the patient to define what he or she means when reporting a history of dizziness. Dizziness is a feeling of faintness experienced within the patient. By contrast, vertigo is a sensation that the environment is whirling around external to the patient. The perception of movement distinguishes dizziness from vertigo (Box 10-2). Nearly all patients who self-report a sensation of motion have vertigo.[4]

Does the dizziness interfere with your normal daily activities? Do you experience these symptoms when driving a car or operating machinery? Have you ever fallen as a result of the dizziness?

Knowing the effect on activities of daily living (ADLs) helps determine the extent to which the dizziness is interfering with the patient's life and the frequency of the problem. Assessing the patient's risk of falling during periods of dizziness is important. If the patient describes symptoms consistent with vertigo, he or she should be advised about the potential hazard of driving or operating machinery.

What have you done to treat the dizziness? Has it been effective?

It is important to note any attempts at self-treatment by the patient.

Difficulty with Vision

What type of difficulty are you having with vision? When did it begin? Did it begin suddenly or gradually? Does the problem affect one eye or both? Is it constant, or does it come and go?

The patient's description is essential in determining the cause of the visual difficulty. A sudden onset of visual symptoms may indicate a detached retina and requires an emergency

Dizziness is a symptom used by many patients to describe a wide range of sensations, including faintness or inability to maintain normal balance in a standing or seated position. Based on the description and findings, a generalized symptom of dizziness can be more specifically classified as presyncope, disequilibrium, vertigo, or light-headedness.

Presyncope: Feeling of faintness and impending loss of consciousness—often a cardiovascular symptom.

Disequilibrium: Feeling of falling—often a locomotor problem.

Vertigo: Sensation of movement, usually rotational motion such as whirling or spinning. Subjective vertigo is the sensation that one's body is rotating in space; objective vertigo is the sensation that objects are spinning around the body. Vertigo is the cardinal symptom of vestibular dysfunction.

Light-headedness: Vague description of dizziness that does not fit any of the other classifications—usually idiopathic or psychogenic.

referral. Involvement of both eyes tends to indicate a systemic problem, whereas involvement of one eye is a local problem.

What other symptoms are you experiencing?
Headaches, dizziness, and nausea are symptoms commonly associated with visual difficulty.

What makes your vision worse? What makes it better? What treatment have you tried for the vision difficulty? How effective was the treatment?
Knowing what makes the vision problem worse may help identify its cause. Determining which therapies have been used successfully or unsuccessfully helps in understanding the problem and guiding current treatment strategies.

Has your vision problem interfered with your daily life? If so, describe how.
Determine the impact that this visual difficulty has had on the patient's quality of life and evaluate the adjustments the patient has made to lifestyle and routines.

Hearing Loss

How long have you had trouble hearing? What tones or sounds are difficult for you to hear?
Establish onset of the problem (sudden or gradual over time). A sudden hearing loss in one or both ears that is not associated with an ear infection or upper respiratory infection requires further evaluation. Hearing loss associated with aging (presbycusis) occurs gradually and increases with advancing age, particularly with high frequencies.

Have you noticed other symptoms associated with the hearing loss?
Explore other symptoms such as fevers, headaches, or visual changes.

To what degree does your hearing loss bother you? Does it interfere with your daily routine or create problems on the job or social interactions?
Hearing loss may cause individuals to withdraw or become isolated because they cannot hear or they are embarrassed. This may lead to reduced interpersonal communication, depression, and exacerbation of coexisting psychiatric conditions.

Ringing in the Ears (Tinnitus)

Describe the noise that you are hearing. Is it ringing, hissing, crackling, or buzzing? When did it first begin?
Ringing of the ears (tinnitus) is a sensation or sound heard only by the affected individual. It can manifest differently with a variety of sounds or sensations.[5]

Does the sound occur all of the time, or does it come and go? If it comes and goes, does it occur with certain activities or at the same time of day?
Establish the pattern of the symptom; this may provide clues to determine the cause of the problem.

Earache

How long have you had an earache? Do you know what might be causing the pain?
Determine the onset of pain. Ear pain can be related to an infection in the mouth, sinuses, or throat.

Describe the location of the pain. Is it constant, or does it come and go? If it comes and goes, how often does it occur, and how long does it last?
Determine the location of the pain. Ear pain can be unilateral or bilateral; it can be internal or external. Also determine the duration of the pain. If it is intermittent, explore possible triggering mechanisms.

What does the pain feel like? On a scale of 0 to 10, how would you rate the severity of your ear pain? Does it hurt when you pull on or touch your ear? Does the pain change when you change your position (e.g., when you lie down)?
Description of the pain may help determine the cause. Pain caused by an ear infection involving the external ear or ear canal increases with movement of the ear; pain caused by otitis media does not change with manipulation of the ear.

Is there any discharge from the ear? If so, what does it look like? Does it have an odor?
A description of ear discharge might help determine the cause of the symptoms.

Nasal Discharge/Nose Bleed

When did the nasal discharge/nose bleed begin? How would you describe the discharge (color, consistency, odor)? Is it on one side of your nose or both?
A thick or purulent green-yellow, malodorous discharge usually results from a bacterial infection. A foul-smelling discharge, especially unilateral discharge, is associated with a foreign body or chronic sinusitis. Profuse watery discharge is

typically seen with allergies. Bloody discharge may result from a neoplasm, trauma, or an opportunistic infection such as a fungal disease. A nose bleed (epistaxis) may occur secondary to trauma, chronic sinusitis, malignancy, or a bleeding disorder; it may also result from cocaine abuse.

What other symptoms do you have?
Associated symptoms consistent with allergic rhinitis include itching, swelling, discharge from the eyes, postnasal drip, and cough.[6] Fatigue, fever, and pain may be associated symptoms for individuals with infections.

What do you do to treat the discharge/bleeding? How effective is the treatment?
Determining what has been used successfully in the past may guide current treatment strategies and provide an opportunity for teaching. If the patient uses nasal spray other than normal saline, alert him or her that it should be used for only 3 to 5 days to avoid causing rebound congestion.

Sore Throat

How long have you had a sore throat? Describe what it feels like (e.g., a lump, burning, scratchy). Does it hurt to swallow? Is your sore throat associated with fever, cough, fatigue, painful lymph nodes?
A sore throat may have many causes, from nasal congestion or sinus drainage to an infection or allergy. Often edema and pain associated with throat infections make it difficult to swallow. Common associated symptoms include fever, fatigue, and pain when swallowing. Nasal congestion that requires mouth breathing during the night may cause a sore throat in the morning.

Are others in your home ill or have they just recovered from a sore throat or cold? Do you inhale dust or fumes at work? Is the air in your home or office dry?
These questions explore possible environmental factors that contribute to sore throat and whether the sore throat may be communicable.

How have you been treating your sore throat? How effective was the treatment?
Determining what has been used successfully in the past may guide current treatment strategies.

Mouth Lesions

Where is the mouth sore? How long has the soreness been present?
Mouth lesions can be caused by many things, including trauma, infection, nutritional deficits, immunologic problem, or cancer.

Which other symptoms have you noticed? Does the sore bother you when eating or talking?
Bleeding, lumps, and thickened areas in the mouth are possible symptoms of oral cancer. Enlarged lymph nodes might be associated with cancer or an infection. Painful ulcerations may impair adequate nutritional intake.

Are there sores anywhere else on your body such as in the vagina? In the urethra? On the penis? In the anus?
Sexually transmitted diseases such as herpes may be transmitted through oral sex.

HEALTH PROMOTION FOR EVIDENCE-BASED PRACTICE
Hearing

An estimated 28 million people in the United States have a hearing impairment. These impairments are caused by a number of factors, including genetics (congenital), exposure to excessive noise (noise-induced hearing loss), trauma, infections (especially otitis media), and certain drugs. Hearing is a necessary component for child development; therefore identification of hearing impairment at an early age is critical. Newborn hearing screening is required by law in many states.

Goals and Objectives—*Healthy People 2020*
The *Healthy People 2020* goal for hearing is to reduce the prevalence and severity of disorders of hearing and balance; smell and taste; and voice, speech, and language. Specific objectives include increasing the number of newborns screened for hearing loss by 1 month of age with appropriate follow-up care (if loss is identified, perform audiologic evaluation by age 3 months and enroll in appropriate intervention services by age 6 months); reducing the incidence of otitis media in children and adolescents; reducing adult hearing loss through enhanced prevention efforts; increasing screening for hearing loss; and increasing the proportion of people with hearing impairments who have hearing assistance.

Recommendations to Reduce Risk (Primary Prevention)
American Speech-Language Hearing Association (ASLHA)
- Wear hearing protection when exposed to loud or potentially damaging noise at work, in the community, or at home.
- Limit periods of exposure to noise.
- Reduce volume when using stereo headsets or listening to amplified music in a confined place such as a car.
- Be aware of and minimize noise in personal environment. Consider noise rating when purchasing recreational equipment, children's toys, household appliances, and power tools; look for those items with lower noise ratings.

Screening Recommendations (Secondary Prevention)
The U.S. Preventive Services Task Force (USPSTF) and the Centers for Disease Control and Prevention recommend screening for hearing loss in all newborn infants. If loss is identified, perform audiologic evaluation by age 3 months and enroll in appropriate intervention services by age 6 months as needed. Screen adults every decade between ages 18 and 50; monitor more frequently after age 50 years.

From American Speech-Language-Hearing Association website, available at www.asha.org; Centers for Disease Control and Prevention: *Hearing detection and intervention program,* available at www.cdc.gov; US Department of Health and Human Services: *Vision and hearing.* In *Healthy People 2020,* available at http://www.healthypeople.gov/2020/.

EXAMINATION

ROUTINE TECHNIQUES	SPECIAL CIRCUMSTANCES OR ADVANCED PRACTICE

Head
- INSPECT the head.
- INSPECT the facial structures.

Eyes
- TEST visual acuity.
- INSPECT the external ocular structures:
  - Eyebrows, eyelids, eyelashes
  - Conjunctiva
- INSPECT the eyes.
- INSPECT the corneal light reflex.
- INSPECT the sclera.
- INSPECT the cornea transparency and surface characteristics.
- INSPECT the iris.
- INSPECT the pupils.

Ears
- ASSESS hearing based on response from conversation.
- INSPECT the external ears.
- INSPECT the external auditory meatus.

Nose
- INSPECT the nose.

Mouth
- INSPECT the lips.
- INSPECT the teeth and gums.
- INSPECT the tongue.
- INSPECT the buccal mucosa and anterior and posterior pillars.
- INSPECT the palate, uvula, posterior pharynx, and tonsils.

Neck
- INSPECT the neck:
  - Appearance
  - Position
  - Skin characteristics

Head
- PALPATE structures of the skull.
- PALPATE the bony structures of the face and jaw.
- PALPATE the temporal arteries.

Eyes
- ASSESS the visual fields for peripheral vision.
- ASSESS eye movement:
  - Six cardinal fields of gaze
  - Cover-uncover test
- PALPATE the eye, eyelids, and lacrimal puncta.
- TEST the corneal reflex.
- INSPECT the anterior chamber.
- INSPECT intraocular structures: ★
  - Red reflex
  - Optic disc
  - Retinal vessels
  - Retinal background
  - Macula

Ears
- PALPATE the external ears and mastoid areas.
- INSPECT the internal ear structures: ★
  - External ear canal
  - Tympanic membrane
- TEST auditory function.

Nose
- PALPATE the nose.
- INSPECT the internal nasal cavity.
- PALPATE the paranasal sinuses.
- TRANSILLUMINATE the sinuses. ★

Mouth
- PALPATE the teeth, inner lips, and gums.
- PALPATE the tongue.

Neck
- INSPECT the neck:
  - Range of motion
- PALPATE the neck:
  - Anatomic structures
  - Tenderness
  - Muscle strength
  - Thyroid gland ★

Lymph Nodes
- PALPATE regional lymph nodes.

EQUIPMENT NEEDED

Ophthalmoscope • Otoscope • Stethoscope • Penlight • Snellen chart or Snellen "E" chart • Handheld vision screener (Rosenbaum or Jaeger) • Cover card (opaque) • Tuning fork • Audioscope • Nasal speculum • Examination gloves • Tongue blade • 4 × 4 gauze

★ Advanced practice.

| PROCEDURES AND TECHNIQUES WITH EXPECTED FINDINGS | ABNORMAL FINDINGS |

ROUTINE TECHNIQUES: HEAD

CLEAN hands.

INSPECT the head for size, shape, skin characteristics.

Look at the head in relation to the neck and shoulders for size and shape. *Normocephalic* is the term designating that the skull is symmetric and appropriately proportioned for the size of the body. The head should be held upright in a straight position. To inspect the scalp, part the hair in various locations. The scalp should be intact, without lesions, redness, or flakes.

Microcephaly is an abnormally small head. *Macrocephaly* is an abnormally large head.
    Lice may be noticed in the scalp. Refer to Fig. 9-43.

INSPECT the facial structures for size, symmetry, movement, skin characteristics, and facial expression.

The facial features (eyes and eyebrows, palpebral fissures, nasolabial folds, and sides of the mouth) should appear symmetric with a calm facial expression (Fig. 10-13). Facial bones should be symmetric and appear proportional to the size of the head.

Note abnormal skin color, uneven skin pigmentation, skin lesions, coarse facial hair (in women), asymmetry, edema, or abnormal facial movements (tics) (Fig. 10-14).

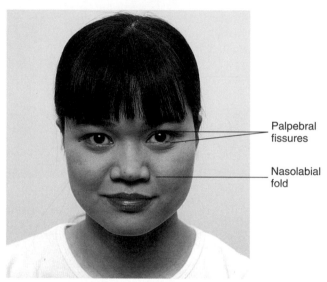

Palpebral fissures

Nasolabial fold

FIG. 10-13 Symmetry of facial features (eyebrows, palpebral fissures, nasolabial folds, and corners of the mouth) is a normal finding.

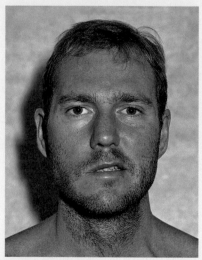

FIG. 10-14 Right facial palsy causing asymmetry of facial features. (From Swartz, 2010.)

SPECIAL CIRCUMSTANCES OR ADVANCED PRACTICE: HEAD

PALPATE the structures of the skull for contour, tenderness, and intactness.

Palpation of the skull is done when there is a suspected injury, observed irregularity or abnormality, or reported pain. Palpate the skull from front to back using a gentle rotary motion. The skull should be symmetric and feel firm without tenderness. The frontal, parietal, and bilateral occipital prominences may be felt. Examination gloves should be worn if the patient has scalp lesions, injury, or poor hygiene.

Lumps, marked protrusions, or tenderness should be differentiated to determine if they are on the scalp or actually part of the skull. Depressions or unevenness of the skull may occur secondary to skull injury.

PROCEDURES AND TECHNIQUES WITH EXPECTED FINDINGS	ABNORMAL FINDINGS

PALPATE the bony structures of the face and jaw, noting tenderness and jaw movement.

Palpation of the face and jaw is done when there is suspected injury, observed irregularity, or a reported problem such as pain or jaw clicking. To palpate jaw movement, place two fingers in front of each ear and ask the patient to slowly open and close the mouth and move the lower jaw from side to side. The jaw should move smoothly and without pain (Fig. 10-15).

Pain associated with palpation of facial structures should be explored further. Limited movement, pain with movement, and a jaw that clicks or catches with movement may indicate temporomandibular joint disease.[7]

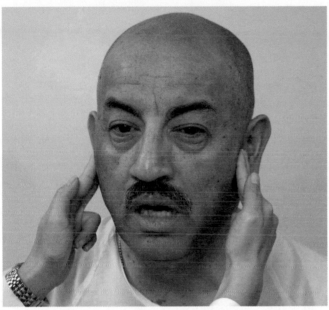

FIG. 10-15 Position fingers in front of each ear to palpate the temporomandibular joint.

PALPATE the temporal arteries for pulsation, texture, and tenderness.

Temporal arteries are examined further if the patient reports headache/pain in the temporal area. Using your fingertips, palpate over the temporal bone on each side of the head lateral to each eyebrow for the temporal artery. See Figs. 12-11 and 12-12 for finger placement. The artery should be smooth and nontender, with pulsation noted. If indicated, use the bell of your stethoscope to auscultate the temporal arteries. An expected finding is that no sound is auscultated.

Tender, edematous, or hardened temporal arteries with redness over the temporal region suggest temporal arteritis. A bruit (a low-pitched blowing sound) heard during auscultation indicates a vascular abnormality.

ROUTINE TECHNIQUES: EYES

TEST visual acuity (distance vision) (tests cranial nerve II).

Procedure: Place Snellen chart on the wall in a well-lighted room. The patient may sit or stand 20 feet (6 m) from the chart. If the patient wears contact lenses or glasses, he or she should leave them in place.

- Have the patient cover one eye with an opaque card and read the line of smallest letters that is possible to read. Test the other eye and then test both eyes using the same procedure.
- Document the line read completely by the patient, using the fraction printed at the end of the line; also indicate if the patient was wearing glasses or contacts.
- Next, to assess perception ask the patient to use both eyes to distinguish which of the two horizontal lines is longer. Finally ask the patient to name the colors of the two horizontal lines to document red and green color perception.

NOTE: Use the "E" chart for patients who cannot read letters. This can be a very sensitive area for adults who do not know how to read. The patient is asked to indicate the direction in which the "E" points (see Fig. 3-13, *B*).

PROCEDURES AND TECHNIQUES WITH EXPECTED FINDINGS	ABNORMAL FINDINGS

Findings: The reading pattern should be smooth. The expected finding is 20/20. A finding of 20/30 means that the patient can read at 20 feet what a person with normal vision can read at 30 feet. If the patient can read all the letters in the 20/30 line and two letters in the 20/20 line, document the finding. as 20/30 + 2.

Note any hesitancy, squinting, leaning forward, blinking, or facial expressions indicating that the patient is struggling to see. The larger the denominator, the poorer the vision. If vision is poorer than 20/30 or if patient is unable to distinguish colors or line length, refer him or her to an ophthalmologist or optometrist. A person is considered legally blind when the best corrected visual acuity is 20/200.

TEST visual acuity (near vision).

Assess near vision for people over 40 years of age or for those who think that they have difficulty reading. Ask the patient to cover one eye, hold a Jaeger or Rosenbaum card or a newspaper about 14 inches from the eyes, and read the smallest line possible (see Fig. 3-14). Repeat the assessment, covering the other eye. Document the line read completely using the fraction at the end of the line. The findings are the same as those for the Snellen chart.

With age there is a loss of elasticity of the lens of the eye; this finding is termed *presbyopia*. As a result, the patient needs to move the Jaeger or Rosenbaum card farther away to see it clearly.

ASSESS visual fields for peripheral vision (confrontation test).

Procedure: Face the patient, standing or sitting at a distance of 2 to 3 feet (60 to 90 cm). Ask the patient to cover one eye with an opaque card and look directly at you as you cover your own eye directly opposite the patient's covered eye.

- Hold a pencil or use your finger and extend it to the farthest periphery and gradually bring the object close to the midline (equal distance between you and the patient). Ask the patient to report when he or she first sees the object; you should see the object at the same time.
- Slowly move the object inward from the periphery in four directions. Move your fingers anteriorly (from above the head down into field of vision), inferiorly (from upper chest up toward field of vision), temporally (move in laterally from behind the patient's ear into field of vision), and nasally (move medially into field of vision) (Fig. 10-16).
- Estimate the angle between the anteroposterior axis of the eye and the peripheral axis when the pencil or finger is first seen.

(NOTE: This test assumes that the nurse has normal peripheral visual fields.)

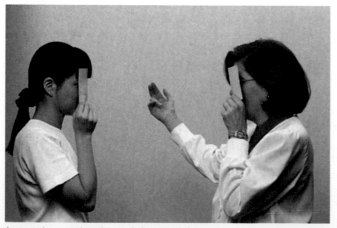

FIG. 10-16 Assessing patient's peripheral vision nasally by moving object medially into field of vision.

PROCEDURES AND TECHNIQUES WITH EXPECTED FINDINGS

Findings: Normal values are 50 degrees anteriorly, 70 degrees inferiorly, 90 degrees temporally, and 60 degrees nasally. The temporal value is greater than the nasal value because of the position of the opaque card covering one of the eyes.

INSPECT the eyebrows, eyelashes, and eyelids for symmetry, skin characteristics, and discharge.

Skin should be intact, and eyebrows symmetric. Note whether the eyebrow extends over the eye. Eyelashes should be distributed equally and curled slightly outward. Palpebral fissures (the opening between eyelids) should be equal bilaterally. The color of the eyelids should correspond to skin color. The eyelid margins should be pale pink and fit flush against the eyeball surfaces; the upper lid should cover part of the iris but not the pupil; the lower lid generally covers to just below the limbus (see Fig. 10-13). Lid closure should be complete, with smooth, easy motion. Blinking is typically frequent and bilateral with involuntary movements, averaging 15 to 20 blinks per minute. No drainage or discharge should be present.

🌐 **ETHNIC, CULTURAL, AND SPIRITUAL VARIATIONS**

Palbebral Fissures

> The palpebral fissures are horizontal in non-Asians, whereas Asians normally have an upward slant to the palpebral fissures (see Fig. 10-13).

🌐 **ETHNIC, CULTURAL, AND SPIRITUAL VARIATIONS**

Eyes

> In Caucasian patients the eyeball does not protrude beyond the supraorbital ridge of the frontal bone. In African American patients it may protrude slightly beyond the supraorbital ridge.

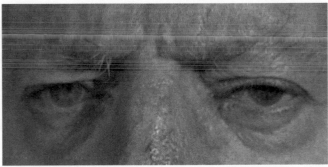

FIG. 10-17 Ptosis. Patient with ptosis to left eye. Note that lid is covering a portion of the pupil. (Courtesy Lemmi and Lemmi, 2013.)

ABNORMAL FINDINGS

If the patient cannot see the pencil or finger at the same time that you see it, peripheral field loss is suspected. Refer the patient to an eye care specialist for more precise testing.

Flakiness, loss of eyebrows or lashes, scaling, and unequal alignment of movement are abnormal as are asymmetrical palpebral fissures. The lid of either eye covering part of the pupil is known as *ptosis* (Fig. 10-17). Sclera is visible between the upper lid and iris in hyperthyroid exophthalmos (Fig. 10-18). Closure of the lid that is incomplete or accomplished only with pain or difficulty may occur with infections. Edema of the lid may occur with trauma or infection. The presence of lesions, nodules, erythema, flaking, crusting, excessive tearing, or discharge should be documented. Note inward deformity of the lid and lashes. This is a finding seen in enophthalmos (Fig. 10-19).

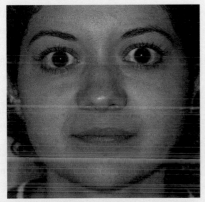

FIG. 10-18 Exophthalmos. (Courtesy Lemmi and Lemmi, 2013.)

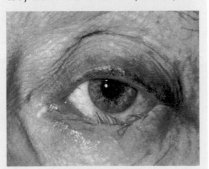

FIG. 10-19 Enophthalmos. The eyelid and lashes are rolled in. (From Bedford, 1986.)

PROCEDURES AND TECHNIQUES WITH EXPECTED FINDINGS	ABNORMAL FINDINGS

INSPECT the conjunctiva for color, drainage, and lesions.

Procedure: Don examination gloves. Ask the patient to look up. Gently separate the lids widely with the thumb and index finger, exerting pressure over the bony orbit surrounding the eye. Have the patient look up, down, and to each side. Next pull down and evert the lower lid; ask the patient to look up (Fig. 10-20).

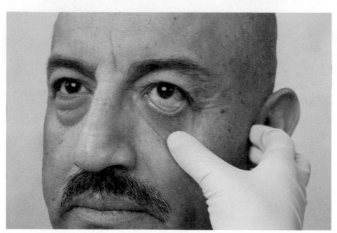

FIG. 10-20 To inspect the palpebral conjunctiva, gently pull down and evert the lower eyelid.

Occasionally eversion of the upper eyelid is necessary when you must inspect the conjunctiva of the upper lid (such as when patients complain of eye pain or a foreign body is suspected). Wearing gloves, gently grasp the upper eyelashes and pull downward gently while the patient is looking down with the eyes slightly open. Place a cotton-tipped applicator stick about 1 cm above the upper lid margin and push gently down with the applicator while still holding the lashes to evert the lid (Fig. 10-21, *A*). Hold the lashes of the everted lid against the upper ridge of the bony orbit, just below the eyebrow, and examine the lid (Fig. 10-21, *B*). Return the lid to its normal position by moving the lashes slightly forward and asking the patient to look up and then blink.

Red conjunctiva, particularly with purulent drainage, may indicate conjunctivitis (see Fig. 10-60). A sharply defined area of blood adjacent to normal-appearing conjunctiva may indicate subconjunctival hemorrhage. Lesions, nodules, and foreign bodies are abnormal findings.

Findings: The bulbar conjunctiva should be pink and clear; tiny red vessels are often noted.

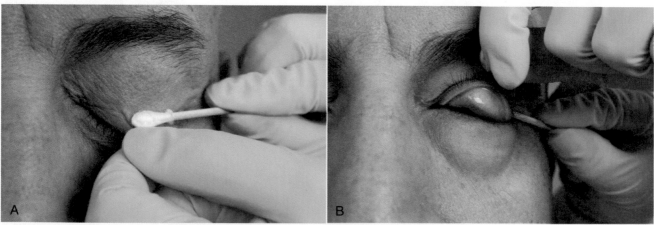

FIG. 10-21 Everting upper eyelid.

PROCEDURES AND TECHNIQUES WITH EXPECTED FINDINGS	ABNORMAL FINDINGS

INSPECT the corneal light reflex for symmetry (Hirschberg's test).

Ask the patient to stare straight ahead with both eyes open. Shine a penlight toward the bridge of the nose at a distance of 12 to 15 inches (30 to 38 cm). Light reflections should appear symmetrically in both corneas (Fig. 10-22). *Note: When an imbalance is found in the corneal light reflex, perform the cover-uncover test (discussed in following sections).*

If light reflections appear at different spots in each eye (asymmetrically), it may indicate weak extraocular muscles.

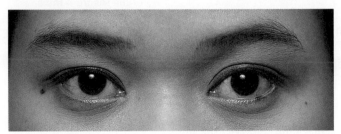

FIG. 10-22 Normal position of eyes and eyelids. The symmetric light reflection in both corneas is a normal finding.

INSPECT the sclera for color and surface characteristics.

Sclera should be white and clear, although slight yellowing may be seen in darkly pigmented individuals.

Yellow sclera may indicate jaundice caused by liver disease or obstruction of the common bile duct. Redness within the sclera suggests inflammation or hemorrhage (Fig. 10-23). A blue tone to the sclera may be caused by osteogenesis imperfecta.

🌐 ETHNIC, CULTURAL, AND SPIRITUAL VARIATIONS
Sclera

The sclera appears white except in darker-skinned patients, in whom it is normally a darker shade. Tiny black dots of pigmentation may be present near the limbus in dark-skinned individuals. In light-skinned individuals there may be a slight yellow cast.

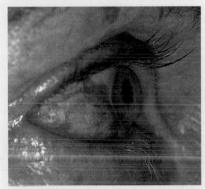

FIG. 10-23 Subconjunctival hemorrhage. Note red patch with sharp edge of demarcation. (Courtesy Lemmi and Lemmi, 2013.)

INSPECT the cornea for transparency and surface characteristics.

Use oblique lighting and slowly move the light reflection over the corneal surface. Observe for transparent quality and a smooth surface that is clear and shiny.

Note opacities, irregularities in light reflections, lesions, abrasions, or foreign bodies. Especially note a white, opaque ring encircling the limbus, termed *corneal arcus,* seen in many patients over 60 years old and individuals with hyperlipidemia.

INSPECT the iris for shape and color.

The iris should be round with consistent coloration. Some people may have a normal variation in color in which each iris is a different color. This is caused by genetic factors.

Patients who have had an iridectomy or iridotomy to correct glaucoma have a section of the iris missing. Coloboma is a congenital defect of the iris. Blunt trauma to the eye can cause an iridodialysis, a circumferential tearing of the iris from the sclera.

INSPECT the pupils for size, shape, reaction to light, accommodation, and consensual reaction.

Procedure: To determine the pupil size, use a pupil gauge like the one found at the bottom of a Rosenbaum pocket vision screener (see Fig. 3-14). To assess reaction to light and consensual reaction, dim the room lights if possible. Ask the patient to hold the eyes open and fix his or her gaze on an object across the room. Approach with a penlight beam from the side and shine it directly on the pupil. Observe the pupil receiving the light for the direct reaction and the other pupil for the consensual reaction. Repeat with the other eye. To test accommodation, ask the patient to fix his or her gaze on a distant object across the room. Then ask the patient to shift his or her gaze to your finger, placed about 6 inches from the patient's nose.

Findings: The pupil diameter is normally between 2 and 6 mm. Pupils should be round and equal in size. The illuminated pupil should constrict (direct response); the other pupil should constrict simultaneously (consensual response). The pupils should dilate when visualizing a distant object and constrict when focusing on a near object. Box 10-3 provides tips used to document expected findings of pupils.

Pupillary abnormalities are described in Table 10-1. Failure of either one or both eyes to constrict to light in speed or magnitude indicates dysfunction of the oculomotor nerve (cranial nerve III). *Mydriasis* is pupil size greater than 6 mm that fails to constrict. *Miosis* is constriction to less than 2 mm. Unequal pupils may be normal, but the inequality may occur as a result of past eye surgery, trauma, or congenital anomalies.

BOX 10-3 **DOCUMENTATION TIPS FOR EYES**	
PERRLA *P*upils are *E*qual and *R*ound and *R*eact to *L*ight and *A*ccommodation.	**Remembering Cs and Ds for Expected Findings for Accommodation** Pupils *C*onstrict when focusing on a *C*lose object Pupils *D*ilate when focusing on a *D*istant object Even the name helps you remember the expected findings. The *C* in a*C*commodation is close to the beginning of the word, whereas the *D* in accommo*D*ation is distant from the beginning of the word.

SPECIAL CIRCUMSTANCES OR ADVANCED PRACTICE: EYE

ASSESS eye movement for the six cardinal fields of gaze (tests cranial nerves III, IV, and VI).

This procedure is done as part of a neurologic exam or when the corneal light reflex is not symmetric.

Procedure: While the patient is looking at you, position your finger 10 to 12 inches (25 to 30 cm) from the patient's nose. Ask the patient to keep the head still and use the eyes only to follow your finger or an object in your hand (Fig. 10-24).

- Move the object from its center position to upper outer extreme, hold there, move back to center, to lower inner extreme, and hold there.
- Move the object to temporal-nasal extremes, holding there momentarily. Move the object to opposite upper outer extreme and back to opposite lower inner extreme.

TABLE 10-1 PUPIL ABNORMALITIES

ABNORMALITY	CONTRIBUTING FACTORS	APPEARANCE
Miosis (pupillary constriction; usually less than 2 mm in diameter)	Miotic eyedrops such as pilocarpine given for glaucoma	
Mydriasis (pupillary dilation; usually more than 6 mm in diameter)	Mydriatic or cycloplegic drops such as atropine; midbrain (reflex arc) lesions or hypoxia; oculomotor (cranial nerve III) damage; acute-angle glaucoma (slight dilation)	
Oval pupil	Sometimes occurs with head injury or intracranial hemorrhage; transitional stage between normal pupil and dilated, fixed pupil with increased intracranial pressure (ICP); in most instances returns to normal when ICP is returned to normal	
Anisocoria (unequal size of pupils)	Congenital (approximately 20% of normal people have minor or noticeable differences in pupil size, but reflexes are normal) or caused by local eye medications (constrictors or dilators), amblyopia, or unilateral sympathetic or parasympathetic pupillary pathway destruction (NOTE: Nurse should test whether pupils react equally to light; if response is unequal, nurse should note whether larger or smaller pupil reacts more slowly [or not at all], since either pupil could be abnormal size)	
Iridectomy	Surgical excision of portion of iris usually done in superior area so upper lid covers additional exposure	

From Thompson JM et al: *Mosby's clinical nursing*, ed 5, St Louis, 2002, Mosby.

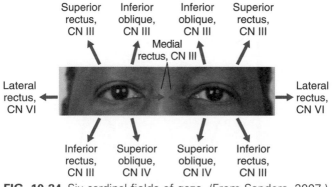

FIG. 10-24 Six cardinal fields of gaze. (From Sanders, 2007.)

PROCEDURES AND TECHNIQUES WITH EXPECTED FINDINGS

An alternative method is to move your finger slowly in a circle to each of the six directions. Stop in each position so the patient can hold the gaze briefly before moving to the next position.

Findings: Normally there will be parallel tracking of the object with both eyes. Mild nystagmus at extreme lateral gaze is also normal.

PERFORM the cover-uncover eye test.

Perform this test if the corneal light reflex is asymmetric.

Procedure: Ask the patient to stare straight ahead at your nose.

- Cover one of the patient's eyes with the opaque card. Observe the uncovered eye. **Findings:** No deviation or movement from a steady, fixed gaze (Fig. 10-25, *A*).
- Remove the card from the covered eye; observe if this eye moves to try to focus. **Findings:** The eye should not move (Fig. 10-25, *B* and *C*).
- Repeat steps with the other eye.

ABNORMAL FINDINGS

Nystagmus is involuntary movement of the eyeball in a horizontal, vertical, rotary, or mixed direction. It may be congenital or acquired (from multiple causes).

If the uncovered eye moves to focus, it is the weaker eye, and strabismus is present (see Fig. 10-61). An eye that moves to focus after being uncovered indicates strabismus.

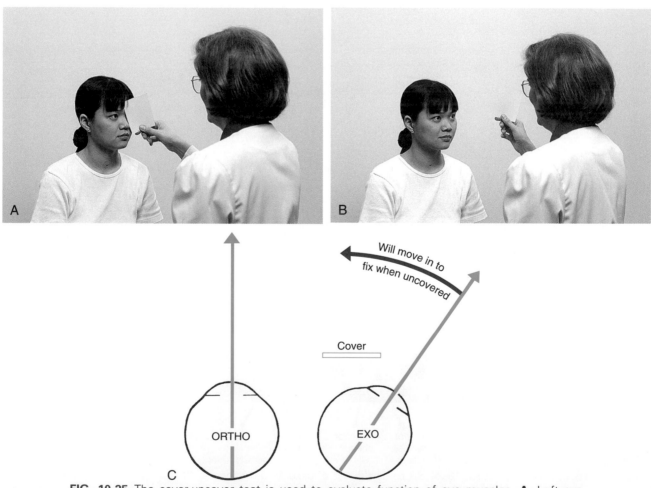

FIG. 10-25 The cover-uncover test is used to evaluate function of eye muscles. **A,** Left eye covered; observe right eye. **B,** Left eye uncovered; observe it for movement. **C,** Exophoria; the right eye shifted from right to center when the eye was uncovered. (**C** from Prior, Silberstein, and Stang, 1981.)

PROCEDURES AND TECHNIQUES WITH EXPECTED FINDINGS	**ABNORMAL FINDINGS**

PALPATE the eye, eyelids, and lacrimal puncta.

This procedure is done when inflammation is observed or pain is reported.

Procedure and Findings: Ask the patient to look down with lids closed so you will not palpate the cornea. Gently palpate the eyeball; it should indent with slight pressure. Palpate the lower orbital rim near the inner canthus. This pressure slightly everts the lower lid. Puncta are seen as small elevations on the nasal side of the upper and lower lid margins. Mucosa should be pink and intact despite pressure. Eyes should be moist, without excessive tears. Gently palpate the upper and lower lids for tenderness or nodules; there should be no pain.

An eyeball that is very firm and resists palpation may occur in glaucoma. Lacrimal puncta that are clogged with mucus or dirt cause inflammation (dacryocystitis). Fluid or purulent material may be discharged from the puncta in response to pressure. Excessive tearing (epiphora) may be caused by blockage of the nasolacrimal duct. Tenderness, nodules, or irregularities to the lids indicate a problem.

TEST the corneal reflex.

Test the corneal reflex *only* in selected cases such as unconscious patients.

Procedure and Findings: Lightly touch the cornea with cotton. The lids of both eyes blink when either cornea is touched. This reflex tests the sensory reception of the ophthalmic branch of the trigeminal nerve (cranial nerve V) and the motor branch of the facial nerve (cranial nerve VII), which creates a blink.

Edema of the brainstem might impair the function of cranial nerves V and VII and may occur after head injury or with cerebral hemorrhage or tumor.

INSPECT the anterior chamber for transparency, iris surface, and chamber depth.

Assessment of transparency for opacities is observed on the cornea. Chamber depth is assessed in patients with a risk for acute angle glaucoma.

Procedure: Using a penlight or an ophthalmoscope, shine light from the side across the iris.
Findings: Anterior chamber is transparent, iris is flat, and chamber depth is noted (Fig. 10-26).

Cloudiness, visible material, or blood should be noted. The iris should not bulge toward the cornea, and the chamber should not be shallow. Also note iris or pupil shapes other than round, inconsistent iris coloration, and unequal pupil sizes.

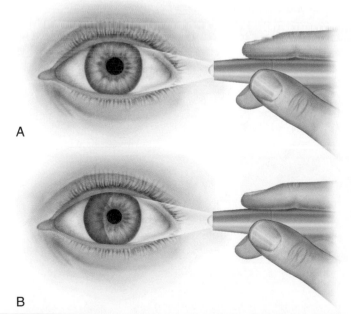

A

B

FIG. 10-26 Evaluation of depth of anterior chambers. **A,** Normal anterior chamber. **B,** Shallow anterior chamber. (From Seidel et al., 2011.)

PROCEDURES AND TECHNIQUES WITH EXPECTED FINDINGS	ABNORMAL FINDINGS

★ INSPECT intraocular structures (ophthalmoscopic examination).

This is an advanced skill and is indicated to assess for the presence of many eye conditions such as cataracts, macular degeneration, and retinopathy.

Procedure: Darken the room to help dilate the patient's pupils. Have the patient remove glasses; contact lenses may be left in. You may leave your glasses or contact lenses in place. Turn on the ophthalmoscope light and set the diopter wheel to 0.

To examine the patient's right eye, hold the ophthalmoscope in your right hand and use your right eye. To examine the patient's left eye, hold the ophthalmoscope in your left hand and use your left eye. Place your index finger on the diopter wheel so you can change the focus as needed to visualize the internal structures. Red numbers (minus) compensate for myopia (nearsighted), and black numbers (positive) compensate for hyperopia (farsighted). With the ophthalmoscope against your eye, your field of vision is reduced. To help orient yourself, place your free hand on the patient's shoulder or forehead.

Direct the patient to continuously gaze at a point across the room and slightly above your shoulder. Begin about 10 inches (25 mm) from patient's eye at a 15-degree angle lateral to his or her line of vision. Shine the light of the ophthalmoscope on the pupil while looking through the viewing lens. If you lose sight of the red reflex, you have moved the light away from the pupil. Reposition the light.

INSPECT for a red reflex.

Procedure and Findings: The red reflex is a red or orange glow over the patient's pupil created by light illuminating the retina. Keep the red reflex in sight and move closer to the eye, adjusting the lens with the diopter wheel as needed to focus; there should be no interruption in the red reflex. Absence of the red reflex may be caused by movement of the light away from the pupil; correct by repositioning the light.

Decreased or irregular red reflex, dark spots, and opacities should be noted. Dark shadows or black dots may indicate opacities that occur with cataracts or may be caused by hemorrhage in the vitreous humor.

INSPECT the optic disc for discrete margin, shape, size, color, and physiologic cup.

Procedure: After seeing the red reflex, continue to move closer until you nearly touch foreheads with the patient (Fig. 10-27). Focus varies, depending on the refractive state of both the nurse and the patient; adjust your focus with the diopter wheel. When you locate a blood vessel, follow it inward toward the nose until you see the optic disc.

Cataracts prevent inspection of the optic disc because the light cannot penetrate the opacity of the lens.

★ Advanced practice.

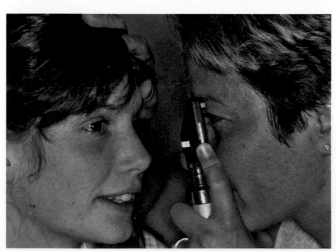

FIG. 10-27 Move close to the patient until you nearly touch foreheads. Adjust focus with the diopter dial. (Courtesy Lemmi and Lemmi, 2013.)

| **PROCEDURES AND TECHNIQUES WITH EXPECTED FINDINGS** | **ABNORMAL FINDINGS** |

Findings: The margin of the disc should be regular and have a distinct, sharp outline. Scattered or dense pigment deposits may be seen at the border. A gray crescent may appear at the temporal border.

Blurred margin may indicate papilledema, which is caused by increased intracranial pressure relayed along the optic nerve.

The optic disc should be round or slightly vertically oval. Marked myopic refractive errors may make the disc appear larger, and hyperopic errors may make it appear smaller. The color of the optic disc should be creamy yellow to pink, lighter than the retina, possibly with tiny blood vessels visible on the surface (Fig. 10-28).

Irregular disc or discs that differ in size or shape between the two eyes should be noted. Impaired blood flow may cause the disc to appear whiter than expected. Hyperemic discs with engorged or tortuous vessels on the surface are abnormal.

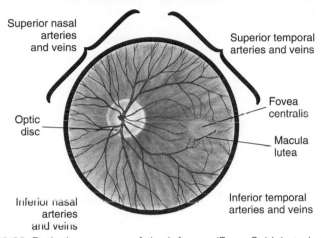

FIG. 10-28 Retinal structures of the left eye. (From Seidel et al., 2011.)

The physiologic cup is a small depression just temporal to the disc center that does not extend to the border. It usually appears lighter than the rest of the disc and occupies less than one half of the diameter of the disc. Vessels entering the disc may drop abruptly into the cup or appear to fade gradually.

The depression of the physiologic cup should not extend to the border of the disc and should not occupy more than one half of the diameter of the disc. The appearance (size or placement) of the physiologic cup should not differ between eyes.

INSPECT the retinal vessels for color, arteriolar light reflex, artery-to-vein ratio, and arteriovenous crossing changes.

Procedure and Findings: From the optic disc follow each of the four sets of retinal vessels from the disc to the periphery. Arteries are on average one fourth narrower than veins; artery-to-vein width should be 2:3 to 4:5. Arteries are light red and may have a narrow band of light in the center. By contrast, veins are larger than arteries and have no light reflex. They are darker, and venous pulsations may be visible (see Fig. 10-28).

Extremely narrow arteries are abnormal. The width of the light reflex should not cover more than one third of the artery. Arteries should not be pale or opaque.

Overall the caliber of both arteries and veins should be regular and uniformly decreasing in size as they branch and move toward the periphery. Artery and vein crossing should give no evidence of constricting either vessel.

Irregularities of caliber, either dilation or constriction, should be noted. Compact areas of tortuous, narrow vessels should be investigated. Indentations or pinched appearances where veins and arteries cross occur with hypertension and are termed *arteriovenous nicking.*

PROCEDURES AND TECHNIQUES WITH EXPECTED FINDINGS	ABNORMAL FINDINGS

INSPECT the retinal background for color, presence of microaneurysms, hemorrhages, and exudates.

Findings: The color is uniform throughout and may be pink, red, or orange; it varies with skin color. The retinal surface should be finely granular, with choroidal vessels possibly visible. Movable light reflections may appear on the surface, usually in young people.

Pale fundus in either general or localized areas, or hemorrhages (linear, flame shaped, round, dark red, large, or small) must be noted. Note microaneurysms, which appear as fine red dots, and any exudates (i.e., soft, hard, fuzzy, or well defined).

INSPECT the macula for color and surface characteristics.

Procedure and Findings: Ask the patient to look directly into the ophthalmoscope light. The macula is about one disc diameter (DD) in size and lies about two DDs temporal to the optic disc. The macula and its center should be slightly darker than the rest of the retina. Tiny vessels may appear on the surface. Fine pigmentation and granular appearance may be visible. The macula may be difficult to see if the patient's pupil has not been dilated chemically.

Drusen bodies are deposits that form within the layer under the retina and appear as small, discrete spots in the retina. They become yellow as the spots enlarge. When drusen bodies increase in size or number, they may contribute to macular degeneration.

ROUTINE TECHNIQUES: EARS

ASSESS hearing based on response from conversation.

As you conduct the history, note the patient's ability to hear by observing communication patterns. A patient's ability to engage in conversation is considered an expected finding. *Note: Perform further tests for hearing if findings suggest a hearing deficit (described in the following Special Circumstances section).*

Subtle indications of hearing loss include the patient who asks you to repeat yourself, repeatedly misunderstands questions you ask, has garbled speech sounds with word distortion, leans forward or tilts his or her head, watches your lips as you speak, or speaks in a loud monotone voice.

INSPECT the external ears for alignment and position.

The top of the pinna of the ear should align directly with the outer canthus of the eye and be angled no more than 10 degrees from a vertical position (Fig. 10-29).

Low-set ears (the pinna is located below the external corner of the eye) or ears that are misaligned (the ear is angled more than 10 degrees from a vertical position) should be considered abnormal. Low-set ears are seen in persons with congenital diseases such as Down syndrome.

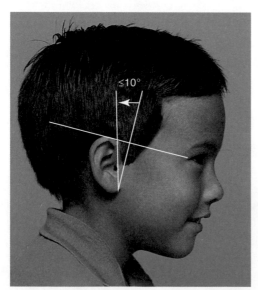

FIG. 10-29 Normal ear position and alignment. (From Hockenberry et al., 2011.)

PROCEDURES AND TECHNIQUES WITH EXPECTED FINDINGS

INSPECT for shape, symmetry, skin color, and skin intactness.

The ears should be between 4 and 10 cm in length and appear the same bilaterally. If the ears are pierced, note the skin around the piercing for skin intactness, edema, or discharge. The skin should be an even skin tone, with color about the same as that noted on the face. It should be intact and without lesions. A small, painless nodule, called *Darwin's tubercle*, is a normal deviation and may be noted at the helix of the ear (Fig. 10-30).

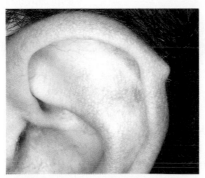

FIG. 10-30 Darwin's tubercle. (From Bingham, Hawke, and Kwok, 1992.)

ABNORMAL FINDINGS

If the ears are smaller than 4 cm in length, they are referred to as *microtia* ears. If the ears are larger than 10 cm in length, they are referred to as *macrotia* ears.

Other abnormal findings include lesions or deformities such as nodules, cancerous lesions, sebaceous cysts, cauliflower ear, hematoma, or edema (Table 10-2).

TABLE 10-2 ABNORMAL FINDINGS OF THE EXTERNAL EAR

CAULIFLOWER EAR

Thickened, disfigured auricle resulting from repeated episodes of minor or major blunt trauma. When observed in infants and young children, child abuse should be suspected.

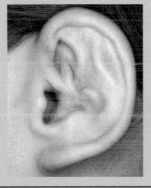

CARCINOMA

Cancer to the skin on the external ear can appear in the form of progressive ulcer (as shown) or a patch of crusty skin (squamous cell) or a waxy bump or flat lesion (basal cell).

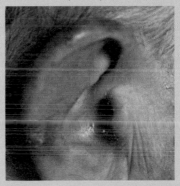

HEMATOMA

Most commonly caused by direct trauma, usually from a contact sport (e.g., football, rugby, wrestling) or a blow to the side of the head (e.g., trauma from a motor vehicle accident, assault). When observed in infants and young children, child abuse should be suspected.

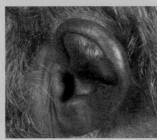

SEBACEOUS CYST

Manifests as a nodule usually found behind the earlobe in the postauricular fold. It is very painful if it becomes infected.

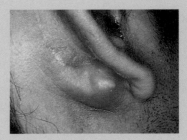

PROCEDURES AND TECHNIQUES WITH EXPECTED FINDINGS

ABNORMAL FINDINGS

INSPECT the external auditory meatus for discharge or lesions.

There should be no lesions or discharge.

Discharge from the ear should be considered abnormal. A bloody or clear discharge from the ear accompanied by a history of head injury should lead to suspicion of possible skull fracture. A purulent or crusty discharge usually indicates infection or the presence of a foreign body.

SPECIAL CIRCUMSTANCES OR ADVANCED PRACTICE: EARS

PALPATE the external ears and mastoid areas for tenderness and edema.

Palpation of the ear is usually done in the presence of deformity, injury, inflammation, and/or reported pain.

The upper part of the ear should be firm and flexible; the earlobe should be soft. All areas should be without tenderness or edema. Gently pull on the helix of the ear to determine if there is any discomfort or pain. There should be none.

Tenderness of the mastoid area may indicate mastoiditis. Pain when the helix of the ear is pulled may indicate an inflammation within the auditory canal.

★ INSPECT the internal ear structures.

Inspection of internal structures is indicated when inflammation, foreign body, or obstruction of the ear canal is suspected.

Procedure: Use an otoscope to inspect the outer and middle ear. If you have a choice of speculum size, always choose the largest speculum that comfortably fits into the external auditory meatus.

Proper technique using the otoscope is necessary to optimize visualization and prevent discomfort or injury.

- When examining the patient's right ear, grasp the top of the pinna with the left hand and gently pull the helix upward and slightly toward the back of the head, and hold the scope in the right hand (Fig. 10-31, *A*). This straightens the S-shaped curve of the auditory canal. (When examining the patient's left ear, grasp the top of the pinna with the right hand and gently pull the helix upward and slightly toward the back of the head, and hold the scope in the left hand.)
- Holding the otoscope with the handle upside down in the right hand, insert the lighted speculum of the otoscope 1 to 1.5 cm into the patient's external auditory canal. Rest the back of the right hand against the patient's temple area to steady the positioning of the otoscope (Fig. 10-31, *B*). Alternatively many nurses hold the otoscope in a handle-down position. Either way, be careful not to insert the otoscope speculum into the canal too far because the bony section of the ear canal is very sensitive.

★ Advanced practice.

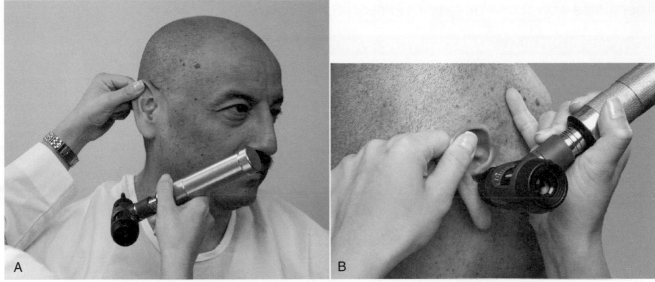

FIG. 10-31 Use of an otoscope. **A,** Pull the patient's helix upward and slightly toward the back of the head. **B,** Hold the otoscope either vertically or upside down (as shown). Stabilize the stethoscope by resting the back of your hand against the patient's temple area.

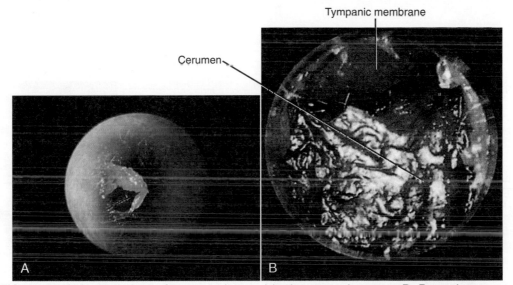

Tympanic membrane

Cerumen

FIG. 10-32 A, Normal piece of cerumen (earwax) in the external meatus. **B,** Excessive earwax in the external auditory canal. (**A** from Bingham, Hawke, and Kwok, 1992. **B** courtesy Dr. Richard A. Buckingham, Abraham Lincoln School of Medicine, University of Illinois, Chicago. From Barkauskas et al., 2002.)

PROCEDURES AND TECHNIQUES WITH EXPECTED FINDINGS

INSPECT the external ear canal for cerumen, edema, erythema, discharge, and foreign bodies.

Once the otoscope is properly positioned, look through the lens to visualize the walls of the canal.

Findings: Cerumen is almost always in the canal (Fig. 10-32, *A*). Note the characteristics of the cerumen. The color may be black, brown, dark red, creamy, or brown-gray. The texture ranges from moist to dry and flaky to hard. There should be no odor, edema, or erythema.

ABNORMAL FINDINGS

Erythema and edema of the auditory canal may be an indication of otitis externa. The infection may cause the canal to become occluded.

PROCEDURES AND TECHNIQUES WITH EXPECTED FINDINGS

🌐 ETHNIC, CULTURAL, AND SPIRITUAL VARIATIONS
Cerumen

White and dark-skinned races have cerumen that is moist, sticky, and dark.
  Asians, Native Americans, and Alaskan Natives have cerumen that is generally sparse, dry, flaky, and lighter.

INSPECT the tympanic membrane for landmarks, color, contour, translucence, and fluctuation.

Findings: Most of the TM is taut and is known as the *pars tensa;* a smaller, less taut part is the *pars flaccida,* and the dense fibrous ring around the membrane is the *annulus.* The cone of light may be seen downward and anteriorly. Using an example of a clock face, the cone of light is seen at the 5 o'clock location in the right ear and the 7 o'clock location in the left ear. Part of the malleus and incus may be visualized through the TM (Fig. 10-33). Note the color and contour. It should be a translucent, pearly gray color.

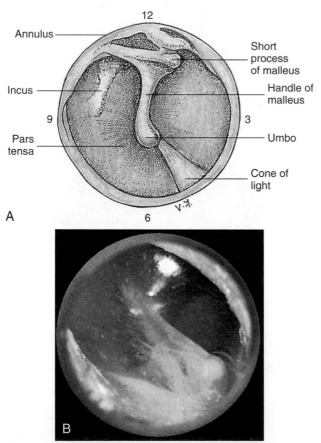

FIG. 10-33 Tympanic membrane. **A,** Landmarks of tympanic membrane with "clock" superimposed (right ear). **B,** Photograph of a normal-appearing tympanic membrane. (**A** from Potter and Perry, 1991. **B** courtesy Dr. Richard A. Buckingham, Clinical Professor, Otolaryngology, Abraham Lincoln School of Medicine, University of Illinois, Chicago. From Barkauskas et al., 2002.)

ABNORMAL FINDINGS

Purulent discharge may occur secondary to otitis externa or with rupture of the tympanic membrane (TM) associated with acute otitis media. Clear fluid or frank bloody drainage following a head injury may indicate a basilar skull fracture. Other abnormal findings in the auditory canal include the presence of foreign bodies, excessive cerumen, or a polyp. If an excessive amount of cerumen is present in the ear, it may occlude the entire ear canal (Fig. 10-32, *B*). The excessive cerumen must be removed before the examination can continue (Box 10-4).

Absence or distortion of the landmarks on the TM should be considered abnormal. A hole in the TM is referred to as a perforation (Fig. 10-34), which occurs with untreated acute otitis media, a blow to the head, or penetration by a foreign body. Variations in the color and characteristics of the TM indicating an abnormality are presented in Box 10-5.

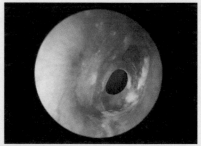

FIG. 10-34 Perforated tympanic membrane. (From Bingham, Hawke, and Kwok, 1992.)

BOX 10-4 REMOVING CERUMEN FROM THE AUDITORY CANAL
To remove cerumen from the auditory canal, first fill the canal with a cerumen-softening agent. Block the opening of the canal with a cotton ball and wait 5 to 10 minutes. The cerumen may then be removed easily from the canal by irrigating the canal with warm water. Some nurses prefer to remove the cerumen with a cerumen spoon. This technique requires skill so as not to scrape the walls of the canal or injure the tympanic membrane.
CAUTION: Do not use water irrigation of the canal if any of the following are suspected: otitis externa, tympanic membrane perforation, or myringotomy tubes in place.

BOX 10-5 ABNORMAL COLOR CHARACTERISTICS OF THE TYMPANIC MEMBRANE AND POSSIBLE CAUSES
• *Yellow/amber:* Serous fluid in the middle ear, which may indicate otitis media with effusion
• *Redness:* Infection in the middle ear such as acute purulent otitis media
• *Chalky white:* Infection in the middle ear such as otitis media
• *Blue or deep red:* Blood behind the tympanic membrane (TM), which may have occurred secondary to injury
• *Red streaks:* Injected/increased vascularization may be caused by allergy
• *Dullness:* Fibrosis or scarring of the TM secondary to repeated infections
• *White flecks/plaques:* Healed inflammation of the TM

PROCEDURES AND TECHNIQUES WITH EXPECTED FINDINGS

ABNORMAL FINDINGS

Procedure: Mobility of the TM is evaluated by attaching a pneumatic bulb to the otoscope. To perform this procedure, make sure that the speculum is fully inserted into the canal and the speculum is large enough to completely occlude the canal. Gently squeeze the bulb so puffs of air are transmitted to the TM.

Findings: The expected response is that the TM slightly fluctuates with the puffs of air. This procedure can be performed with any age-group but is most commonly done when examining infants and young children because they are unable to provide a history regarding the pain they are experiencing.

Bulging of the TM with no mobility indicates pus or fluid behind the TM. Retraction of the TM with no mobility with negative pressure indicates obstruction of the eustachian tube.

Increased mobility of only one part of the TM (as determined with the pneumatic bulb) indicates an area of healed TM perforation.

TEST the acoustic cranial nerve (VIII) to evaluate auditory function.

The following tests are indicated when hearing loss is suspected.

Whispered Voice Test

Procedure: Stand 1 to 2 feet in front of or to the side of the patient. Instruct the patient to cover one ear with his or her hand so one ear may be tested at a time. Shield your mouth so the patient cannot read your lips. Softly whisper several monosyllabic (e.g., ball, chair, cat) and disyllabic (e.g., streetcar, baseball, highchair) words and ask the patient to repeat what is heard. Repeat the procedure with the other ear. Although this test is simple, standardization of the results is difficult because of variance of the loudness of whispers among nurses.

Findings: The patient should be able to hear and repeat at last 50% of all words whispered.

When the patient cannot repeat at least 50% of the spoken words, the findings are considered abnormal. Consider each ear separately.

Finger-Rubbing Test

Another simple hearing screening test may be done by holding your hand 3 to 4 inches from the patient's ear and briskly rubbing your index finger against your thumb. The patient should be able to hear the noise generated by rubbing the fingers together. Repeat the technique with the other ear.

Patients with a high-frequency hearing loss may not be able to hear the noise generated by your fingers.

PROCEDURES AND TECHNIQUES WITH EXPECTED FINDINGS

Weber's Test

Procedure: This test uses a tuning fork to assess hearing. Activate the tuning fork by holding it by the base stem and striking the forked section against the base of the palm. Immediately place the base of the fork on the midline of the patient's skull. Ask the patient to indicate in which ear the sound is heard louder.

Findings: Because sound is transmitted along the skull to the inner ear, the patient should hear the tone equally in both ears (Fig. 10-35).

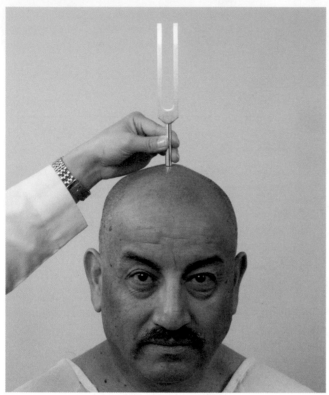

FIG. 10-35 Weber's test. The tuning fork is placed on the midline of the skull.

ABNORMAL FINDINGS

If the sound lateralizes to one side (i.e., the patient hears the tone better in one ear than the other), the test should be considered abnormal. Lateralization of sound to the affected ear suggests conductive hearing loss (Fig. 10-36, *A*). Lateralization of sound to the unaffected ear suggests sensorineural hearing loss (Fig. 10-36, *B*).

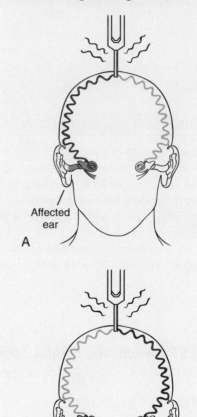

FIG. 10-36 A, Patient with conduction loss; sound lateralizes to the defective ear because the sound transmits through the bone rather than air. **B,** Patient with sensorineural loss; sound lateralizes to the unaffected ear.

PROCEDURES AND TECHNIQUES WITH EXPECTED FINDINGS

ABNORMAL FINDINGS

Rinne Test

The Rinne test also uses a tuning fork to assess hearing by comparing air conduction (AC) of sound to bone conduction (BC) of sound. The AC route through the ear canal is a more sensitive route.

Procedure: Explain the procedure and ask the patient to indicate when the sound is no longer heard when the tuning fork is placed on the bone and when it is placed in the front of the ear.

- Activate the tuning fork by holding it by the base stem and striking the forked section against the base of the palm of your hand. Immediately place the base of the tuning fork directly on the patient's mastoid process (Fig. 10-37, *A*).
- Use a watch with a second hand to time the seconds. The patient should be able to hear the tone. Instruct the patient to tell you when the tone can no longer be heard.
- When the patient indicates the tone can no longer be heard, note the number of seconds counted; quickly remove the fork from the mastoid process, invert the fork, and hold the vibrating section of the tuning fork in front of the patient's ear (Fig. 10-37, *B*).
- Begin timing again. The patient should be able to hear the tone again. Instruct the patient to tell you when the vibration is no longer heard.
- When the patient no longer hears the tone, note the time.

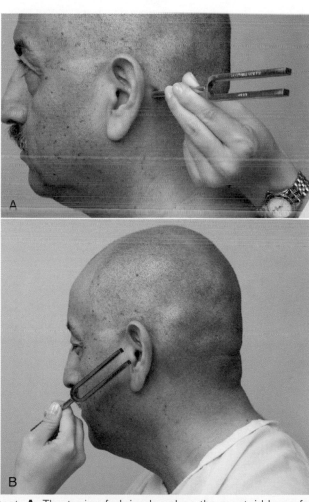

FIG. 10-37 Rinne test. **A,** The tuning fork is placed on the mastoid bone for bone conduction. **B,** The tuning fork is placed in front of the ear for air conduction.

PROCEDURES AND TECHNIQUES WITH EXPECTED FINDINGS

Findings: The tone heard in front of the ear should last twice as long as the tone heard when the fork was on the mastoid process (AC > BC by 2:1). This is the expected (positive) response. Repeat the test with the other ear.

Audioscope

Each of the screening tests described previously may identify an individual with decreased hearing, but none of these tests measures the degree of hearing loss. An audioscope provides a measurement of hearing (see Fig. 3-26).

Procedure: Select a speculum that best fits the ear canal (a snug fit is desired to screen out surrounding noise). Attach the speculum to the probe and insert in the ear, sealing the external auditory canal. As tones are delivered at each frequency, the patient indicates if the tone can be heard, thus providing objective measurement of hearing. Because of the high degree of accuracy and ease of use, the audioscope is often used for hearing screening in primary care.[8]

Findings: The patient who hears well is able to hear all tones at all frequencies delivered by the audioscope.

ABNORMAL FINDINGS

Consider the test abnormal when the sound is heard longer by bone conduction than air conduction (BC > AC). Patients with conductive hearing loss have bone conduction longer than air conduction in the affected ear (Fig. 10-38, *A*). Patients with sensorineural hearing loss have air conduction longer than bone conduction (AC > BC) in the affected ear, but it will be less than a 2:1 ratio (Fig. 10-38, *B*).

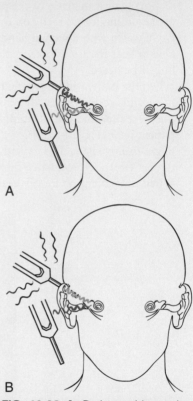

A

B

FIG. 10-38 A, Patient with conduction loss hears bone conduction longer than air conduction (BC > AC). **B,** Patient with sensorineural loss hears air conduction longer than bone conduction (AC > BC).

A 20-dB loss in high frequencies results in difficulty hearing high-pitched consonants. A 40-dB loss in all frequencies causes moderate difficulty in hearing normal speech.

PROCEDURES AND TECHNIQUES WITH EXPECTED FINDINGS	ABNORMAL FINDINGS

ROUTINE TECHNIQUES: NOSE

INSPECT the nose for general appearance, symmetry, and discharge.

The skin should be smooth and intact, with the color matching the rest of the face. It should appear symmetric and midline. The nostrils should be symmetric, not flaring or narrowed. There should be no nasal discharge present.

Lesions, erythema, and discoloration are abnormal and may be signs of a systemic illness. Marked asymmetry of the nose may be the result of current or past injury.

Edema, nasal discharge, and crusting are possible signs of infection, allergy, or injury. Watery, unilateral nasal discharge following a history of head injury may indicate skull fracture. Unilateral, purulent, thick nasal drainage may indicate a foreign body.

SPECIAL CIRCUMSTANCES OR ADVANCED PRACTICE: NOSE

PALPATE the nose for tenderness and to assess patency.

This is done in the presence of injury or reported pain or obstruction.

Apply pressure to occlude one nostril; ask the patient to close his or her mouth and sniff through the opposite nostril; repeat on the other side. There should be noiseless, free exchange of air on each side. The nose should not be tender with palpation

Narrowing of the nostrils when the patient inhales may be associated with chronic obstruction that may necessitate mouth breathing. Noisy or obstructed breathing may occur secondary to nasal congestion, trauma to the nasal passage, polyps, or allergies. Instability or tenderness from trauma or inflammation may be noted on palpation.

INSPECT the internal nasal cavity for surface characteristics, lesions, erythema, discharge, and foreign bodies.

This is done in the presence of injury or reported pain or obstruction.

Procedure: The internal nasal cavity is inspected using a nasal speculum and a light source. Hold the speculum in the palm of the hand and use your index finger to stabilize it against the side of the nose. Insert the speculum slowly and cautiously; open it on a slightly oblique axis (not horizontally) because direct pressure on the septum is painful. Use your other hand to hold the light source. Alternatively, an otoscope with a nasal speculum attached may be used for the examination, as shown in Fig. 10-39.

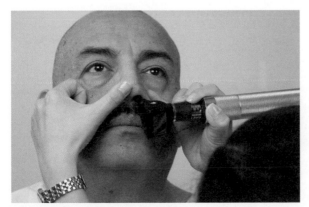

FIG. 10-39 Inspect the nasal cavity with a light source.

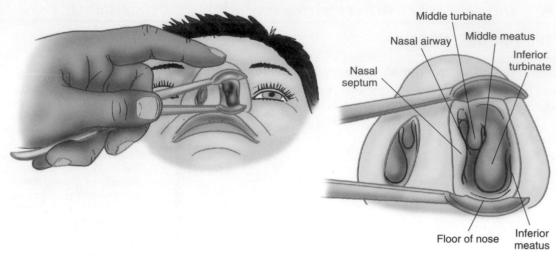

Middle turbinate
Nasal airway   Middle meatus
Inferior turbinate
Nasal septum
Floor of nose   Inferior meatus

FIG. 10-40 View of the nasal mucosa through the nasal speculum. (From Seidel et al., 2006.)

PROCEDURES AND TECHNIQUES WITH EXPECTED FINDINGS

Findings: With the patient's head erect, note the floor of the nose, inferior turbinate, nasal hairs, and mucosa, which should be slightly darker red than the oral mucosa. The patient's nasal septum should be straight, intact, and midline. With the patient's head back, inspect the middle meatus and middle turbinate (Fig. 10-40). Turbinates and meatus should be a deep pink color, similar to the color of the surrounding tissue.

PALPATE the frontal and maxillary paranasal sinus areas for tenderness.

This is done in the presence of injury or reported pain over the sinuses.

Procedure: To palpate the frontal sinuses, press upward on the frontal sinuses with your thumbs on the supraorbital ridge just below the eyebrows. Be careful not to press directly over the eyeballs. To palpate the maxillary sinuses, press over the sinus area above the cheekbones (Fig. 10-42).
Findings: There should be no tenderness or pain with palpation over the sinuses.

ABNORMAL FINDINGS

There should be no perforations, bleeding, or crusting. A perforation is often associated with cocaine use (Fig. 10-41). A deviated nasal septum with a decrease in airflow is abnormal. Increased redness may occur secondary to infection, whereas localized erythema and edema in the vestibule may indicate a furuncle or localized infection.

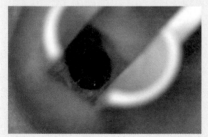

FIG. 10-41 Perforation of nasal septum from cocaine use. (Courtesy Lemmi and Lemmi, 2013.)

Tenderness on palpation may indicate sinus congestion or infection. If the patient complains of sinus pain or shows signs of sinus congestion, transilluminate the sinuses (described in the next section).

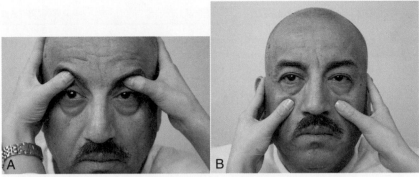

FIG. 10-42 Palpation of sinuses. **A,** Frontal. **B,** Maxillary.

PROCEDURES AND TECHNIQUES WITH EXPECTED FINDINGS	ABNORMAL FINDINGS

★ TRANSILLUMINATE the sinus area.

If the patient complains of sinus pain or shows signs of sinus congestion, transilluminate the sinuses using a transilluminator or bright penlight.

Procedure: After darkening the room, place the source of light lateral to the nose, just beneath the medial aspect of the eye. Look through the patient's open mouth for illumination of the hard palate. Transilluminate the frontal sinuses by placing the light source against the medial aspect of each supraorbital rim.
Findings: A dim red glow is transmitted above the eyebrows.

An absence of a glow during transillumination of the sinuses may indicate that the sinus is congested and filled with secretions or that it never developed.

ROUTINE TECHNIQUES: MOUTH

INSPECT the lips for color, symmetry, moisture, and texture.

Lips should appear pink and symmetric both vertically and laterally. They should be smooth and moist and have slight vertical linear markings. There should be a distinct border between the lips and the facial skin (vermillion border).

Pale lips may indicate anemia or shock. Cyanotic (bluish) lips and circumoral cyanosis (bluish tint surrounding the mouth) may indicate hypoxemia or hypothermia. Dry, flaking, or cracked lips may be caused by dehydration or exposure to dry air or wind. Cracks and erythema in the corners of the mouth may be caused by vitamin B deficiencies.[9] Lesions, plaques, vesicles, nodules, or ulcerations may be signs of infection, irritation (such as lip biting), or skin cancer. Lips may be edematous because of an allergic reaction.

INSPECT the teeth and gums for condition, color, surface characteristics, stability, and alignment.

The teeth should be white, yellow, or gray, with smooth edges. Inspect the condition of the teeth, making note of caries and broken, loose, and missing teeth.

Observe alignment by asking the patient to clench the teeth and smile. The upper back teeth should rest directly on the lower back teeth, with the upper incisors slightly overriding the lower ones. The teeth should be evenly spaced and firmly anchored.

The gingiva around the base of the teeth should have a pink, moist appearance with a clearly defined margin at each tooth. For patients who wear dentures, observe the gum line beneath the dentures.

Missing teeth may occur secondary to tooth extraction or trauma. Darkened or stained teeth may occur secondary to coffee, medications, poor dental care, or frequent vomiting. Brown spots in the crevices or between the teeth may indicate caries.

★ Advanced practice.

PROCEDURES AND TECHNIQUES WITH EXPECTED FINDINGS

⊕ ETHNIC, CULTURAL, AND SPIRITUAL VARIATIONS

Variations in the Number and Size of Teeth

About 30% of Asian Americans, 15% of Native Americans, and 10% of Caucasians have a congenital absence of the third molar and thus have only 28 teeth as adults. This pattern is rare in African Americans.

Caucasians have the smallest teeth; African Americans tend to have larger teeth than Caucasians; Asians and Native Americans have the largest teeth.

⊕ ETHNIC, CULTURAL, AND SPIRITUAL VARIATIONS

Mucous Membranes

Darker-skinned persons often have darker oral pigmentation and may have a patchy brown pigmentation of the gums. There may also be a dark melanotic line along the gingival margin.

ABNORMAL FINDINGS

Excessively exposed tooth neck (the narrowed part of the tooth between the crown and the root) with receding gums may occur secondary to aging or gingival disease.

Malocclusion refers to a misalignment of teeth. Common variations of malocclusion include protrusion of the upper incisors (also known as overbite) (Fig. 10-43), protrusion of the lower jaw (known as prognathism) (Fig. 10-44), or misalignment of teeth (Fig. 10-45).

Presence of debris usually occurs because of poor dental hygiene. Redness, edema, and bleeding of the gums may occur secondary to gingivitis, systemic disease, hormonal changes, and drug therapy (see Fig. 10-70).

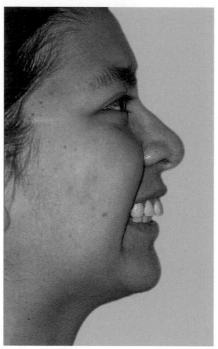

FIG. 10-43 Malocclusion of teeth: overbite. (Courtesy Lemmi and Lemmi, 2013.)

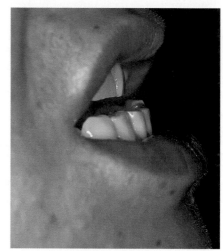

FIG. 10-44 Malocclusion of teeth: prognathism. (Courtesy Lemmi and Lemmi, 2013.)

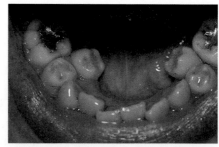

FIG. 10-45 Misalignment of teeth in lower jaw. (Courtesy Lemmi and Lemmi, 2013.)

| PROCEDURES AND TECHNIQUES WITH EXPECTED FINDINGS | ABNORMAL FINDINGS |

INSPECT the tongue for movement, symmetry, color, and surface characteristics.

Ask the patient to stick out his or her tongue. (This maneuver also tests cranial nerve XII—the hypoglossal nerve.) The forward thrust should be smooth and symmetric, and the tongue itself should appear symmetric. The tongue should be pink and moist with a glistening surface dorsally and laterally. The surface may appear slightly rough because of the papillae on the dorsal surface of the tongue. Also note any edema or variation in size, color, coating, or ulceration.

Atrophy of the tongue on one side or deviation of the tongue may be a sign of a neurologic disorder. A smooth or beefy-red–colored, edematous tongue with a slick appearance may indicate B vitamin deficiency.[10] A tongue with irregular patches with a maplike appearance is referred to as a geographic tongue (Fig. 10-46). A hairy tongue with yellow-brown–to-black, elongated papillae may occur secondary to antibiotic therapy, superinfection, or pipe smoking. An enlarged tongue may be seen in patients with Down syndrome or hypothyroidism. Lesions and sores are always considered abnormal.

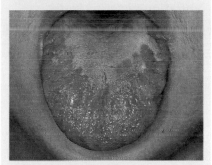

FIG. 10-46 Geographic tongue. (Courtesy Lemmi and Lemmi, 2013.)

INSPECT the buccal mucosa and anterior and posterior pillars for color, surface characteristics, and odor.

Ask the patient to open the mouth widely to allow you to inspect the buccal mucosa with gloved hands using a penlight and tongue blade. Inspect the anterior and posterior pillars. Note the color of the mucosa and the symmetry of the pillars. The color of the tissue should be pale coral or pink with slight vascularity. Using a tongue blade, gently pull the buccal mucosa away from the molars. It should be smooth, with a transverse occlusion line appearing adjacent to where teeth meet. Clear saliva should cover the surface. The parotid gland duct opening (also known as Stensen's duct) is on the buccal mucosa adjacent to the upper second molar. It appears as a slightly elevated pinpoint red mark. Also note the odor of the breath. The mouth should have a slightly sweet odor or none at all.

Aphthous ulcers on the buccal mucosa appear as white, round, or oval ulcerative lesions with a red halo (see Fig. 10-73). Leukoplakia is a white patch or plaque found on the oral mucosa that cannot be scraped off. Erythroplakia is a red patch found on the oral mucosa. An excessively dry mouth or excessive salivation may indicate salivary gland blockage or may occur secondary to medications, dehydration, or stress.

An acetone odor on the breath may indicate diabetic ketoacidosis. A fetid odor may occur secondary to gum disease, caries, poor dental care, or sinusitis.

PROCEDURES AND TECHNIQUES WITH EXPECTED FINDINGS

INSPECT the palate, uvula, posterior pharynx, and tonsils for texture, color, surface characteristics, and movement.

Instruct the patient to tilt his or her head back so the palate and uvula can be inspected. The hard palate should be smooth, pale, and immovable with irregular transverse rugae. The soft palate and uvula should be smooth and pink, with the uvula in a midline position. Instruct the patient to say "ah." If necessary, depress the tongue with a tongue depressor. (This tests cranial nerve X, the vagus nerve.) Observe if the soft palate rises symmetrically with the uvula remaining in the midline position. (This tests cranial nerve IX, glossopharyngeal nerve.)

Using a tongue depressor to hold the tongue down, examine the posterior wall of the pharynx (Fig. 10-47). The tissue should be smooth and have a glistening pink coloration. The tonsils extend beyond the posterior pillars. They should appear slightly pink with an irregular surface. Enlarged, noninflamed tonsils are a normal variation among adolescents as shown in Fig. 10-48.

🌐 ETHNIC, CULTURAL, AND SPIRITUAL VARIATIONS

Variations in the Uvula

A split uvula occurs in up to 10% of Asians and 18% of some Native American groups.

From Giger JN, Davidhizar RE: *Transcultural nursing*, ed 5, St Louis, 2008, Mosby.

ABNORMAL FINDINGS

Nodules observed on the palate may indicate a tumor. Lesions associated with Kaposi's sarcoma may be present on both the hard and soft palates. Opportunistic infections may occur when an individual has been on antibiotics or is immunosuppressed. Failure of the soft palate to rise bilaterally and uvula deviation during vocalization may indicate a neurologic problem.

Exudate or mucoid film on the posterior pharynx may be present secondary to postnasal drip or infection. A grayish tinge to the membrane may occur with allergies or diphtheria. Edematous, erythematous tonsils with or without exudate may indicate infection. Tonsil enlargement is graded from 1+ to 4+ (Fig. 10-49).

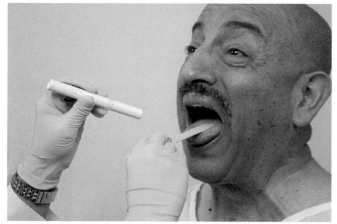

FIG. 10-47 Displace the tongue with a tongue depressor for inspection of the pharynx.

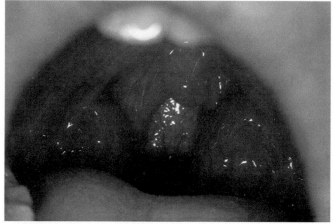

FIG. 10-48 Tonsil enlargement in healthy adolescent. (Courtesy Lemmi and Lemmi, 2013.)

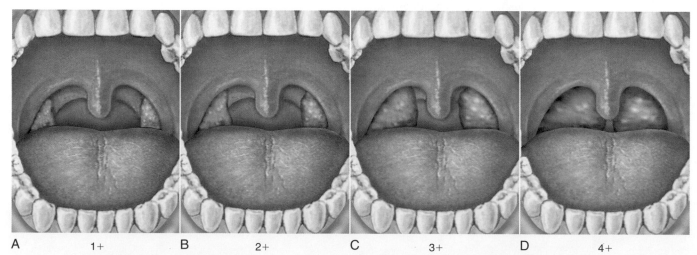

A   1+   B   2+   C   3+   D   4+

FIG. 10-49 Grading tonsil enlargement. **A,** 1+, visible; **B,** 2+, halfway between tonsillar pillars and uvula; **C,** 3+, nearly touching the uvula; **D,** 4+, touching one another. (From Seidel et al., 2011.)

PROCEDURES AND TECHNIQUES WITH EXPECTED FINDINGS	ABNORMAL FINDINGS

SPECIAL CIRCUMSTANCES OR ADVANCED PRACTICE: MOUTH

PALPATE the teeth, inner lips, and gums for condition and tenderness.

This technique is indicated in the presence of injury, lesions, or reported pain.

Wearing examination gloves, palpate the teeth and inner aspects of the lips and upper and lower gingivobuccal fornices and gingivae (gums). The teeth should be anchored firmly.

Marked movement of the teeth may be secondary to either periodontal disease or trauma. Gum tenderness with palpation or thickening may indicate that the dentures do not fit well or the presence of lesions.

PALPATE the tongue for texture.

Wearing examination gloves, grasp the tongue with a 4 × 4–inch gauze pad, and palpate all sides (Fig. 10-50). During palpation note any lumps, nodules, or areas of thickening. The tongue should feel relatively smooth and even. Papillae create slight roughness on the dorsum of the tongue.

Lumps, nodules, or masses may indicate local or systemic disease or oral cancer.

ROUTINE TECHNIQUES: NECK

INSPECT the neck position in relation to the head and trachea.

The neck should be centered, and the trapezius and sternocleidomastoid muscles should be bilaterally symmetric (Fig. 10-51). The trachea should be midline.

Note rhythmic movements or tremor of the neck and head. Observe also for tics or spasms. Tracheal deviation suggests displacement by a mass in the chest.

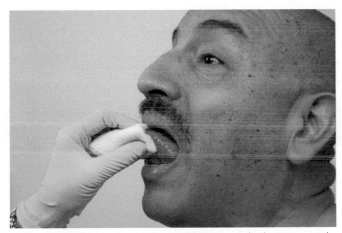

FIG. 10-50 Grasp the tongue with a 4 × 4–inch gauze pad.

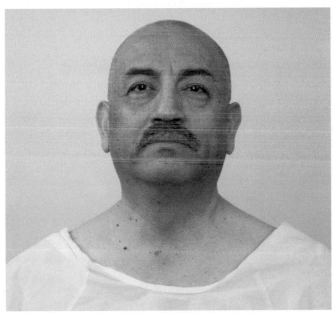

FIG. 10-51 Bilateral symmetry of neck muscles.

PROCEDURES AND TECHNIQUES WITH EXPECTED FINDINGS	ABNORMAL FINDINGS

INSPECT the neck for skin characteristics, presence of lumps, masses.

The skin color should match other skin areas. In some individuals (particularly thin men) the thyroid cartilage may protrude enough to be visible. The thyroid gland is usually not visualized clearly.

Lesions or masses on the neck are abnormal. A goiter (enlarged thyroid) may be seen as fullness in the neck (Fig. 10-52).

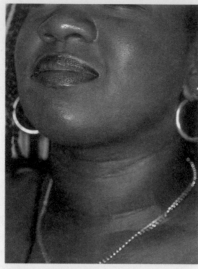

FIG. 10-52 Goiter. Note visible enlargement over the anterior neck. (Courtesy Lemmi and Lemmi, 2013.)

SPECIAL CIRCUMSTANCES OR ADVANCED PRACTICE: NECK

The following procedures are indicated if abnormalities are observed or if the patient reports pain, masses, or reduced range of motion.

INSPECT the neck for range of motion.

Ask the patient to move the neck forward (chin to chest, 45 degrees), backward (toward ceiling, 55 degrees), and side to side (ear to shoulder, 40 degrees). The shoulders should remain stationary during assessment. Next ask the patient to rotate the head laterally to the right and left (70 degrees in both directions). All movements should be controlled, smooth, and painless.

Limited range of motion or pain during movement may indicate either a systemic infection with meningeal irritation, a musculoskeletal problem such as muscle spasm, or degenerative vertebral disks. Note weakness of muscles or tremors. Note if the patient complains of pain throughout the movement or at particular points.

PALPATE the neck for anatomic structures and trachea.

Palpate the neck and trachea just above the suprasternal notch. Palpate for the tracheal rings, cricoid cartilage, and thyroid cartilage. All structures should be midline and nontender.

Assess sternocleidomastoid muscle strength by asking the patient to turn his or her head from side to side against the resistance of your hand. Assess trapezius muscle strength by asking the patient to shrug the shoulders against the resistance of your hands pressing down on his or her shoulders. By doing this you are also assessing the spinal accessory nerve (cranial nerve XI). Palpation of the neck muscles helps assess for areas of muscle tenderness. The muscles should be firm and nontender with palpation.

Abnormalities include tenderness or masses on palpation or location of the structures away from the midline position.

Unilateral or bilateral muscle weakness is an abnormal finding.

Tenderness, muscle spasms, and edema are abnormal findings and may suggest injury.

| **PROCEDURES AND TECHNIQUES WITH EXPECTED FINDINGS** | **ABNORMAL FINDINGS** |

PALPATE the thyroid gland for size, shape consistency, tenderness, and presence of nodules.

This procedure is indicated when patients report an enlarged mass in their neck or when they display symptoms of hyperthyroidism or hypothyroidism.

Procedure: The thyroid may be palpated using either an anterior or a posterior approach. The technique used is the choice of the nurse. Use a gentle touch to palpate the thyroid. Your fingernails should be well trimmed at or below the fingertips. Nodules and asymmetric position are more difficult to detect if the pressure is too hard. In either technique the patient should flex the neck slightly forward and toward the side being examined to relax the sternocleidomastoid muscle.

Posterior approach (Fig. 10-53, *A*): Stand behind the patient. Have him or her sit straight with the head slightly flexed. Reach from behind around the patient's neck and place your fingers on either side of the trachea below the cricoid cartilage. Use two fingers of the left hand to push the trachea to the right. Instruct the patient to swallow while using the finger pads of your right hand to feel for the right lobe of the thyroid gland, the right sternocleidomastoid muscle, and the trachea. Repeat the technique using the right hand to push the trachea to the left. Instruct the patient to swallow while your left hand feels for the left lobe of the thyroid.

Anterior approach (Fig. 10-53, *B*): Stand in front of the patient. Ask him or her to sit up straight and bend the head slightly forward and to the right. Push the patient's trachea to the right with your left thumb. Palpate the thyroid gland below the cricoid process. Instruct the patient to swallow; the patient's displaced right thyroid lobe may be palpated between the sternocleidomastoid muscle and the trachea by the finger pads of your left index and middle fingers. Use the same examination techniques with reversed hand position to examine the left thyroid lobe.

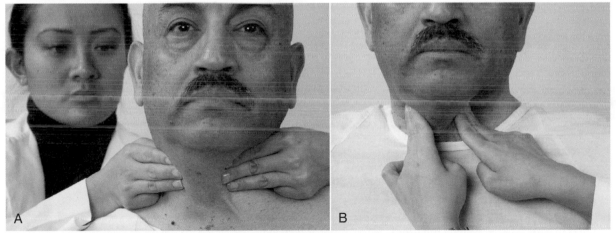

FIG. 10-53 Palpation of thyroid gland. **A,** Posterior approach. **B,** Anterior approach.

PROCEDURES AND TECHNIQUES WITH EXPECTED FINDINGS

Findings: The thyroid gland is a little larger than the size of your thumb pad. It often is not detected, and this is considered a normal finding. If the thyroid is felt, it should feel small, smooth, and soft; and the gland should move freely during swallowing. The thyroid should be nontender.

SPECIAL CIRCUMSTANCES OR ADVANCED PRACTICE: LYMPH NODES

PALPATE lymph nodes for size, consistency, mobility, borders, tenderness, and warmth.

Lymph nodes are palpated as a general screening measure, when an inflammatory process or malignancy is suspected, or if the patient reports pain. Regional lymph nodes include occipital nodes (at base of skull), preauricular nodes (in front of the ear), postauricular nodes (behind the ear), anterior and posterior cervical chain nodes (within the neck), parotid nodes (along the angle of the jaw), retropharyngeal (tonsillar), submental (above posterior cervical chain), and submandibular nodes (under the mandible), and supraclavicular nodes (under the clavicle).

Procedure: Palpate the nodes using your fingertips. You may want to use both hands, one on each side of the head and neck, to compare the findings. However, the submental nodes are easier to palpate with one hand.

Begin by palpating the preauricular nodes (Fig. 10-55), followed by the parotid, postauricular, occipital, retropharyngeal, submandibular, and submental nodes. Next examine the anterior and posterior cervical chain by tipping the patient's head toward the side being examined (Fig. 10-56); palpate the anterior chain on either side of the sternocleidomastoid muscle and the deep posterior cervical nodes at the anterior border of the trapezius muscle. Palpate the supraclavicular nodes by having the patient hunch the shoulders forward and flex the chin toward the side being examined. Place your fingers into the medial supraclavicular fossa. Ask the patient to take a deep breath while you press deeply behind the clavicles to detect nodes.

Findings: Lymph nodes may or may not be palpable. If they are palpable, they should be soft, mobile, nontender, and bilaterally equal.

ABNORMAL FINDINGS

A thyroid that is easily palpable before swallowing is enlarged—a common finding in hyperthyroidism (Fig. 10-54). If the thyroid gland is enlarged, use the bell of the stethoscope to auscultate it for vascular sounds. A bruit indicates an abnormally large volume of blood flow and suggests a goiter. Lumps, nodules, or tenderness are abnormal findings.

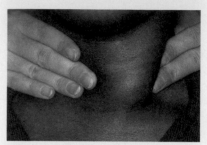

FIG.   10-54 Multinodular goiter visible with palpation. (Courtesy Lemmi and Lemmi, 2013.)

Lymph nodes that are enlarged, tender, and firm but freely movable may suggest an infection of the head or throat. Malignancy may be suspected when nodes are unilateral, hard, asymmetric, fixed, and nontender.

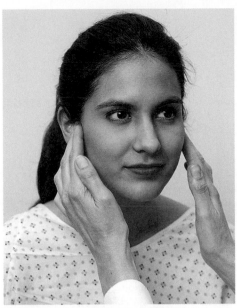

FIG. 10-55 Palpation of preauricular nodes.

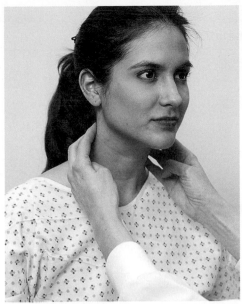

FIG. 10-56 Palpation of posterior superficial cervical chain nodes.

DOCUMENTING EXPECTED FINDINGS

Head: Head symmetric and proportioned for body size. Scalp clean, intact with male-pattern balding. Face and jaw symmetric and proportional. TMJ moves smoothly. Temporal arteries palpable bilaterally with a regular rate and rhythm, 2+.

Eyes: Distance and near vision 20/20 both eyes with contact lens. Horizontal and color perceptions intact. Eyebrows symmetric, with eyelashes evenly distributed and curled upward. Palpebral fissures equal bilaterally, and eyelid color appropriate for race. Eyelid margins pale pink and cover top of the brown iris. Lid closure complete with frequent, bilateral, and involuntary blinking. Bulbar conjunctiva pink and clear. Corneal light reflex symmetric. Sclera white, clear, and moist; corneas transparent. PERRLA, consensual reaction present. Peripheral vision present. EOM intact. Eyeballs indent with slight pressure, no tenderness of eyelids. Irises are clear, with no shadow noted. *Ophthalmic examination:* Red reflex present; disc margins distinct; round, yellow, physiologic cup temporal to disc center; artery-to-vein ratio 2:3, retina red uniformly; macula and fovea slightly darker.

Ears: Hearing present with conversation. Pinna aligned with outer canthus of eyes. Upper part of ear firm, flexible, and soft without discomfort; aligned with eyes; ears symmetric. Cerumen in auditory canal; TM pearly gray, cone of light reflex present. Whispered words repeated correctly, tone heard bilaterally in Weber's test, AC:BC = 2:1.

Nose: Skin smooth, intact, and oily. Nasal passages patent, turbinates pink without exudate, septum midline, sinuses nontender.

Mouth, Throat, and Neck: Breath without odor. Lips symmetric, moist, smooth; 32 white, smooth, aligned teeth. Tongue symmetric, pink, moist, and movable. Gingiva pink and moist, symmetric pillars, clear saliva. Hard palate smooth, pale; soft palate smooth, pink, and rises as expected; uvula midline; posterior pharynx pink, smooth tonsils pink with irregular surface. Trachea midline; thyroid smooth, soft, moves freely with swallow. Neck is centered with full ROM, no palpable lymph nodes.

CLINICAL REASONING: THINKING LIKE A NURSE
Inflammation

A 17-year-old Native American woman brings her 5-month-old son to a medical clinic reporting that he is fussy and his skin is very hot. She also reports that the baby has low energy and is not sleeping or eating well.

Interpreting

Early in the encounter the nurse knows that the two most common causes of fever in an infant this age are a respiratory or ear infection. To determine if either has any probability of being correct, the nurse gathers additional data.
- Are there signs of respiratory involvement? No evidence of nasal flaring or discharge, cough, stridor, grunting, or retractions is observed; lung sounds are clear; the left tympanic membrane is red.
- Has the infant had a recent cough or nasal drainage? Has he been pulling at his ear? The mother denies cough or nasal drainage but reports ear rubbing. The experienced nurse not only recognizes infection by the clinical signs (red tympanic membrane, fever) and symptoms (fussy, poor sleeping, eating, rubbing the ear) but also interprets this information in the context of his age.

Nurse's Background, Experience, Perspective

The experienced nurse immediately has a perceptual grasp of the situation at hand. Extensive practical knowledge about what to expect with this age-group and diagnoses allows the nurse to recognize risk factors of inflammation given the age of the infent and symptoms reported by the mother.

Noticing

Extensive practical knowledge about what to expect with infants allows the experienced nurse to recognize that these are common findings associated with fever. This background knowledge sets up the possibility of noticing when there are signs of a prevalent complication (such as respiratory compromise and dehydration) in an infant presenting with fever and considering possible causes of fever. The nurse observes an infant who is crying with adequate air exchange and appears well hydrated; the nurse confirms that the infant has a fever when the temperature is measured at 100.7° F (38° C). His respiratory rate is 40 breaths/min.

Responding

The experienced nurse initiates appropriate initial interventions, determines the type of health care provider for the baby, and ensures that the infant receives appropriate immediate and follow-up care, including family teaching about otitis media and fever management.

Reflecting

The nurse evaluates the presentation and outcomes of interventions (reflection-in-action); this experience contributes to and deepens the expertise on which to draw again (reflection-on-action) when encountering a similar situation.

AGE-RELATED VARIATIONS

This chapter discusses assessment techniques with adult patients. These data are important to assess for individuals of all ages, but the approach and techniques used to collect the information may vary depending on the patient's age.

INFANTS AND CHILDREN

The nurse should be aware of several important differences when conducting an assessment of the head, eyes, ears, nose, and throat of infants and young children. These differences include interview questions to ask, anatomical differences,

examination procedures, and findings. Refer to Chapter 19 for a detailed discussion related to assessment for this age-group.

OLDER ADULTS

Multiple changes occur as a consequence of advancing age; many of these age-related changes impact assessment findings presented within this chapter. See Chapter 21 for further information about the differences of assessment for this age-group.

COMMON PROBLEMS AND CONDITIONS

RISK FACTORS

Vision, Hearing, Mouth Cancer

Hearing Loss

- Age: Increased incidence after age 50
- Environmental noise (repeated exposure to loud noise >80 dB) (M)
- Ototoxic medications (aminoglycosides, salicylates, furosemide) (M)
- Family history (sensorineural hearing loss)
- Autoimmune disorders (sensorineural hearing loss)
- History of congenital hearing loss

Cataracts

- Age: Between 65 and 74 years 70% of adults had opaque areas, and 18% had cataracts; between 75 and 84 years, 90% of adults had opaque areas, and about 50% had cataracts.
- Gender: Women have a higher risk than men.
- Ethnicity: African Americans have highest risk.
- Smokers: Those who smoke 20 or more cigarettes daily have twice the risk. (M)
- Alcohol: Chronic drinkers of alcohol have increased risk. (M)
- Light exposure: Exposure to low-level ultraviolet B (UVB) or occupational exposure such as arc welding increases risk. (M)
- Medication: People who take corticosteroids may have increased risk. (M)
- Chronic disease: Diabetes mellitus increases risk.

Glaucoma

- Age: Risk increases each year over age 50.
- Family history: Those with a history of glaucoma in a first-degree relative have three times the risk.

- Ethnicity: African Americans are more likely to develop open-angle glaucoma than Caucasians. Asians and Eskimos have an increased risk for closed-angle glaucoma.
- Medication: People who take corticosteroids (including inhaled steroids) on a regular, long-term basis have increased risk. (M)
- Chronic disease: Diabetes mellitus and hypertension significantly increase risk.

Macular Degeneration

- Age: Macular degeneration exists in 25% of those between ages 65 and 74 years and 33% of those above age 75 years.
- Smoking: Cigarette smokers have twice the risk. (M)
- Chronic disease: Hypertension is associated with increased risk.
- Diet: High intake of monosaturated, polyunsaturated, and vegetable fats have increased risk. (M)

Oropharyngeal Cancer

- Age: Incidence is increased after age 40, with peak incidence between ages 64 and 74.
- Gender: There is a 2:1 male-to-female incidence.
- Race: African Americans have highest incidence.
- Tobacco: 90% of individuals who develop oral cancer are tobacco users. (M)
- Alcohol: 75% to 80% of individuals who develop oral cancer consume excessive amounts of alcohol. (M)
- Exposure to sunlight: 30% of those who have cancer on the lip have an outdoor occupation with prolonged exposure to the sun. (M)
- History of previously diagnosed cancer increases risk.
- Immunosuppression increases risk.

From National Eye Institute, available at www.nei.nih.gov/health/; American Cancer Society, available at www.cancer.org; National Institute on Deafness and Communication Disorders, available at www.nidcd.nih.gov/.

M, Modifiable risk factor.

HEAD AND NECK

Headaches

Headaches are one of the most common medical complaints of humans. Most recurrent headaches are symptoms of a chronic primary headache disorder; but they can also be associated with other problems such as ophthalmologic problems, dental problems, sinusitis, infections, adverse effects from medications, cerebral hemorrhage, or tumors. The pain associated with headaches can be mild or severe. Typically headaches can be classified based on the symptoms and history.

Migraine Headache

Migraine headache is the second most common headache syndrome in the United States. These headaches can occur in childhood, adolescence, or early adult life; young women are most susceptible. **Clinical Findings:** The headache generally starts with an aura caused by a vasospasm of intracranial arteries and is described as a throbbing unilateral distribution of the headache pain.[11] Accompanying signs may include feelings of depression, restlessness or irritability, photophobia, and nausea or vomiting. The headache may last up to 72 hours.

Cluster Headache

A cluster headache is considered to be the most painful of primary headaches. Cluster headaches are most common from adolescence to middle age. **Clinical Findings:** This type of headache is characterized by intense episodes of excruciating unilateral pain. A cluster headache may last from 30 minutes to 1 hour but may repeat daily for weeks at a time (hence the term *cluster*) followed by periods of remission, during which the person is completely free from the attacks. On average a cluster period lasts from 6 to 12 weeks; and remissions last for an average of 12 months, although they

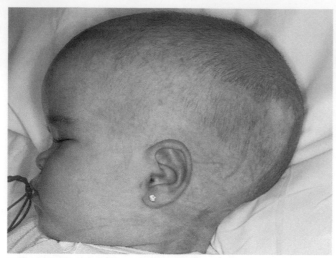

FIG. 10-57 Three-month-old infant with hydrocephalus. (From Bowden, 1998.)

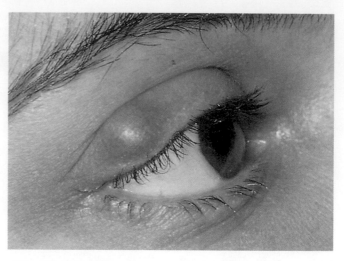

FIG. 10-58 Chalazion (right upper eyelid). (From Newell, 1992.)

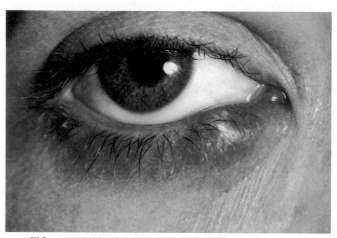

FIG. 10-59 Hordeolum (sty). (From Bedford, 1986.)

may last for years.[12] The pain is described as "burning," "boring," or "stabbing" pain behind one eye and may be accompanied by unilateral ptosis, ipsilateral lacrimation, and nasal stuffiness and drainage. Generally the headaches occur without warning, although some report a vague premonitory warning such as slight nausea.

Tension Headache

A tension headache is the most common type of headache experienced by adults between 20 and 40 years of age. **Clinical Findings:** It is usually bilateral and may be diffuse or confined to the frontal, temporal, parietal, or occipital area. The onset may be very gradual and may last for several days. The headache may be accompanied by contraction of the skeletal muscles of the face, jaw, and neck. Patients frequently describe this headache as feeling a tight band around their head.[12]

Posttraumatic Headache

This headache occurs secondary to a head injury or concussion. **Clinical Findings:** A posttraumatic headache is characterized by a dull, generalized head pain. Accompanying symptoms may be a lack of ability to concentrate, giddiness, or dizziness.

Hydrocephalus

Hydrocephalus is abnormal accumulation of cerebrospinal fluid (CSF) that may develop from infancy to adulthood. In infants hydrocephalus is usually a result of an obstruction of the drainage of CSF in the head. In adults it may be caused by obstruction of CSF circulation or resorption. **Clinical Findings:** In infants a gradual increase in intracranial pressure occurs, leading to an actual enlargement of the head (Fig. 10-57). As the head enlarges, the facial features appear small in proportion to the cranium; fontanels may bulge, and the scalp veins dilate. In adults the signs of increased intracranial pressure (decreased mental status, headache) are noted because the skull is unable to expand.

EYES

External Eye
Chalazion

A chalazion is a nodule of the meibomian gland in the eyelid. It may be tender if infected and often follows hordeolum or chronic inflammation such as conjunctivitis, blepharitis, or meibomian cyst (Fig. 10-58). **Clinical Findings:** A firm, nontender nodule is observed in the eyelid.

Hordeolum (Sty)

An acute infection originating in the sebaceous gland of the eyelid is termed a *hordeolum*. It is usually caused by *Staphylococcus aureus* (Fig. 10-59). **Clinical Findings:** The affected area usually is painful, red, and edematous.

Conjunctivitis

An inflammation of the palpebral or bulbar conjunctiva is termed *conjunctivitis*. It is caused by local infection of bacteria or virus and by an allergic reaction, systemic infection, or chemical irritation (Fig. 10-60). **Clinical Findings:** The eye

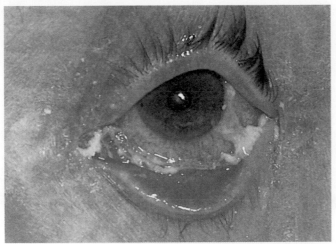

FIG. 10-60 Acute conjunctivitis. (From Newell, 1996.)

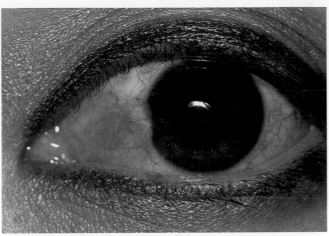

FIG. 10-62 Pterygium. (Courtesy Lemmi and Lemmi, 2013.)

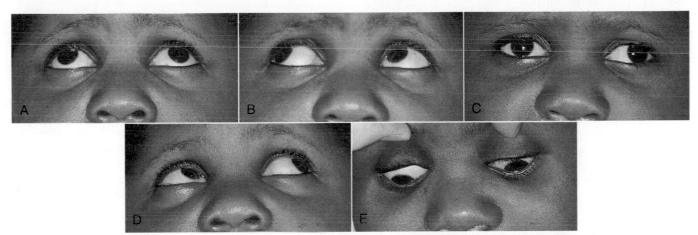

FIG. 10-61 This child has a form of strabismus called *exotropia* as seen by the outward turning of the eyes as they move in various fields of gaze. (From Yanoff and Duker, 2009.)

appears red, with thick, sticky discharge on the eyelids in the morning.

Corneal Abrasion or Ulcer

Disruptions of the corneal epithelium and stroma create a corneal abrasion or ulcer. It is caused by fungal, viral, or bacterial infections or desiccation (dryness) because of incomplete lid closure or poor lacrimal gland function. It can also be caused by scratches, foreign bodies, or contact lenses that are poorly fitted or overworn. **Clinical Findings:** The patient feels intense pain, has a foreign body sensation, and reports photophobia. Tearing and redness are observed.

Strabismus

An abnormal ocular alignment in which the visual axes do not meet at the desired point is termed *strabismus* (Fig. 10-61). Nonparalytic strabismus is caused by muscle weakness, focusing difficulties, unilateral refractive error, or anatomic differences in eyes. Paralytic strabismus is a motor imbalance caused by paresis or paralysis of an extraocular muscle. **Clinical Findings:** Two of the most common types of strabismus are esotropia and exotropia. Esotropia is an inward-turning eye and is the most common type of strabismus in infants. Exotropia is an outward-turning eye.

Pterygium

A pterygium is a noncancerous growth within the conjunctiva (the transparent tissue overlying the sclera). Although the exact cause is unknown, it is often associated with excessive exposure to sunlight and wind. This condition is most often seen among adults and older adults and rarely among children. **Clinical Findings:** The pterygium is usually painless; but it may cause inflammation or irritation or create a feeling of a foreign body in the eye. It appears as an area of raised white tissue, with blood vessels on the inner or outer edge of the cornea (Fig. 10-62).

Internal Eye
Cataract

A cataract is an opacity of the crystalline lens. It most commonly occurs from denaturation of lens protein caused by aging, but it can also be congenital or caused by trauma

(Fig. 10-63). **Clinical Findings:** Patients report cloudy or blurred vision; glare from headlights, lamps, or sunlight; and diplopia. They also report poor night vision and frequent changes in their glasses prescriptions.[13] A cloudy lens can be observed on inspection. The red reflex is absent because the light cannot penetrate the opacity of the lens.

Diabetic Retinopathy

Visual alteration caused by diabetes mellitus is termed *diabetic retinopathy*. It is caused by a deterioration of the retinal vasculature as a consequence of hyperglycemia and is the leading cause of blindness in working Americans.[14] Diabetic retinopathy can be nonproliferative and proliferative. **Clinical Findings:** Patients report decrease in vision. In nonproliferative diabetic retinopathy microaneurysms and hemorrhages are seen. Exudates may also be seen around the macula. Patients with proliferative diabetic retinopathy have elaborate vessel formation (i.e., vessels appear where they should not be) (Fig. 10-64, *A* to *C*).

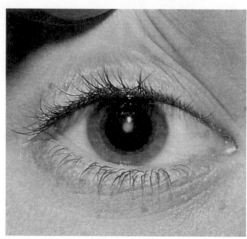

FIG. 10-63 Cataract. Note cloudy white spot over pupil. (From Zitelli, McIntire, and Nowalk, 2012.)

Glaucoma

Glaucoma is a group of diseases characterized by an increase in intraocular pressure. Untreated it causes damage to the optic nerve and leads to blindness.[15] Types of glaucoma include open-angle (most common), closed-angle, congenital, and glaucoma caused by drugs or other medical conditions (leads to open or closed glaucoma). **Clinical Findings:** No specific symptoms accompany open-angle glaucoma. Patients may report gradual and painless loss of peripheral vision, and the eye may be very firm to palpation. The most reliable indicator is an intraocular pressure measurement. Patients with closed-angle glaucoma complain of sharp eye pain and seeing a halo around lights. Clinical findings associated with congenital glaucoma usually begin during infancy within the first few months of life and include cloudiness over the pupil, red-appearing eye, eye enlargement (compared to other eye), and light sensitivity.

EARS

Foreign Body

A foreign body within the ear is most frequently seen in children, although it may occur in all age-groups. A foreign body can be any small object such as a small stone, a small part of a toy, or even an insect. **Clinical Findings:** The patient feels a sense of fullness in the ear and experiences decreased hearing. If the foreign body is a live insect, the patient may report hearing the insect move and often experiences severe pain. In this case symptoms may also include fever. Inspection of the auditory canal reveals the foreign body (Fig. 10-65).

Infection
Acute Otitis Media

Acute otitis media (AOM) is an infection of the middle ear. It can occur at any age but is one of the most common of all childhood infections.[16] **Clinical Findings:** The major

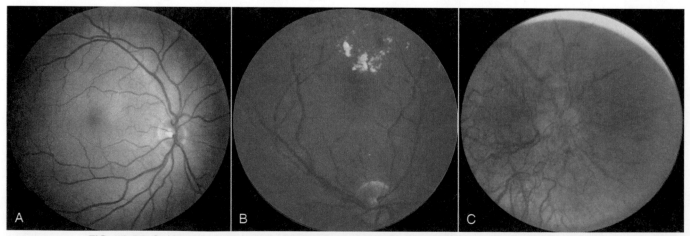

FIG. 10-64 A, Normal appearance of retinal structures. **B,** Nonproliferative diabetic retinopathy. **C,** Proliferative diabetic retinopathy. (**A** courtesy Lemmi and Lemmi, 2013. **B** from Bedford, 1986. **C** courtesy John W. Payne, MD, The Wilmer Ophthalmological Institute, The Johns Hopkins University and Hospital, Baltimore, MD. From Seidel et al., 2011.)

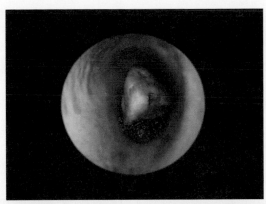

FIG. 10-65 Patient inserted a small stone into the deep part of the external ear canal. It is lying against the tympanic membrane. (From Bingham, Hawke, and Kwok, 1992.)

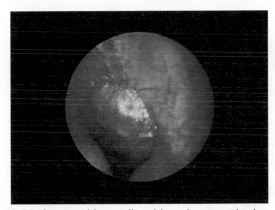

FIG. 10-66 Acute otitis media with redness and edematous swelling of the pars flaccida, shown in the central part of the illustration (left ear). (From Bingham, Hawke, and Kwok, 1992.)

symptom associated with AOM is ear pain (otalgia). Infants unable to verbally communicate pain may demonstrate irritability, fussiness, crying, lethargy, and pulling at the affected ear. Associated manifestations include fever, vomiting (infants), and decreased hearing (older children and adults). On inspection in the early stages, the TM appears inflamed; it is red and may be bulging and immobile (Fig. 10-66). Later stages may reveal discoloration (white or yellow drainage) and opacification to the TM. Purulent drainage from the ear canal with a sudden relief of pain suggests perforation.

Otitis Media with Effusion

Otitis media with effusion (OME) is an inflammation of the middle ear space resulting in accumulation of serous fluid in the middle ear. **Clinical Findings:** Common symptoms include a clogged sensation in the ears and problems with hearing and balance. Some report clicking or popping sounds within the ear. Because OME is not associated with acute inflammation (as with AOM), fever and ear pain are absent. On examination the TM is often retracted and is yellow or gray with limited mobility (Fig. 10-67).

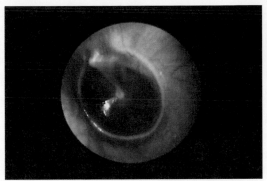

FIG. 10-67 Otitis media with effusion. (From Bingham, Hawke, and Kwok, 1992.)

Hearing Loss
Conductive Hearing Loss

Conductive hearing loss is caused by the interference of air conduction to the middle ear. It can result from blockage of the external auditory canal (such as a cerumen impaction), problems with the TM (perforations, retraction pockets, or tympanosclerosis), or problems within the middle ear (otitis media with effusion, otosclerosis, trauma, or cholesteatoma).[17] **Clinical Findings:** Typically the chief complaint is a decreased ability to hear and the report of muffled tones. Other findings depend on the cause; obstructions within the auditory canal or problems with the TM may be visible with otoscopic examination, whereas problems within the middle ear may not be visible. During a Weber's test, the patient reports sound heard in the affected ear. During a Rinne test, the patient hears bone conduction longer than air conduction.

Sensorineural Hearing Loss

Sensorineural hearing loss (SNHL) is caused by structural changes, disorders of the inner ear, or problems with the auditory nerve. SNHL accounts for over 90% of hearing loss cases.[8] Presbycusis, the most common cause of SNHL, is caused by atrophy and deterioration of the cells in the cochlea or atrophy, degeneration, and stiffening of cochlear motion. **Clinical Findings:** Presbycusis usually manifests as a gradual and progressive bilateral deafness with a loss of high-pitched tones. Patients with presbycusis have difficulty filtering background noise, making listening difficult. During a Weber's test, the patient reports sound in the unaffected ear. During a Rinne test, the patient hears air conduction longer than bone conduction, but it will be less than a 2 : 1 ratio.

NOSE
Epistaxis

The term *epistaxis* means bleeding from the nose. Epistaxis occurs in all age-groups but most commonly affects the elderly and is one of the most common conditions of the nose.[18] Common causes of nosebleeds include forceful sneezing or coughing, trauma, picking the nose, or heavy exertion. Some nosebleeds occur spontaneously without an obvious causative event. **Clinical Findings:** The primary sign and symptom is bleeding from the nose. Bleeding can be mild or heavy. Because of the high vascularity, most nosebleeds occur from Kiesselbach's area, which is located in the anterior aspect of the septum; however, bleeds from the posterior septum may also occur and tend to be more severe.

Inflammation/Infection
Allergic Rhinitis

The term *rhinitis* refers to inflammation of the nasal mucosa. Chronic rhinitis affects millions of individuals and is usually caused by an inhalant allergy, which may be a seasonal allergy or a year-round sensitivity to dust and molds. A strong family history is associated with allergic rhinitis. **Clinical Findings:** After exposure to the allergen the individual experiences sneezing, nasal congestion, and nasal drainage. Other symptoms can include itchy eyes, cough, and fatigue.[6] Turbinates are often enlarged and may appear pale or darker red.

Acute Sinusitis

This is an infection of the sinuses that typically occurs as a result of pooling of secretions within the sinuses, which often occurs after an upper respiratory infection. These pooled secretions provide a medium for bacterial growth. **Clinical Findings:** The most common symptom is throbbing pain within the affected sinus. The sinus is tender to palpation. The patient may also have fever; thick purulent nasal discharge; and edematous, erythematous nasal mucosa. If transillumination is performed, absence of a red glow is noted in the affected sinus.[19]

MOUTH

Inflammation/Infection
Herpes Simplex

A cold sore is a highly contagious, common viral infection caused by the herpes simplex type 1 virus. It is spread by direct contact. Recurrent infections occur following a stimulus of sun exposure, cold temperature, fever, or allergy. Herpes simplex lesions also can occur in the mouth. **Clinical Findings:** The patient typically has a prodromal burning, tingling, or pain sensation before the outbreak of the lesions.[20] They usually appear on the lip-skin junction as groups of vesicular lesions with an erythematous base. Like other herpes infections, the lesions progress from vesicles, to pustules, and finally to crusts (Fig. 10-68). Herpes simplex lesions in the mouth appear as white ulcerations (Fig. 10-69).

Gingivitis

A common condition among adults, gingivitis is an inflammation of the gingivae (gums). It can be acute, chronic, or recurrent. The most common cause is poor dental hygiene, leading to the formation of bacterial plaque on the tooth surface at the gum line, resulting in inflammation. **Clinical Findings:** Hyperplasia of the gums, erythema, and bleeding with manipulation are the most common signs[21] (Fig. 10-70). Edema of the gum tissue deepens the crevice between

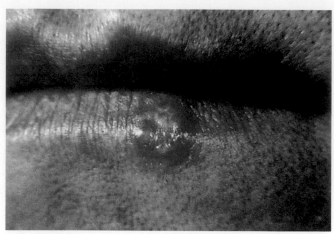

FIG. 10-68 Herpes simplex lesion (cold sore) of the lower lip. (From Grimes, 1991.)

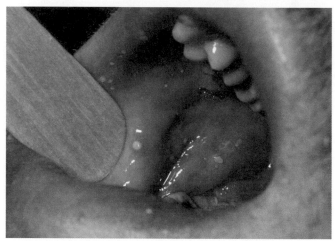

FIG. 10-69 Herpes simplex lesions on the mucous membranes of the mouth. (Courtesy Lemmi and Lemmi, 2013.)

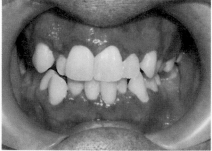

FIG. 10-70 Gingivitis. Note enlargement of gums. (From Bingham, Hawke, and Kwok, 1992.)

the gingivae and teeth, allowing for the formation of gingival pockets where food particles collect, causing further inflammation. Periodontitis occurs when the inflammatory process causes erosion of the gum tissue and loosening of the teeth.

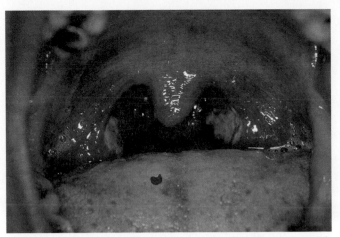

FIG. 10-71 Tonsillitis. (Courtesy Lemmi and Lemmi, 2013.)

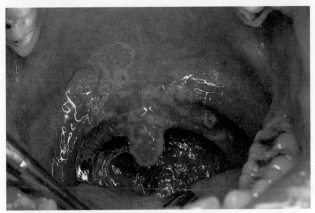

FIG. 10-72 Candidiasis. (From Regezi, Sciubba, and Jordan, 2012.)

Tonsillitis

Tonsillitis is infection of the tonsils. Common bacterial pathogens include beta-hemolytic and other streptococci. **Clinical Findings:** The classic presentation of tonsillitis includes sore throat, pain with swallowing (odynophagia), fever, chills, and tender cervical lymph nodes. Some patients may also complain of ear pain.[22] On inspection the tonsils appear enlarged and red and may be covered with white or yellow exudates (Fig. 10-71).

Candidiasis (Thrush)

Candidiasis is an opportunistic infection typically caused by *Candida albicans.* Thrush is commonly seen among individuals who are chronically debilitated, in patients who are immunosuppressed, or as a result of antibiotic therapy. **Clinical Findings:** Oral candidiasis appears as soft, white plaques on the tongue, buccal mucosa, or posterior pharynx (Fig. 10-72). If the membrane is peeled off, a raw, bleeding, erythematous, eroded, or ulcerated surface results.

Lesions
Aphthous Ulcer (Canker Sore)

A canker sore is a common oral lesion with an unknown etiology that affects up to 66% of the population.[23] **Clinical Findings:** These lesions are very painful and appear on the buccal mucosa, the lips, the tongue, or the palate as round or oval ulcerative lesions with a yellow-white center and an erythematous halo (Fig. 10-73). The ulcers may last up to 2 weeks.

Oral Cancer

Oral cancers can occur on the lip or within the oral cavity and oropharynx. An estimated 39,400 new cases of new cases were diagnosed in 2011.[24] **Clinical Findings:** Oral cancer lesions are often subtle and asymptomatic in early stages; premalignant changes of the oral mucosa such as white or red patches (leukoplakia and erythroplakia) may be seen. These lesions progress to painless, nonhealing ulcers (Fig. 10-74, *A* and *B*). Later-stage signs and symptoms include enlarged, hard, nontender cervical chain or submental lymph nodes;

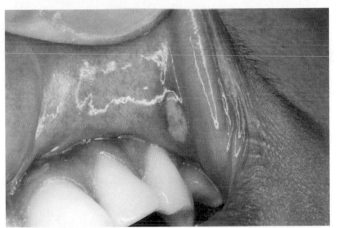

FIG. 10-73 Small aphthous ulcer (canker sore) on the lower lip (From Bingham, Hawke, and Kwok, 1992.)

noticeable mass; bleeding; loosening of teeth; difficulty wearing dentures; and difficulty swallowing.

NECK

Thyroid Disorders
Hyperthyroidism

Hyperthyroidism is a condition associated with excessive production and secretion of thyroid hormone. Of the several diseases that can cause hyperthyroidism, Graves' disease, a familial autoimmune disorder, is the most common cause.[25] **Clinical Findings:** Because thyroid hormone affects all body tissue, most body systems are affected. The signs and symptoms reflect increased metabolism and may include enlargement of the thyroid gland and exophthalmos (see Fig. 10-18). Auscultation of the goiter may reveal a bruit.

Hypothyroidism

Hypothyroidism, the most common problem associated with thyroid function, is characterized by a decreased production

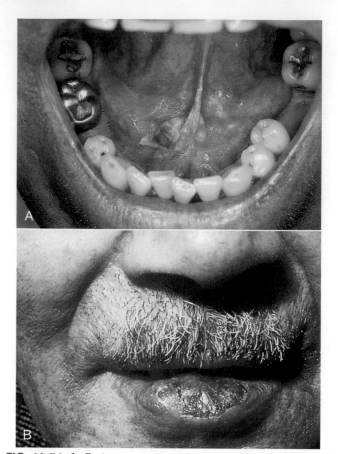

FIG. 10-74 A, Early squamous cell carcinoma on the floor of the mouth. **B,** Squamous cell carcinoma on the lip. (**A** from Regezi, Sciubba, and Jordan, 2012. **B** from Hill, 1994.)

of thyroid hormone by the thyroid gland. Several etiologies have been linked to hypothyroidism, including autoimmune thyroiditis, decreased secretion of thyroid-releasing hormone from the hypothalamus, congenital defects, a result of treatment for hyperthyroidism (i.e., antithyroid drugs or surgical resection of thyroid tissue), atrophy of the thyroid gland, and iodine deficiency.[26] **Clinical Findings:** Clinical findings reflect an overall decreased metabolism; patients seem to be in "slow motion," with a depressed affect. Goiter may be seen with hypothyroidism because of increases in thyroid-stimulating hormone (see Fig. 10-52).

Thyroid Cancer

Thyroid cancer is the most common type of endocrine malignancy. **Clinical Findings:** Thyroid cancer frequently does not cause symptoms. Typically it is first discovered as a small nodule on the thyroid gland. As the tumor grows, changes in the voice and problems with swallowing or breathing may be experienced because of invasion of the tumor into the larynx, esophagus, and trachea, respectively.

Lymphoma

Lymphomas are a group of disorders characterized by malignant neoplasms of the lymph tissue. They occur in adolescents, young adults, and people over 50 years of age. **Clinical Findings:** Malignant lymphomas cause lymph nodes to be large, discrete, nontender, and firm to rubbery. Enlarged nodes usually are unilateral and localized; however, chronic lymphocytic leukemia causes generalized lymphadenopathy. Hodgkin's disease is a malignant lymphoma characterized by a painless, progressive enlargement of lymphoid tissue, usually first evident by the cervical lymph nodes, splenomegaly, and atypical macrophages.

CLINICAL APPLICATION AND CLINICAL REASONING

See Appendix D for answers to exercises in this section.

REVIEW QUESTIONS

1. A patient describes a recent onset of frequent and severe unilateral headaches that last about 1 hour. Based on these symptoms, the nurse suspects which type of headache?
   1. Cluster headaches
   2. Migraine headaches
   3. Tension headache
   4. Sinus headache

2. During a physical examination the nurse is unable to feel the patient's thyroid gland with palpation. What is the appropriate action of the nurse at this time?
   1. Recognize that this is an expected finding.
   2. Auscultate the thyroid area.
   3. Percuss the anterior neck for thyroid span.
   4. Refer the patient for follow-up with an endocrinologist.

3. A 24-year-old female patient has a 2-day history of clear nasal drainage. Based on these data, which question is the most logical for the nurse to ask?
   1. "Is there a foul odor coming from your nose?"
   2. "Have you recently had nosebleeds?"
   3. "Do you snore when sleeping?"
   4. "Do you have allergies?"

4. A 32-year-old woman has a 4-day history of sore throat and difficulty swallowing. The nurse observes tonsils covered with yellow patches. The tonsils are so large that they fill the entire oropharynx and appear to be touching. How does the nurse document these findings?
   1. "Tonsils yellow and swollen."
   2. "Enlarged tonsils 4+ with yellow exudate."
   3. "Strep infection to tonsils with 3+ swelling."
   4. "1+ edema of tonsils with pus."

5. A nurse is obtaining a health history from a 52-year-old male patient with a red lesion at the base of the tongue. What additional data does the nurse specifically collect about this patient?
   1. Alcohol and tobacco use
   2. The date of his last dental examination
   3. The presence of dentures
   4. A history of pyorrhea

6. While talking with a patient, the nurse suspects that he has hearing loss. Which examination technique is most accurate for assessing hearing loss?
   1. Whispered voice test
   2. Rinne test
   3. Weber's test
   4. Audiometry test

7. Which data from the health history of a 42-year-old man should be evaluated further as a possible risk for hearing loss?
   1. "I watch TV in the evenings with my wife and children."
   2. "When I was younger, I wore an earring."
   3. "My primary hobby is carpentry work."
   4. "I have been an accountant for 16 years for an insurance agency."

8. The nurse examines a patient's auditory canal and tympanic membrane with an otoscope. Which finding is considered abnormal?
   1. Presence of cerumen
   2. Yellow or amber color to the tympanic membrane
   3. Presence of a cone of light
   4. Shiny, translucent tympanic membrane

9. During the history the patient indicates that her eyes have been red and itching. Which additional question does the nurse ask?
   1. "Have you ever had a detached retina?"
   2. "Have you had the pressure in your eyes checked?"
   3. "Do you have seasonal allergies?"
   4. "Do you also have double vision?"

10. How does the nurse assess a patient's consensual reaction?
    1. By touching the cornea with a small piece of sterile cotton and observing the change in the pupil size
    2. By observing the patient's pupil size when she or he looks at an object 2 to 3 feet away and then looks at an object 6 to 8 inches away
    3. By shining a light into the patient's right eye and observing the pupillary reaction of the left eye
    4. By covering one eye with a card and observing the pupillary reaction when the card is removed

11. What are the characteristics of lymph nodes in patients who have an acute infection?
    1. They are enlarged and tender.
    2. They are round, rubbery, and mobile.
    3. They are hard, fixed, and painless.
    4. They are soft, mobile, and painless.

12. Which technique is used for palpating lymph nodes?
    1. Apply firm pressure over the nodes with the pads of the fingers.
    2. Apply gentle pressure over the nodes with the tips of the fingers.
    3. Apply firm pressure anterior to the nodes with the tips of the fingers.
    4. Apply gentle pressure over the nodes with the pads of the fingers.

CASE STUDY

Trudy Neinto is a 25-year-old Native American (Navajo) female who was brought to the clinic by her sister. The following data are collected by the nurse during an interview and assessment.

Interview Data

The patient tells the nurse, "My ear is hurting very badly, and I'm hot." She adds, "I wanted to go to the clinic yesterday, but my grandmother told me I shouldn't." Trudy tells the nurse, "I have been treated many times for this problem over the last several years by the medicine man. Last night I had drainage from my ears. Grandmother told me that this was a sign that the illness was being chased from my body. I did not know what it was, but I felt scared."

Examination Data

- *General survey:* Healthy-appearing adult female. Temperature: 101.8° F (38.8° C).

- *External ear examination:* Typical position of ears bilaterally. Left ear pinna red. Dried purulent drainage noted on left external ear and in left external canal. Grimaces when left ear is touched. Right ear unremarkable.
- *Internal canal and tympanic membrane:* Dried drainage noted in left ear canal. TM perforated. Right ear unremarkable.
- *Hearing examination:* Whisper test in right ear 80%; whisper test in left ear 0%.

Clinical Reasoning

1. Which data deviate from normal findings, suggesting a need for further investigation?
2. For which additional information should the nurse ask or assess?
3. Based on the data, which risk factors for hearing loss does Trudy have?
4. With which additional health care professionals should you consider collaborating to meet her health care needs?

Lungs and Respiratory System

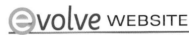
CONCEPT OVERVIEW

The feature concept for this chapter is *Oxygenation*. This concept represents processes that facilitate and impair oxygenation to and from tissues. Several concepts are interrelated with oxygenation and are shown in the following illustration.

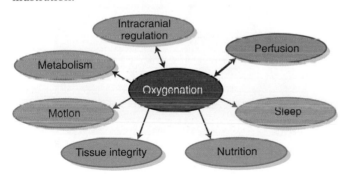

Because adequate perfusion is necessary to deliver oxygenated blood to and remove metabolic wastes from tissues, this interrelationship is foundational to all others. Intracranial regulation supports respiratory function, and adequate oxygenation is needed to support intracranial function. Metabolism, motion, tissue integrity, sleep, and nutrition all require

adequate oxygenation for optimal function. Having an understanding of the interrelationship of these concepts helps the nurse recognize risk factors and thus increases awareness when conducting a health assessment.

The following case provides a clinical example featuring several of these interrelated concepts.

> John Armstrong is a 59-year-old man who has smoked a pack of cigarettes each day for 41 years. He has chronic obstructive pulmonary disease, which affects his lungs in two ways. Obstructed bronchi increase the work needed to get air into his lungs, and destruction of alveoli impairs diffusion of oxygen into pulmonary capillaries and leads to trapping of air. These changes in oxygenation result in hypoxemia. Low arterial oxygen causes dyspnea, which limits his motion (because of activity intolerance), especially when he walks upstairs or any distances over two blocks. Not only does hypoxemia reduce appetite, but Mr. Armstrong often becomes short of breath when eating; thus he has experienced unintentional weight loss and has become malnourished. Because he becomes dyspneic when fully reclined, Mr. Armstrong props himself up with three pillows or sleeps in his recliner. He reports that he has not slept more than a few hours at a time for several months.

ANATOMY AND PHYSIOLOGY

The primary purpose of the respiratory system is to supply oxygen to cells and remove carbon dioxide. This purpose is accomplished using the processes of ventilation and diffusion. *Ventilation* is the process of moving gases in and out of

the lungs by inspiration and expiration. *Diffusion* is the process by which oxygen and carbon dioxide move from areas of high concentration to areas of lower concentration. For example, at the end of inspiration the concentration of

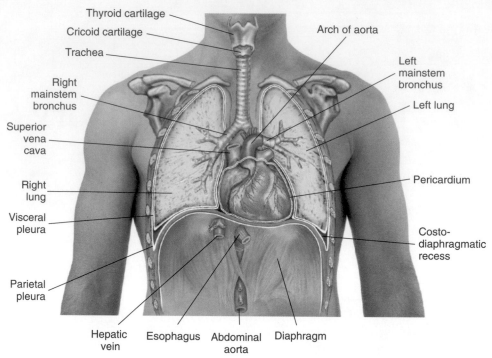

FIG. 11-1 Structures within the thoracic cavity. (From Seidel et al., 2011.)

oxygen is higher in the alveoli than it is in pulmonary capillaries. This difference in concentration causes oxygen to move or diffuse from alveoli across the alveolar-capillary membrane to the adjacent pulmonary capillaries, where it is carried by erythrocytes to cells. At the cellular level oxygen diffuses into the cells; and carbon dioxide diffuses from the cells into the capillaries, where it is carried by erythrocytes to alveoli. Carbon dioxide diffuses from the pulmonary capillaries to the alveoli and is exhaled. The cardiovascular system provides transportation of oxygen and carbon dioxide between alveoli and cells.

STRUCTURES WITHIN THE THORAX

There are three main structures within the thorax or chest: the mediastinum and the right and left pleural cavities. The mediastinum is positioned in the middle of the chest. Within it lie the heart, the arch of aorta, the superior vena cava, the lower esophagus, and the lower part of the trachea. The pleural cavities contain the lungs. These cavities are lined with two types of serous membranes: the parietal and visceral pleurae. The chest wall and diaphragm are protected by the parietal pleura, and the lungs are protected by the visceral pleura. A small amount of fluid lubricates the space between the pleurae to reduce friction as the lungs move during inspiration and expiration (Fig. 11-1). The right lung has three lobes, and the left has two. Each lobe has a major, oblique fissure dividing the upper and lower portions; however, the right lung has a lesser horizontal fissure dividing the upper lung into upper and middle lobes (Fig. 11-2). Each lung

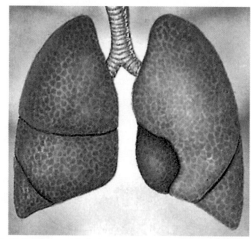

FIG. 11-2 Right and left lung. Note fissures dividing lobes of the lungs.

extends anteriorly about 1.5 inches (4 cm) above the first rib into the base of the neck in adults and posteriorly approximately to the level of T1 (first thoracic vertebra). The base or lower border of each lung expands approximately down to T12 during deep inspiration and rises approximately to T9 on expiration (Fig. 11-3, *A* and *B*).

EXTERNAL THORAX

Most of the respiratory system is protected by the thoracic cage consisting of 11 thoracic vertebrae, 12 pairs of ribs, and

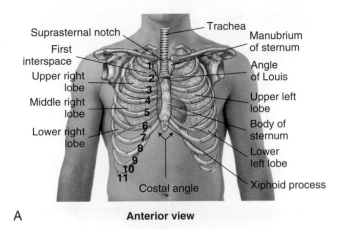

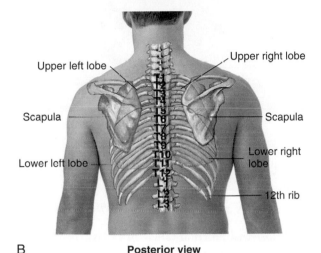

FIG. 11-3 Thorax and underlying structures. **A,** Anterior view. **B,** Posterior view.

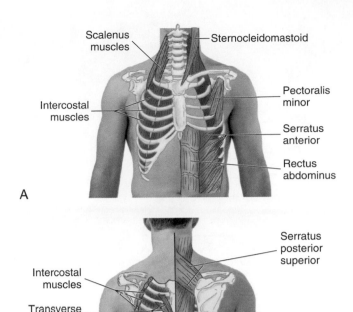

FIG. 11-4 Muscles involved in ventilation. **A,** Anterior view. **B,** Posterior view. (From Seidel et al., 2011.)

the sternum. All the ribs are connected to the thoracic vertebrae posteriorly. The first seven ribs are also connected anteriorly to the sternum by the costal cartilages. The costal cartilages of the eighth to tenth ribs are connected immediately superior to the ribs. The eleventh and twelfth ribs are unattached anteriorly and are called *floating ribs.* The tips of the eleventh ribs are located in the lateral thorax, and those of the twelfth ribs are located in the posterior thorax (see Fig. 11-3).

The adult sternum is about 7 inches (17 cm) long and has three components: the manubrium, the body, and the xiphoid process. The manubrium and the body of the sternum articulate with the first seven ribs; the manubrium also supports the clavicle. The intercostal space (ICS) is the area between the ribs. The ICS is named according to the rib immediately above it. Thus the first ICS is located between the first and second ribs (see Fig. 11-3, *A*).

MECHANICS OF BREATHING

The diaphragm and the intercostal muscles are the primary muscles of inspiration. During inspiration the diaphragm

contracts and pushes the abdominal contents down while the intercostal muscles help to push the chest wall outward. These combined efforts decrease the intrathoracic pressure, which creates a negative pressure within the lungs compared with the pressure outside the lungs. This pressure difference causes the lungs to fill with air. During expiration the muscles relax, expelling the air as the intrathoracic pressure rises. Accessory muscles that may contribute to respiratory effort include anteriorly the sternocleidomastoid, scalenus, pectoralis minor, serratus anterior, and rectus abdominis muscles and posteriorly the serratus posterior superior, transverse thoracic, and serratus posterior inferior muscles (Fig. 11-4, A and B).

During inspiration air is drawn in through the mouth or nose and passes through the pharynx and the larynx to reach the trachea, a flexible tube approximately 4 inches (10 cm) long in the adult. These structures (i.e., the nose, pharynx, larynx, and trachea) make up the upper airway (Fig. 11-5), which has three functions in respiration: to conduct air to the lower airway; to protect the lower airway from foreign matter; and to warm, filter, and humidify inspired air. The lower airway consists of the right and left main-stem bronchi, the segmental and subsegmental bronchi, the terminal bronchioles, and alveoli (Fig. 11-6). The trachea splits into a left and right main-stem bronchus at about the level of T4 and T5. The right bronchus is shorter, wider, and more vertical

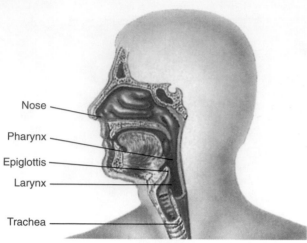

FIG. 11-5 Structures of the upper airway.

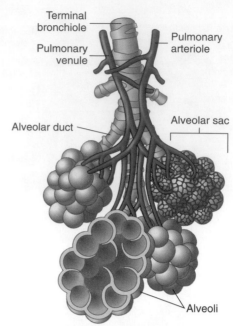

FIG. 11-7 Alveolar sac. (From Patton and Thibodeau, 2010.)

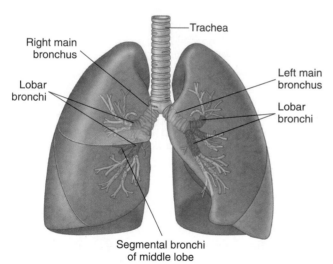

FIG. 11-6 Structures of the lower airway. (From Drake, Vogl, and Mitchell, 2010.)

than the left bronchus. The bronchi are further subdivided into increasingly smaller bronchioles. Each bronchiole opens into an alveolar duct and terminates in multiple alveoli, where gas exchanges occur (Fig. 11-7).

TOPOGRAPHIC MARKERS

Surface landmarks are helpful in locating underlying structures and describing the exact location of physical findings (Fig. 11-8, *A* to *C*).

Anterior Chest Wall

- Nipples
- Suprasternal notch: The depression at the anterior aspect of the neck, just above the manubrium
- Manubriosternal junction (angle of Louis): The junction between the manubrium and sternum; useful for rib identification
- Midsternal line: Imaginary vertical line through the middle of the sternum
- Costal angle: Intersection of the costal margins, usually no more than 90 degrees. The costal margins are the medial margins formed by the false ribs, from the eighth to the tenth ribs (see Fig. 11-8, *A*)
- Clavicles: Bones extending out both sides of the manubrium to the shoulder; they cover the first ribs
- Midclavicular lines: Imaginary vertical lines on the right and left sides of the chest that are "drawn" through the clavicle midpoints parallel to the midsternal line

Lateral Chest Wall

- Anterior axillary lines: Imaginary vertical lines on the right and left sides of the chest "drawn" from anterior axillary folds through the anterolateral chest, parallel to the midsternal line
- Posterior axillary lines: Imaginary vertical lines on the right and left sides of the chest "drawn" from the posterior axillary folds along the posterolateral thoracic wall with abducted lateral arm
- Midaxillary lines: Imaginary vertical lines on the right and left sides of the chest "drawn" from axillary apices; midway between and parallel to the anterior and posterior axillary lines (see Fig. 11-8, *B*)

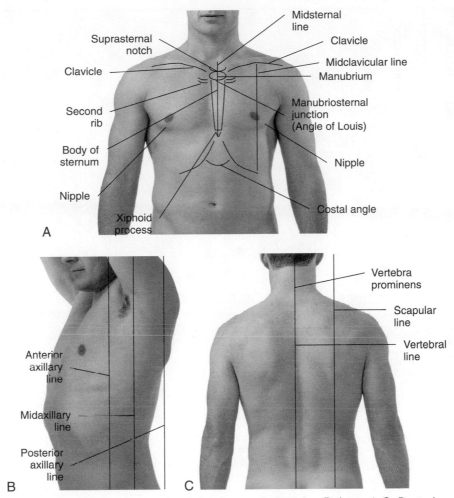

FIG. 11-8 Topographic landmarks of the thorax. **A,** Anterior. **B,** Lateral. **C,** Posterior.

Posterior Chest Wall
- Vertebra prominens: Spinous process of C7; visible and palpable with the head bent forward
- Vertebral line: Imaginary vertical line "drawn" along the posterior vertebral spinous processes
- Scapular lines: Imaginary vertical lines on the right and left sides of the chest "drawn" parallel to the mid-spinal line; they pass through inferior angles of the scapulae in the upright patient with arms at sides (see Fig 11-8, *C*)

HEALTH HISTORY

GENERAL HEALTH HISTORY

Nurses interview patients to collect subjective data about their present health and any past medical experiences. In addition to present health status, past medical history, family history, and personal and psychosocial history, nurses ask patients about their home environment, occupational environment, and travel, which may affect the functions of the their lungs and respiratory system. Quality Improvement Competencies for Nurses are shown in Table 11-1 on p. 196, which presents knowledge, skills, and attitudes to use when demonstrating patient-centered care and interdisciplinary teamwork with health care providers and respiratory therapists.

Present Health Status
Do you have any chronic illnesses?
Many chronic illnesses can cause symptoms that affect the respiratory system, including heart disease or renal disease, which may cause pulmonary edema.

TABLE 11-1 QUALITY IMPROVEMENT COMPETENCIES FOR NURSES: LUNGS AND RESPIRATORY ASSESSMENT

KNOWLEDGE	SKILLS	ATTITUDES
Patient-Centered Care		
Integrate understanding of multiple dimensions of patient-centered care: • Patient/family/community preferences, values • Information, communication, and education • Involvement of family and friends	Elicit patient values, preferences, and expressed needs as part of clinical interview. Communicate patient values, preferences, and expressed needs to other members of health care team.	Value seeing health care situations "through patients' eyes." Respect and encourage individual expression of patient values, preferences, and expressed needs. Value patient's expertise with own health and symptoms.
Describe how diverse cultural, ethnic, and social backgrounds function as sources of patient, family, and community values.	Provide patient-centered care with sensitivity and respect for the diversity of human experience	Recognize personally held attitudes about working with patients from different ethnic, cultural, and social backgrounds.
Demonstrate comprehensive understanding of the concepts of pain and suffering, including physiologic models of pain and comfort.	Assess presence and extent of pain and suffering, Assess levels of physical and emotional comfort.	Recognize personally held values and beliefs about the management of pain or suffering.
Discuss principles of effective communication.	Discuss principles of effective communication.	Value continuous improvement of own communication.
Interdisciplinary Teamwork		
Describe own strengths, limitations, and values in functioning as a member of a team.	Demonstrate awareness of own strengths and limitations as a team member. Act with integrity, consistency, and respect for differing views.	Acknowledge own potential to contribute to effective team functioning. Appreciate importance of intraprofessional and interprofessional collaboration.
Recognize contributions of other individuals and groups in helping patient/family achieve health goals.	Function competently within own scope of practice as a member of the health care team. Initiate requests for help when appropriate to situation.	Respect the centrality of the patient/family as core members of any health care team. Respect the unique attributes that members bring to a team, including variations in professional orientations and accountabilities.

Available at www.qsen.org, Competency KSA Prelicensure.

Do you have allergies? If so, to what are you allergic? Describe your symptoms. How frequently do you have these symptoms?

The severity of allergies can range from mild seasonal allergies to an anaphylactic allergic reaction. Respiratory symptoms can range from runny nose, nasal congestion, and cough to wheezes and dyspnea. An increased frequency may indicate the onset of new allergies or ineffective therapy for respiratory disease.

Do you have difficulty breathing during your daily activities? If so, describe the difficulty.

Individuals who have no difficulty breathing until they are active may have pulmonary or heart disease that limits the availability of oxygen needed during exertion. The nurse may need to collect additional data from this individual as described in the next section under the heading "Shortness of breath."

Do you have difficulty breathing when you're lying flat? Do you prop yourself up with pillows to make your breathing easier?

When the body is lying flat, the abdominal contents push against the diaphragm. Individuals with pulmonary disease may experience an increased work of breathing because of pressure of the abdominal contents against the diaphragm. They may prop themselves up with pillows, which moves the abdominal contents away from the diaphragm, to make it easier to breathe.

Are you currently taking any oral medications for a respiratory disorder? If so, which medications are you taking and how effective are they?

Medications taken to treat respiratory disorders and their effectiveness need to be documented.

Do you use an inhaler? If yes, which medication is in the inhaler, what is the purpose of the medication, and how often do you use the inhaler?

Individuals with asthma may use inhalers to prevent symptoms, treat bronchial inflammation, and dilate bronchi. How frequently they use their inhalers is an indication of how well their symptoms are controlled. These questions also assess their understanding of the reason for taking the medications. Individuals may report ineffective response to medications delivered by their inhaler because they are using them incorrectly.

Do you use oxygen at home? If yes, describe which equipment you use, how much oxygen you use, and how often you use it. Does the oxygen relieve your symptoms?

Many individuals with chronic pulmonary disease use oxygen at home. The frequency, amount, and effect help determine the adequacy of this therapy.

Past Health History

Have you ever had any problems with your lungs? If yes, describe.

Asking this question may encourage individuals to describe symptoms they may be experiencing. These symptoms may or may not have been diagnosed and treated in the past.

Have you been diagnosed with a respiratory disease such as asthma, bronchitis, bronchiectasis, emphysema, cystic fibrosis, lung cancer, tuberculosis, or pneumonia? If yes, please describe.

Background information regarding respiratory problems tells which types of problems the person is likely to experience and which clinical findings to anticipate.

Have you ever had an injury to your chest? Surgery to your chest? If yes, describe.

The incidence of injury or surgery may provide additional information about a possible respiratory or lung problem.

Family History

Is there a family history of lung disease? Cancer? Tuberculosis? Cystic fibrosis? Emphysema? Asthma? If yes, which family member and what is the condition?

Family history may be used to determine risk for this individual.

Personal and Psychosocial History

Do you smoke or have you been a smoker in the past? If yes, what do (did) you smoke (cigarettes, cigar, pipe)? How long have you smoked (did you smoke)? How often do you (did you) smoke? Have you ever tried to quit smoking? If yes, describe. What helped you quit? Why do you think your attempt was unsuccessful?

These questions determine the patient's smoking history and if there is an interest in quitting. If the individual is or has been a smoker, determine the number of pack-years that the individual has smoked (Box 11-1).

Home Environment

Are there environmental conditions that may affect your breathing at home? If yes, what are they and how do they affect your breathing? Common things to consider include the following:

- **Air pollution (near factory, on a busy street, new construction in area)**
- **Possible allergens in home such as pets**
- **Type of heating or air conditioning, including filtering system, humidification, and ventilation**

BOX 11-1 RECORDING TOBACCO USE

Cigarette use is documented by *pack-years*. A pack-year is the number of years that a patient has smoked multiplied by the number of packs of cigarettes smoked each day. If a patient tells you that he or she smoked one-half pack of cigarettes a day for 40 years, it would be recorded as a 20 pack-year smoking history.

Use of pipes, cigars, marijuana, chewing tobacco, or snuff is usually recorded in the amount used daily.

- **Hobbies: Woodworking, plants, metal work**
- **Exposure to the smoke of others in your home**

A number of respiratory irritants found in or near the home may cause temporary or permanent lung damage. Environmental tobacco smoke (also known as secondhand smoke) has been shown to affect nonsmokers.[1]

Occupational Environment

Where do you work? Are you frequently exposed to respiratory irritants at work? Dust? Vapors? Chemicals? Paint fumes? Irritants such as asbestos? Known allergens?

The person may be exposed to respiratory irritants in the workplace. These irritants may be risk factors for pulmonary diseases. The person may or may not be aware of the presence of irritants.

If you are exposed to respiratory irritants, do you wear a mask or a respirator mask? Does your work area have a special ventilatory system to clear out pollutants? Do you wear a monitor to evaluate exposure? Do you have periodic health examinations, pulmonary function tests, or x-ray examinations?

Individuals may not be able to alter the presence of environmental irritants that are in the work environment. Instead they must use protective equipment such as masks, respirators, or ventilation hoods to reduce the amount of exposure to respiratory irritants. Regulatory agencies such as the Occupational Safety and Health Administration (OSHA) have guidelines and regulations to reduce the amount of occupational exposure to respiratory irritants.[2]

Travel

Have you recently traveled to foreign countries or areas of the United States where you may have been exposed to uncommon respiratory diseases (e.g., histoplasmosis in the Southeast and Midwest; schistosomiasis or sudden acute respiratory syndrome [SARS] in Southwest Asia, the Caribbean, and Asia)?

Travel to other areas of the country or world may expose people to infections to which they have little or no resistance, increasing their susceptibility to infection.

PROBLEM-BASED HISTORY

Commonly reported problems related to the lungs are cough, shortness of breath, and chest pain with breathing. As with symptoms in all areas of health assessment, a symptom analysis is completed using the mnemonic OLD CARTS, which includes the *Onset, Location, Duration, Characteristics, Aggravating* factors, *Related* symptoms, *Treatment,* and *Severity* (see Box 2-3).

Cough

When did you first notice the cough? Is it constant or does it come and go? Has it changed since you first noticed it?

A cough can be acute (sudden onset and usually lasting less than 3 weeks) or chronic (lasting longer than 3 weeks).

Common causes of acute cough are viral infections, allergic rhinitis, acute asthma, acute bacterial sinusitis, or environmental irritants. Chronic cough is commonly caused by postnasal drip, gastroesophageal reflux disease (GERD), asthma, infections such as chronic bronchitis, and blood pressure drugs. Angiotensin-converting enzyme (ACE) inhibitors such as captopril, commonly prescribed for high blood pressure and heart failure, are known to cause chronic cough in some people.[3]

Describe your cough. Is it dry? Productive? Hacking? Hoarse?

A description of the cough may provide clues to the cause. For example, viral pneumonia causes a dry cough, whereas bacterial pneumonia causes a productive cough.

How often do you cough up sputum (all of the time or periodically)? How much sputum do you cough up?

The frequency of sputum production and the time of day most sputum is produced should be explored. Increased sputum in the morning implies an accumulation of sputum during the night and is common with bronchitis. Sputum production with a change in position suggests lung abscess and bronchiectasis. The amount of sputum production can vary from a few teaspoons to a copious amount (a pint or more).

What is the color of the sputum?

Documenting the appearance of the sputum is important. Some conditions have characteristic sputum production; for example, white or clear sputum may occur with colds, viral infections, or bronchitis; yellow or green sputum may occur with bacterial infections; black sputum may occur with smoke or coal dust inhalation; or rust-colored sputum may occur with tuberculosis or pneumococcal pneumonia. *Hemoptysis* is the expectoration of sputum containing blood. It may vary in severity from slight streaking of blood to frank bleeding.

What is the consistency of the sputum (thick, thin, frothy)?

The consistency of sputum may be described as thin, thick, gelatinous, sticky, or frothy. Pink, frothy sputum with dyspnea is associated with pulmonary edema. Thick sputum is commonly associated with cystic fibrosis.

Have you noticed if the sputum has an odor?

Foul-smelling (fetid) sputum is typically associated with bacterial pneumonia, lung abscess, or bronchiectasis.

Have you noticed any other symptoms along with the cough such as shortness of breath, chest pain or tightness with breathing, fever, stuffy nose, noisy respiration, hoarseness, or gagging? Does the cough tire you out? Does it keep you awake at night?

A cough may be a symptom of pulmonary problems, or it may exist in conjunction with other problems. Associated signs and symptoms are important factors to assess when trying to determine the underlying cause of the cough. For example, a cough associated with a fever, shortness of breath, and noisy breath sounds may indicate a lung infection; whereas tightness of the chest associated with shortness of breath and a nonproductive cough is more likely to be associated with a problem such as asthma.

Have you done anything to treat the cough yourself such as medications, fluids, or a vaporizer? Have these measures been effective?

Determining what has been used to relieve symptoms may help you understand the problem and may guide current treatment strategies.

Shortness of Breath

How long have you had shortness of breath? Are you short of breath all the time, or does it come and go?

Shortness of breath, or dyspnea, occurs when breathing becomes difficult. Some conditions such as pneumonia may cause sudden onset of shortness of breath; other conditions such as heart failure may be associated with a more gradual onset. Some people may experience shortness of breath at intervals over a period of time. When taking a history from a person who has dyspnea, notice how many words the person can say between breaths. Box 11-2 contains information about how to document this finding.

How would you describe your shortness of breath? Is it harder to inhale or exhale or are both equally affected? Do the symptoms interfere with your activities?

Knowing the person's perception of the severity and the extent of disablement, if any, helps understand the extent to which the dyspnea is interfering with the daily activities.

Does anything seem to trigger these episodes or make the shortness of breath worse such as activity or environmental factors? If they occur when you are lying flat, such as during sleep, in which position do you sleep? How many pillows do you use to prop behind you? Do you sleep in a recliner? Does changing your position affect the problem?

Causative factors for the dyspnea should be determined. If it is brought on by activity, find out how much exercise precipitates the episode (e.g., number of steps climbed, blocks walked). Positions or other conditions may also initiate dyspnea. *Orthopnea* is difficulty breathing when the individual is lying down. People may describe using several pillows to prop themselves up in bed to relieve the dyspnea so they can sleep. The term *three-pillow orthopnea* means that the person needs to prop up with three pillows to relieve the dyspnea. *Paroxysmal nocturnal dyspnea* is shortness of breath that awakens the individual in the middle of the night, usually in a panic with the feeling of suffocation. Asthma attacks may be triggered by a specific allergen, which may be external or extrinsic such as a pet or internal or intrinsic such as stress or emotions.

Have you noticed any other problems when you're short of breath? Cough? Chest pain? Breaking out in a sweat? Swelling of the feet, ankles, or legs?

Shortness of breath may be a problem of the respiratory system, or it may be a symptom associated with the cardiovascular system such as a severe heart murmur or heart failure that may produce peripheral edema.

When these episodes of shortness of breath occur, what do you do to relieve the symptoms?

Assess the effectiveness of treatment and any progression that the person has noted. Determining what has been used successfully or unsuccessfully helps in understanding the problem and may guide current treatment strategies.

Chest Pain with Breathing

How long have you had pain in your chest when you breathe? When did it start? Did it start suddenly or gradually? Where do you feel it? Does it radiate to other areas such as the neck or arms?

Chest pain caused by respiratory disease is usually associated with chest wall or parietal pleura (e.g., pneumonia). In contrast, chest pain associated with heart disease (primarily in men) is usually associated with radiating pain to the jaw, left arm, and back.

How does the pain feel (viselike, tight, sharp, burning)? On a scale of 0 to 10, how would you rate the intensity of the pain? Is it constant or does it come and go?

A sharp, abrupt pain associated with deep breathing may be an indication of pleural lining irritation, also called *pleuretic chest pain.*

When it started, was the pain associated with an injury to your ribs or a respiratory infection? Is it worse with deep inspiration? Does it interfere with your getting enough air?

Injured ribs cause pain when the individual breathes in; as a result, the person is likely to have shallow breathing, which may lead to respiratory congestion.

Is there anything that seems to make the pain worse such as movement or coughing?

Assess for aggravating factors.

Have you done anything to treat the pain such as applying heat or using pain medication? Have any measures been effective?

Assess self-care behaviors and successful treatment to relieve the pain.

BOX 11-2 CLINICAL NOTES

An indirect way to assess the severity of dyspnea is to count the words that the patient can say between breaths. Usually a person can say 10 to 14 words before taking a breath. A patient who has severe dyspnea may take a breath after every third word. This is documented as "three-word dyspnea."

HEALTH PROMOTION FOR EVIDENCE-BASED PRACTICE

Tobacco Use

Cigarette smoking is the single most preventable cause of death and disease in the United States. The majority of all cancers of the lung, trachea, bronchus, larynx, pharynx, oral cavity, and esophagus are caused by tobacco products. Smoking is a leading risk factor for cardiovascular diseases, including myocardial infarction, coronary artery disease, stroke, and peripheral vascular disease. Smoking is also an important risk factor for lung disease, including chronic obstructive pulmonary disease. During pregnancy, smoking may increase the risk for premature birth, low birth weight, stillbirth, and infant death. There is no safe tobacco alternative to cigarettes.

Environmental smoke (secondhand smoke) affects the health of nonsmokers, particularly children. Secondhand smoke causes heart disease and lung cancer in adults and a number of health problems in infants and children, including severe asthma attacks, respiratory infections, ear infections, and sudden infant death syndrome (SIDS).

Smokeless tobacco causes a number of serious oral health problems, including cancer of the mouth and gums, periodontitis, and tooth loss. Cigar use causes cancer of the larynx, mouth, esophagus, and lung.

Goals—Healthy People 2020

The goal for tobacco use is to reduce illness, disability, and death related to tobacco use and secondhand smoke exposure.

Recommendations to Reduce Risk (Primary Prevention)

NOTE: All major health care organizations recommend routine counseling for smoking cessation and recommend against the use of smokeless tobacco.

Clinical Recommendations

U.S. Preventive Services Task Force

- Clinicians ask all adults about tobacco use and provide tobacco cessation interventions for those who use tobacco products.
- Clinicians ask all pregnant women about tobacco use and provide augmented, pregnancy-tailored counseling for those who smoke.

Available at www.healthypeople.gov/2020/topicsobjectives2020/default.aspx?topicid=41, accessed August 30, 2001; and www.uspreventiveservicestaskforce.org/uspstf/uspstbac2.htm, April, 2009, accessed August 30, 2011.

EXAMINATION

ROUTINE TECHNIQUES

- INSPECT patient's general appearance, posture, and breathing effort.
- OBSERVE respirations.
- INSPECT patient's nails, skin, and lips.
- INSPECT the anterior and posterior thorax.
- AUSCULTATE the anterior, posterior, and lateral thorax.

SPECIAL CIRCUMSTANCES OR ADVANCED PRACTICE

- PALPATE the trachea.
- PALPATE the thoracic muscles.
- PALPATE the thoracic wall for expansion.
- PALPATE the thoracic wall for vocal (tactile) fremitus. ★
- PERCUSS the thorax for tone and diaphragmatic excursion. ★
- AUSCULTATE the thorax for vocal sounds (vocal resonance). ★

EQUIPMENT NEEDED

Stethoscope • Ruler and tape measure • Marking pen to mark diaphragmatic excursion

★ Advanced practice.

PROCEDURES AND TECHNIQUES WITH EXPECTED FINDINGS

ABNORMAL FINDINGS

ROUTINE TECHNIQUES

CLEAN hands.

INSPECT patient for general appearance, posture, and breathing effort.

The patient's general appearance and posture should be relaxed. The posture should be upright. Breathing should be quiet, effortless, and at a rate appropriate for the patient's age (Fig. 11-9).

Indications of respiratory distress include an appearance of apprehension with restlessness, nasal flaring, supraclavicular or intercostal retractions, and bulging with expiration and use of accessory muscles. *Paradoxical chest wall movement* may occur after chest trauma when the chest wall moves in on inspiration and out on expiration *Tripod position* (leaning forward with the arms braced against the knees, a chair, or a bed) also suggests respiratory distress. Tripod position enhances accessory muscle use (Fig. 11-10).

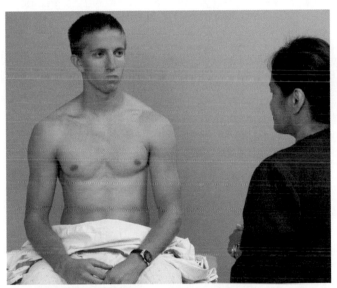

FIG. 11-9 Observing patient for breathing effort.

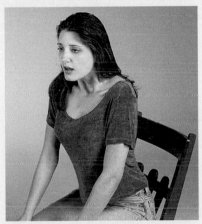

FIG. 11-10 Tripod position. (From Shade et al., 2012.)

OBSERVE respirations for rate, breathing pattern, and chest expansion.

Notice the respiratory rate. In the adult passive breathing should occur at a rate of 12 to 20 breaths/min (this range in respiratory rate is referred to as *eupnea*). The pattern of breathing should be smooth, with an even respiratory depth (Fig. 11-11). The chest wall should rise and expand symmetrically and then relax without effort. An expected variation is the abdominal breathing pattern. Men tend to use abdominal breathing (or diaphragmatic breathing), whereas women tend to use more thoracic breathing.

A sigh is another expected variation observed with breathing. It is an occasional interspersed deep breath associated with an expected breathing pattern (Fig. 11-12).

Abnormal breathing patterns are described in Fig. 11-13.

Chest retraction appears when intercostal muscles are drawn inward between the ribs and indicates airway obstruction that may occur during an asthma attack or pneumonia.

Frequent sighing is considered an abnormal finding and may indicate fatigue or anxiety.

Normal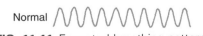

FIG. 11-11 Expected breathing pattern.

Sighing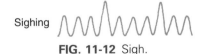

FIG. 11-12 Sigh.

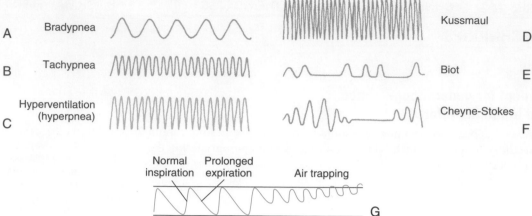

FIG. 11-13 Abnormal breathing patterns. **A,** *Bradypnea* is a respiratory rate less than 11 breaths/min. The rate and depth remain smooth and even. **B,** *Tachypnea* is a respiratory rate greater than 20 breaths/min. The rate and depth remain smooth and even. Tachypnea can be caused by a number of factors, including fever, fear, or activity. **C,** *Hyperventilation* is characterized by increased rate and depth of respiration. **D,** When hyperventilation occurs with ketoacidosis, it is very deep and laborious and is termed *Kussmaul* breathing. **E,** *Biot breathing pattern* is characterized by irregularly interspersed periods of apnea in a disorganized and irregular pattern, rate, or depth. It may be associated with persistent intracranial pressure, respiratory distress, or damage to the medulla. **F,** *Cheyne-Stokes* is characterized by intervals of apnea interspersed with a deep and rapid breathing pattern. This may be seen in patients with severe illness, brain damage, or drug overdose. **G,** *Air trapping* is an abnormal respiratory pattern frequently seen in patients with chronic obstructive pulmonary disease. It is characterized by rapid inspirations with prolonged, forced expirations. Air is not fully exhaled; thus it becomes trapped in the lungs, which eventually leads to a barrel chest. (Adapted from Seidel et al., 2011.)

PROCEDURES AND TECHNIQUES WITH EXPECTED FINDINGS	ABNORMAL FINDINGS

INSPECT patient's nails, skin, and lips for color.

Nail beds should be pink, with an angle of 160 degrees at the nail bed. Skin tones vary among individuals; therefore the general color should be consistent with skin and lip color for that individual. Specifically notice the presence of cyanosis or pallor (see Chapters 9 and 12 for details). If there is any question about adequate oxygenation, measure the person's oxygen saturation level using pulse oximetry (see Chapter 3).

Cyanosis or pallor of the nails, skin, or lips may be a sign of inadequate oxygenation of tissues caused by an underlying respiratory or cardiovascular condition. Clubbing of the nails is associated with chronic hypoxia observed in patients with cystic fibrosis or chronic obstructive pulmonary disease (see Figs. 9-10 and 12-21 for finger clubbing).

ROUTINE TECHNIQUES: POSTERIOR THORAX

Move behind the individual who is seated on an examination table or on a bed with the back of the gown open (especially for women) or removed.

INSPECT the posterior thorax for shape, symmetry, and muscle development.

The ribs should slope down at about 45 degrees relative to the spine. The thorax should be symmetric. The spinous processes should appear in a straight line. The scapulae should be bilaterally symmetric. Muscle development should be equal.

Asymmetry or unequal muscle development is abnormal. Skeletal deformities such as scoliosis or kyphosis may limit the expansion of the chest. Patients with COPD may have a barrel-shaped chest.

PROCEDURES AND TECHNIQUES WITH EXPECTED FINDINGS	ABNORMAL FINDINGS

AUSCULTATE the posterior and lateral thoraxes for breath sounds.

Procedure: Instruct the person to sit upright and breathe deeply and slowly through the mouth. Ask the person periodically about feeling dizzy from frequent deep breaths. If dizziness is reported, wait for it to subside before proceeding. Place the diaphragm of the stethoscope against the person's skin to auscultate breath sounds. Use a systematic pattern to listen over the posterior and lateral chest walls (Fig. 11-14, *A* and *B*). Move from the apex (above the clavicle) to the base (at the 11th rib). Leave the stethoscope in each location during at least one respiratory cycle so you can hear breath sounds during both inspiration and expiration. Compare one side with the other following the landmarks (Fig. 11-15, *A* and *C*). When auscultating over the lateral thorax, ask the patient to fold the arms in front to give you better access.

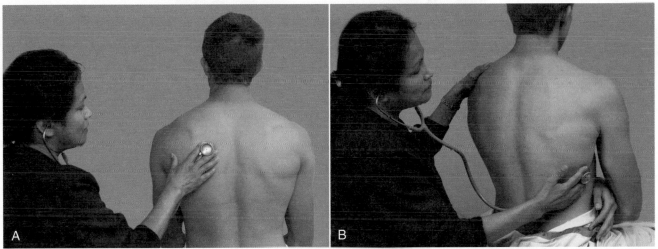

FIG. 11-14 Auscultating the posterior and lateral chest. **A,** Posterior thorax. **B,** Lateral thorax.

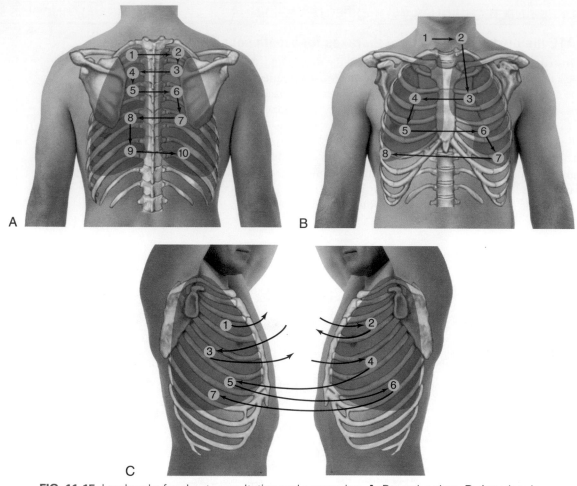

FIG. 11-15 Landmarks for chest auscultation and percussion. **A,** Posterior view. **B,** Anterior view. **C,** Lateral view. (From Seidel et al., 2011.)

PROCEDURES AND TECHNIQUES WITH EXPECTED FINDINGS

Findings: Breath sounds should be clear over the posterior and lateral thoraxes. Three types of breath sounds are expected in various parts of the thorax: *vesicular, bronchovesicular,* and *bronchial* (Fig. 11-16, *B,* and Table 11-2). If an adventitious sound is heard, have the patient cough; repeat the auscultation to see if the sound has changed or disappeared (Box 11-3).

BOX 11-3 CLINICAL NOTES

Before you decide that the patient has an adventitious sound, remember that the following may also be causes of sound distortion:
- If you bump the stethoscope tubing against something or if the patient touches the tubing, the sound will be distorted.
- If the patient is cold and shivering, the sound will be distorted.
- The stethoscope placed and unintentionally moved on a patient's excess chest hair may give a false finding of crackles or pleural friction rub.
- Extraneous environmental noises such as the rustling of a paper gown or drape may sound like crackles or pleural friction rub.

ABNORMAL FINDINGS

Expected breath sounds can be considered abnormal if heard over areas of the lungs where they are not expected. Bronchial breath sounds are abnormal if heard anywhere over the posterior or lateral thorax and may indicate consolidation of the lung, as may be found with pneumonia. (The sound heard is loud and high pitched. It sounds as if the air source is just under the stethoscope.) Bronchovesicular breath sounds should be considered abnormal when heard over the peripheral lung areas.

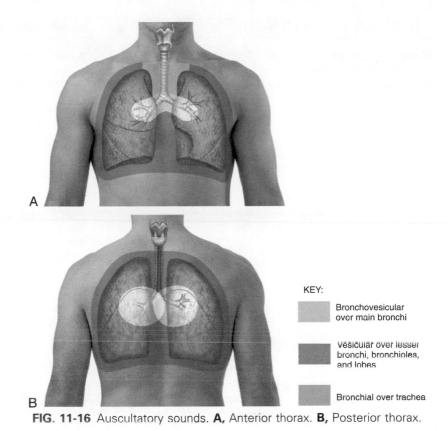

FIG. 11-16 Auscultatory sounds. **A,** Anterior thorax. **B,** Posterior thorax.

KEY:

Bronchovesicular over main bronchi

Vesicular over lesser bronchi, bronchioles, and lobes

Bronchial over trachea

TABLE 11-2   CHARACTERISTICS OF BREATH SOUNDS

	BRONCHIAL	BRONCHOVESICULAR	VESICULAR
Pitch	High	Moderate	Low
Intensity	Loud	Medium	Soft
Duration: Inspiration and expiration	Insp < Exp 1:2	Insp – Exp 1:1	Insp > Exp 2.5:1
	1 2	1 1	2.5 1
Expected location	Over trachea	First and second intercostal spaces at sternal border anteriorly; posteriorly at T4 medial to scapula	Peripheral lung fields
Abnormal location	Over peripheral lung fields	Over peripheral lung fields	Not applicable

PROCEDURES AND TECHNIQUES WITH EXPECTED FINDINGS

Vesicular breath sounds should be heard over almost all of the posterior and lateral thoraxes. *Bronchovesicular breath sounds* are the expected sounds heard over the posterior thorax, over the upper center area of the back on either side of the spine between the scapulae.

ABNORMAL FINDINGS

Adventitious breath sounds (crackles, wheezing, and rhonchi) are extraneous sounds that are superimposed on the breath sounds (Table 11-3). If you hear adventitious sounds, identify the type of sound, the location (i.e., right lung, left lung, or bilaterally; upper lobes or lower lobes; anterior or posterior), and the phase of breathing in which it is heard (i.e., inspiration or expiration). The term *respiratory stridor* is used to describe a harsh, high-pitched sound associated with breathing that is often caused by laryngeal or tracheal obstruction.

Diminished breath sounds may be heard in patients whose alveoli have been destroyed, which may occur in patients with emphysema. Diminished or absent breath sounds may be heard in patients with collapsed alveoli, which may occur in patients who have atelectasis or are having a severe asthma attack.

TABLE 11-3 CHARACTERISTICS OF ADVENTITIOUS SOUNDS

ADVENTITIOUS SOUNDS	CHARACTERISTICS	CLINICAL EXAMPLES
Crackles (previously called *rales*)		
Fine crackles	Fine, high-pitched crackling and popping noises (discontinuous sounds) heard during the end of inspiration; not cleared by cough	May be heard in pneumonia, heart failure, asthma, and restrictive pulmonary diseases
Medium crackles	Medium-pitched, moist sound heard about halfway through inspiration; not cleared by cough	Same as for fine crackles, but condition is worse
Coarse crackles	Low-pitched, bubbling, or gurgling sounds that start early in inspiration and extend into the first part of expiration	Same as for fine crackles, but condition is worse or in terminally ill patients with diminished gag reflex; also heard in pulmonary edema and pulmonary fibrosis
Wheeze (also called *sibilant wheeze*)	High-pitched, musical sound similar to a squeak; heard more commonly during expiration but may also be heard during inspiration; occurs in small airways	Heard in narrowed airway diseases such as asthma
Rhonchi (also called *sonorous wheeze*)	Low-pitched, coarse, loud, low snoring or moaning tone; actually sounds like snoring; heard primarily during expiration but may also be heard during inspiration; coughing may clear	Heard in disorders causing obstruction of the trachea or bronchus such as chronic bronchitis
Pleural friction rub	Superficial, low-pitched, coarse rubbing or grating sound; sounds like two surfaces rubbing together; heard throughout inspiration and expiration; loudest over the lower anterolateral surface; not cleared by cough	Heard in individuals with pleurisy (inflammation of the pleural surfaces)

PROCEDURES AND TECHNIQUES WITH EXPECTED FINDINGS

ROUTINE TECHNIQUES: ANTERIOR THORAX

Move in front of the person to assess the anterior thorax.

INSPECT the anterior thorax for shape and symmetry, muscle development, and costal angle.

When examining women, limit the time of exposure as much as possible. The ribs should slope down at approximately 45 degrees relative to the spine. The thorax should be symmetric. Muscle development should be equal. Anteriorly, the costal angle should be less than 90 degrees (Fig. 11-17, *A* to *C*).

Asymmetry or unequal muscle development is abnormal. The costal angle is greater than 90 degrees (Fig. 11-18, *A* to *C*). Other chest wall skeletal deformities include scoliosis, pectus carinatum (Fig. 11-19), and pectus excavatum (Fig. 11-20).

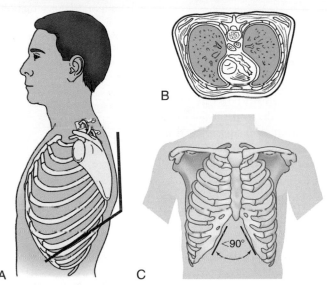

FIG. 11-17 Expected chest findings. **A,** Angulation of ribs. **B,** Anteroposterior diameter is about one half the lateral diameter. **C,** Costal angle less than 90 degrees. (**A** from Urden, Stacy, and Lough, 2010. **B** from Salvo, 2009.)

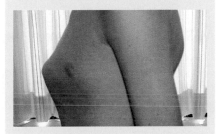

FIG. 11-19 Pectus carinatum, or pigeon chest. Note prominent sternum. (From Townsend et al., 2008.)

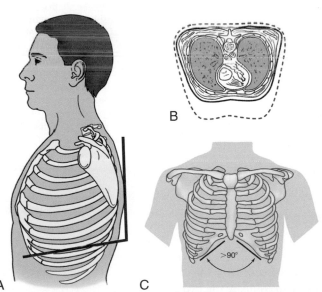

FIG. 11-18 Barrel chest. **A,** Horizontal ribs. **B,** Increased anteroposterior diameter. **C,** Costal angle greater than 90 degrees. (**A** From Urden, Stacy, and Lough, 2010. **B** from Salvo, 2009.)

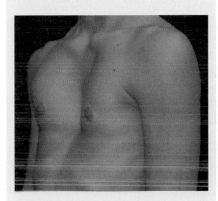

FIG. 11-20 Pectus excavatum, or funnel chest. Note that sternum is indented above xiphoid. (From Townsend et al., 2008.)

| PROCEDURES AND TECHNIQUES WITH EXPECTED FINDINGS | ABNORMAL FINDINGS |

INSPECT the anterior thorax for anteroposterior to lateral diameter.

Procedure: The AP diameter can be visualized or indirectly determined by using the distance between hands as a "measure." Standing in front of the patient, place your hands on either side of his or her anterior chest, noting the distance between your hands. Next, maintaining the distance between hands, move to the side of the patient to compare the distance from front to back with the distance between the hands.

Findings: The anteroposterior (AP) diameter of the chest should be approximately one half the lateral diameter—or about a 1 : 2 ratio of AP to lateral diameter. Thus the distance from the front to the back of the chest should be half the distance from one side of the chest to the other.

In disorders that cause lung hyperinflation such as emphysema, the chest wall may have a barrel-chest appearance because of an increased AP diameter. In this situation the ribs are more horizontal, and the chest looks as if it is held in constant inspiration.

AUSCULTATE the anterior thorax for breath sounds.

Procedure: Follow the same procedure as used to auscultate the posterior thorax. When examining women, you may reach under the gown with the stethoscope to auscultate while maintaining her modesty. Using the diaphragm of the stethoscope, listen to the patient's breath sounds in a systematic pattern over the anterior thorax. Auscultate from the apex of the lungs (above the clavicles) to the base (at the 11th rib). Leave the stethoscope in each location during at least one respiratory cycle so you can hear breath sounds during both inspiration and expiration. Compare one side to the other (see Fig. 11-15, *B*; Fig. 11-21, *A* to *C*). Ask the person periodically about the feeling of dizziness from frequent deep breathing. If dizziness is reported, wait for it to subside before proceeding.

Findings: *Vesicular breath sounds* should be heard throughout the periphery of the anterior thorax, including the apex of the lungs above the clavicles. *Bronchovesicular breath sounds* are expected sounds heard over the central area of the anterior thorax around the sternal border. These sounds are heard in an area that approximates the area where the bronchi split off from the trachea. *Bronchial breath sounds* are the expected sounds heard over the trachea and the area immediately above the manubrium.

Adventitious breath sounds (crackles, wheezing, and rhonchi) are extraneous sounds that are superimposed on the breath sounds (see Table 11-2). If you hear adventitious sounds, identify the type of sound, the location (i.e., right lung, left lung, or bilaterally; upper or lower lobes; anterior or posterior), and the phase of breathing in which it is heard (i.e., inspiration or expiration).

Diminished breath sounds may be heard in patients whose alveoli have been destroyed, which may occur in patients with emphysema. Diminished or absent breath sounds may be heard in patients with collapsed alveoli, which may occur in patients who have atelectasis or are having a severe asthma attack.

SPECIAL CIRCUMSTANCES OR ADVANCED PRACTICE: POSTERIOR THORAX

PALPATE posterior thoracic muscles for tenderness, bulges, and symmetry.

Procedure: With the palmar surface of your fingers, feel the texture and consistency of the skin over the chest and the alignment of vertebrae. Identify areas that the patient reports as tender or painful. Use both hands simultaneously to compare the two sides of the posterior chest wall.

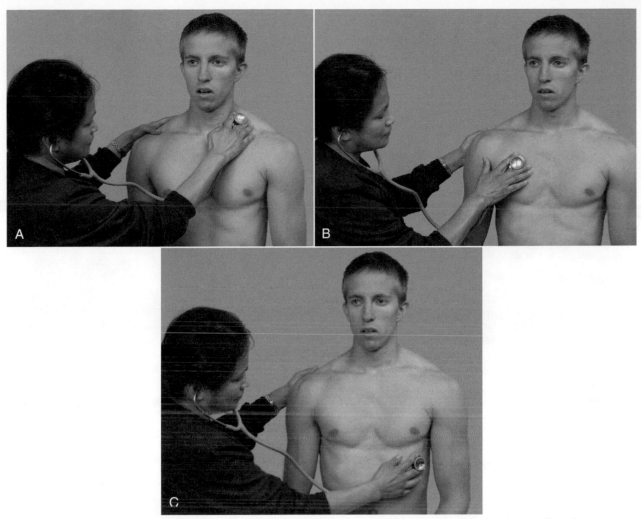

FIG. 11-21 Auscultating the anterior chest. **A,** Left apex. **B,** Right middle anterior thorax. **C,** Left lower anterior thorax.

PROCEDURES AND TECHNIQUES WITH EXPECTED FINDINGS

Findings: The vertebrae should be straight and nontender from C7 through T12. The scapulae should be symmetric, and the surrounding musculature well developed. The posterior ribs should be stable and nontender. The posterior rib cage should be symmetric and firm.

PALPATE the posterior thoracic wall for expansion.

Procedure: After inspecting the thorax, assess the patient's thoracic expansion if you suspect asymmetry. Stand behind the patient and place both thumbs on either side of the spinal processes at about the level of T9 or T10. While maintaining the thumb position, extend the fingers of both hands laterally (outward) over the posterior chest wall. Instruct the patient to take several deep breaths. Observe for lateral movement of both thumbs during the patient's inspirations (Fig. 11-22, *A* and *B*).

ABNORMAL FINDINGS

Note any crepitus, which feels like a crackly sensation under your fingers. This abnormal finding indicates air in the subcutaneous tissue caused by an air leak from somewhere in the respiratory tree. Pleural friction rub may be felt as a coarse, grating sensation during inspiration. It occurs secondary to inflammation of the pleural surface. Muscular development that is asymmetric or an unstable chest wall may indicate a thoracic disorder such as fractured ribs.

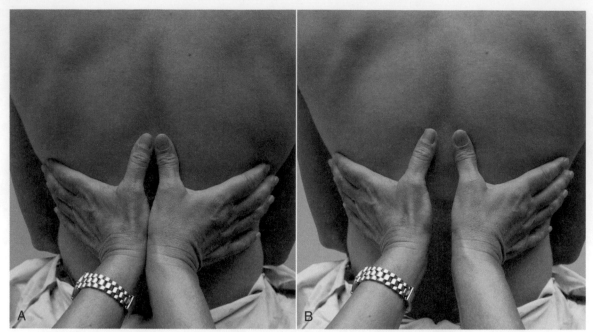

FIG. 11-22 Assessing for posterior thoracic expansion. **A,** With thumbs together on either side of patient's spinal process, extend fingers and ask patient to take deep breaths through the mouth. **B,** As patient takes deep breaths, observe lateral movement of both thumbs.

PROCEDURES AND TECHNIQUES WITH EXPECTED FINDINGS

Findings: Both thumbs should move apart symmetrically on the posterior chest wall with each breath.

PALPATE the posterior thoracic wall for vocal (tactile) fremitus.

Procedure: Fremitus provides information about the density of underlying lung tissue and thorax.[4] Vocal fremitus is a vibration resulting from verbalizations. You can feel this vibration using the palmar surface of your hand and fingers or the ulnar surfaces of your hands. Place your hands on the posterior thorax over the right and left lung fields following the landmarks shown in Figure 11-23, *A*. Instruct the patient to recite "one-two-three" or "ninety-nine" while you systematically palpate the chest wall (from apices to bases (Fig. 11-23, *B*).

Findings: The fremitus should feel bilaterally equal, although the quality of the vibrations may vary from person to person because of chest wall density and relative location of the bronchi to the chest wall.

ABNORMAL FINDINGS

A unilateral or unequal movement of your thumbs suggests asymmetry of expansion, which may be caused by pain, or localized pulmonary disease, such as fractured ribs or chest wall injury, pneumonia, and atelectasis or collapsed lung. If unequal chest wall movement is noted, further evaluation is warranted.

Vibrations feel unequal when comparing sides. Decreased or absent fremitus is felt unilaterally when the vibrations are blocked, which may occur in patients with pneumothorax, pleural effusion, atelectasis, or bronchial obstruction. Decreased fremitus is felt bilaterally in patients with chronic obstructive pulmonary disease, massive pulmonary edema, or excess fat tissue on the chest.[4,5] Increased fremitus is detected when the vibrations feel enhanced— sometimes described as rougher or coarser vibrations. This occurs when lung tissues are congested or consolidated, which may occur in patients who have pneumonia or a tumor.

PROCEDURES AND TECHNIQUES WITH EXPECTED FINDINGS

ABNORMAL FINDINGS

★ PERCUSS the posterior and lateral thorax for tone.

If necessary, review the techniques of performing percussion in Chapter 3. The sound heard during percussion of the lung depends on the air-tissue ratio. Perform percussion when you suspect overinflation of the lung or fluid or consolidation in the lung.[4]

Procedure: Systematically percuss the posterior thoracic wall following the same pattern that was used for auscultation (see Fig. 11-15, *A* and *C*). Begin with the patient in a sitting position with arms folded in front with head bent forward to move the scapulae laterally, exposing more lung field. Stand behind the patient and percuss between the ribs from above the scapula to the bottom of the ribs, comparing the two sides as you go (Fig. 11-24). Next compare percussion tones between the left and right lateral thoraxes.

Findings: The sound should be resonant, which is loud in intensity, low in pitch, long in duration, and hollow in quality (Table 11-4 and Fig. 11-25, *B*).

Hyperresonance is heard when there is overinflation of the lungs. It has a very loud resonance of low pitch that sounds "booming." This may be found in individuals with emphysema. Dull tones may be heard in patients with pneumonia, pleural effusion, or atelectasis.

★ Advanced practice

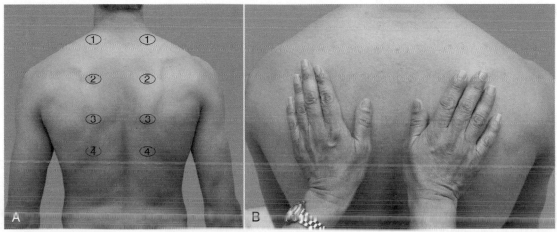

FIG. 11-23 Assessing for posterior vocal (tactile) fremitus. **A,** Hand position for assessment. **B,** Position hands over both lung fields, making bilateral comparisons.

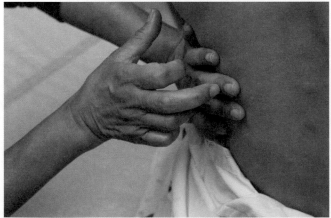

FIG. 11-24 Percussing the posterior thorax using the tip of the middle finger of the right hand to strike the middle finger of the left hand.

TABLE 11-4	**PERCUSSION TONES OVER THE LUNGS**	
	DESCRIPTION	**ADULT PERIPHERAL LUNG**
Tone	Description of tone	Resonance
Intensity	Loudness or softness of tone heard	Loud
Pitch	Number of vibrations per second: Fast vibrations—high pitch Slow vibrations—low pitch	Low
Duration	Length of time that a vibration note is sustained	Long
Quality	Subjective assessment of characteristics of tone	Hollow

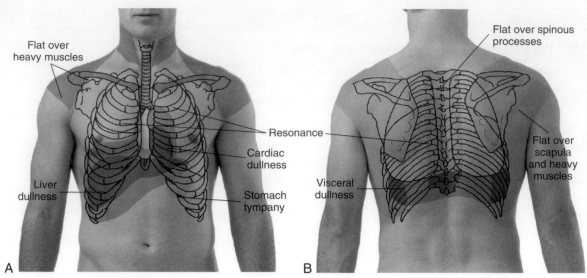

FIG. 11-25 Percussion tones of the chest. **A,** Anterior chest. **B,** Posterior chest.

PROCEDURES AND TECHNIQUES WITH EXPECTED FINDINGS	ABNORMAL FINDINGS

★ PERCUSS the thorax for diaphragmatic (respiratory) excursion.

Diaphragmatic excursion measures the movement of the diaphragm with maximum inspiration and expiration. This allows the nurse to estimate the lower lung border during inspiration and expiration. Perform this procedure when you suspect patients have increased or decreased downward lung expansion.

Procedure: To measure diaphragmatic excursion, follow these steps:

1. Stand behind the patient. Instruct the patient to sit upright, inhale deeply, and hold his or her breath. *(Hold your breath at the same time so you can determine the pace of your percussion.)*
2. While the patient is holding the breath, quickly percuss down the posterior chest wall along the midscapular line to determine the lower border of the lungs. (The percussion tone should change from resonant to dull.)
3. Using a marking pen, make a small line at the level where the percussion tone changed.
4. Tell the patient to breathe as usual. When ready, instruct the patient to *exhale* as much as possible and hold the breath.
5. Repeat the sequence during the patient's exhalation. Mark the point along the chest wall where the sound changes from resonant to dull at the bottom of the lungs. The difference between the two marks on each side is termed *diaphragmatic excursion* (Fig. 11-26). Repeat the sequence on the other side of the chest.

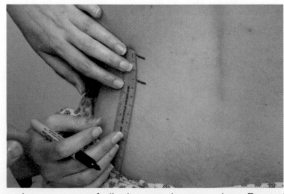

FIG. 11-26 Measuring amount of diaphragmatic excursion. Excursion usually measures 3 to 5 cm.

★ Advanced practice

PROCEDURES AND TECHNIQUES WITH EXPECTED FINDINGS	ABNORMAL FINDINGS

Findings: The diaphragmatic excursion should be equal bilaterally and measure at least 1 to 2 inches (3 to 5 cm); in well-conditioned individuals it may measure as much as 3 inches (7 to 8 cm).

Any pathologic condition limiting downward lung expansion or diaphragmatic movement results in a decreased diaphragmatic excursion. Examples include pleural effusion, emphysema, atelectasis, abdominal tumor or ascites, and severe pain with injured or fractured ribs.

★ AUSCULTATE the thorax for vocal sounds (vocal resonance).

When there is an indication of consolidation within the lung or if there was an abnormal finding when tactile fremitus was performed, evaluate for vocal resonance. Three techniques are included: testing for absence of bronchophony, whispered pectoriloquy, and egophony. The spoken voice vibrates and transmits sounds through the lung fields. These sounds are usually muffled and cannot be understood clearly. The sound is louder medially and softer at the periphery of the lung.

Bronchophony

Procedure: Instruct the patient to repeat one of the following phrases: "ninety-nine," "e-e-e," or "one-two-three." While the patient is speaking, use the diaphragm of the stethoscope to systematically auscultate the posterior thorax to listen for the response.

Findings: The expected response is a muffled tone such as "nin-nin" or muffled "one-two-three."

Bronchophony is present and abnormal if the sound is loud and clear. Presence of consolidation or compression of the lung creates a sound like "ninety-nine" or "one-two-three."

Whispered Pectoriloquy

Procedure: Perform this procedure when there is a positive finding of bronchophony. It is used to more clearly specify the problem and is referred to as an exaggerated bronchophony. Ask the patient to whisper "one-two-three." Systematically auscultate the posterior thorax, listening for the quality of the whispered tones.

Findings: The expected response is a muffled "one-two-three."

Whispered pectoriloquy is present and abnormal if the sound is loud and clear, which may be found in consolidation or compression of the lung.

Egophony

Egophony is the final test for vocal resonance. It evaluates the intensity of the spoken voice.

Procedure: Instruct the patient to say "e-e-e" as you auscultate the posterior thorax.

Findings: The expected response is the sound of a muffled "e-e-e."

If there is consolidation of the lung, you may hear changes in intensity and pitch so the sound is heard as "a-a-a," a positive indication of egophony.

SPECIAL CIRCUMSTANCES OR ADVANCED PRACTICE: ANTERIOR THORAX

PALPATE the trachea for position.

Perform this procedure when you suspect tracheal deviation.

Procedure: Stand facing the patient. Using the thumbs of both hands (or index finger and thumb of one hand), palpate the trachea on the anterior aspect of the neck by placing the thumbs on either side (Fig. 11-27).

★ Advanced practice

PROCEDURES AND TECHNIQUES WITH EXPECTED FINDINGS	ABNORMAL FINDINGS

Findings: The trachea should be palpable, midline, and slightly movable.

If the trachea is not midline, it may be an indication of a thorax mass, mediastinal shift, or some degree of lung collapse.

PALPATE the anterior thoracic muscles for tenderness, bulges, and symmetry.

Procedure: Repeat the same procedure as used for the posterior thorax. With the palmar surface of your fingers, feel the texture and consistency of the skin over the anterior chest. Identify areas that the patient reports as tender or painful. Use both hands simultaneously to compare the two sides of the posterior chest wall.

Findings: The clavicles should be symmetric, and the surrounding musculature well developed. The anterior ribs should be stable and nontender. The rib cage should be symmetric and firm. The sternum and xiphoid should be relatively inflexible.

Note any crepitus, which feels like a crackly sensation under your fingers. This abnormal finding indicates air in the subcutaneous tissue caused by an air leak from somewhere in the respiratory tree. Pleural friction rub may be felt as a coarse grating sensation during inspiration. Muscular development that is asymmetric or an unstable chest wall may indicate a thoracic disorder such as fractured ribs.

PALPATE the anterior chest wall for thoracic expansion.

Procedure: Repeat the same technique as used for the posterior thorax. Facing the patient, place both thumbs along the coastal margin and the xiphoid process with your palms against the anterolateral chest wall (Fig. 11-28). Instruct the patient to take several deep breaths. Observe for lateral movement of both thumbs during the patient's deep breaths.

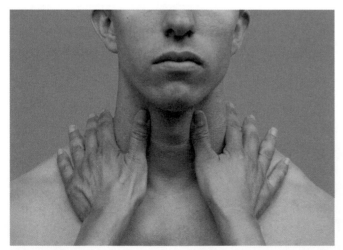

FIG. 11-27 Palpating to evaluate midline position of trachea.

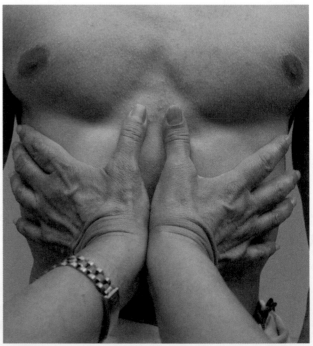

FIG. 11-28 Assessing for anterior thoracic expansion.

| PROCEDURES AND TECHNIQUES WITH EXPECTED FINDINGS | ABNORMAL FINDINGS |

Findings: Both thumbs should move apart symmetrically on the anterior chest walls with each breath.

A unilateral or unequal movement of your thumbs suggests asymmetry of expansion, which may be caused by pain, fractured ribs or chest wall injury, pneumonia, and atelectasis or collapsed lung.

★ PALPATE the anterior thoracic wall for vocal (tactile) fremitus.

Procedure: Repeat the same procedure used for the posterior thorax. Place the palmar side of your hands and fingers or ulnar side of your hands on the anterior thorax over the right and left lung fields. Instruct the patient to recite "one-two-three" or "ninety-nine" while you systematically palpate the chest wall following the landmarks shown in Fig. 11-29.

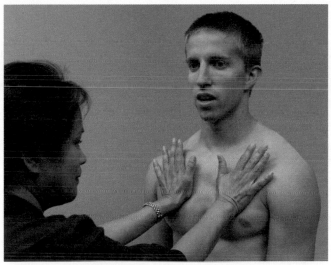

FIG. 11-29 Assessing for anterior vocal (tactile) fremitus.

Findings: The fremitus should feel equal bilaterally, although the quality of the vibrations may vary from person to person because of chest wall density and relative location of the bronchi to the chest wall.

Vibrations feel unequal when comparing sides. Decreased or absent fremitus is felt unilaterally when the vibrations are blocked, which may occur in patients with pneumothorax, pleural effusion, atelectasis, or bronchial obstruction. Decreased fremitus is felt bilaterally in patients with chronic obstructive pulmonary disease, a massive pulmonary edema, or excess fat tissue on the chest.[4,5] Increased fremitus is detected when the vibrations feel enhanced—sometimes described as rougher or coarser vibrations. This occurs when lung tissues are congested or consolidated, which may occur in patients who have pneumonia or a tumor.

★ PERCUSS the anterior thorax for tone.

Procedure: Repeat the same procedure as used for percussion of the posterior thorax. Systematically percuss the anterior chest wall following the same pattern that was used for auscultation (see Fig. 11-15, *B*). Stand in front of the patient. Percuss down the anterior aspects of the thorax, moving from side to side to compare findings.

★ Advanced practice

PROCEDURES AND TECHNIQUES WITH EXPECTED FINDINGS

Findings: There should be a resonant tone, which is loud in intensity, low in pitch, long in duration, and hollow in quality as shown in Fig. 11-25, *A.*

ABNORMAL FINDINGS

Hyperresonance is heard when there is overinflation of the lungs. It has a very loud resonance of low pitch that sounds "booming." This may be found in individuals with emphysema. Dull tones may be heard in patients with pneumonia, pleural effusion, or atelectasis.

? CLINICAL REASONING: THINKING LIKE A NURSE
Respiratory System

At the beginning of a shift, the husband of a 52-year-old woman tells the nurse that something seems to be wrong with his wife. She had a nephrectomy for renal cell carcinoma 14 hours ago. She can have nothing by mouth, and her last set of vital signs was stable. The man indicates that his wife was fine when she came back from surgery, but she has become progressively less responsive over the last few hours.

Interpreting
Early in the encounter the nurse considers two possible causes of these findings: medication reaction or hypovolemia. To determine if either have any probability of being correct, the nurse gathers additional data. *How much intravenous (IV) fluid has been administered?* The woman has an IV of $D_5\frac{1}{2}NS$ (5% dextrose in normal saline) infusing at 125 mL/hour. According to the intake and output record, 950 mL of IV fluid infused with 620 mL of urine output during the last shift. *What pain medication is she taking?* The woman has a patient-controlled analgesia (PCA) delivering morphine sulfate 1 mg every 10 minutes on demand. The PCA has delivered a total of 15 mg in the last 2½ hours.

The experienced nurse recognizes the adverse effects of morphine (hypotension, respiratory depression, and hypoxia as evidenced by low oxygenation saturation and changes in cognition) and interprets this information in the context of a patient 14 hours after a nephrectomy.

Nurse's Background, Experience, Perspective
The experienced nurse immediately has a grasp of the situation at hand. Extensive practical knowledge about what to expect with this age-group, diagnoses, and treatment allows the nurse to recognize risk factors, given the patient's age and postoperative status and the surgical procedure.

Noticing
This background knowledge sets up the possibility of noticing signs of a prevalent complication in an individual presenting with these data. The experienced nurse with extensive postoperative care experience knows that 14 hours following a surgical procedure such as this, the patient should be more responsive. The woman is difficult to arouse, and vital signs are taken: blood pressure, 100/60; pulse, 118 beats/min (thready); temperature, 97.2° F (36.2° C); and respiratory rate, 10 breaths/min with an oxygen saturation of 88% on 2 L of oxygen. Her lungs are clear bilaterally; her respirations are shallow. The nurse notices that her skin is warm, dry, and pale and that her surgical dressing is dry and intact.

Responding
The nurse initiates appropriate initial interventions (increases the oxygen delivery and turns off the PCA) and contacts the attending health care provider to discuss the situation, ensuring that the patient receives appropriate immediate and follow-up care.

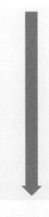

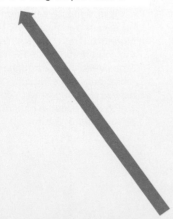

Reflecting
The nurse evaluates this patient's assessment data and outcomes of interventions (reflection-in-action); this experience contributes to and deepens the expertise on which to draw again (reflection-on-action) when encountering a similar situation.

DOCUMENTING EXPECTED FINDINGS

Breathing quiet and effortless at a rate of 16 breaths/min. Skin, nails, and lips appropriate color for individual's ethnic background. Thorax symmetric, with ribs sloping downward at about 45 degrees relative to the spine. Muscle development of the thorax equal bilaterally without tenderness. Thoracic expansion symmetric bilaterally. Spinous processes in alignment; scapulae, bilaterally symmetric. The anteroposterior (AP) diameter of the chest approximately a 1:2 ratio of AP to lateral diameter. Trachea midline. Breath sounds clear, with vesicular breath sounds heard over most lung fields, bronchovesicular breath sounds in the posterior chest over the upper center area of the back and around the sternal border, and bronchial breath sounds heard over the trachea.

AGE-RELATED VARIATIONS

Nurses adapt their examinations of the lungs and respiratory system when assessing patients at either end of the life span. Assessing neonates and infants requires use of different equipment and an unhurried approach. When assessing older adults, the nurse also uses an unhurried approach and may find expected variations from adults, such as changes in the musculoskeletal system that affect respiratory function.

examination while the infant is calm if possible; examination of a crying infant is difficult. By the ages of 2 or 3 years the child is usually cooperative during the respiratory examination. Before that age you need to develop a relationship with the child to improve cooperation during the examination. Chapter 19 presents further information regarding the respiratory assessment of infants, children, and adolescents.

INFANTS, CHILDREN, AND ADOLESCENTS

Assessing the respiratory status of an infant, child, or adolescent usually follows the same sequence as for an adult, although there are a few differences worth noting. Use a pediatric stethoscope when examining an infant or child. The infant must be undressed at least to the diaper to perform an adequate assessment. Keep the infant covered when you are not performing the examination to prevent exposure and cooling. Conduct the

OLDER ADULTS

Assessing the respiratory status of an older adult follows the same procedures as for an adult, although structural and functional differences may be noted. Posterior thoracic stooping or bending or kyphosis may alter the thorax wall configuration and make thoracic expansion more difficult. Chapter 21 presents further information regarding the respiratory assessment of an older adult.

COMMON PROBLEMS AND CONDITIONS

RISK FACTORS

Lung Cancer

- *Tobacco smoking:* Smoking is the most important risk factor for lung cancer. (M)
- *Secondhand smoke:* Smoke from other people's cigarettes causes lung cancer in people and animals. (M)
- *Asbestos:* People who work with asbestos are approximately seven times more likely to die of lung cancer. (M)
- *Environmental exposure in the workplace:* Carcinogens in the workplace include radioactive ores such as radon; arsenic; uranium; coal products; and chemicals such as vinyl chloride, nickel chromates, mustard gas, and chloromethyl ethers. (M)
- *Marijuana:* Marijuana contains more tar than cigarettes and is usually inhaled deeply, and the smoke is held in the lungs for a longer time. (M)
- *Personal and family history:* People who have lung cancer are at a higher risk of developing another lung cancer.

Brothers, sisters, and children of people who have lung cancer have a slightly higher risk of lung cancer themselves. However, it is difficult to say how much of the excess risk is the result of genetic factors versus environmental tobacco smoke.
- *Gender:* Women's lungs may have a genetic predisposition to developing cancer when they are exposed to tobacco smoke.
- *Air pollution:* In some cities air pollution may slightly increase the risk for lung cancer; however, this risk is far less than that caused by smoking. (M)
- *Cancers in other organs:* Cigarette smoking causes cancer of the esophagus, larynx, mouth, throat, kidney, bladder, pancreas, stomach, and cervix and acute myeloid leukemia.

Available at *www.cdc.gov/cancer/lung* 2011, www.cancer.org, 2011.
M, Modifiable risk factor.

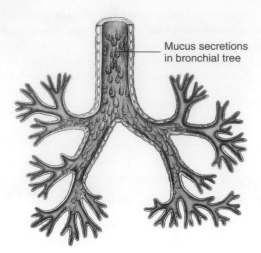

FIG. 11-30 Bronchitis. Irritation of the bronchi causes inflammation.

INFLAMMATION/INFECTION

Acute Bronchitis

An inflammation of the mucous membranes of the bronchial tree caused by viruses or bacteria is called *acute bronchitis*. **Clinical Findings:** The cough initially is nonproductive, but it may become productive after a few days. Patients may complain of substernal chest pain that is aggravated by coughing. Other clinical manifestations include fever, malaise, and tachypnea. Rhonchi are heard on auscultation, with wheezing heard after coughing (Fig. 11-30).

Pneumonia

An inflammation of the terminal bronchioles and alveoli is called *pneumonia*. It may be caused by bacteria, fungi, viruses, mycoplasma, or aspiration of gastric secretions. **Clinical Findings:** Viral pneumonia tends to produce a nonproductive cough or clear sputum, whereas bacterial pneumonia causes a productive cough that may produce white, yellow, or green sputum. Other clinical findings include fever, malaise, and pleuritic chest pain. Signs of pulmonary consolidation may be noted such as inspiratory crackles, increased tactile fremitus, egophony, and whispered pectoriloquy (Fig. 11-31).

Tuberculosis

This contagious, bacterial infecti on caused by *Mycobacterium tuberculosis* is transmitted by airborne droplets. This infection is primarily in the lungs; but kidney, bone, lymph node, and meninges can also be involved. **Clinical Findings:** The patient is usually asymptomatic during the early stages of the disease. The initial clinical manifestations may consist of fatigue, anorexia, weight loss, night sweats, and fever. A characteristic finding later in the disease is a cough that becomes increasingly frequent, producing a mucopurulent sputum (Fig. 11-32).

Pleural Effusion

An accumulation of serous fluid in the pleural space between the visceral and parietal pleurae is called *pleural effusion*.

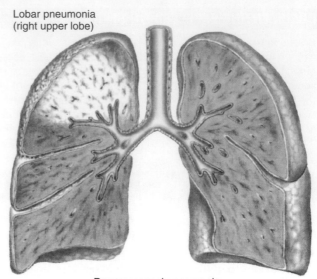

Lobar pneumonia
(right upper lobe)

Pneumococcal pneumonia
FIG. 11-31 Right upper lobe pneumonia.

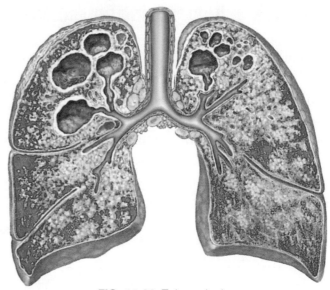

FIG. 11-32 Tuberculosis.

Clinical Findings: Manifestations depend on the amount of fluid accumulation and the position of the patient. If the effusion occurs rapidly and if it is large, there may be dyspnea, intercostal bulging, or decreased chest wall movement (Fig. 11-33).

CHRONIC PULMONARY DISEASE

Asthma

This hyperreactive airway disease is characterized by bronchoconstriction, airway obstruction, and inflammation. Causes of asthma include inhalation of allergens or pollutants, infection, cold air, vigorous exercise, or emotional stress. **Clinical Findings:** Signs include increased respiratory rate with prolonged expiration, audible wheeze, dyspnea, tachycardia, anxious appearance, possible use of accessory

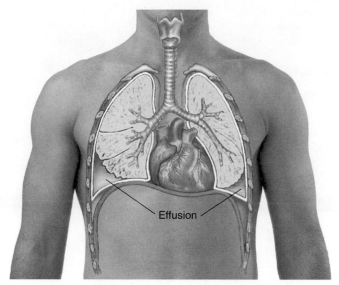

FIG. 11-33 Pleural effusion.

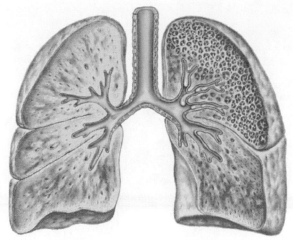

FIG. 11-35 Emphysema in upper left lobe. (From Seidel et al., 2011.)

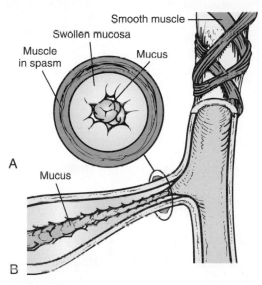

FIG. 11-34 Factors causing airway obstruction in asthma. **A,** Cross-section of a bronchiole occluded by muscle spasm, mucosal edema, and mucus. **B,** Longitudinal section of a bronchiole. (From Lewis et al., 2011. Redrawn from Price and Wilson, 2003.)

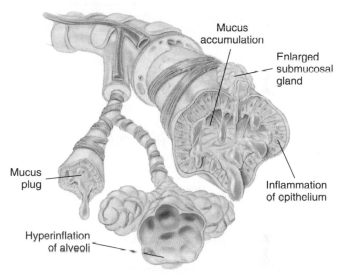

FIG. 11-36 Chronic bronchitis. (From McCance and Huether, 2002. Modified from Des Jardins and Burton, 1995.)

muscles, and cough. Expiratory and occasionally inspiratory wheeze and diminished breath sounds are common findings (Fig. 11-34).

Emphysema

Destruction of the alveolar walls causes permanent abnormal enlargement of the air spaces in emphysema. The major cause is cigarette smoking; however, a small percentage of cases result from an inherited deficiency of the enzyme alpha$_1$ antitrypsin (α_1a). **Clinical Findings:** The classic general appearance of a patient with advanced emphysema is an underweight individual with a barrel chest who becomes short of breath with minimal exertion. When the patient is short of breath, pursed-lip breathing and tripod position are frequently observed. Other clinical findings typically reveal diminished breath and voice sounds, possible wheezing or crackles on auscultation, and decreased diaphragmatic excursion (Fig. 11-35).

Chronic Bronchitis

This disorder is characterized by hypersecretion of mucus by the goblet cells of the trachea and bronchi, resulting in a productive cough for 3 months in each of 2 successive years. It is caused by irritants such as cigarette smoke and air pollution or by infection. **Clinical Findings:** Symptoms of chronic bronchitis are productive cough, increased mucus production, and dyspnea. Findings are rhonchi, sometimes cleared by coughing. When there is sufficient mucus to occlude alveoli, crackles may be heard (Fig. 11-36).

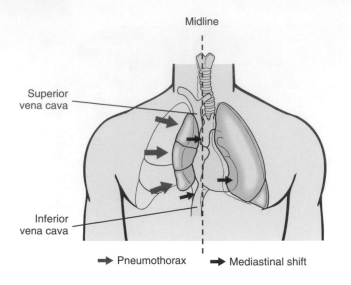

FIG. 11-37 Tension pneumothorax. (From Lewis et al., 2011.)

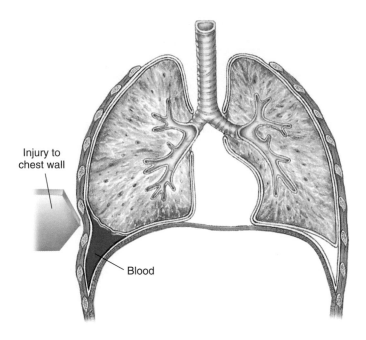

FIG. 11-38 Hemothorax.

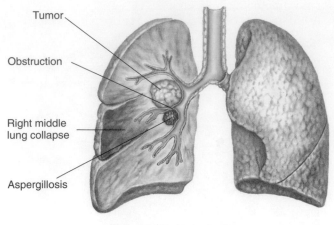

FIG. 11-39 Atelectasis.

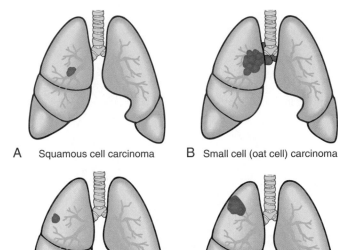

A   Squamous cell carcinoma   B   Small cell (oat cell) carcinoma

C   Adenocarcinoma   D   Large cell carcinoma

FIG. 11-40 Cancer of the lung. **A,** Squamous cell carcinoma. **B,** Small cell (oat cell) carcinoma. **C,** Adenocarcinoma. **D,** Large cell carcinoma. (From Lewis et al., 2004.)

ACUTE OR TRAUMATIC CONDITIONS

Pneumothorax

Air in the pleural spaces results in a pneumothorax. There are three types of pneumothorax: (1) closed, which may be spontaneous, traumatic, or iatrogenic; (2) open, which occurs following penetration of the chest by either injury or surgical procedure; and (3) tension, which develops when air leaks into the pleura and cannot escape. **Clinical Findings:** The signs vary, depending on the amount of lung collapse. If there is very minor collapse, the patient may be slightly short of breath, anxious, and report chest pain. If a large amount of lung collapses, the patient may experience severe respiratory

distress, including dyspnea, tachypnea, and cyanosis. Distant and hyperresonant breath sounds over the affected area are heard. Decreased chest wall movement on the affected side may be noted. The patient may also have paradoxical chest wall movement, when the chest wall moves in on inspiration and out on expiration. If severe, there may be tracheal displacement toward the unaffected side with a mediastinal shift, termed a *tension pneumothorax* (Fig. 11-37).

Hemothorax

Blood in the pleural space caused by chest injury results in hemothorax, but it also may be a complication of thoracic surgery. **Clinical Findings:** Signs are similar to those described for pneumothorax, although it is common to note distant muffled breath sounds and dullness with percussion over the affected area (Fig. 11-38).

OTHER PULMONARY CONDITIONS

Atelectasis

This disorder refers to collapsed alveoli caused by external pressure from a tumor, fluid, or air in the pleural space (compression atelectasis) or by lack of air from hypoventilation or obstruction by secretions (absorption atelectasis). **Clinical Findings:** The affected area has diminished or absent breath sounds. The oxygen saturation may decrease to less than 90% (Fig. 11-39).

Lung Cancer

An uncontrolled growth of anaplastic cells in the lung describes lung cancer. Agents such as tobacco smoke, asbestos, ionizing radiation, and other noxious inhalants can be causes. **Clinical Findings:** The most common initial symptom reported is a persistent cough. Weight loss, congestion, wheezing, hemoptysis, labored breathing, and dyspnea are other manifestations that occur with advanced disease. Lung sounds may sound as expected or be diminished over the affected area. If there is a partial obstruction of airways from the tumor, wheezes may be heard. Percussion tones may sound as expected or may be dull over the tumor, particularly if the cancer is large or the patient has associated atelectasis (Fig. 11-40).

CLINICAL APPLICATION AND CLINICAL REASONING

See Appendix D for answers to exercises in this section.

REVIEW QUESTIONS

1. A nurse suspects a viral infection or upper respiratory allergies when the patient describes the sputum as being which color?
   1. White
   2. Clear
   3. Yellow
   4. Pink tinged

2. During inspection of the respiratory system the nurse documents which finding as abnormal?
   1. Skin color consistent with patient's ethnicity
   2. 1:2 ratio of anteroposterior to lateral diameter
   3. Anterior costal angle is 85 degrees
   4. Patient leaning forward with arms braced against the knees

3. A patient has an infection of the terminal bronchioles and alveoli that involves the right lower lobe of the lung. Which abnormal findings are expected?
   1. Dyspnea with diminished breath sounds bilaterally
   2. Asymmetric chest expansion on the right side
   3. Fever and tachypnea with crackles over the right lower lobe
   4. Prolonged expiration with an occasional wheeze in the right lower lobe

4. On auscultation of a patient's lungs, the nurse hears a low-pitched, coarse, loud, and low snoring sound. Which term does the nurse use to document this finding?
   1. Rhonchi
   2. Wheeze
   3. Crackles
   4. Pleural friction rub

5. Which question gives the nurse further information about the patient's complaint of chest pain?
   1. "Have you had your influenza immunization this year?"
   2. "Are there environmental conditions that may affect your breathing at home?"
   3. "How would you describe the chest pain?"
   4. "Has the chest pain been interrupting your sleep?"

6. Which finding does the nurse expect when performing tactile fremitus?
   1. A vibration of sounds that are equal bilaterally
   2. A change in muscle tone when the patient inhales and exhales, indicating weakness
   3. The symmetric rise of the thorax as the patient speaks, indicating equal expansion
   4. Coughing triggered by patient speech, indicating bronchial irritation

7. How does the nurse palpate the chest for tenderness, bulges, and symmetry?
   1. Uses the fist of the dominant hand to gently tap the anterior, lateral, and posterior chest, comparing one side with another
   2. Uses the ulnar surface of one hand to palpate the anterior, posterior, and lateral chest, comparing one side with another
   3. With the tips of the fingers, palpates the skin over the chest and the alignment of vertebrae
   4. With the palmar surface of fingers of both hands, feels the consistency of the skin over the chest and the alignment of vertebrae

8. Which breath sounds are expected over the posterior chest of an adult?
   1. Vesicular
   2. Bronchovesicular
   3. Bronchial
   4. Bronchoalveolar

9. Narrowing of the bronchi creates which adventitious sound?
   1. Wheeze
   2. Crackles
   3. Rhonchi
   4. Pleural friction rub

10. Which finding may indicate abnormal thoracic expansion?
    1. A 4-cm diaphragmatic excursion
    2. A 1:2 ratio anteroposterior to lateral diameter
    3. An S-shaped curvature of the spine
    4. A costal angle of 85 degrees

CASE STUDY

Ms. Martinez is a 66-year-old woman complaining of shortness of breath. The following initial data are collected.

Interview Data

Ms. Martinez says that she has had breathing problems "for years" but her breathing is getting worse. She tells the nurse that she gets short of breath with activity, adding that she can do things around the house for only a few minutes before she has to sit down to catch her breath. She says that she can sleep for only a couple of hours at a time. She sleeps best using two pillows to prop up, but on some nights she just sits in a chair. Ms. Martinez does not currently use oxygen, but she thinks oxygen would help. She admits to smoking 1.5 packs of cigarettes a day. She has never quit because she says she "just can't do it."

Examination Data

- *General survey:* Alert and slightly anxious female, sitting slightly forward, with moderately labored breathing. Skin pale with slight cyanosis around the lips and in nail beds. Appears extremely thin.

- *Chest and lungs:* Chest is round shaped and symmetric with increased AP diameter and costal angle greater than 90 degrees. Small muscle mass is noted over chest; ribs protrude. Respiratory rate is 24 breaths/min and labored. Chest wall expansion with respirations is reduced but symmetric. Sibilant wheezes are heard on expiration throughout lung fields. Lung sounds are diminished in lung bases bilaterally. Vocal sounds are muffled bilaterally.

Clinical Reasoning

1. Which data deviate from expected findings, suggesting a need for further investigation?
2. For which additional information should the nurse ask or assess?
3. Based on the data, which risk factors does Ms. Martinez have for lung cancer?
4. With which health care team member would you collaborate to meet this patient's needs?

Heart and Peripheral Vascular System

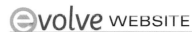 WEBSITE

http://evolve.elsevier.com/Wilson/assessment

CONCEPT OVERVIEW

The feature concept for this chapter is *Perfusion*. This concept represents mechanisms that facilitate and impair perfusion of oxygenated blood throughout the body. Because all tissues require perfusion of oxygenated blood, all of these physiologic concepts are interrelated; but oxygenation is foundational to all others. Nutrition plays an important interrelated role because of the impact on cardiovascular health. The most important concepts are represented in the following model.

This model shows the interrelationship of concepts associated with perfusion. Understanding this interrelationship helps the nurse recognize risk factors and thus increases awareness when conducting a health assessment. Blood flow supplies oxygen and nutrients continuously to tissues so they can perform their functions. These tissues include skin, the kidneys to produce urine, the brain for intracranial regulation, the gastrointestinal tract for metabolism, and muscles and nerves for motion. Pain results when perfusion is interrupted.

The following case provides a clinical example featuring several of these interrelated concepts.

Eva Schmanski is a 79-year-old woman who has heart failure resulting from long-standing hypertension. Reduced cardiac output from the left ventricle has resulted in a back-up of blood into the pulmonary vascular system. The increased pressure has caused fluid to leak out of the vascular space that surrounds the alveoli, thus interfering with gas exchange and oxygenation. Furthermore, poor perfusion of oxygenated blood limits motion (because of activity intolerance and fatigue) and elimination (caused by poor perfusion of blood to the kidneys) and potentially results in confusion as a result of poor perfusion of oxygenated blood to the brain.

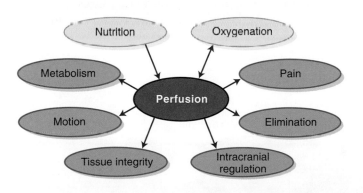

ANATOMY AND PHYSIOLOGY

The cardiovascular system transports oxygen, nutrients, and other substances to body tissues and metabolic waste products to the kidneys and lungs. This dynamic system is able to adjust to changing demands for blood by constricting or dilating blood vessels and altering the cardiac output.

THE HEART AND GREAT VESSELS

The heart is a pump about the size of a fist that beats 60 to 100 times a minute without rest, responding to both external and internal demands such as exercise, temperature changes, and stress. Each side of the heart has two chambers, an atrium and a ventricle. The right side receives blood from the superior and inferior venae cavae and pumps it through the pulmonary arteries to the pulmonary circulation; the left side receives blood from the pulmonary veins and pumps it through the aorta into the systemic circulation.

The upper part of the heart is called the *base,* and the lower left ventricle is called the *apex.* The heart lies behind the sternum and above the diaphragm in the mediastinum. It lies at an angle so the right ventricle makes up most of the anterior surface and the left ventricle lies to the left and posteriorly. The right atrium forms the right border of the heart, and the left atrium lies posteriorly. The pulmonary arteries and aorta are termed the *great vessels.* The aorta curves upward out of the left ventricle and bends posteriorly and downward just above the sternal angle. The pulmonary arteries emerge from the superior aspect of the right ventricle near the third intercostal space (Fig. 12-1).

Pericardium and Cardiac Muscle

The heart wall has three layers: pericardium, myocardium, and endocardium (Fig. 12-2). The heart is encased in the

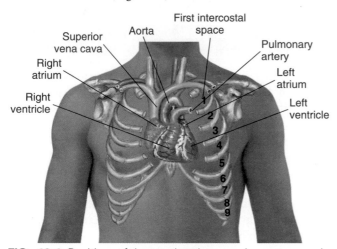

FIG. 12-1 Position of heart chambers and great vessels. Intercostal spaces 1 to 9 are numbered.

pericardium, which has a fibrous layer and two serous layers. The fibrous layer, termed the *fibrous pericardium* or *parietal layer,* is a fibrous sac of elastic connective tissue that shields the heart from trauma and infection. One of the serous layers lies next to the fibrous pericardium, and the other lies next to the myocardium. Between the fibrous pericardium and the serous pericardium is the pericardial space, which contains a small amount of pericardial fluid to reduce friction as the myocardium contracts and relaxes. The serous pericardium, also termed the *visceral layer* or *epicardium,* covers the heart surface and extends to the great vessels. The middle layer, or myocardium, is thick muscular tissue that contracts to eject blood from the ventricles. The endocardium lines the inner chambers and valves.

Blood Flow Through the Heart: The Cardiac Cycle

Four valves govern blood flow through the four chambers of the heart. The tricuspid valve on the right and mitral valve on the left are termed the *atrioventricular (AV)* valves because they separate the atria from the ventricles (Fig. 12-3). The aortic valve opens from the left ventricle into the aorta; the pulmonic valve opens from the right ventricle into the pulmonary artery. The aortic and pulmonic valves are termed *semilunar* valves because of their half-moon shape.

Diastole

During diastole the ventricles are relaxed and fill with blood from the atria. The movement of blood from the atria to the ventricles is accomplished when the pressure of the blood in the atria becomes higher than the pressure in the ventricles. The higher atrial pressures passively open the AV valves, allowing blood to fill the ventricles (Fig. 12-4). Approximately 80% of the blood from the atria flows into relaxed ventricles. A contraction of the atria forces the remaining 20% into the ventricles. This added atrial thrust is termed the *atrial kick.* At the end of diastole the ventricles are filled with blood.

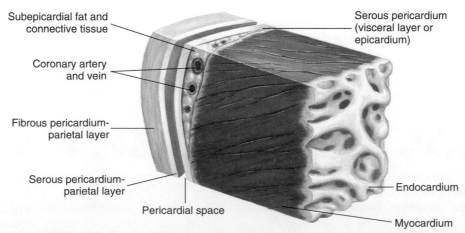

FIG. 12-2 Cross-section of cardiac muscle. (From Canobbio, 1990.)

Systole

During systole the ventricles contract, creating a pressure that closes the AV valves, preventing the backflow of blood into the atria. This ventricular pressure also forces the semilunar valves to open, resulting in ejection of blood into the aorta (from the left ventricle) and the pulmonary arteries (from the right ventricle) (Fig. 12-5). As blood is ejected, the ventricular pressure decreases, causing the semilunar valves to close. The ventricles relax to begin diastole.

Cardiac Cycle

Events in the cardiac cycle showing the venous pressure waves, electrocardiogram, and heart sounds in systole and diastole are shown in Fig. 12-6. Further discussion about using the electrocardiogram to assess cardiac conduction is found at the end of the examination section (see Fig. 12-34 later in this chapter). The S_3 and S_4 heart sounds are abnormal; however, they are shown in Fig. 12-6 at the point in the cardiac cycle where they would be heard if present.

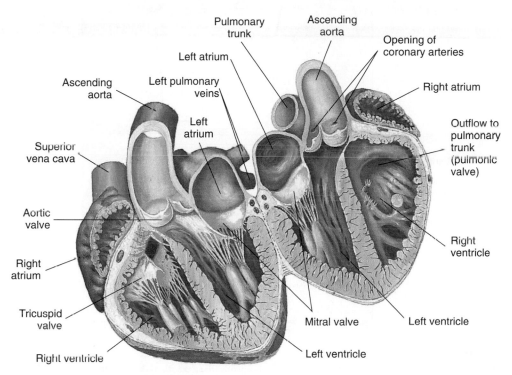

FIG. 12-3 Anterior cross-section showing valves and chambers of the heart. (From Seidel et al., 2011.)

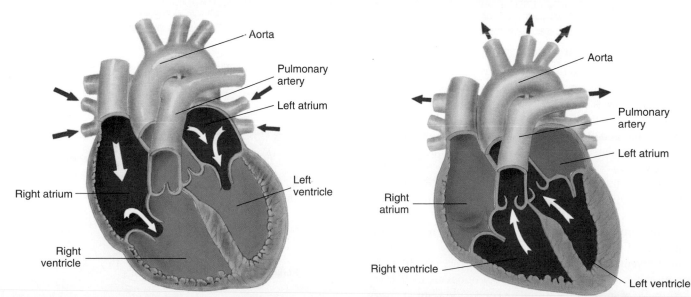

FIG. 12-4 Blood flow during diastole. (From Canobbio, 1990.)

FIG. 12-5 Blood flow during systole. (From Canobbio, 1990.)

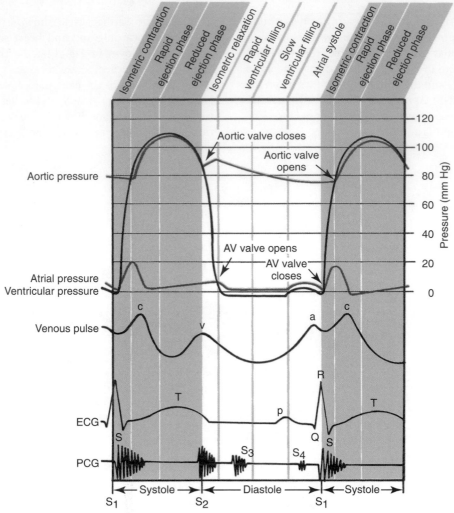

FIG. 12-6 Events of the cardiac cycle showing venous pressure waves, electrocardiograph, and heart sounds in systole and diastole. *a,* Atrial contraction; *AV,* atrioventricular; *c,* carotid artery; *ECG,* electrocardiogram; *PCG,* phonocardiogram; *p,* p wave (atrial contraction); *QRS,* QRS complex (ventricular contraction); *S₁,* first heart sound; *S₂,* second heart sound; *S₃,* third heart sound; *S₄,* fourth heart sound; *T,* T wave (ventricular repolarization); *v,* venous return coming into the atrium. (From Seidel et al., 2011. Modified from Guzetta and Dossey, 1992.)

Electric Conduction

The heart is stimulated by an electric impulse that originates in the sinoatrial (SA) node in the superior aspect of the right atrium and travels in internodal tracts to the AV node. The SA node, termed the *cardiac pacemaker,* normally discharges between 60 and 100 impulses per minute. The electric impulses stimulate contractions of both atria and then flow to the AV node in the inferior aspect of the right atrium. The impulses are then transmitted through a series of branches (bundle of His) and Purkinje fibers in the myocardium, which results in ventricular contraction (Fig. 12-7). The AV node prevents excessive atrial impulses from reaching the ventricles. If the SA node fails to discharge, the AV node can generate ventricular contraction at a slower rate, 40 to 60 impulses per minute. If both SA and AV nodes are ineffective, the bundle branches may stimulate contraction but at a very slow rate of 20 to 40 impulses per minute.

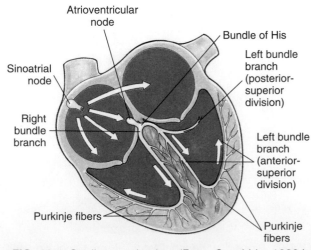

FIG. 12-7 Cardiac conduction. (From Canobbio, 1990.)

PERIPHERAL VASCULAR SYSTEM

Arteries, capillaries, and veins provide blood flow to and from tissues. The tough and tensile arteries and their smaller branches, the arterioles, are subjected to remarkable pressure generated from the myocardial contractions. They maintain blood pressure by constricting or dilating in response to stimuli. The veins and their smaller branches, the venules, are less sturdy but more expansible, enabling them to act as a reservoir for extra blood, if needed, to decrease the workload on the heart. Pressure within the veins is low compared with arterial circulation. The valves in each vein keep blood flowing in a forward direction toward the heart. A comparison of the structures of arteries and veins is shown in Fig. 12-8.

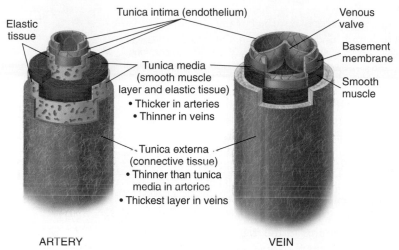

FIG. 12-8 Schematic drawing of artery and vein. Shown is the comparative thickness of three layers: fibrous connective tissue (tunica externa), muscle layer (tunica media), and lining of endothelium (tunica intima). Note that the muscle and outer coats are much thinner in the veins than in the arteries and that veins have valves. (From Thibodeau and Patton, 2010.)

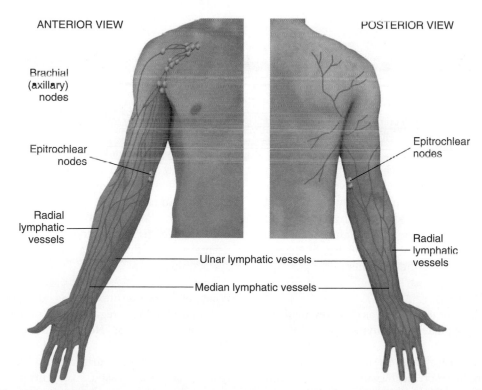

FIG. 12-9 System of deep and superficial collecting ducts carrying lymph from upper extremity to subclavian lymphatic trunk. The only peripheral lymph center is the epitrochlear, which receives some of the collecting ducts from the pathway of the ulnar and radial vessels. (From Seidel et al., 2011.)

LYMPH SYSTEM

The lymph system works in collaboration with the peripheral vascular system in removing fluid from the interstitial spaces. As blood flows from arterioles into venules, oxygen and nutrient-rich fluid are forced out at the arterial end of the capillary into the interstitial space and then into cells. Waste products from cells flow through the interstitial spaces to the venous end of the capillary.

Excess fluid left in the interstitial spaces is absorbed by the lymph system and carried to lymph nodes throughout the body. Lymphatic fluid is clear, composed mainly of water and a small amount of protein, mostly albumin. Lymph nodes are tiny oval clumps of lymphatic tissue, usually located in groups along blood vessels. In the peripheral vascular system the lymph node locations of interest are the arm, groin, and leg. The epitrochlear nodes on the medial surface of the arm above the elbow are palpable (Fig. 12-9). These lymph nodes receive fluid via the radial, ulnar, and median lymph vessels. In the upper thigh the inguinal lymph nodes are superficial; they receive most of the lymph drainage from the great and small saphenous lymphatic vessels in the legs. In men lymph from the penile and scrotal surfaces drains to the inguinal nodes, but nodes of the testes drain into the abdomen. In the posterior surface of the leg behind the knee are the popliteal nodes, which receive lymph from the medial portion of the lower leg (Fig. 12-10). Ducts from the lymph nodes empty into the subclavian veins.

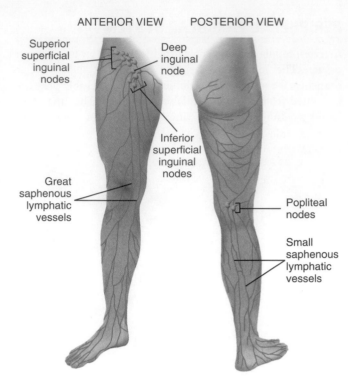

FIG. 12-10 Lymphatic drainage of lower extremity. (From Seidel et al., 2011.)

HEALTH HISTORY

GENERAL HEALTH HISTORY

Nurses interview patients to collect subjective data about their present health and any past medical experiences. These data include the present health status, past medical history, family history, and personal and psychosocial history as they relate to the functions of the heart and blood vessels. Quality Improvement Competencies for Nurses include providing patient-centered care and interdisciplinary teamwork with dietitians and personnel in cardiac rehabilitation applies to assessment of the heart and peripheral vascular system. Refer to Table 11-1 on p. 196 for specific competencies.

Present Health Status

Do you have any chronic illnesses such as diabetes mellitus, renal failure, chronic hypoxemia, or hypertension? If yes, describe.
Chronic illnesses can cause symptoms affecting the cardiovascular system when they increase the workload of the heart by narrowing peripheral vessels (diabetes, hypertension), the fluid volume to be pumped (diabetes, renal failure), or the heart rate and cause pulmonary capillary vasoconstriction (chronic hypoxemia).

Are you taking any medications? If yes, what are you taking, and when did you start taking them? Have you had any adverse effects from them? Do you take them as prescribed?
Medications may be taken to treat cardiovascular problems, or they may be taken to treat another disorder, but have adverse effects on the cardiovascular system. For example, tricyclic antidepressants, phenothiazines, or lithium can cause dysrhythmias; hormonal contraceptives can cause thrombophlebitis; corticosteroids can cause sodium and fluid retention; and theophylline can cause tachycardia and dysrhythmias.

What over-the-counter drugs do you take? Do you take an aspirin on a regular basis to help thin your blood? Do you take herbs? How often do you use herbs or drugs?
These nonprescription drugs may affect the cardiovascular system. For example, aspirin prevents platelet aggregation to reduce clot formation. Decongestants containing pseudoephedrine may aggravate hypertension. Ayurvedic herbs can act as a cardiac stimulant, whereas other herbs act as a cardiac depressant.

Past Health History

As a child did you have congenital heart disease or heart defect?
Data from past medical history gives information about clinical findings to anticipate.

During childhood did you have "growing pains" (i.e., unexplained joint pains)? Recurrent tonsillitis? Rheumatic fever? Heart murmur?
These questions relate to diagnosis of rheumatic fever, which may have contributed to rheumatoid arthritis or rheumatic heart disease, which gives information about clinical findings to anticipate.

Have you been told that you have high levels of cholesterol or elevated triglycerides?
High levels of serum lipids line the arteries, which may impede blood flow to tissues and increase workload on the heart.

Have you ever had surgery on your heart? On your blood vessels? If so, which procedure was done? When was it done? How successful was the surgery?
Knowledge of past surgical procedures may provide additional information about possible cardiovascular problems. These data also explain the presence of scars that you will observe on examination.

Have you ever had any tests on your heart? Electrocardiogram (EKG or ECG), stress ECG, or other heart tests? What did the tests reveal? What, if any, treatment did you receive?
These tests provide baseline data on the health of the patient's heart.

Family History

Does anyone in your family have a history of diabetes, heart disease, hyperlipidemia, or hypertension, especially young and middle-age relatives? Is so, who?
These conditions are risk factors for heart disease and have familial tendencies, especially among first-degree relatives.

Personal and Psychosocial History

Do you exercise? If yes, what kind of exercise? How often do you exercise? How much time do you spend exercising? If no, have you ever exercised? What motivated you to start in the past? What influenced you to stop exercising?
Physical activity for at least 30 minutes five times weekly increases energy; improves self-esteem; and prevents coronary artery disease, hypertension, and obesity.

Patients who no longer exercise should be encouraged to resume an exercise program. Exploring reasons for stopping can begin the problem-solving process to determine what can motivate them to start again.

How would you describe your personality type? How do you deal with stress?

Stress and persistent intensity are risk factors for heart disease. (Observe the patient as he or she responds and throughout the examination to detect stress or intensity.) Patients who are frequently in stressful environments should be encouraged to use several strategies to relieve stress and change their perceptions of the situations so they are perceived as less stressful.

How often do you take time to relax? What do you do to relax? Hobbies? Sports? Meditation? Yoga? Music?
Physical relaxation can relieve stress and reduce blood pressure.

Describe your usual eating habits. How often do you eat red meat? How much red meat do you eat at a meal? Do you monitor your fat and salt intake? Do you eat whole grains each day?
Selecting foods consistent with the MyPlate guide provides balanced nutrition. Calories from fat should be limited to 20% of daily calories, with 10% limited to saturated fat. Frequent consumption of large servings of red meat is associated with high cholesterol. A serving of red meat is 4 oz and should be limited to three times weekly. Whole grains (e.g., cereals) have been found to reduce heart disease.

Do you drink alcoholic beverages? What type of alcohol do you drink? How much? How often?
Excessive alcohol intake has been associated with hypertension and the development of cardiomyopathy. Moderate alcohol intake is defined as two drinks per day for men and one drink per day for women and those over 65 years of age. One drink is defined as 12 oz of beer, 5 oz of wine, or 1.5 oz of 80-proof distilled spirits.

Do you use cocaine? Other street drugs? How often do you use these drugs?
Cocaine use has been associated with myocardial infarction and stroke.

Do you consume caffeine? In coffee? Chocolate? Soft drinks? How much caffeine do you consume? How often?
Excessive caffeine intake can cause tachycardia, which can increase the workload of the heart.

Do you smoke or have you been a smoker in the past? If yes, what forms of tobacco do (did) you use (cigarettes, cigars, pipe, marijuana, smokeless or chewing tobacco)? How often do you use tobacco? Have you ever quit smoking? If yes, how did you accomplish it, and for what length of time? Are you interested in quitting smoking?
Nicotine in tobacco causes vasoconstriction, which may decrease blood flow to extremities and increase blood pressure, both of which increase the workload on the heart. Patients who previously were successful at stopping their tobacco use may be more easily convinced to repeat their success. Patients must be interested in stopping tobacco use; otherwise there is little motivation to change behavior.

Perhaps educating them about the negative effects of nicotine on the cardiovascular system provides some motivation.

PROBLEM-BASED HISTORY

The focus of the history includes descriptions of chest pain, shortness of breath, cough, urinating during the night (nocturia), fatigue, fainting (syncope), swelling of the extremities, leg pain, and enlarged lymph nodes. As with symptoms in all areas of health assessment, a symptom analysis is completed using the mnemonic OLD CARTS, which includes the Onset, Location, Duration, Characteristics, Aggravating factors, Related Symptoms, Treatment, and Severity (see Box 2-3).

Chest Pain

Where are you feeling the chest pain? What does it feel like? Does it radiate to any location? How severe is it on a scale of 0 to 10?
The origin of chest pain may be pulmonary, musculoskeletal, or gastrointestinal rather than cardiac. Table 12-1 describes different types of chest pain. If patients indicate that they are having active chest pain, the nurse assesses quickly to determine the need for immediate treatment.

Angina is an important symptom of coronary artery disease, which indicates myocardial ischemia caused by a lack of oxygen to meet the demand of the myocardium. Women may experience pain or discomfort in the center of the chest or in the arms, back, neck, jaw, or stomach.[1]

The patient's description of the pain is important to help distinguish stable angina versus unstable angina. Patients, especially men, report the chest pain of stable angina as pressure or an ache in the chest and often describe the sensation as squeezing, heavy, or choking. In contrast, unstable angina is new-onset chest pain, occurs at rest, or is a worse pattern than previously experienced. The pain is described as a crushing, severe, burning, or constricting sensation that is not relieved by rest or nitroglycerin. In addition, patients may report the pain as radiating to the neck, jaw, or arms.

When did the pain start? Is it intermittent or constant? If intermittent, how long does it last?
These questions help distinguish different types of chest pain (see Table 12-1). Stable angina often has a gradual onset, whereas unstable angina may have a sudden onset.

Which symptoms have you noticed along with the pain? Sweating? Turning pale or gray? Heart skipping beats or racing? Shortness of breath? Nausea or vomiting? Dizziness? Anxiety?
These associated symptoms frequently accompany a myocardial infarction in men. The symptoms reported initially by women with heart disease may include discomfort of the neck, shoulder, upper back, or abdomen; sweating; nausea or vomiting; light-headedness; and unusual fatigue or shortness of breath as warning signs of a myocardial infarction.[2]

Which factors preceded the pain? Exercise? Rest? Highly emotional situations? Eating? Sexual intercourse?
Chest pain that begins during exertion such as exercise and diminishes after exertion may indicate an inability of the coronary arteries to provide adequate blood to the myocardium during exertion.

What makes the pain worse? Moving the arms or neck? Deep breathing? Lying flat? Exercise?
The chest pain from pericarditis is aggravated by deep breathing, coughing, or lying supine. Chest pain from muscle strain may be aggravated by movement of arms.

What relieves the pain? Rest? Nitroglycerin? How many nitroglycerin tablets does it take to relieve chest pain?
These questions assess for alleviating factors. Chest pain that is relieved by nitroglycerin may be caused by myocardial ischemia (stable angina), whereas chest pain that is not relieved by four or more nitroglycerin tablets taken 5 minutes apart may be caused by myocardial necrosis (unstable angina), which may lead to myocardial infarction.

Shortness of Breath

How long have you had shortness of breath? Do you feel short of breath now?
Dyspnea may be caused by respiratory or cardiac problems. A gradual onset may be caused by heart failure that develops slowly from backup of fluid from the left heart into the alveoli.

When does the shortness of breath happen? How often does it occur? How long does it last?
These questions determine the frequency and duration of dyspnea.

Does the shortness of breath interfere with your daily activities? How many level blocks can you walk before you become short of breath? How many blocks could you walk 6 months ago?
Dyspnea that interferes with activities of daily living may require the patient to use supplemental oxygen. If the distance the patient can walk is decreased, it is a sign that the dyspnea is getting worse. Notice if the patient has to take a breath in the middle of sentences (see Box 11-2).

Do you have any other symptoms with the shortness of breath (e.g., do your feet swell during the day when you are sitting or standing)?
Dependent edema seen in the ankles or feet may develop from retained fluid because of right-sided heart failure.

What makes the shortness of breath worse? Walking upstairs? Lying down? How many pillows do you require when you lie down? Do you breathe easier when in a recliner?
Walking up stairs increases the workload of the heart. When dyspnea becomes worse on lying down, the term *orthopnea* is

TABLE 12-1 DIFFERENTIATION OF CHEST PAIN

CAUSE	LOCATION	QUALITY OF PAIN	QUANTITY OF PAIN	CHRONOLOGY	ASSOCIATED MANIFESTATIONS	AGGRAVATING FACTORS	ALLEVIATING FACTORS
Stable angina	Precordial or retrosternal, radiates to L>R arm, jaw, interscapular or epigastrium not above C3 or below T10	Pressure, burning, dull, or sharp	Variable, usually worse with activity	>1 min or <1 hr	Dyspnea, diaphoresis, palpitations, nausea, weakness	Physical exertion, emotional stress, cold	Rest, nitroglycerin, beta-blocker, calcium channel blocker
Unstable angina/myocardial infarction (MI)	Precordial or retrosternal, radiates to L>R arm, jaw, interscapular or epigastrium not above C3 or below T10	Pressure, squeezing, crushing; burning, dull, or sharp	10 of 10 on pain scale	Sudden onset or progressing <30-40 min for unstable angina, >1 hr to 2-3 days for MI	Dyspnea, diaphoresis, palpitations, nausea, weakness	Chest pain during exercise or at rest	Beta-blocker, aspirin, heparin, oxygen
Cocaine-induced chest pain	Similar to myocardial infarction	Sharp, pressurelike, squeezing	Severe, 8 to 10 of 10 on pain scale	Gradual onset over minutes, lasting minutes to hours	Tachycardia, tachypnea, hypertension	During and shortly after cocaine use	Nitroglycerin or calcium channel blockers
Mitral valve prolapse	Anywhere in chest, localized or diffuse; does not radiate	Variable, often sharp or "kick"	Variable within same patient	Sudden, recurrent onset; lasts seconds or persists for days	Often asymptomatic; palpitations when lying on left side, dyspnea, dizziness	Usually nonexertional, occasionally positional	Position change, nitroglycerin, analgesics
Acute pericarditis	Precordial, posterior neck, trapezius muscle	Boring, oppressive, pleuritic, or positional	Moderate, 4 to 6 of 10 pain scale	Onset hours to days, lasts hours to weeks	Fever, dyspnea, orthopnea, friction rub	Reclining	Leaning forward
Panic disorder	Localized retrosternally, abdomen	Tightness, vague, diffuse, unrelated to exertion	May be described as disabling	Lasts 30 min or more	Hyperventilation, fatigue, anorexia, emotional strain	Emotional strain	Variable by patient
Peptic ulcer disease	Epigastric radiating to lower bilateral chest (T6 to T10)	Burning, gnawing	Moderate, 4 to 6 of 10 cm pain scale	Gradual, recurrent onset, lasts hours	Nausea, abdominal tenderness	Empty stomach	Food, antacids, histamine₂ (H₂) blocker, proton pump inhibitor
Esophageal reflux	Midepigastric to xiphoid; C7 to T12; radiates to neck, ear, or jaw	Burning, pressurelike, squeezing	Moderate to severe	Spontaneous onset, lasts min to days	Dysphagia	Spicy or acidic meal, alcohol, lying supine	Oral fluids, belching, antacids, nitroglycerin, H₂ blocker
Costochondritis (inflammation of rib or cartilage)	Second to fourth costochondral junction, xiphoid, radiates to precordium, arms, shoulders	Variable	Variable	Gradual onset, constant pain, lasts for days	None	Coughing, deep breathing, laughing, sneezing	Localized heat, analgesics, antiinflammatories

Adapted with permission from Hill B, Geraci SA: A diagnostic approach to chest pain based on history and ancillary evaluation, *Nurse Pract* 23(4):20-45, 1998, ©Springhouse Corporation/www.springnet.com.

used. Orthopnea occurs when a person must sit up or stand to breathe easily. The number of pillows necessary to relieve the orthopnea is documented (e.g., *two-pillow orthopnea* means that the patient must elevate his or her chest with two pillows to breathe easily). Some patients use a recliner for elevation rather than using pillows.

When these episodes of shortness of breath occur, what do you do to breathe more easily?
Determine the effectiveness of the action(s) to relieve dyspnea. This information may be helpful in planning future treatment strategies.

Cough

When did your cough start? How often do you cough? Do you cough up anything? What does it look like?
Coughing up blood (hemoptysis) is a symptom of mitral stenosis and pulmonary disorders. White, frothy sputum may be a sign of pulmonary edema that occurs with left-sided heart failure.

Is your cough associated with position (more coughing when lying down), anxiety, or talking or activity? What makes it worse? Which actions do you take to relieve the cough?
Coughing more when lying down may indicate heart failure. Knowing how the patient relieves the cough may help to identify treatment strategies.

Urinating During the Night

How long have you been getting up during the night to urinate? How many times a night do you get up to urinate?
Nocturia occurs with heart failure in persons who are ambulatory during the day. Lying down at night creates a fluid shift and increases the need to urinate. Taking a diuretic before bedtime may also contribute to nocturia.

What have you done to prevent this from happening? How successful have your efforts been?
Stopping fluid intake within a few hours of bed or changing the time for taking a diuretic may help prevent nocturia. This information may guide future teaching and treatment strategies.

Fatigue

When do you notice fatigue? Was the onset sudden or gradual? Is the fatigue worse in the morning or evening? Are you too tired to take part in your usual activities?
Fatigue may be experienced during daily activities such as shopping, climbing stairs, carrying groceries, or walking because the heart cannot pump enough blood to meet the body tissue needs. The body diverts blood from less vital organs such as muscles of extremities to the heart and brain.[3] Fatigue from other causes (e.g., psychogenic [depression or anxiety]) occurs all day or is worse in the morning and varies by location. Fatigue from anemia lasts all day. Fatigue from anemia and heart disease occurs

gradually, whereas fatigue from acute blood loss occurs more rapidly.

Do you take iron pills? Do you eat foods with iron such as green leafy vegetables and liver? For women: Do you have a heavy menstrual flow?
These questions relate to iron deficiency anemia, which can cause fatigue. Women may have iron deficiency from monthly blood loss.

Have you had any other symptoms associated with the fatigue such as rapid heart rate, headache, pale skin, sore tongue or lips, or changes in your nails?
Fatigue and exertional dyspnea are manifestations of mild anemia and heart failure. Additional signs of tachycardia, headache, pallor, brittle, spoon-shaped nails, glossitis (inflammation of the tongue), and cheilitis (inflammation of the lips) occur with moderate-to-severe anemia.

Have you noticed any unusual feelings in your feet and hands, muscle weakness, or trouble thinking?
Neurologic symptoms in addition to those described previously may indicate anemia from vitamin B_{12} deficiency.

Fainting

What were you doing just before you fainted? Did you feel dizzy? Did you lose consciousness?
A brief lapse of consciousness is termed *syncope*. When syncope occurs with activity or position changes and causes dizziness, it may be the result of hypotension or inadequate blood flow to the brain.

Has this happened to you before? How often has this occurred?
These questions determine frequency of syncope.

Was fainting preceded by any other symptoms? Nausea? Chest pain? Headache? Sweating? Rapid heart rate? Confusion? Numbness? Hunger? Ringing in your ears?
These questions attempt to determine whether the cause of fainting is a cardiovascular, a neurologic, or an inner ear problem. It may be caused by small emboli in the cerebral circulation. Emboli may be the result of atrial fibrillation, valvular disease, or cardiac dysrhythmias. Cerebral emboli may cause a stroke, resulting in reports of headache, confusion, and numbness. Ask about tinnitus to rule out Meniere's disease, an inner ear disorder.

Swelling of Extremities

Where is the swelling located? Arms or Legs? Unilateral or bilateral?
Edema of both legs may be caused by fluid overload from systemic disease (e.g., heart failure, renal failure, or liver disease). Unilateral edema of an extremity may be lymphedema caused by occlusion of lymph channels (e.g., elephantiasis or trauma) or surgical removal of lymph channels (e.g., after mastectomy). Localized edema of one leg may

be caused by venous insufficiency from varicosities or thrombophlebitis.

What makes the swelling go away? Does elevating your arms or feet reduce the swelling? Does the swelling disappear after a night's sleep?

Edema that increases during the day and decreases at night or with elevation may be related to venous stasis, which may occur with right-sided heart failure. Compression garments for the arms or legs may reduce lymphedema or venous insufficiency.

Are any symptoms associated with the swelling? Shortness of breath? Weight gain? Warmth? Discoloration?

Dyspnea may be caused by heart failure. Weight gain occurs anytime there is fluid retention, regardless of cause. Warmth and redness of the legs may indicate an inflammatory process, whereas discoloration and ulceration may indicate ischemia.

For women: Is the swelling associated with your menstrual period?

Hormonal contraceptives may be associated with thrombophlebitis, which may cause unilateral leg edema. Changes in estrogen and progesterone blood levels can contribute to fluid retention, resulting in dependent edema.

Leg Cramps or Pain

Describe the pain and its location. Feet? Calf? Thighs? Buttocks? How severe is the pain on a scale of 0 to 10? What makes it worse? What relieves it?

Pain from arterial insufficiency is commonly felt in the calf but may occur in other locations mentioned. Arterial insufficiency produces pain that worsens with activity, especially prolonged walking. Leg pain that occurs while walking and that is relieved by rest is termed *intermittent claudication.* This occurs when the artery is about 50% occluded. As the insufficiency becomes worse, the patient reports pain when walking that is not relieved after rest. This is termed *rest pain.*

HEALTH PROMOTION FOR EVIDENCE-BASED PRACTICE

Cardiovascular Disease

Cardiovascular disease is the leading cause of death and a major cause of disability in the United States, contributing to increases in health care costs. These diseases include coronary artery disease and myocardial infarction, stroke, hypertension, hyperlipidemia, and peripheral vascular diseases.

Goals and Objectives—*Healthy People 2020*
The overall *Healthy People 2020* goal related to cardiovascular disease is to improve cardiovascular health and quality of life through the prevention, detection, and treatment of risk factors; early identification and treatment of heart attacks and strokes; and prevention of recurrent cardiovascular events.

Recommendations to Reduce Risk (Primary Prevention)
American Heart Association
Smoking cessation (see Health Promotion: Tobacco Use in Chapter 11).
Diet: (a) Limit intake of high-cholesterol, saturated fats; (b) promote diet high in fruits, vegetables, and grains; (c) limit salt intake to less than 1500 mg/day.
Blood lipid management. Total cholesterol less than 200 mg/dL
Fasting serum glucose. less than 100 mg/dL
Weight: Achieve and maintain a desirable body weight (body mass index [BMI] between 18.5 and 24.9).
Physical activity: At least 150 minutes a week of at least moderate-intensity physical activity such as brisk walking.

Screening Recommendations (Secondary Prevention)
U.S. Preventive Services Task Force
Blood Pressure Screening
Screening for hypertension is recommended for all adults age 18 and older. Optimal interval for screening has not been determined and is left to clinical discretion. For normotensive adults blood pressure measurement is suggested at least every 2 years; for adults with known hypertension more frequent intervals are recommended.

Lipid-level Screening
Screening for lipid disorders is strongly recommended for men age 35 and older and women age 45 and older.
  Screening for lipid disorders is recommended for younger adults (men ages 20 to 35 years and women ages 20 to 45 years) if they have other risk factors for heart disease (family history of cardiovascular disease before age 50 in male relatives or age 60 in female relatives, family history of hyperlipidemia, diabetes mellitus, and multiple other risk factors, including tobacco use, hypertension).
  Optimal interval for screening is uncertain; reasonable options include every 5 years (more frequently for individuals who have lipid levels warranting therapy and less frequently for individuals at low risk who have repeatedly low or normal lipid levels).

Use of Aspirin
The use of aspirin is recommended for men ages 45 to 79 years and women ages 55 to 79 years when the potential benefit from reduction of myocardial infarction outweighs the potential harm caused by an increase in gastrointestinal hemorrhage.

Data from www.uspreventiveservicestaskforce.org/adultrec.htm#heartvasc, accessed September 17, 2011; US Department of Health and Human Services: *Healthy People 2020,* available at http://www.healthypeople.gov/2020; Lloyd-Jones DM et al: Defining and setting national goals for cardiovascular health promotion and disease reduction: the American Heart Association's strategic impact goal through 2020 and beyond, *Circulation* 121:586-613, 2010: originally published January 20, 2010, doi:10.1161/CIRCULATIONAHA.109.192703, accessed September 19, 2011.

Leg pain caused by arterial insufficiency is worse when legs are elevated and improves when they are in a dependent position. By contrast, pain caused by venous insufficiency intensifies with prolonged standing or sitting in one position. Pain is worse when legs are in a dependent position and is relieved when they are elevated. Discomfort increases throughout the day, being worse at the end of the day.

Have you noticed any changes in the skin of your legs such as coldness, pallor, hair loss, sores, redness or warmth over the veins, or visible veins?
These signs may indicate arterial insufficiency of the legs.

EXAMINATION

ROUTINE TECHNIQUES

General Appearance
• INSPECT for general appearance, skin color, and breathing effort.

Peripheral Vascular System
• PALPATE the temporal and carotid pulses.
• INSPECT the jugular vein.
• MEASURE blood pressure.
• INSPECT and PALPATE the upper extremities.
• PALPATE upper-extremity pulses.
• INSPECT and PALPATE the lower extremities.
• PALPATE lower-extremity pulses.

Heart
• INSPECT the anterior chest wall.
• PALPATE the apical pulse.
• AUSCULTATE heart sounds.
• INTERPRET the electrocardiogram of the conduction of the heart

SPECIAL CIRCUMSTANCES OR ADVANCED PRACTICE

Peripheral Vascular System
• AUSCULTATE the carotid arteries.
• ESTIMATE jugular venous pressure. ★
• PALPATE the epitrochlear lymph nodes.
• PALPATE the lower extremities.
• PALPATE the inguinal lymph nodes.
• CALCULATE the ankle-brachial index.
• ASSESS for varicose veins. ★

Heart
• PALPATE the precordium. ★
• PERCUSS the heart borders. ★

EQUIPMENT NEEDED
Stethoscope • Sphygmomanometer • Tape measure • Penlight • Tongue blade and ruler • Marking pen or pencil and centimeter ruler (optional) • Doppler and conductivity gel

★ Advanced practice.

PROCEDURE AND TECHNIQUES WITH EXPECTED FINDINGS

ROUTINE TECHNIQUES: GENERAL APPEARANCE

CLEAN hands.

INSPECT the patient for general appearance, skin color, and breathing effort.
Observe the patient. He or she should appear at ease and relaxed with skin color appropriate for race and regular, unlabored respirations.

ROUTINE TECHNIQUES: PERIPHERAL VASCULAR SYSTEM

PALPATE temporal and carotid pulses for amplitude.
Procedure: For the temporal pulse, palpate over the temporal bone on each side of the head lateral to each eyebrow to assess perfusion and pain (Figs. 12-11 and 12-12).

For the carotid pulse, palpate along the medial edge of the sternocleidomastoid muscle in the lower third of the neck to assess perfusion. Palpate one carotid pulse at a time to avoid reducing blood flow to the brain (Figs. 12-13 and 12-14; also see Fig. 12-12).

ABNORMAL FINDINGS

Dyspnea, cyanosis, pallor, and use of accessory muscles to breathe are abnormal findings.

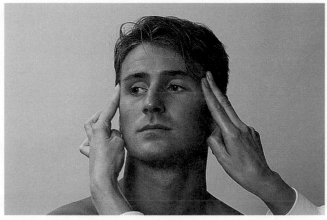

FIG. 12-11 Palpating temporal pulses lateral to each eyebrow.

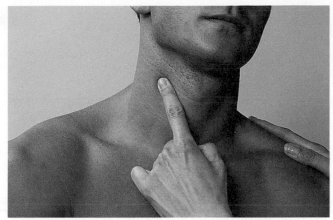

FIG. 12-13 Palpating carotid pulse in lower third of the neck.

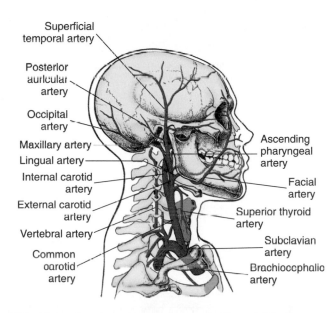

FIG. 12-12 Arteries of head and neck. (From Thibodeau and Patton, 1999.)

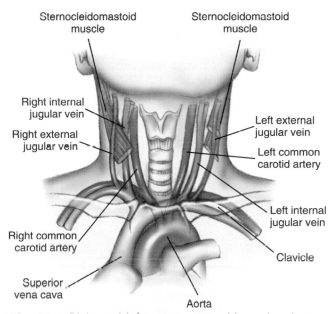

FIG. 12-14 Right and left common carotid arteries that are palpated. (From Barkauskas et al., 2002.)

PROCEDURE AND TECHNIQUES WITH EXPECTED FINDINGS	**ABNORMAL FINDINGS**

Findings: See Box 12-1.

INSPECT the jugular vein for pulsations.

The external jugular vein provides information about the right atrial pressure.

Procedure: Elevate the head of the bed until venous pulsation in the external jugular vein is seen above the clavicle, close to the insertion of the sternocleidomastoid muscles. The angle may be 30 to 45 degrees or as high as 90 degrees if venous pressure is elevated. Elevate the patient's chin slightly and tilt the head away from the side being examined. Use a penlight to create tangential light across the jugular veins and observe for pulsations (Fig. 12-15).

Tenderness and edema may be found in temporal arteritis. See Box 12-1, right column.

BOX 12-1 PALPATING PULSES

Palpate arteries using the finger pads of the first two fingers and applying light pressure. If you press too hard, you obscure the pulse. Note the rate, rhythm, amplitude, and contour of each pulse. Comparing pulses on each side of the body is customary. When you are unable to palpate a pulse, use a Doppler to amplify the sounds of the pulse (see Fig. 3-22).

EXPECTED FINDINGS	ABNORMAL FINDINGS
Rate	
60 to 100 beats/min (athletes may be as low as 50 beats/min). Pulse rates in women tend to be 5 to 10 beats/min faster than men.	Rates above 100 beats/min (tachycardia) or below 60 beats/min (bradycardia) are typically abnormal, although recent exertion, smoking, or anxiety elevates the rate.
Rhythm	
Regular (i.e., equal spacing between beats).	Irregular rhythms without any pattern should be noted. Coupled beats (two beats that occur close together) are abnormal also.
	When you palpate an irregular pulse rhythm, note whether there is a pattern to the irregularity. For example, pulses of patients who have premature ventricular contractions may have a pattern to the irregularity such as an extra beat every third heartbeat. This is documented as a *regular irregularity*. By contrast, pulses of patients who have atrial fibrillation may not have any pattern to the irregularity. This is documented as an *irregular irregularity*.
Amplitude	
Easily palpable, smooth upstroke. Compare the strength of upper-extremity with lower-extremity pulses and the left with the right.	Note any exaggerated or bounding upstroke or, conversely, pulses that are weak, small, or thready or when the peak is prolonged. Upstrokes should not vary (seen in pulsus alternans). The force of the beat should not be reduced during inspiration (paradoxical pulse).

Pulse Amplitude Ratings
- 0+ Absent
- 1+ Diminished, barely palpable
- 2+ Normal
- 3+ Full volume
- 4+ Full volume, bounding hyperkinetic

Contour (Outline of the Pulse That Is Felt)
Smooth and rounded, a series of unvaried, symmetric pulse strokes
NOTE: There may be a slight transient increase in rate during inspiration, especially in patients younger than 40.

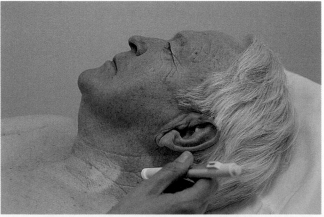

FIG. 12-15 Tangential light to view jugular veins and pulsations.

| PROCEDURE AND TECHNIQUES WITH EXPECTED FINDINGS | ABNORMAL FINDINGS |

Findings: Pulsations of the vein are visible, but not the vein itself.

Note any fluttering or oscillating of the pulsations. Note irregular rhythms or unusually prominent waves (Fig. 12-16). These may indicate right-sided heart failure.

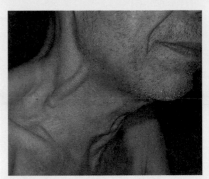

FIG. 12-16 Neck vein distention. (From Swartz, 2010.)

MEASURE blood pressure.

(See Chapter 4 for procedure.) For comparison the blood pressure frequently is taken in both arms during an initial visit. Blood pressure varies with gender, body weight, and time of day; but the upper limits for adults are less than 120 mm Hg systolic, less than 80 mm Hg diastolic, and 30 to 40 mm Hg pulse pressure. The pressure should not vary more than 5 to 10 mm Hg systolic between the two arms (Fig. 12-17).

Note elevated systolic or diastolic pressures (hypertension) and lowered systolic or diastolic pressures (hypotension). Also note significant discrepancies in measurements between the two arms.

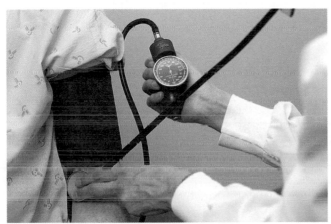

FIG. 12-17 Assessing blood pressure.

If the patient offers a history of dizziness or is taking antihypertensive medications, measure his or her blood pressure and heart rate while he or she is supine, sitting, and standing. The blood pressure is usually lower in the supine position than sitting. The blood pressure taken when standing may be lower than it is when sitting by 10 to 15 mm Hg systolic and 5 mm Hg diastolic.

A decrease in systolic blood pressure greater than 20 mm Hg and symptoms such as dizziness indicate orthostatic (postural) hypotension. Diastolic pressure may also decrease. This may be caused by a fluid volume deficit, drugs (e.g., antihypertensives), or prolonged bed rest.

INSPECT and PALPATE the upper extremities for symmetry and skin turgor.

Procedure: Inspect the upper extremities comparing the size and proportion. Pinch an area of the skin between your finger and thumb and release the skin. It should immediately fall back into place.

PROCEDURE AND TECHNIQUES WITH EXPECTED FINDINGS

Findings: The arms should appear symmetric. Skin turgor should be elastic (see Fig. 9-4).

TABLE 12-2 PITTING EDEMA SCALE

SCALE	DESCRIPTION	"MEASUREMENT"*
1+	Barely perceptible pit	2 mm (³⁄₃₂ in)
2+	Deeper pit, rebounds in a few seconds	4 mm (⁵⁄₃₂ in)
3+	Deep pit, rebounds in 10-20 seconds	6 mm (¼ in)
4+	Deeper pit, rebounds in >30 seconds	8 mm (⁵⁄₁₆ in)

1+   2   2+   4   3+   6   4+   8
mm   mm   mm   mm

Description column data from Kirton C: Assessing edema, *Nursing 96* 26(7):54, 1996.
Illustration from Seidel HM et al: *Mosby's guide to physical examination,* ed 7, St Louis, 2011, Mosby.
*"Measurement" is in quotation marks because depth of edema is rarely actually measured but is included as a frame of reference.

INSPECT and PALPATE the upper extremities for skin integrity, color, and temperature; capillary refill; and color and angle of the nail beds.

Procedure: As you inspect, notice the skin integrity and color. Use the back of your hand to assess skin temperature (Fig. 12-19). Assess capillary refill by gently squeezing pads of fingers or nails until they blanche. Release pressure and observe capillary refill (i.e., how many seconds it takes for the original color to appear) (Fig. 12-20). Inspect the nail color and the nail base angle.

ABNORMAL FINDINGS

Asymmetric upper extremities are abnormal. When one arm is larger in circumference than the other, it could be caused by lymphedema. When the skin does not immediately fall back into place, it is termed *tenting* and is an indication of reduced fluid in the interstitial space from fluid volume deficit (see Fig. 9-5). When the indentation of the thumb or finger remains in the skin, it is termed *pitting edema* and is an indication of excess fluid in the interstitial space (Fig. 12-18). Refer to Table 12-2 for an interpretation of edema.

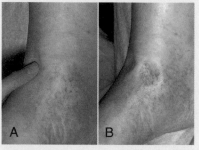

FIG. 12-18 Technique for testing for pitting edema. **A,** The nurse presses into the shin area. **B,** An indentation remains after the fingers are lifted when pitting edema is present. (From Forbes and Jackson, 2003.)

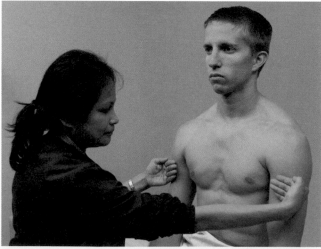

FIG. 12-19 Assess for skin temperature comparing sides using the back of the hand.

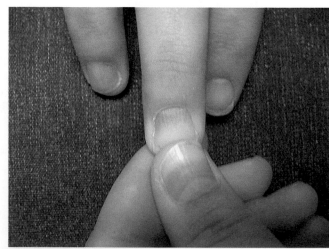

FIG. 12-20 Assessing capillary refill. (From Cummings, Stanley-Green, and Higgs, 2009.)

PROCEDURE AND TECHNIQUES WITH EXPECTED FINDINGS

Findings: The skin should be intact, with color appropriate for race. The skin should feel warm bilaterally. Capillary refill should be 2 seconds or less. Nail beds should be pink, with an angle of 160 degrees at the nail bed (see Fig. 9-10, *A*).

ABNORMAL FINDINGS

Thickening skin, skin tears, and ulceration are abnormal findings. Note marked pallor or mottling when the extremity is elevated or any ulcerated fingertips. Arterial insufficiency may cause cold extremities in a warm environment and is abnormal. A capillary refill time greater than 2 seconds indicates poor perfusion. Clubbing of fingers (angle of nail disappears, becoming greater than 160 degrees) indicates chronic hypoxemia (Fig. 12-21).

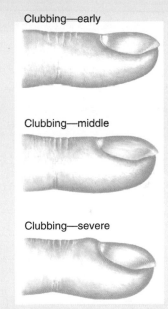

Clubbing—early

Clubbing—middle

Clubbing—severe

FIG. 12-21 Clubbing of fingers. (From Canobbio, 1990.)

PALPATE brachial and radial pulses for rate, rhythm, amplitude, and contour. When indicated, palpate ulnar pulses.

Procedure: Recall from Chapter 4 that pulses are palpated with the pads of the index and second fingers using pressure that is firm but not so hard as to occlude the pulsations. For the brachial pulse palpate in the groove between the biceps and triceps muscle just medial to the biceps tendon at the antecubital fossa (in the bend of the elbow) (Figs. 12-22 and 12-24).

For the radial pulses palpate at the radial or thumb sides of the forearm at the wrist. Often both radial pulses are palpated at the same time to assess for equality (Fig. 12-23; see Fig. 12-24).

When palpating the radial artery is difficult or it has been injured, palpate the ulnar pulses located on the medial side of the forearm (Fig. 12-25).

Findings: Box 12-1, left column, has expected findings for pulses.

See Box 12-1, right column, for abnormal findings. Patients who take certain medications such as beta-adrenergic antagonists and digoxin may have slow pulse rates because of the medication.

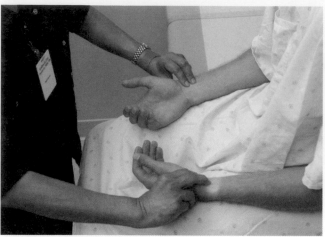

FIG. 12-22 Palpating brachial pulse at antecubital fossa.

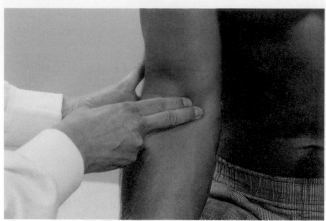

FIG. 12-23 Palpating radial pulse on thumb side of forearm at the wrist. Often both radial pulses are palpated at the same time to assess for equality.

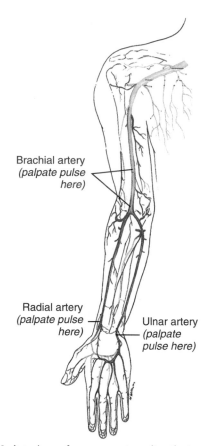

Brachial artery
(palpate pulse here)

Radial artery
(palpate pulse here)

Ulnar artery
(palpate pulse here)

FIG. 12-24 Arteries of upper extremity that are palpated. (Modified from Francis and Martin, 1975.)

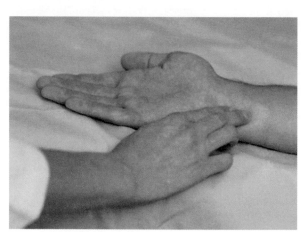

FIG. 12-25 Palpating ulnar pulse on medial side of forearm. (From Potter et al., 2013.)

PROCEDURE AND TECHNIQUES WITH EXPECTED FINDINGS	**ABNORMAL FINDINGS**

INSPECT and PALPATE the lower extremities for symmetry and skin turgor.

Procedure: Inspect the lower extremities, comparing the size and proportion. Pinch an area of the skin between your finger and thumb and release the skin as was performed on the upper extremities. It should immediately fall back into place, indicating elasticity.

Findings: Legs should appear symmetric. Skin turgor should be elastic (see Fig. 9-4).

Abnormalities are similar to those described for the upper extremities.

INSPECT and PALPATE the lower extremities for skin integrity, color, and temperature; capillary refill; hair distribution; color and angle of nail beds; superficial veins; and gross sensation.

Procedure: Follow the same procedures performed on the upper extremities for assessment of skin integrity, color, temperature; capillary refill; and color and angle of nail beds. Observe the hair distribution. Some women shave leg hair, but others do not. With the patient's legs dependent, observe for superficial veins that appear dilated. Palpate the legs lightly for tenderness or numbness.

Findings: The skin should be intact, with color appropriate for race. The skin should feel warm. Capillary refill should be 2 seconds or less. Nails should be pink, with an angle of 160 degrees at the nail bed. Men and women who do not shave their legs should have hair evenly distributed on upper and lower legs. Veins should not be visible. Sensation of the legs should be present without tenderness or numbness.

Abnormalities of integrity, color, temperature, capillary refill, and nail color and angle are similar to those described for the upper extremities. Note marked pallor or mottling when the extremity is elevated or any ulcerated digit tips. Arterial insufficiency may cause a decrease in or lack of hair peripherally or skin that appears thin, shiny, and taut. Varicose veins appear as dilated, often tortuous veins when legs are in a dependent position. Note if there is tenderness on palpation or the sensation of "stocking anesthesia," wherein the legs feel numb in a pattern resembling stockings

PALPATE femoral, popliteal, posterior tibial, and dorsalis pedis pulses for amplitude.

Procedure:

- To locate the *femoral pulse*, palpate below the inguinal ligament, midway between the symphysis pubis and anterior superior iliac, and move your fingers inward toward the pubic hair. You can locate the anatomy using the mnemonic NAVEL: *N*, nerve; *A*, artery; *V*, vein; *E*, empty space; *L*, lymph. Firm compression may be needed for obese patients (Fig. 12-26; see Fig. 12-30).
- For the *popliteal pulse*, palpate the popliteal artery behind the knee in the popliteal fossa to assess perfusion (Fig. 12-27; see Fig. 12-30). This pulse may be difficult to find. Having the patient in the prone position and flexing the leg slightly may help to find it.
- For the *posterior tibial pulse*, palpate on the inner aspect of the ankle below and slightly behind the medial malleolus (ankle bone) to assess for perfusion (Fig. 12-28; see Fig. 12-30).
- For the *dorsalis pedis pulse*, palpate lightly over the dorsum of the foot between the extension tendons of the first and second toes to assess for perfusion (Figs. 12-29 and 12-30). Often both dorsalis pedis pulses are palpated at the same time to assess for equality.

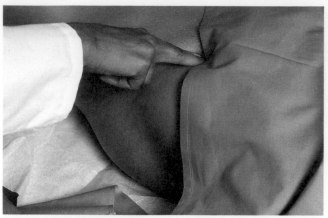

FIG. 12-26 Palpating femoral pulse below inguinal ligament between symphysis pubis and anterior-superior iliac crest. (From Canobbio, 1990.)

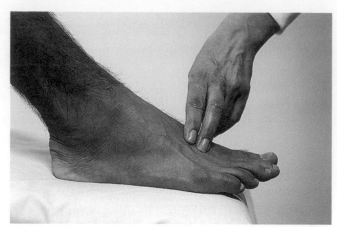

FIG. 12-29 Palpating dorsalis pedis pulse on top of foot between first and second toes.

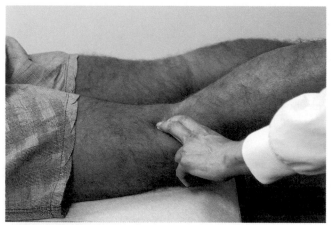

FIG. 12-27 Palpating popliteal pulse behind the knee.

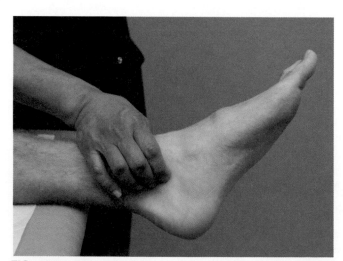

FIG. 12-28 Palpating posterior tibial pulse on inner aspect of the ankle.

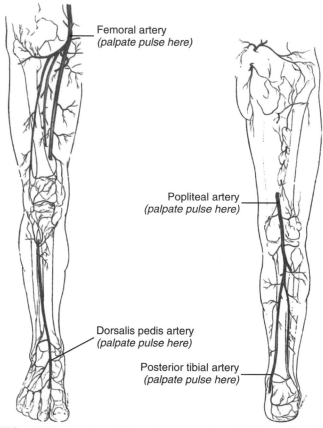

Femoral artery
(palpate pulse here)

Popliteal artery
(palpate pulse here)

Dorsalis pedis artery
(palpate pulse here)

Posterior tibial artery
(palpate pulse here)

FIG. 12-30 Arteries of leg that are palpated. (From Francis and Martin, 1975.)

| **PROCEDURE AND TECHNIQUES WITH EXPECTED FINDINGS** | **ABNORMAL FINDINGS** |

Findings: See Box 12-1, left column.

See Box 12-1, right column. Impaired peripheral pulses may indicate arterial insufficiency.

ROUTINE TECHNIQUES: HEART

INSPECT the anterior chest wall for contour, pulsations, lifts, heaves, and retractions.

Provide modesty and privacy while inspecting the female patient's unclothed chest. Use tangential light to inspect the patient's chest at eye level. The chest should be rounded and symmetric. Slight retraction medial to the left midclavicular line at the fourth or fifth intercostal space is expected; this is the apical pulse. This location may be documented as LMCL 5ICS. See Box 12-2 for abbreviations of topographic landmarks.

Note any sternal depression or asymmetry. A retraction is noted when some of the tissue is pulled into the chest on the precordium. Marked retraction of apical space may indicate pericardial disease or right ventricular hypertrophy. Box 12-3 has definitions of lifts, heaves, thrills, and retraction.

The apical pulse may be visible only when the patient sits up and leans forward, bringing the heart closer to the anterior chest. It may be obscured by obesity, large breasts, or muscularity.

Apical pulsation may be observed after exertion, in hyperthyroidism, or in left ventricular hypertrophy. Pulsations may be displaced left, right, or downward because of cardiac anomalies or change in heart size.

PALPATE apical pulse for location.

Procedure: With the patient in a sitting position, palpate over the apex of the heart at the fifth intercostal space, left midclavicular line, using the fingertips (Fig. 12-31). This is the point of maximal impulse (PMI) that corresponds to the left ventricular apex. If the PMI cannot be palpated in this position, repeat the procedure with the patient lying supine and also on the left side.

| BOX 12-2 | **ABBREVIATIONS FOR TOPOGRAPHIC LANDMARKS** |

ICS	Intercostal space	LSB	Left sternal border
RICS	Right intercostal space	MCL	Midclavicular line
LICS	Left intercostal space	RMCL	Right midclavicular line
SB	Sternal border		
RSB	Right sternal border	LMCL	Left midclavicular line

| BOX 12-3 | **DEFINITIONS OF LIFT, HEAVE, THRILL, AND RETRACTION** |

A *lift* feels like a more sustained thrust than an expected apical pulse and is felt during systole. A *heave* is a more prominent thrust of the heart against the chest wall during systole. Lifts and heaves may occur from left or right ventricular hypertrophy caused by increased workload. A *thrill* is a palpable vibration over the precordium or artery: it feels like a fine, palpable, rushing vibration. A thrill is associated with a loud murmur. *Retraction* of the chest is a visible sinking in of tissues between and around the ribs. Retraction begins in the intercostal spaces. It occurs with increased respiratory effort. If additional effort is needed to fill the lungs, supraclavicular and infraclavicular retraction may be seen.

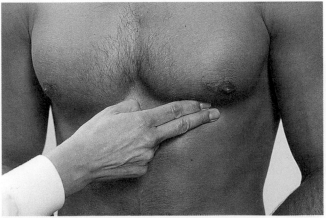

FIG. 12-31 Palpating apical pulse at fourth or fifth intercostal space, left midclavicular line.

PROCEDURE AND TECHNIQUES WITH EXPECTED FINDINGS

Findings: The apical pulse or PMI is expected in the fifth intercostal space at the left midclavicular line.

AUSCULTATE S_1 and S_2 heart sounds for rate, rhythm, pitch, and splitting.

Procedure:

- Box 12-4 describes a technique for locating intercostal spaces for auscultation of the heart. All five areas should be auscultated, first with the diaphragm using firm pressure and then with the bell using light pressure. The sounds are generated by valve closure and are best heard where blood flows away from the valve instead of directly over the valve area (Fig. 12-32). Heart sounds may be low pitched, making them difficult to hear (Box 12-5). When first learning heart sounds, you may want to close your eyes to concentrate on each sound (i.e., selective listening).
- Clean the bell and diaphragm of your stethoscope.
- Begin with the patient sitting upright. Use a systematic approach to listen in the five auscultatory areas, with the patient breathing normally and then holding the breath in expiration. This allows you to hear the heart sounds better.
- Using the diaphragm, begin with the aortic valve area (second ICS, RSB) (see Box 12-2 for abbreviations) (Fig. 12-33, *A*), then the pulmonic valve area (second ICS, LSB) (Fig. 12-33, *B*), then Erb's point (third ICS, LSB) (Fig. 12-33, *C*), then the tricuspid valve area (fourth ICS, LSB) (Fig. 12-33, *D*), and finally the mitral valve area/apical pulse (fifth ICS, LMCL) (Fig. 12-33, *E*). Repeat the auscultation of the five areas using the bell of the stethoscope. Box 12-6 has tips to help you remember to which valves you are listening.

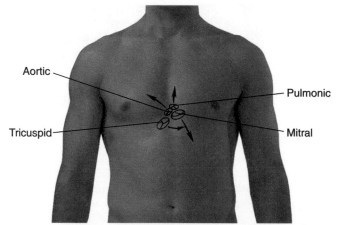

FIG. 12-32 Transmission of closure sounds from heart valves.

ASSESS heart rate.

Count the number of heartbeats (S_1 and S_2) heard for 1 minute for the apical rate. First heart sound (S_1) is made by the closing of the mitral (M1) and tricuspid (T1) valves. (When the heart sounds are described as *lubb-dubb*, the *lubb* represents S_1.) S_1 indicates the beginning of systole. The second heart sound (S_2) is made by the closing of the aortic (A2) and pulmonic (P2) valves. It is described as the "dub" of *lubb-dubb* and indicates the beginning of diastole.

ABNORMAL FINDINGS

If the patient has ventricular hypertrophy, the myocardium is enlarged, which may move the PMI laterally. Patients who have chronic obstructive lung disease have overinflated lungs, which may displace the PMI downward and to the right.[4]

BOX 12-4 TECHNIQUE FOR LOCATING INTERCOSTAL SPACES FOR AUSCULTATION OF THE HEART

- A systematic approach is needed for this assessment. Some nurses begin at the apex and proceed upward toward the base of the heart, whereas others begin at the base and proceed downward toward the apex. The sequence is irrelevant as long as the assessment is systematic. Listen first with the diaphragm to hear high-pitched sounds and then with the bell to hear low-pitched sounds.
- When auscultating from base to apex, begin at the second intercostal space (ICS). Locate this ICS by palpating the right sternoclavicular joint (where the right clavicle joins the sternum).
- Palpate the first rib and then move down to palpate the space between the first and second ribs: this is the first ICS.
- Continue palpating downward to the space between the second and third ribs. This is the second ICS at the right sternal border (RSB), the auscultatory site for the aortic valve area. This is not the anatomic site of the aortic valve but the site on the chest wall where sounds produced by the valve are heard best.
- Moving to the left side of the sternum at the second ICS, the area for auscultating the pulmonic valve area is found.
- Remaining at the left sternal border (LSB), move the stethoscope down to the third ICS, which is called Erb's point, an area to which pulmonic or aortic sounds frequently radiate. The fourth ICS, the LSB is over the tricuspid valve area.

- At the fifth ICS, move the stethoscope laterally to the left midclavicular line (LMCL), where the mitral valve area is located.

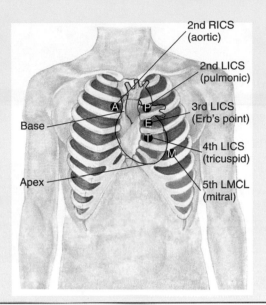

2nd RICS (aortic)
2nd LICS (pulmonic)
3rd LICS (Erb's point)
Base
4th LICS (tricuspid)
Apex
5th LMCL (mitral)

BOX 12-5 LOW- AND HIGH-PITCHED SOUNDS OF THE HEART

In Chapter 4 you read that the heart had low-pitched (low frequency) sounds best heard with the bell of the stethoscope and that breath sounds were high pitched (high frequency), best heard with the diaphragm of the stethoscope. In this chapter you read that S_1 is lower in pitch than S_2 or that S_2 is higher in pitch than S_1 and that bruits are low pitched. How can both statements be true? The pitch of the sounds is relative, depending on which sounds you are comparing. When comparing breath sounds with heart sounds, heart sounds are low pitched. However, when comparing the sounds of S_1 with S_2, the pitch of S_1 is lower than S_2. Now, if you compared the pitch of breath sounds to the pitch of S_2, you would find that S_2 is low pitched. These sounds could be put on a continuum from high to low pitch. Breath sounds would be high pitched, S_2 would be a lower pitch than breath sounds but higher than S_1, and S_1 would be the lowest pitch of all three sounds.

BOX 12-6 TIPS TO REMEMBER

To help you remember to which valve you are listening (aortic, pulmonic, tricuspid, or mitral), use the mnemonic:

Apartment M or APT M:
Aortic
Pulmonic
Tricuspid
Mitral

Or

APE TO MAN:
Aortic
Pulmonic
Erb's point
To tricuspid
Mitral

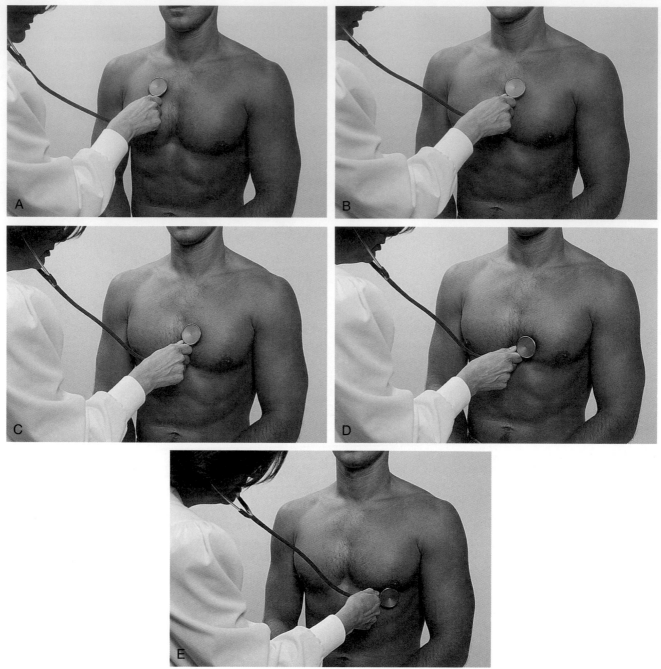

FIG. 12-33 Position for cardiac auscultation. **A,** Aortic area. **B,** Pulmonic area. **C,** Erb's point. **D,** Tricuspid area. **E,** Mitral area.

PROCEDURE AND TECHNIQUES WITH EXPECTED FINDINGS

Findings: This heart sound should be heard at all sites. S_1 is louder than S_2 at the apex over the tricuspid valve (fourth left ICS) and the mitral valve (fifth left MCL). S_1 is usually lower in pitch than S_2; it is almost synchronous with the carotid pulse.

Expected range is 60 to 100 beats/min; conditioned athletes may have slower rates.

ABNORMAL FINDINGS

Rates greater than 100 or less than 60 beats/min are abnormal. Note any irregular rhythm, sporadic or extra beats, or pauses between beats.

See Box 12-1, right column, for abnormal findings.

PROCEDURE AND TECHNIQUES WITH EXPECTED FINDINGS	ABNORMAL FINDINGS

ASSESS rhythm.

When listening to each heartbeat, notice the spacing between beats. Normally the heart rate is regular (i.e., an equal space between beats).

See Box 12-1, right column, for abnormal findings. Table 12-3 describes abnormal heart sounds.

ASSESS pitch.

Note the pitch of the heart sounds. Pitch is the quality of the sound dependent on the relative speed of the vibrations by which it is produced. The first and second heart sounds have low and high pitches, respectively (see Box 12-5).

An abnormality may be present when the first heart sound seems accented, diminished, or muffled or when intensity varies with different beats.

TABLE 12-3 ABNORMAL HEART SOUNDS

Abnormal heart sounds and murmurs are described by where they occur in the cardiac cycle. The normal sequence of events in the cardiac cycle can be diagrammed as follows:

$$S_1 \rightarrow systole \rightarrow S_2 \rightarrow diastole \rightarrow S_1 \rightarrow etc.$$

To determine if an abnormal sound occurs in systole or diastole, determine if the sound occurs after S_1 or after S_2.

- During diastole, when 80% of the blood in the atria rapidly fills the ventricles, a third heart sound may be heard (S_3). It is often heard at the apex. An S_3 occurs just after the S_2 and lasts about the same time as it takes to say "me too." The "me" is the S_2, and the "too" is the S_3. An S_3 is normal in children and young adults. However, when an S_3 is heard in adults over 30 years of age, it signifies fluid volume overload to the ventricle that may be caused by heart failure or mitral or tricuspid regurgitation.[4]
- At the end of diastole, when atrial contraction completes the filling of the ventricle, a fourth heart sound may be heard (S_4). An S_4 occurs just before the S_1 and lasts about the same time as it takes to say "middle." The "mi" is the S_4, and the "ddle" is the S_1. An S_4 is normal in children and young adults. However, when an S_4 is heard in adults over 30 years of age, it signifies a noncompliant or "stiff" ventricle. Hypertrophy of the ventricle precedes a noncompliant ventricle. Coronary artery disease is also a major cause of a stiff ventricle. Useful mnemonics for remembering the cadence and pathophysiology of the third and fourth heart sounds[5] are as follows.

SLOSH'ing-in	SLOSH'ing-in	SLOSH'ing in
$S_1\ S_2\ S_3$	$S_1\ S_2\ S_3$	$S_1\ S_2\ S_3$
a-STIFF'-wall	a-STIFF'-wall	a-STIFF'-wall
$S_4\ S_1\ S_2$	$S_4\ S_1\ S_2$	$S_4\ S_1\ S_2$

Another way to remember the cadence of the S_3 and S_4 heart sounds is to use the words "Kentucky" and "Tennessee."

Ken-tuck-y	Ken-tuck-y	Ken-tuck-y
$S_1\ S_2\ S_3$	$S_1\ S_2\ S_3$	$S_1\ S_2\ S_3$
Ten-ness-ee	Ten-ness-ee	Ten-ness-ee
$S_4\ S_1\ S_2$	$S_4\ S_1\ S_2$	$S_4\ S_1\ S_2$

Thus the third and fourth heart sounds can be abnormal when they occur in adults over 30. Both sounds occur in diastole.

The opening *snap* caused by the opening of the mitral or tricuspid valves is another abnormal sound heard in diastole when either valve is thickened, stenotic, or deformed. The sounds are high pitched and occur early in diastole.

- In systole *ejection clicks* may be heard if either the aortic or pulmonic valve is stenotic or deformed. The aortic valve ejection click is heard at either the apex or base of the heart and does not change with respiration. The less common pulmonic valve ejection click is heard over the second or third left intercostal space. It increases with expiration and decreases with inspiration.
- *Pericardial friction rubs* are caused by inflammation of the layers of the pericardial sac. A rubbing sound is usually present in both diastole and systole and is best heard over the apical area.

PROCEDURE AND TECHNIQUES WITH EXPECTED FINDINGS

ASSESS splitting.

Notice whether there is one sound or two for each S_1 and S_2 sound. Although the closing of two valves creates each heart sound, you should hear only one sound indicating that the valves are closing at the same time.

TABLE 12-4	LISTENING TO MURMURS
When you identify a heart murmur, consider the following variables for documentation:	
Timing and duration	At what part of the cycle is the murmur heard? Is it associated with S_1 or S_2, or is it continuous?
Pitch	Is it a low or high pitch? Low pitches are best heard with the bell of the stethoscope.
Quality	Quality refers to the type of sound, including a harsh sound; a raspy, machinelike sound; or a vibratory, musical, or blowing sound.
Intensity	Murmur intensity refers to how loud the murmur is: • Grade I is barely audible in a quiet room. • Grade II is quiet but clearly audible. • Grade III is moderately loud. • Grade IV is loud and associated with a thrill. • Grade V is very loud, and a thrill is easily palpable. • Grade VI is very loud, and a thrill is palpable and visible.
Location	Where is the sound heard loudest? Most often it is over one of the five anatomic landmarks used to auscultate heart sounds.
Example of documentation	S_1, grade II, low-pitch murmur auscultated at fifth ICS, MCL. No thrill palpable.

ICS, Intercostal space; *MCL*, midclavicular line.

INTERPRET the electrocardiogram of the conduction of the heart.

The electrical conduction of the heart can be seen on an electrocardiogram (ECG) to assess rate and rhythm. When spoken, the abbreviation for this assessment tool is called an EKG rather than an ECG to avoid errors because the sound of ECG is similar to that of EEG (electroencephalogram). Fig. 12-34, *A*, shows the ECG reflections of one cardiac cycle. The P wave represents the atrial contraction or depolarization. The QRS complex represents the ventricular contraction or depolarization. The atrial repolarization occurs at the same time but is overshadowed by the ventricular contraction. The T wave represents the repolarization of the ventricle. Fig. 12-34, *B*, shows the time intervals of each part of the cardiac cycle. Fig. 12-34, *C*, shows which part of the heart is represented by the wave or complex.

ABNORMAL FINDINGS

When the mitral and tricuspid valves do not close at the same time, S_1 sounds as if it were split into two sounds instead of one. Splitting is heard infrequently in the tricuspid area with deep inspiration and varies from beat to beat, occasionally heard as a narrow split. Note that the fourth heart sound is sometimes mistaken for the splitting of the first heart sound.

Table 12-4 describes variables when a murmur is heard. Table 12-5 describes murmurs caused by valvular defects.

Systolic Murmur

A murmur occurring during the ventricular ejection phase of the cardiac cycle is termed a *systolic murmur*. Most systolic murmurs are caused by obstruction of the outflow of the semilunar valves or by incompetent atrioventricular (AV) valves. The vibration is heard during all or part of systole. Other causes of systolic murmurs are structural deformities of the aorta or pulmonary arteries, anemia, and thyrotoxicosis (hyperthyroidism). A ventricular septal defect results in a murmur classified as *pansystolic* or *holosystolic* because it occupies all of systole.

Diastolic Murmur

A murmur occurring in the filling phase of the cardiac cycle is termed a *diastolic murmur*. Incompetent semilunar valves or stenotic AV valves create diastolic murmurs. These murmurs almost always indicate heart disease. Early diastolic murmurs usually result from insufficiency of a semilunar valve or dilation of the valvular ring. Mid- and late-diastolic murmurs are generally caused by stenosed mitral and tricuspid valves that obstruct blood flow.

TABLE 12-5 MURMURS CAUSED BY VALVULAR DEFECTS

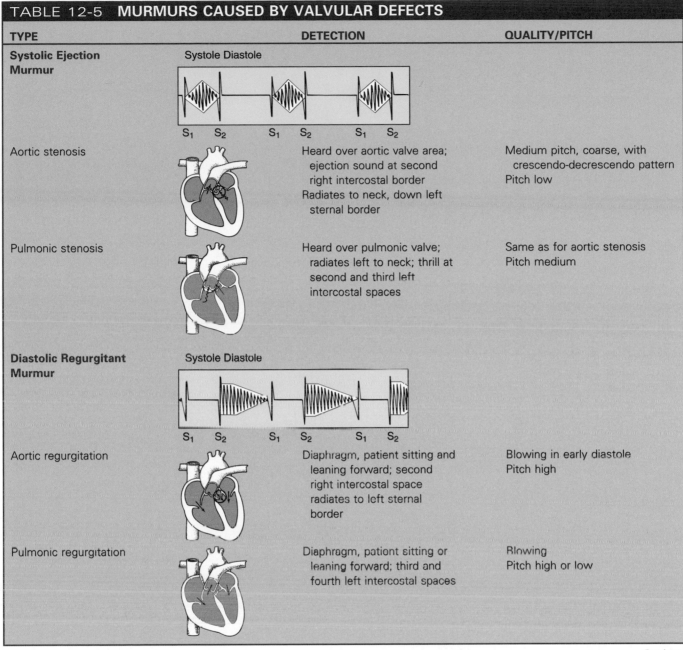

TYPE	DETECTION	QUALITY/PITCH
Systolic Ejection Murmur	Systole Diastole S₁ S₂ S₁ S₂ S₁ S₂	
Aortic stenosis	Heard over aortic valve area; ejection sound at second right intercostal border Radiates to neck, down left sternal border	Medium pitch, coarse, with crescendo-decrescendo pattern Pitch low
Pulmonic stenosis	Heard over pulmonic valve; radiates left to neck; thrill at second and third left intercostal spaces	Same as for aortic stenosis Pitch medium
Diastolic Regurgitant Murmur	Systole Diastole S₁ S₂ S₁ S₂ S₁ S₂	
Aortic regurgitation	Diaphragm, patient sitting and leaning forward; second right intercostal space radiates to left sternal border	Blowing in early diastole Pitch high
Pulmonic regurgitation	Diaphragm, patient sitting or leaning forward; third and fourth left intercostal spaces	Blowing Pitch high or low

Continued

TABLE 12-5 MURMURS CAUSED BY VALVULAR DEFECTS—cont'd

TYPE	DETECTION	QUALITY/PITCH
Diastolic Murmur	Systole Diastole	
Mitral stenosis	Bell at apex with patient in left lateral decubitus position	Low rumble more intense in early and late diastole Pitch low
Tricuspid stenosis	Bell over tricuspid area.	Similar to mitral stenosis but louder on inspiration Pitch low
Holosystolic Murmur	Systole Diastole	
Mitral regurgitation	Diaphragm at apex, radiates to left axilla or base	Harsh blowing quality Pitch high
Tricuspid regurgitation	Fifth intercostal space, left lower sternal border	Blowing Pitch high

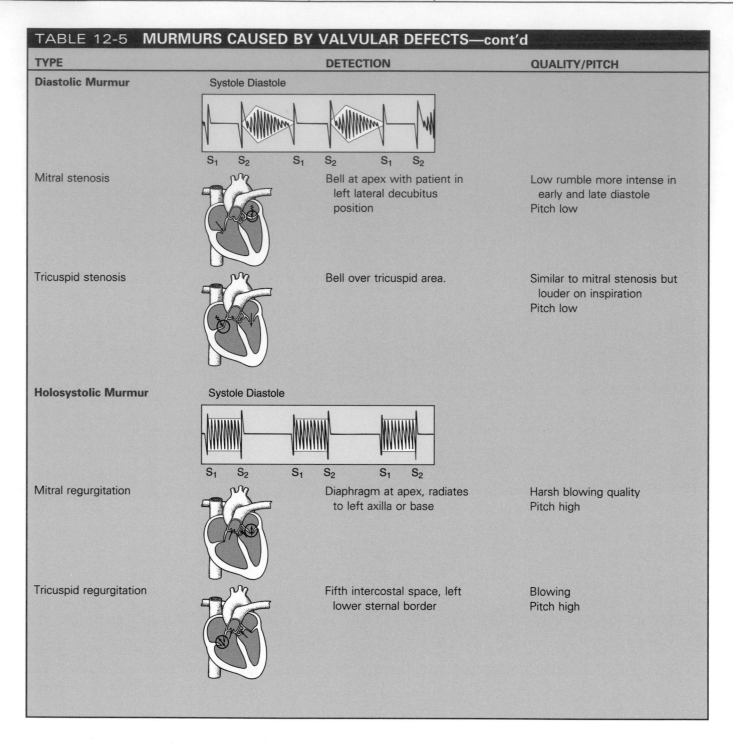

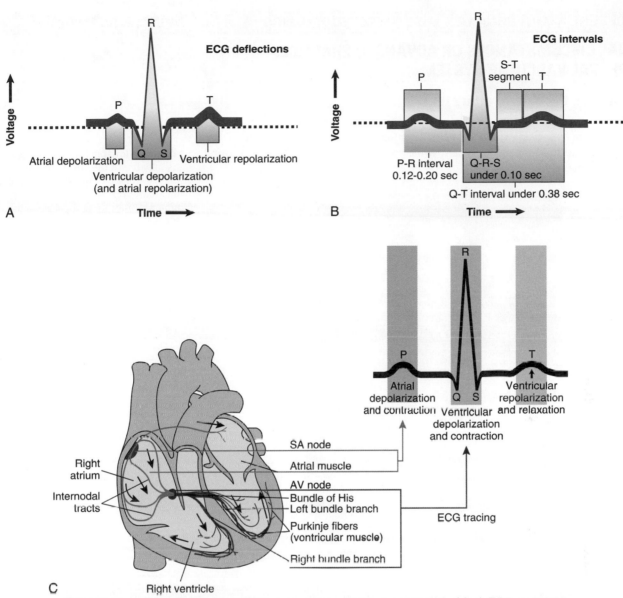

FIG. 12-34 Electrocardiogram (ECG) and cardiac electrical activity. **A,** Ideal ECG deflections represent depolarization and repolarization of cardiac muscle tissue. **B,** Principal ECG interval among P, QRS, and T waves. Note that the P-R interval is measured from the start of the P wave to the end of the Q wave. **C,** Schematic representation of ECG and its relationship to the cardiac electrical activity. *AV,* Atrioventricular; *LA,* left atrium; *LBB,* left bundle branch; *LV,* left ventricle; *RA,* right atrium; *RBB,* right bundle branch; *RV,* right ventricular, *SA,* sinoatrial. (**A** and **B** from Patton and Thibodeau, 2010. **C** from Gould and Dyer, 2011.)

| PROCEDURE AND TECHNIQUES WITH EXPECTED FINDINGS | ABNORMAL FINDINGS |

SPECIAL CIRCUMSTANCES OR ADVANCED PRACTICE: PERIPHERAL VASCULAR SYSTEM

AUSCULTATE the carotid artery for bruits.

Listen for carotid bruits when the patient has a history of atherosclerosis or reports dizziness or syncope. Using the bell of the stethoscope, auscultate the carotid artery. Ask the patient to hold his or her breath while you listen. You should hear no sound over these arteries (Fig. 12-35).

Bruits are low-pitched blowing sounds usually heard during systole that indicate occlusion of the vessel. Occlusion of a carotid artery may impair perfusion of the brain and increase the risk for transient ischemic attack (TIA).

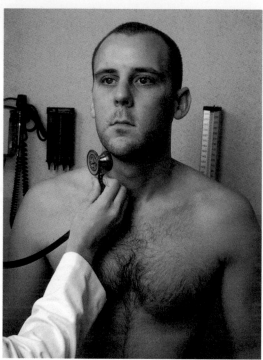

FIG. 12-35 Auscultating carotid artery. (From Harkreader, Hogan, and Thobaben, 2007.)

★ ESTIMATE jugular venous pressure for pulsations.

Jugular venous pressure estimates the pressure in the right side of the heart. Estimate this pressure when the patient has fluid retention or right-sided heart failure.

Procedure: With the patient's head elevated, identify the highest level at which jugular vein pulsations are visible and identify the manubriosternal joint (angle of Louis). Use a tongue blade or ruler to create an imaginary line from the highest venous pulsation to the manubriosternal angle. Measure the vertical distance between the tongue blade and the manubriosternal angle to estimate jugular venous pressure in centimeters (Fig. 12-36). This pressure should not rise more than 1 inch (2.5 cm) above the sternal angle. (NOTE: If you cannot find the jugular vein, have the patient lie down flat for a few minutes so it will distend.)

★ Advanced practice.

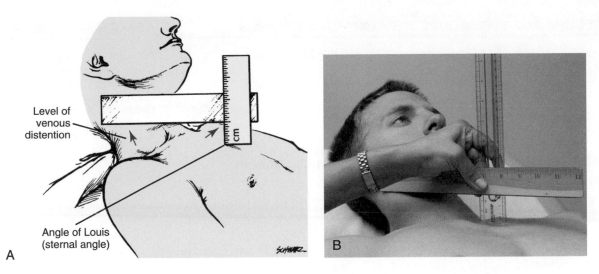

Level of venous distention

Angle of Louis (sternal angle)

A

B

FIG. 12-36 Measuring jugular venous pressure. (**A** from Barkauskas et al., 2002.)

PROCEDURE AND TECHNIQUES WITH EXPECTED FINDINGS

Findings: Pulsations should be regular, soft, and of a wavelike quality. The level of pulsation decreases with inspiration, and the pulsation increases in recumbent position.

PALPATE epitrochlear lymph nodes for size, consistency, mobility, borders, tenderness, and warmth.

These lymph nodes are palpated when the patient has an acute infection of the ulnar aspect of the arm or a malignancy such as non-Hodgkin's lymphoma.[4]

Procedure: Flex the patient's arm to a 90-degree angle and palpate below the elbow posterior to the medial condyle of the humerus (Fig. 12-37). Compare the sizes of the upper and lower arms for symmetry.

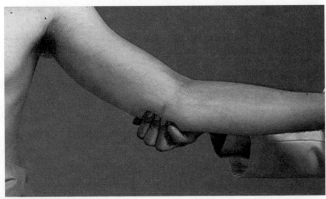

FIG. 12-37 Palpation for epitrochlear lymph nodes is performed in the depression above and posterior to the medial condyle of the humerus. (From Seidel et al., 2011.)

ABNORMAL FINDINGS

Note if the jugular venous pressure exceeds 1 inch (2.5 cm) above the level of the manubrium. **Note:** If venous pressure is elevated (meaning that the vein is distended up to the neck), raise the patient's head until the highest jugular pulsation can be detected. The distance in inches above the sternal angle and the angle at which the patient is reclining should be recorded. Also note if other veins in the neck, shoulder, or upper chest are distended. Note any fluttering or oscillating of the pulsation. Note irregular rhythms or unusually prominent waves.

PROCEDURE AND TECHNIQUES WITH EXPECTED FINDINGS	ABNORMAL FINDINGS

Findings: The arms should be symmetric with no palpable lymph nodes.

Enlarged, firm, warm, movable, and tender nodes may be associated with infection of the ulnar aspect of the forearm and the fourth and fifth fingers. When one arm is larger in circumference than the other, it could be caused by lymphedema.

PALPATE inguinal lymph nodes for size, consistency, mobility, borders, tenderness, and warmth.

Palpate these nodes when an inflammatory process is suspected or the patient complains of pain.

Procedure: With the patient in the supine position, lightly palpate with finger pads in the area just below the inguinal ligament and on the inner aspect of the thigh at the groin (Fig. 12-38). It may not be possible to palpate them at all, but they should be smooth and soft if they can be felt. Moving inward toward the genitalia, you can locate the anatomy using the mnemonic NAVEL: *N*, nerve; *A*, artery; *V*, vein; *E*, empty space; *L*, lymph nodes. Compare the sizes of the upper and lower legs for symmetry.

Findings: The inguinal nodes are small, mobile nodes, some of which may be nontender. The upper and lower legs should be symmetric.

Enlarged, tender, firm, warm, and freely movable nodes indicate an inflammatory process distal to these nodes such as in the leg, vulva, penis, or scrotum. When one leg is larger in circumference than the other, it could be caused by lymphedema.

MEASURE leg circumferences to assess symmetry.

When one of the patient's thighs or calves looks bigger than the other or the patient complains of pain in these areas, measure the circumferences of the affected area and the other leg to compare values.

Procedure: Place a tape measure around the enlarged area (in the thigh or calf) and note the circumference (Fig. 12-39). To measure the other leg in the same location, measure the distance from the end of the patella to the affected area. Note the distance and measure the same distance from the end of the patella on the other leg; at that location measure the circumference and compare. To ensure consistent location for measurement, you can use a marker to note the area measured on the affected leg.

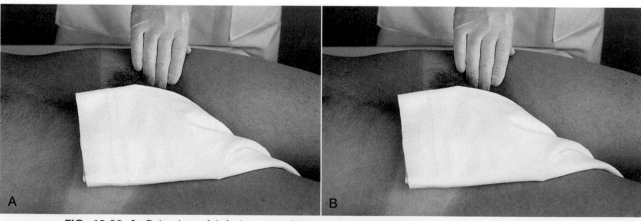

FIG. 12-38 A, Palpation of inferior superficial inguinal (femoral) lymph nodes. **B,** Palpation of superior superficial inguinal lymph nodes. (From Seidel et al., 1999.)

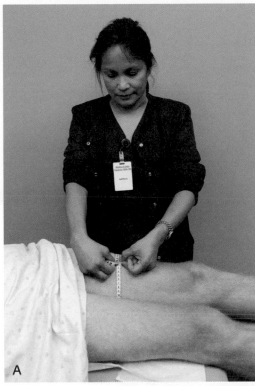

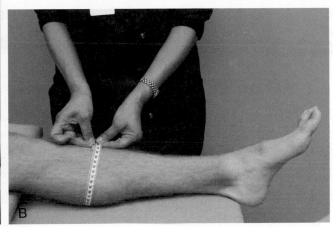

FIG. 12-39 Measurement of thigh **(A)** and calf circumference **(B)**.

PROCEDURE AND TECHNIQUES WITH EXPECTED FINDINGS

Findings: Both leg measurements should be the same.

ABNORMAL FINDINGS

Although signs and symptoms of deep vein thromboses are often silent, an increase in thigh or calf circumference may be an early indicator of a venous blood clot. Other indicators may be differences in the color or temperature of the legs. Some patients report pain at the site.[5] Chronic venous stasis may produce increases in circumferences bilaterally (Fig. 12-40).

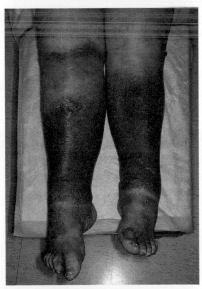

FIG. 12-40 Chronic venous stasis. (From Swartz, 2010.)

PROCEDURE AND TECHNIQUES WITH EXPECTED FINDINGS	ABNORMAL FINDINGS

★ PERFORM Trendelenburg's test to evaluate competence of venous valves.

This test is performed when patients have varicose veins. With the patient in a supine position, lift one leg above the level of the heart to allow veins to empty and help the patient stand. If veins are competent, veins fill slowly. Repeat the test on the other leg.

If the veins fill rapidly, the valves may be incompetent, and varicose veins may be present.

CALCULATE the ankle brachial index (ABI) to estimate arterial occlusion.

Calculate the ABI when the patient has peripheral arterial disease.

Procedure: The ABI is calculated by dividing the ankle systolic pressure by the brachial systolic pressure. With the patient in a supine position, take the brachial blood pressure in both arms using Doppler sound (Fig. 12-41). Apply the blood pressure cuff above the ankle to measure the systolic pressure of the posterior tibialis pulses using the Doppler. Divide the posterior tibial (ankle) systolic pressure by the brachial systolic blood pressure for each side.

Findings: The expected value of ABI is 0.95 to 1.2.

The patient who has peripheral artery disease (PAD) has impaired peripheral perfusion that is reflected in a lower systolic pressure in the leg than the arm, which reveals an ABI less than normal.
- Less than 0.80 indicates mild PAD.
- 0.40-0.80 indicates moderate PAD.
- Less than 0.40 indicates severe PAD.

Severe PAD may lead to ischemia.[6]

★ Advanced practice.

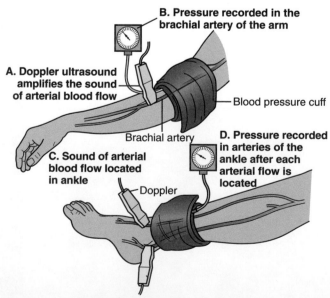

B. Pressure recorded in the brachial artery of the arm

A. Doppler ultrasound amplifies the sound of arterial blood flow

Blood pressure cuff

Brachial artery

D. Pressure recorded in arteries of the ankle after each arterial flow is located

C. Sound of arterial blood flow located in ankle

Doppler

FIG. 12-41 Measuring systolic pressures in arms and legs for ankle-brachial index. (From Roberts and Hedges, 2009.)

PROCEDURE AND TECHNIQUES WITH EXPECTED FINDINGS	ABNORMAL FINDINGS

SPECIAL CIRCUMSTANCES OR ADVANCED PRACTICE: HEART

★ PALPATE the precordium for pulsations, thrills, lifts, and heaves.

Palpate for pulsations when you suspect an aneurysm. Thrills may occur with a valvular disorder. Palpate for lifts and heaves when the patient has ventricular hypertrophy.

Procedure: Supine is the preferred position for cardiac palpation; however, the sitting position may be necessary to feel impulses. Using the palmar surface of your hand and finger pads, gently palpate the anterior chest, allowing the movements of the chest to lift the hands. Palpate systematically from the base to the apex or from the apex to the base.

Palpate the base of the heart (Fig. 12-42, *A*). No pulsations or thrills should be felt.

Observe whether the entire chest seems to lift or heave with the heartbeat. A lift or heave may indicate left ventricular enlargement.

Pulsations may indicate an aortic aneurysm. A thrill may be associated with a murmur from a disorder of the aortic or pulmonic valve.

★ Advanced practice.

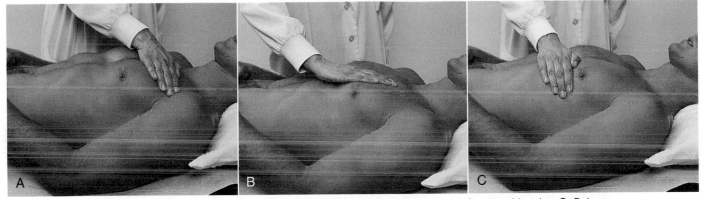

FIG. 12-42 Palpation of precordium. **A,** Palpating base. **B,** Palpating left sternal border. **C,** Palpating apex.

PROCEDURE AND TECHNIQUES WITH EXPECTED FINDINGS

Palpate the left sternal border (LSB) (Fig. 12-42, *B*) with the heel of the hand over the third, fourth, and fifth left intercostal spaces (ICSs) (see Box 12-3). No pulsations, thrills, or lifts should be felt.

Palpate the apex of the heart at the fifth ICS midclavicular line (Fig. 12-42, *C*). The apical impulse has small amplitude, is of brief duration, and is no larger than 2 to 3 cm in diameter. No forceful pulsations or thrills should be palpated.

Palpate the epigastric area for pulsations. There may be an aortic pulsation.

ABNORMAL FINDINGS

Sustained lifts or palpations may indicate right ventricular hypertrophy; pulsations may indicate pulmonary hypertension. A thrill is associated with pulmonic valve stenosis.

Forceful pulsation, displaced laterally or downward, is associated with increased cardiac output or left ventricular hypertrophy. Presence of a thrill may indicate a murmur.

Bounding pulsations may indicate abdominal aortic aneurysm or aortic valve regurgitation.

❓ CLINICAL REASONING: THINKING LIKE A NURSE
Cardiovascular System

A 67-year-old man with a long-standing history of emphysema and hypertension presents to the emergency department with a history of shortness of breath and productive cough that has progressed over the last 2 days. He also complains of being very tired and having no appetite. The nurse obtains a set of vital signs, which include: blood pressure 128/92, pulse 122 beats/min, temperature 99.2° F (37.3° C), and respiratory rate, 26 breaths/min and labored.

Interpreting
Early in the encounter the nurse considers two possible causes of the shortness of breath and cough: pneumonia, heart failure, or both. To determine if either have any probability of being correct, the nurse gathers additional data: *What is the color and character of the sputum?* The man tells the nurse that it is "whitish and bubbly."

Is there evidence of excessive fluid? The man has 2+ pitting edema in his legs and feet; he is wearing house slippers. When asked about this, he tells the nurse that he can't put on his shoes. *The nurse proceeds to auscultate his heart and lung sounds.* His lungs have crackles bilaterally; an S$_3$ heart sound is auscultated.

The experienced nurse not only recognizes heart failure by the clinical signs (increased respiratory rate and effort, bilateral crackles, S$_3$ heart sound, peripheral edema) and symptoms (fatigue, shortness of breath) but also interprets this information in the context of an older adult with hypertension and emphysema.

Nurse's Background, Experience, Perspective
The experienced nurse immediately has a perceptual grasp of the situation at hand. Extensive practical knowledge about what to expect with this age-group and diagnoses allows the nurse to recognize risk factors given his situation: age, emphysema, and hypertension.

Noticing
Although an experienced nurse would expect a patient with emphysema to be dyspneic and have a cough, this patient reports increasing shortness of breath and a productive cough, both apparent changes from his baseline. The experienced nurse understands that patients with chronic obstructive pulmonary disease are at increased risk for pneumonia and congestive heart failure; either of these might result in decreased PO$_2$, and indeed the nurse measures his oxygen saturation at 84% on room air. The nurse notices that the patient's skin is warm and slightly diaphoretic.

Responding
The nurse initiates appropriate initial interventions (oxygen delivery and obtaining intravenous access), and notifies the emergency department health care provider of the situation, ensuring that the patient receives appropriate immediate and follow-up care.

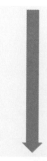

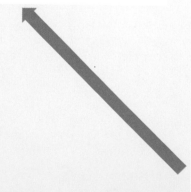

Reflecting
The nurse evaluates the presentation and outcomes of interventions (reflection-in-action); this experience contributes and deepens the expertise on which to draw again (refection-on-action) when encountering a similar situation.

PROCEDURE AND TECHNIQUES WITH EXPECTED FINDINGS

★ PERCUSS the heart borders for the heart size.

(NOTE: This is an optional assessment technique because echocardiogram provides more precise information.) Percussion is performed at the third, fourth, and fifth ICS from the left anterior axillary line to the right anterior axillary line. The expected finding is a change from resonance to dullness about 6 cm lateral to the left of the sternum. The areas of dullness are marked with a pencil, and the distance from the sternum measured with a ruler. Percussion of the heart may be difficult with obese or large-breasted patients.

ABNORMAL FINDINGS

Deviation of the left border further to the left is associated with dilated left ventricle, right pneumothorax, or pericardial effusion. Deviation of the left border to the right is associated with dextrocardia or left pneumothorax.

★ Advanced practice.

DOCUMENTING EXPECTED FINDINGS

Patient sitting in a relaxed position, with regular respirations; BP 120/68, jugular pulsations visible without distention; extremities symmetric in size; skin intact with elastic turgor, warm with color appropriate for patient without pallor or redness; pulses 70 beats/min, regular rhythm, smooth contour with pulse amplitude 2+; capillary refill <2 seconds in all extremities; nail beds pink with angle 160 degrees. Hair distribution even on upper and lower legs (unless purposefully removed). Chest rounded and symmetric. PMI at 5th ICS, MCL, S_1 louder at the apex, and S_2 louder at the base, regular rate and rhythm without murmurs or extra sounds.

No pulsations, lifts, heaves, or thrills palpated.

AGE-RELATED VARIATIONS

Nurses adapt their examinations of the heart and peripheral vascular system when assessing patients at either end of the life span. Assessing neonates and infants requires the use of different equipment and an unhurried approach. When assessing older adults, the nurse also uses an unhurried approach and may find expected variations from adults, such as increases in blood pressure.

older child and adolescent follows the same procedures and reveals similar expected findings. One exception in the examination is the electrocardiogram, which is not typically performed. Chapter 19 presents further information regarding the cardiovascular assessment of infants, children, and adolescents.

INFANTS, CHILDREN, AND ADOLESCENTS

There are several differences in the assessment of the cardiovascular system for infants and young children. For example, the equipment used to measure blood pressure is smaller, the sequence of the examination may be different, and findings may differ based on anatomical differences. Assessment of the

OLDER ADULTS

Assessing the cardiovascular status of an older adult usually follows the same procedures as for an adult. Expected variations may be found in heart rate and blood pressure. Chapter 21 presents further information regarding the cardiovascular assessment of an older adult.

COMMON PROBLEMS AND CONDITIONS

CARDIAC DISORDERS

Valvular Heart Disease

An acquired or congenital disorder of a heart valve is called *valvular heart disease (VHD)*. It can be characterized by a heart valve that does not either open completely (stenotic valve) or close completely (incompetent valve). Rheumatic fever and endocarditis account for most cases of acquired VHD. **Clinical Findings:** See Table 12-5.

Angina Pectoris

Chest pain that is caused by ischemia of the myocardium is called *angina pectoris*, or *stable angina*. It is usually caused by

atherosclerosis within the coronary arteries. Angina can occur during activity, stress, or exposure to intense cold because of an increased demand on the heart. It can also occur during rest as a result of spasms of the coronary arteries. **Clinical Findings:** Patients with stable angina describe the pain as a pressure in the chest, often a squeezing, suffocating, or constricting sensation. Stable angina usually lasts from 5 to 15 minutes and commonly subsides when the precipitating factor is relieved or when treated with nitroglycerin.

Acute Coronary Syndrome

When ischemia is prolonged and not immediately relieved, it is called unstable angina, from which acute coronary

RISK FACTORS
Hypertension and Coronary Artery Disease

Hypertension

- *Family history:* When parents have hypertension, their children have a greater risk.
- *Race:* African Americans are twice as likely to develop high blood pressure as Caucasians.
- *Gender:* Men have a greater risk than women.
- *Age:* Risk increases with age.
- *Obesity:* Overweight people are more likely to develop hypertension. (M)
- *Tobacco smoking:* Nicotine constricts blood vessels. (M)
- *Elevated serum lipids:* Lipid plaques accumulate in arteries, contributing to hypertension. (M)
- *Alcohol:* Excessive alcohol intake is strongly associated with hypertension (M)
- *Excessive sodium intake:* Sodium retains water, increasing blood volume. (M)
- *Physical inactivity:* Inactivity contributes to obesity and elevated serum lipids. (M)
- *Diabetes mellitus:* Atherosclerosis, which obstructs arteries, is a common complication of diabetes mellitus. (M)

Coronary Artery Disease

- *Family history:* When parents have coronary artery disease, their children have a greater risk.
- *Race:* African Americans have more severe high blood pressure than Caucasians and higher risk of heart disease.
- *Gender:* Men have a greater risk than women.
- *Age:* Risk increases with age.
- *Obesity:* People who have excess body fat, especially at the waist, are more likely to develop heart disease, even if they have no other risk factors. (M)
- *Smoking:* Smokers' risk of developing coronary artery disease is 2 to 4 times that of nonsmokers. Exposure to other people's smoke increases the risk of heart disease for nonsmokers. (M)
- *High blood cholesterol:* Risk of coronary artery disease increases as blood cholesterol rises. (M)
- *Diabetes mellitus:* Diabetes increases the risk of heart disease, but the risks are greater if blood glucose is not well controlled.
- *Hypertension:* High blood pressure increases the workload of the heart, causing the myocardium to thicken and become stiffer. It also increases the risk for myocardial infarction and heart failure. When hypertension exists with obesity, smoking, high blood cholesterol, or diabetes, the risk of heart attack increases several times. (M)

Data from *www.cdc.gov/cancer/lung* 2011, www.cancer.org, 2011.
M, Modifiable risk factor.

syndrome (ACS) may develop. This syndrome includes a spectrum from unstable angina to myocardial infarction.[7]

Unstable Angina

Unstable angina is chest pain described as a new onset, experienced at rest, or a worsening pattern than previously experienced. Patients describe their chest pain as occurring with increased frequency, with increased intensity, without a precipitating event, or at rest. Manifestations reported by women with unstable angina may be different from those reported by men. Women describe fatigue, shortness of breath, indigestion, and anxiety.[7]

Myocardial Infarction

This condition occurs when myocardial ischemia is sustained, resulting in death of myocardial cells (necrosis). The left ventricle is more commonly affected, but the right ventricle may also be affected. **Clinical Findings:** Patients describe the pain as the worst chest pain ever experienced, a pain that lasts longer than 5 minutes. It may radiate to the left shoulder, jaw, arm, or other areas of the chest; and it is not relieved by rest or nitroglycerin. Dysrhythmias are common. Heart sounds may be distant with a thready pulse.

Heart Failure

When either ventricle fails to pump blood efficiently into the aorta or pulmonary arteries, the condition is termed *heart*

failure. Heart failure may occur in the left or right ventricle or both.

Left Ventricular Failure

This cardiac condition is caused by (1) increased resistance that occurs with aortic stenosis or hypertension when the ventricle can no longer compensate effectively for the increased workload, or (2) weakening of the left ventricular contraction that occurs after a myocardial infarction when the death of myocardial cells causes an ineffective contraction. Because the left ventricle cannot pump sufficient blood forward, some of the blood backs up into the left atrium and eventually into the pulmonary capillaries, causing pulmonary edema. **Clinical Findings:** The patient complains of fatigue and shortness of breath, including orthopnea, dyspnea on exertion, and paroxysmal nocturnal dyspnea. Findings may reveal precordial movement; displaced apical pulse; and palpable thrill, S_3 heart sound, and systolic murmur at apex. In the acute phase the patient usually has crackles bilaterally from pulmonary edema.

Right Ventricular Failure

This cardiac condition is caused by hypertrophy from pulmonary hypertension or necrosis from a myocardial infarction. The failure of the right ventricle to pump blood into the pulmonary arteries causes a backflow of blood into the inferior and superior venae cavae. Right ventricular failure caused by pulmonary disease, termed *cor pulmonale,* is discussed in

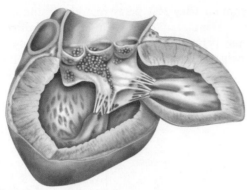

FIG. 12-43 Bacterial endocarditis. (From Seidel et al., 2011. Modified from Canobbio, 1990.)

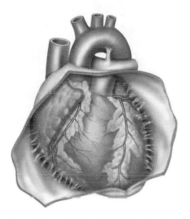

FIG. 12-44 Pericarditis. (From Seidel et al., 2011. Modified from Canobbio, 1990.)

Chapter 11. **Clinical Findings:** Findings may include precordial movement at the xiphoid or left sternal border, elevated jugular venous pressure, dependent peripheral edema, S₃ heart sound at lower left sternal border, systolic murmur, and weight gain.

Infective Endocarditis

An infection of the endothelial layer of the heart, including the cardiac valves, is called *infective endocarditis*. This infection develops when the endocardial surface is damaged by turbulent blood flow as a result of valvular heart disease; congenital lesions; or direct injury from intravenous lines or injections, cardiac catheterization, or artificial valves (Fig. 12-43). **Clinical Findings:** Heart sounds are normal during the early infection. In late infection a murmur is heard if valve damage occurs.

Pericarditis

Inflammation of the parietal and visceral layers of the pericardium and outer myocardium is termed *pericarditis*. It may be idiopathic or the result of myocardial infarction, uremia, cancer, trauma, infections, cardiac surgery, or an autoimmune reaction (Fig. 12-44). **Clinical Findings:** Two classic findings are pericardial friction rub and chest pain. A pericardial friction rub develops as the inflamed layers of pericardium move against one another. The friction rub is best

BOX 12-7	CLASSIFICATION OF BLOOD PRESSURE FOR ADULTS AGE 18 AND OLDER		
CATEGORY*	**SYSTOLIC (mm Hg)**		**DIASTOLIC (mm Hg)**
Normal	<120	and	<80
Prehypertension	120-139	or	80-89
Stage 1 hypertension	140-159	or	90-99
Stage 2 hypertension	>160	or	>100

Modified from National Heart, Lung, and Blood Institute: The seventh report of the Joint Commission on Prevention, Detection, Evaluation and Treatment of High Blood Pressure (JNC VII), available at *www.nhlbi.nih.gov/guidelines*, May 2003.

heard with the patient leaning forward so the heart is closer to the chest wall. Listen in the second, third, or fourth intercostal spaces at the left sternal border or at the apex; it is louder during inspiration. The chest pain is described as a sharp pleuritic pain that is aggravated by deep breathing, lying supine, or coughing.

PERIPHERAL VASCULAR DISEASE

Hypertension

A diagnosis of hypertension is based on the mean of two or more properly measured seated blood pressure readings on each of two or more occasions that are above 120/80 mm Hg in an adult over 18 years of age. Pressure in the arteries can become elevated as a result of constriction of the blood vessels, fluid volume overload, or both. **Clinical Findings:** Expected blood pressure values are less than 120 mm Hg systolic and less than 80 mm Hg diastolic. Criteria for hypertension are shown in Box 12-7. Since there are no specific symptoms of hypertension, periodic screening is important.

Venous Thrombosis and Thrombophlebitis

When a thrombus (clot) develops within a vein it is called a *venous thrombosis* or *venous thrombotic event*. In contrast, thrombophlebitis is inflammation of a vein that may or may not be accompanied by a clot. The triad of venous stasis, damage to the inner layer of veins, and hypercoagulability usually is responsible for both venous thrombosis and thrombophlebitis. Either may occur in the lower extremity, usually in deep veins. **Clinical Findings:** Thromboses are sometimes recognized by dilated superficial veins, edema and redness of the involved extremity, and increased circumference of the involved leg. In the upper extremity venous thrombosis and thrombophlebitis may occur in superficial veins and are recognized by redness, warmth, and tenderness over the affected area. Veins may be visible and palpable (Fig. 12-45).

Aneurysm

A localized dilation of an artery caused by weakness in the arterial wall is referred to as an *aneurysm*. It occurs anywhere along the aorta and iliac and cerebral vessels (Fig. 12-46). **Clinical Findings:** Clinical findings depend on the location of the aneurysm. Thoracic aneurysms are usually asymptomatic, with deep, diffuse chest pain reported by some patients. Aneurysms of the aorta and aortic arch can produce hoarseness from pressure on the laryngeal nerve or dysphagia from pressure on the esophagus. Abdominal aortic aneurysms are most common. They may be asymptomatic and discovered on routine examination or with an ultrasound or computed tomography performed for another reason. A pulsatile mass may be palpated in the periumbilical area. A thrill or bruit may be noted over the aneurysm.[8] Cerebral aneurysms can cause intracranial hemorrhages and the manifestations directly related to the size and location of the bleed.

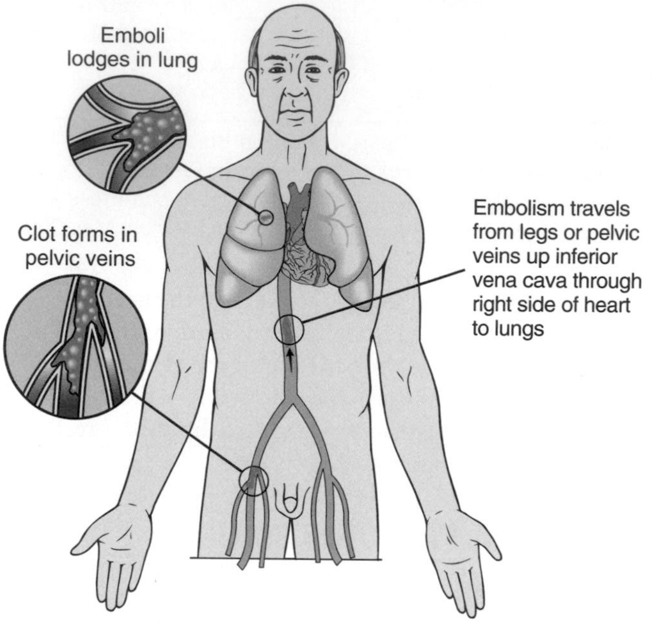

FIG. 12-45 Sites of venous thrombosis. (From Frazier and Drzymkowski, 2008.)

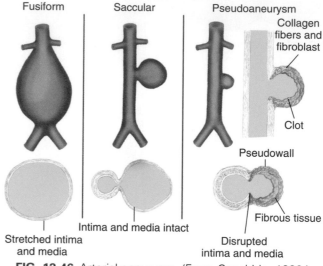

FIG. 12-46 Arterial aneurysm. (From Canobbio, 1990.)

CLINICAL APPLICATION AND CLINICAL REASONING

See Appendix D for answers to exercises in this section.

REVIEW QUESTIONS

1. The nurse is listening to the patient's heart at the left sternal border (LSB) at the second intraclavicular space (ICS). Which area is being auscultated?
   1. Erb's point
   2. Mitral area
   3. Aortic area
   4. Pulmonic area

2. A patient complains of pain in the calf when walking. Which question should the nurse ask for further data?
   1. "Does your calf also swell when this pain occurs?"
   2. "Does the pain go away when you stop walking?"
   3. "Do you become short of breath when you're walking?"
   4. "Do you feel dizzy when the pain occurs?"

3. Which patient has the greatest risk for hypertension?
   1. An Asian man who is 5 ft 5 in (165 cm) tall, weighs 125 lbs (56.7 kg), and complains of a headache over his forehead and eyes
   2. A Cheyenne Indian woman who complains of a gnawing, burning epigastric pain radiating to her neck and jaw
   3. An African American man who has type 2 diabetes mellitus, exercises once a month, and drinks two-to-three alcoholic drinks a night with dinner
   4. A Caucasian woman who has a family history of heart disease and complains of pain in her chest when she takes a deep breath

4. When a patient complains of chest pain, which question is pertinent to ask to gain additional data?
   1. "What were you doing when the pain first occurred?"
   2. "What does the pain feel like?"
   3. "Do you have episodes of shortness of breath?"
   4. "Has anyone in your family ever had a similar pain?"

5. How does a nurse determine jugular vein pulsations?
   1. Elevates the head of the bed about 90 degrees and looks for the jugular vein pulsation parallel to the sternocleidomastoid muscle as the head of the bed is slowly lowered
   2. Looks for jugular vein pulsations at the jaw line as the patient turns from supine to a side-lying position
   3. Elevates the head of the bed until the external jugular vein pulsation is seen above the clavicle
   4. Positions the patient supine and asks him or her to cough; looks for jugular vein pulsations during the cough

6. Where does a nurse palpate to assess the posterior tibial pulse?
   1. Behind the knee in the popliteal fossa
   2. The inner aspect of the ankle below and slightly behind the medial malleolus
   3. Over the dorsum of the foot between the extension tendons of the first and second toes
   4. The outer side of the ankle below and slightly behind the lateral malleolus

7. On auscultation of the heart, the nurse recognizes which expected finding?
   1. A low-pitched blowing sound is heard over the abdominal aorta.
   2. A high-pitched vibration is heard over the base of the heart.
   3. The S_1 heart sound is louder at the apex of the heart.
   4. The S_3 heart sound sounds like "Ken-tucky."

8. What is the most accurate technique for detecting a deep vein thrombosis at the bedside?
   1. Dorsiflex the calf and note if the patient complains of pain.
   2. Elevate one leg above the level of the heart to determine if the veins empty.
   3. Palpate the pulses distal to the areas of the suspected thrombosis.
   4. Measure the thigh circumference to detect an increase from the baseline.

9. Each patient has had consistent blood pressure readings during the last three clinic visits. Which patient has a blood pressure consistent with expected findings?
   1. Mr. P, whose blood pressure has been 110/78
   2. Ms. J, whose blood pressure has been 140/90
   3. Mr. Q, whose blood pressure has been 130/76
   4. Ms. Y, whose blood pressure has been 120/80

10. While inspecting the legs of a male patient, the nurse notes that the skin is shiny and taut with little hair growth. Which additional data would the nurse find to indicate that this patient has peripheral arterial disease?
    1. Pitting edema of one or both feet or legs
    2. Increased circumference in the thighs bilaterally
    3. Pale, cool legs with diminished-to-absent dorsalis pulses
    4. Pain when legs are dependent that is relieved when legs are elevated

CASE STUDY

Mr. Tao is a 56-year-old man complaining of difficulty breathing. The following initial data are collected.

Interview Data

Mr. Tao does not know exactly when his breathing difficulty started, but it has gotten noticeably worse the last couple of days. His father died of a heart attack at age 60. Mr. Tao plays golf twice a week; however, he tells the nurse that this last week he has "just felt too tired to do anything." He says that he has not been able to sleep very well at night because of his breathing difficulty. He adds, "I keep coughing out this bubbly-looking phlegm." He denies taking any medications. He says that he does not smoke or drink alcoholic beverages.

Examination Data

- *General survey:* Alert, anxious, cooperative, well-groomed male. Appears stated age. Breathing labored.
- *Vital signs:* BP, 142/112 mm Hg, right arm; 144/110 mm Hg, left arm; temperature, 98.8° F (37.1° C); pulse, 120 beats/min; respiration, 26 breaths/min.
- Pulses: All pulses palpable 2+. No carotid bruits bilaterally.
- Neck. Jugular distention and pulsation noted with patient in supine position.
- *Lower extremities:* Skin warm and dry, without cyanosis. Even hair distribution. 2+ pitting edema noted bilaterally. No lesions present.

Clinical Reasoning

1. Which data deviate from normal findings, suggesting a need for further investigation?
2. For which additional information should the nurse ask or assess?
3. Based on these data, which risk factors for coronary artery disease does Mr. Tao have?
4. With which health care team member would you collaborate to meet this patient's needs?

Abdomen and Gastrointestinal System

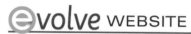 WEBSITE

http://evolve.elsevier.com/Wilson/assessment

ANATOMY AND PHYSIOLOGY

The abdominal cavity, the largest cavity in the human body, contains the stomach, small and large intestines, liver, gallbladder, pancreas, spleen, kidneys, ureters, bladder, adrenal glands, and major vessels (Figs. 13-1 and 13-2). In women the uterus, fallopian tubes, and ovaries are located within the abdominal cavity. Lying outside the abdominal cavity, but a vital part of the gastrointestinal (GI) system, is the esophagus.

PERITONEUM, MUSCULATURE, AND CONNECTIVE TISSUE

The abdominal lining, called the *peritoneum,* is a serous membrane forming a protective cover. It is divided into two layers: the parietal peritoneum and the visceral peritoneum. The parietal peritoneum lines the abdominal wall, and the visceral peritoneum covers organs. The space between the parietal peritoneum and visceral peritoneum is the peritoneal cavity. It usually contains a small amount of serous fluid to reduce friction between abdominal organs and their membranes.

The rectus abdominis muscles form the anterior border of the abdomen, and the vertebral column and lumbar muscles form the posterior border. Lateral support is provided by the internal and external oblique muscles. The external oblique aponeurosis is a strong membrane that covers the entire ventral surface of the abdomen and lies superficial to the rectus abdominis. Fibers from both sides of the aponeurosis interlace in the midline to form the linea alba. The linea alba is a tendinous band that protects the midline of the abdomen between the rectus abdominis muscles. This band extends from the xiphoid process to the symphysis pubis. The abdomen is bordered superiorly by the diaphragm and inferiorly by the superior aperture of the lesser pelvis (Fig. 13-3).

ALIMENTARY TRACT

From the mouth to the anus the adult alimentary tract extends 27 feet (8.2 m) and includes the esophagus, stomach, small intestine, large intestine, rectum, and anal canal (see Fig. 13-1). Its main functions are to ingest and digest food; absorb nutrients, electrolytes, and water; and excrete waste products. Products of digestion are moved along the digestive tract by peristalsis, under the control of the autonomic nervous system.

Esophagus

The alimentary tract begins with the esophagus, a tube about 10 inches (25.4 cm) long connecting the pharynx to the stomach and extending just posterior to the trachea through the mediastinal cavity and diaphragm. The usual pH of the esophagus is between 6.0 and 8.0.

Stomach

The stomach is a hollow, flask-shaped, muscular organ located directly below the diaphragm in the left upper quadrant. Contents from the esophagus enter the stomach through the lower esophageal sphincter and mix with digestive enzymes and hydrochloric acid. Gastric acid continues the breakdown of carbohydrates that began in the mouth. Pepsin breaks down proteins, converting them to peptones and amino acids; and gastric lipase acts on emulsified fats to

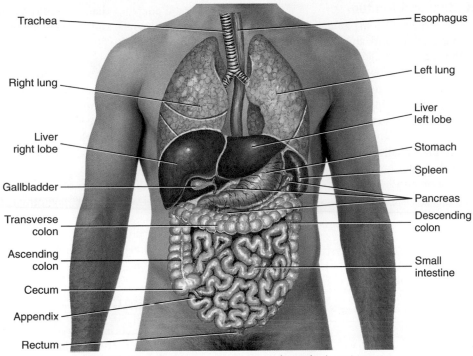

FIG. 13-1 Anatomy of the gastrointestinal system.

Labels (clockwise): Trachea, Esophagus, Right lung, Left lung, Liver left lobe, Liver right lobe, Stomach, Spleen, Gallbladder, Pancreas, Descending colon, Transverse colon, Ascending colon, Small intestine, Cecum, Appendix, Rectum

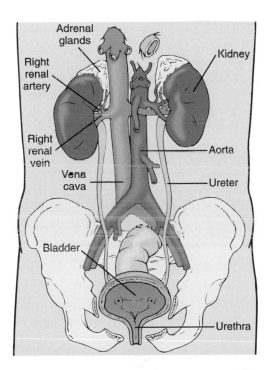

FIG. 13-2 Anatomy of the urinary system and major vessels of the abdominal cavity. (From Lewis et al., 2000.)

Labels: Adrenal glands, Kidney, Right renal artery, Right renal vein, Aorta, Vena cava, Ureter, Bladder, Urethra

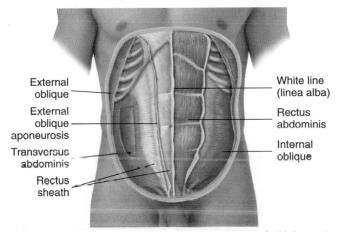

FIG. 13-3 Muscles of the abdomen. (From Seidel et al., 2011.)

Labels: External oblique, White line (linea alba), External oblique aponeurosis, Rectus abdominis, Transversus abdominis, Internal oblique, Rectus sheath

convert triglycerides to fatty acids and glycerol. The stomach also liquefies food into chyme and propels it into the duodenum of the small intestine. The usual pH of the stomach ranges from 2.0 to 4.0. The pyloric sphincter regulates the outflow of chyme into the duodenum.

Small Intestine

The longest section of the alimentary tract, the small intestine, is about 21 feet (6.4 m) long, beginning at the pyloric orifice and joining the large intestine at the ileocecal valve. In the small intestine ingested food is mixed, digested, and absorbed. The small intestine is divided into three segments: the duodenum, jejunum, and ileum. The duodenum occupies the first 1 foot (30 cm) of the small intestine and forms a C-shaped curve around the head of the pancreas. Absorption occurs through the intestinal villi of the duodenum, jejunum (8 feet [2.4 m] long), and ileum (12 feet [3.6 m] long). The ileocecal valve between the ileum and the large intestine prevents backward flow of fecal material (see Fig. 13-1).

Large Intestine (Colon) and Rectum

The large intestine is about 5 feet (1.5 m) long, consisting of cecum, appendix, colon, rectum, and anal canal. The ileal contents empty into the cecum through the ileocecal valve; the appendix extends from the base of the cecum. The colon is divided into three parts: ascending, transverse, and descending. The end of the descending colon turns medially and inferiorly to form the S-shaped sigmoid colon. The rectum extends from the sigmoid colon to the pelvic floor, where it continues as the anal canal, terminating at the anus. The large intestine absorbs water and electrolytes. Feces are formed in the large intestine and held until defecation (see Fig. 13-1).

ACCESSORY ORGANS

Accessory organs of the GI tract are the salivary glands, liver, gallbladder, and pancreas. Salivary glands are described in Chapter 10.

Liver

The liver is the largest organ in the body, weighing about 3.5 pounds (1.6 kg). It lies under the right diaphragm, spanning the upper quadrant of the abdomen from the fifth intercostal space to slightly below the costal margin (see Fig. 13-1). The rib cage covers a substantial portion of the liver; only the lower margin is exposed beneath it. The liver is divided into right and left lobes.

This complex organ has a variety of functions, including the following:
- Bile production and secretion
- Transfer of bilirubin from the blood (conjugated or direct) to the gallbladder (unconjugated or indirect)
- Protein, carbohydrate, and fat metabolism
- Glucose storage in the form of glycogen
- Production of clotting factors and fibrinogen
- Synthesis of most plasma proteins (albumin and globulin)
- Detoxification of a variety of substances, including drugs and alcohol
- Storage of certain minerals (iron and copper) and vitamins (A, B_{12}, and other B-complex vitamins)

Gallbladder

The gallbladder is a pear-shaped sac, 3 inches (7.6 cm) long, attached to the inferior surface of the liver (see Fig. 13-1). It concentrates and stores bile produced in the liver. The cystic duct combines with the hepatic duct to form the common bile duct, which drains bile into the duodenum. Bile contained in feces creates the characteristic brown color.

Pancreas

The pancreas lies in the upper left abdominal cavity, immediately under the left lobe of the liver, behind the stomach (see Fig. 13-1). It has both endocrine and exocrine functions. Endocrine secretions include the secretion of insulin, glucagon, somatostatin, and gastrin for carbohydrate metabolism. Exocrine secretions contain bicarbonate and pancreatic enzymes that flow into the duodenum to break down proteins, fats, and carbohydrates for absorption.

Spleen

The spleen is a highly vascular, concave, encapsulated organ about the size of a fist, situated in the upper left quadrant of the abdomen between the stomach and diaphragm. It is composed of two systems: the white pulp (consisting of lymphatic nodules and diffuse lymphatic tissue) and the red pulp (consisting of venous sinusoids) (see Fig. 13-1). Its main functions include the following:
- Storage of 1% to 2% of erythrocytes and platelets
- Removal of old or agglutinated erythrocytes and platelets
- Activation of B and T lymphocytes
- Production of erythrocytes during bone marrow depression

URINARY TRACT

The urinary tract includes the kidneys, ureters, urinary bladder, and urethra. Together they remove water-soluble waste materials.

Kidneys

The kidneys are located in the posterior abdominal cavity on either side at the spinal levels T12 through L3, where they are covered by the peritoneum and attached to the posterior abdominal wall. Each kidney is partially protected by the ribs and a cushion of fat and fascia. The right kidney is slightly lower than the left because of displacement by the liver (see Fig. 13-2). Additional kidney functions include the following: (1) secretion of erythropoietin to stimulate red blood cell production; (2) secretion of renin to activate the renin-angiotensin-aldosterone system; and (3) production of a biologically active form of vitamin D. The nephron regulates fluid and electrolyte balance through an elaborate microscopic filter and pressure system that eventually produces urine.

Ureters

The urine formed in the nephrons flows from the distal tubes and collecting ducts into the ureters and on into the bladder through peristaltic waves. Each ureter is composed of long, intertwining muscle bundles that extend for approximately 12 inches (30 cm) to insertion points at the base of the bladder (see Fig. 13-2).

Bladder

The bladder, a sac of smooth muscle fibers, is located behind the symphysis pubis in the anterior half of the pelvis (see Fig. 13-2). It contains an internal sphincter, which relaxes in response to a full bladder. Generally, when the urine volume of the bladder reaches about 300 mL, moderate distention is felt; a level of 450 mL causes discomfort. For voiding to occur, the external sphincter relaxes voluntarily; and urine exits through the urethra, which extends out of the base of the bladder to the external meatus.

VASCULATURE OF THE ABDOMEN

In the abdomen, the descending aorta travels through the diaphragm just to the left of midline until it branches into the two common iliac arteries approximately at the level of the umbilicus. Perfusion of the kidneys is provided by the right and left renal arteries, which branch off of the descending aorta. Blood is returned to the right side of the heart from the abdomen in the inferior vena cava, which parallels the abdominal aorta (see Fig. 13-2). Several veins empty into the inferior vena cava. These include the hepatic portal system, which is composed of veins that drain the intestines, pancreas, stomach, and gallbladder; and the renal veins, which drain the kidneys and ureters.

HEALTH HISTORY

Nurses interview patients to collect subjective data about their present health and any past medical experiences. They ask questions about the patient's present health status, past health history, family history, and personal and psychosocial history that may affect the functions of the abdomen and GI system. Questions regarding patient's nutrition and eating habits are asked in the health history in Chapter 8.

GENERAL HEALTH HISTORY

Present Health Status

Do you have any chronic diseases that affect your GI or urinary systems? If yes, describe.
Some chronic diseases such as diabetes mellitus may affect the GI or urinary systems. Diseases such as chronic hepatitis or cirrhosis may impair the ability of the liver to metabolize nutrients and drugs. Quality Improvement Competencies for Nurses include providing patient-centered care and interdisciplinary teamwork. See Table 11-1 on p. 196 for examples of competencies.

Do you take any medications? If yes, what do you take and how often? Are you taking the medications as they were prescribed?
Both prescription and over-the-counter medications should be documented. Medications may cause adverse GI effects. Since drugs are metabolized in the liver, patients with liver diseases may not metabolize drugs well, which causes increased blood levels of these drugs.

How often do you have a bowel movement? When was your last bowel movement? Describe the color and consistency of the stool.
Frequency of bowel movements is individual for each person. The frequency, color, and consistency of stool are documented as baseline data. These questions also give the patient an opportunity to describe disorders of the colon such as diarrhea, constipation, dark or light stools, or blood in stool.

Past Health History

Have you had problems with your abdomen or digestive system in the past? Esophagus? Stomach? Intestines? Liver? Gallbladder? Pancreas? Spleen? If yes, describe.

History of GI disorders may provide insight into findings to anticipate at this visit. These data give clues to patient's education needs about reducing risk for other diseases involving these body systems such as cancers.

Have you had surgery of your abdomen or urinary tract? If yes, describe. Has the surgery required that you change any of your former routines such as the food you can eat or bowel or urinary elimination? How have you been able to cope with having an ostomy?
Patients who have had gastrectomies may have changed the foods they eat and the amount and frequency of meals. Patients may have a colostomy or an ileostomy after surgery for such disorders as colon cancer or ulcerative colitis. Patients who have had bladder cancer may have an ileal conduit as an alternative route for urine excretion. Any of these surgeries requires that the patient change an appliance over the stoma. These questions convey concern about their adjustment to this change in their body.

Have you had problems with your urinary tract in the past? If yes, describe.
History of urinary disorders may provide insight into findings to anticipate at this visit. These data also give clues to patient's education needs about reducing risk for other diseases involving these body systems such as urinary tract infection and cancers.

Do you ever experience the leaking of urine? When does this occur? Do you ever use pads, tissue, or cloth in your underwear to catch urine?
Many patients do not report incontinence unless asked about it, often because of embarrassment. *Stress incontinence* is the most common type and is characterized by involuntary loss of small amounts of urine caused by physical exertion such as coughing, sneezing, jogging, and lifting. Many women with urinary stress incontinence can be diagnosed from the history data alone.[1] *Urge incontinence* is associated with a sudden strong urge to void. People can have both types of incontinence.

Family History

In your family is there a history of diseases of the GI system such as gastroesophageal reflux disease (GERD)? Peptic ulcer disease? Stomach cancer? Colon cancer?
Family history may be used to determine patients' risk factors for GI disorders.

In your family is there a history of diseases of the urinary tract such as kidney stones? Kidney cancer? Bladder cancer?

Family history may be used to determine patients' risk factors for urinary disorders.

Personal and Psychosocial History

Do you drink alcohol? If so, how much? How often? When was your last drink (of alcohol)?

Alcohol is a risk factor for peptic ulcer disease; esophageal, stomach, and colon cancer; pancreatitis; and cirrhosis. Alcoholism may damage the liver, the organ that metabolizes alcohol.

Do you smoke? If so, how much and for how long? Have you considered stopping or cutting down?

Cigarette smoking is a risk factor for peptic ulcer disease and most cancers of the GI system.

PROBLEM-BASED HISTORY

Specific areas of assessment of the abdomen and GI system include abdominal pain, nausea and vomiting, indigestion, abdominal distention, change in bowel habits, jaundice, and problems with urination. As with symptoms in all areas of health assessment, a symptom analysis is completed using the mnemonic OLD CARTS, which includes the *Onset, Location, Duration, Characteristics, Aggravating factors, Related symptoms, Treatment,* and *Severity* (see Box 2-3).

Abdominal Pain

How long have you had abdominal pain? Where is it located? When did you first feel it? What were you doing when it occurred?

Time, location, and activity when pain occurs are important to determine. Sudden, severe pain that awakens the patient may be associated with acute perforation, inflammation, or torsion of an abdominal organ.

Describe the pain. Is it constant or does it come and go? Have you had episodes of this pain before? Did it start suddenly?

Table 13-1 differentiates various types of abdominal pain. Pain description is helpful in determining its cause. Intense pain may be caused by a stone in the biliary tract or ureter, rupture of a fallopian tube from an ectopic pregnancy, or inflammation such as peritonitis following perforation of a gastric ulcer. Visceral pain arises from the GI tract and pancreas and may be described as an ache and well-defined as a result of tumor growth; or it may be cramping, diffuse, and poorly localized because of obstruction.

Has the pain changed its location since it started? Do you feel it in any other parts of your body?

Pain radiation patterns are shown in Table 13-1. Pain from acute appendicitis starts around the umbilicus and radiates to the right lower quadrant. Back pain is associated with

abdominal aneurysms or duodenal ulcers. Pain from gallbladder disease may be felt in the right shoulder.

Is the pain worse when your stomach is empty? Is it affected by eating? Is it worse at night or during the day?

Patterns of GI pain may help identify the cause. For example, the pain of duodenal ulcer may awaken the patient from sleep. Pain in gastroenteritis and irritable bowel disease is worse in the presence of food because peristalsis is stimulated, which causes pain.

What relieves the pain? Is there any particular position that relieves it?

A particular position may relieve abdominal pain (e.g., pain from pancreatitis may be relieved in the knee-chest position). Colicky pain from a gallbladder or kidney stone may be relieved with restless movement. The pain of appendicitis is relieved by lying very still.

Is the pain associated with other symptoms such as stress, fatigue, nausea and vomiting, gas, fever, chills, constipation, diarrhea, rectal bleeding, frequent urination, or vaginal or penile discharge?

Identifying symptoms associated with pain may assist in determining the cause.

For females: Is the pain associated with your menstrual period? When was your last menstrual period? Could you be pregnant?

Dysmenorrhea (pain associated with menstruation) may cause lower abdominal pain and vomiting because of the increase in prostaglandin. An ectopic pregnancy may cause abdominal pain.

Nausea and Vomiting

How long have you been experiencing nausea or vomiting? How often does this occur?

Vomiting has many causes, and gaining additional details helps determine the cause.

How much do you vomit? What does the vomitus look like? Does it contain blood? Does it have an odor?

The characteristics of the vomitus may help determine its cause. Acute gastritis leads to vomiting of stomach contents; obstruction of the bile duct results in greenish-yellow vomitus; and an intestinal obstruction may have a fecal odor to the vomitus. Stomach or duodenal ulcers or esophageal varices may cause blood in vomitus (hematemesis).

For females: Could you be pregnant?

Pregnancy should be ruled out as a cause of nausea and vomiting. Pregnant women have high serum levels of chorionic gonadotropin, which stimulates vomiting.

Do you have nausea without vomiting?

Nausea without vomiting is a common symptom of pregnant patients or those with metastatic disease.

TABLE 13-1 DIFFERENTIATION OF ABDOMINAL PAIN

CAUSE	PATIENT CHARACTERISTICS	QUALITY	LOCATION	ASSOCIATED SYMPTOMS	AGGRAVATED BY	ALLEVIATED BY	FINDINGS
Gastroesophageal reflux	Any age	Gnawing, burning	Midepigastric; may radiate to jaw	Weight loss	Recumbency, bending, stooping	Antacids, sitting up	
Gastroenteritis	Any age	Cramping	Diffuse	Nausea and vomiting, fever, diarrhea	Food	Some relief with vomiting, diarrhea	Hyperactive bowel sounds
Gastritis	Alcoholism	Constant, burning	Epigastric	Hemorrhage, nausea and vomiting, diarrhea, fever	Alcohol, food, salicylates	Antacids	
Peptic ulcer	30-50 years; more males than females	Gnawing, burning	Epigastric, back, and upper abdomen Gastric 1-2 hr after meals Duodenal 2-4 hr after meals, midmorning, midafternoon, and middle of the night	Nausea, vomiting, weight loss	Stress, alcohol; gastric ulcer aggravated by food; duodenal ulcers by empty stomach	Food, antacids—duodenal ulcers only	Epigastric tenderness on palpation or percussion
Pancreatitis	Alcoholism, cholelithiasis	Steady, severe to mild, knifelike, sudden onset	LUQ and epigastric; radiates to back	Nausea and vomiting, diaphoresis	Lying supine	Leaning forward	Abdominal distention, ↓ bowel sounds, LUQ tenderness
Appendicitis	Any age; peak 10-20 yr	Colicky, progressing to constant	Umbilicus, moving to RLQ	Vomiting, constipation, fever	Worse with moving, coughing	Lying still	Rebound tenderness RLQ, positive obturator, positive iliopsoas
Cholecystitis or cholelithiasis	Adults; more females than males	Colicky, progressing to constant	RUQ radiates to right scapula	Nausea and vomiting, dark urine, light stools, jaundice	Fatty foods, drugs		Tender to palpation or percussion of RUQ
Ectopic pregnancy	History of menstrual irregularity	Sudden onset persistent pain	Lower quadrant	Tender adnexal mass, vaginal bleeding			Palpable mass on affected side
Diverticular disease	Older adults	Intermittent cramping	LLQ	Constipation, diarrhea	Eating	Bowel movement, passing flatus	Palpable mass in LLQ
Irritable bowel disease	Young women	Cramping, recurrent, sharp, burning	LLQ	Mucus in stools		May be relieved by defecation	Colon tender on palpation
Intestinal obstruction	Older adults; those with prior abdominal surgery	Colicky, sudden onset	May be localized or generalized	Vomiting, constipation			Hyperactive bowel sounds in small obstruction

LLQ, Left lower quadrant; *LUQ*, left upper quadrant; *RLQ*, right lower quadrant; *RUQ*, right upper quadrant.

Which foods have you eaten in the last 24 hours? Where did you eat? How long after you ate did you vomit? Has anyone else who ate with you had these symptoms over the same time period?

These questions are asked to detect food poisoning or stomach influenza.

Do you have other symptoms with the nausea or vomiting? Pain? Constipation? Diarrhea? Change in color of stools? Change in color of urine? Fever or chills?

Knowing associated symptoms may help determine the cause of nausea and vomiting. For example, liver disease may change stool color from brown to tan. Infection such as hepatitis may cause fever and chills.

Indigestion

How long after eating do you have indigestion or heartburn? Where do you feel the discomfort? In your stomach? Chest? How long has this been happening? How often does this occur?

Heartburn felt in the chest, over the esophagus, or in the stomach that occurs after eating may indicate GERD.

What makes the symptoms worse? Does a change in position such as lying down affect your indigestion?

Heartburn caused by GERD or hiatal hernia is often worse when the patient lies down because the gastric acids move by gravity toward the esophagus.

What relieves these symptoms?

When acid-reducing drugs relieve the indigestion, excessive acid may be the cause.

Are there any other symptoms associated with the heartburn? Radiating pain? Sweating? Light-headedness?

Knowing associated symptoms may help determine the cause of indigestion. Angina or myocardial infarction may be the cause of the "indigestion-like" symptoms. Questions about radiating pain to the arms or jaw, along with other questions, are asked with these cardiovascular disorders in mind.

Abdominal Distention

How long has your abdomen been distended? Does it come and go? Is it related to eating? What relieves the distention?

Distention associated with eating is intermittent and relieved by passing gas. Constipation contributes to distention and develops slowly but is not relieved without bowel movement. Distention caused by ascites is a progressive process and increases abdominal girth.

Are other symptoms associated with the abdominal distention? Vomiting? Loss of appetite? Weight loss? Change in bowel habits? Shortness of breath? Abdominal pain?

Vomiting may indicate intestinal obstruction as a cause of distention. Loss of appetite is associated with cirrhosis and malignancy. Shortness of breath is associated with heart failure and with ascites that occurs with chronic liver disease.

Change in Bowel Habits

Describe the change in your bowel movements. Change in frequency? Change in consistency of feces?

Changes in bowel habits can be related to a number of factors, including changes in diet, activity, stress, and medications. A change in bowel habits is one of the seven warning signs of cancer

When did you first notice the change? What does the stool look like: bloody, mucoid, fatty, watery?

Answers to these questions may help determine the cause of the change in bowel function.

Watery diarrhea containing blood, mucus, and pus may indicate ulcerative colitis. A greater-than-expected amount of fat in the stool (steatorrhea) may indicate pancreatitis.

Are other symptoms such as increased gas, pain, fever, nausea, vomiting, abdominal cramping, or diarrhea associated with the change in bowel habits? Is there a time of day when the change occurs such as after eating or at night?

Knowing associated symptoms may help determine the cause of the change in bowel function. Some foods cause increased gas, fever suggests inflammation or infection, and abdominal cramping with diarrhea may indicate gastroenteritis.

Yellow Discoloration of Eyes or Skin (Jaundice)

When did you first notice the yellow discoloration of your skin or eyes?

Jaundice indicates elevated serum bilirubin that can be caused by liver disease or obstruction of bile flow from gallstones.

Is the yellow discoloration of your skin or eyes associated with abdominal pain? Loss of appetite? Nausea? Vomiting? Fever?

Fever, nausea, vomiting, and loss of appetite are also symptoms of hepatitis.

In the last year have you had a blood transfusion or tattoos? Are you using any intravenous drugs? Do you eat raw shellfish (e.g., oysters)? Have you traveled abroad in the last year? Where? Did you drink unclean water?

These are possible sources of transmission of the hepatitis virus.

Has the color of your urine or stools changed?

Urine changing from amber to brown and stools changing from brown to tan colored suggest high serum bilirubin that occurs with liver disease or obstruction of the common bile duct.

Problems with Urination

Describe the change in your urination. What is your usual pattern of urination? Have you felt any pain or burning when urinating? Are you urinating frequently in small

amounts (frequency) or feeling you cannot wait to urinate (urgency)? If yes, when did this begin?

Pain, burning, or frequency may indicate a bladder infection. Loss of muscle tone may cause incontinence, particularly in women. Men who have an enlarged prostate may have some of these same symptoms (see Chapter 17).

Have you had associated symptoms such as fever, chills, and back pain?

These symptoms may indicate a kidney disorder such as pyelonephritis or kidney stones.

Describe the color of the urine. Is there blood in the urine?

Dark amber urine is associated with kidney or liver disease. Blood in the urine is associated with menstrual periods in women or with kidney disease.

Have you had an unexpected weight gain? Have you noticed swelling in your ankles at the end of the day or shortness of breath? Are you urinating less?

These clinical manifestations may indicate renal failure when kidney dysfunction causes fluid retention.

HEALTH PROMOTION FOR EVIDENCE-BASED PRACTICE

Colorectal Cancer

Goals and Objectives—*Healthy People 2020*
The goal for all cancers is to reduce the number of new cancer cases and illness, disability, and death by cancer. There are three objectives specific to colon cancer: reduce the colorectal cancer death rate, reduce invasive colon cancer, and increase the proportion of adults who receive a colorectal cancer screening based on the most recent guidelines.

Recommendations to Reduce Risk of Colorectal Cancer (Primary Prevention)
American Cancer Society
An individual can lower risk of developing colorectal cancer by managing controllable risk factors such as diet and physical activity. Information to share with patients includes the following:

- Consume diet high in fruits, vegetables, and whole-grain foods; limit intake of high-fat foods.
- Participate in moderate to vigorous activity for 30 minutes 5 days or more a week.
- Attain and maintain a healthy weight.

For individuals with average risk: Beginning at age 50, both men and women should have one of the following screening tests:

- Fecal occult blood test (FOBT) annually
- Flexible sigmoidoscopy every 5 years
- Double-contrast barium enema every 5 years
- Colonoscopy every 10 years

Digital rectal examination is recommended to be done in conjunction with a sigmoidoscopy, colonoscopy, or double-contrast barium enema.

For individuals with higher risk, screening should begin earlier.

Data from US Department of Health and Human Services: *Healthy people 2020,* available at http://www.healthypeople.gov/2020/; www.cancer.org, 2011.

EXAMINATION

ROUTINE TECHNIQUES

- OBSERVE patient's general behavior and position.
- INSPECT the abdomen.
- AUSCULTATE the abdomen.
- PALPATE the abdomen lightly.
- PALPATE the abdomen deeply

SPECIAL CIRCUMSTANCES OR ADVANCED PRACTICE

- PERCUSS the abdomen.★
- PERCUSS the liver.★
- PERCUSS the spleen.★
- PALPATE the liver.★
- PALPATE the gallbladder.★
- PALPATE the spleen.★
- PALPATE the kidneys.★
- PERCUSS the kidneys.
- ASSESS the abdomen for fluid.★
- ELICIT abdominal reflexes.★
- ASSESS for abdominal pain caused by inflammation.★
- ASSESS the abdomen for floating mass.★

EQUIPMENT NEEDED
Stethoscope • Penlight • Tape measure • Small ruler • Marking pen

★ Advanced practice.

PROCEDURES AND TECHNIQUES WITH EXPECTED FINDINGS	ABNORMAL FINDINGS

ROUTINE TECHNIQUES: ABDOMEN

CLEAN hands.
OBSERVE patient's general behavior and position.

The patient should appear relaxed, sitting or lying quietly with slow, even respirations.

Note abnormal findings such as emaciation, obesity, distended abdomen, marked restlessness, a rigid posture, knees drawn up; facial grimacing, and rapid, uneven, or grunting respirations. Patients with pancreatitis may prefer the knee-chest position; those with peritonitis or appendicitis may lie very still; those with colicky gallstones or ureteral stones may rock back and forth.

INSPECT the abdomen for skin color, surface characteristics, venous patterns, contour, symmetry, and surface movements.

Direct a light source at a right angle to the patient's long axis. Skin color may be paler than other parts of the skin because of lack of exposure.

Jaundice indicates elevated serum bilirubin, erythema may indicate inflammation, bruises may indicate trauma or low platelet count, and striae may indicate abdominal distention.

Surface characteristics should be smooth. Silver-white striae; scars; and a very faint, fine vascular network may be present. The umbilicus should be centrally located (Fig. 13-4). The pattern of veins of the abdomen is usually barely visible.

The umbilicus should not be displaced upward, downward, or laterally; nor should a hernia be visible around or slightly above the umbilicus. An inverted umbilicus is often a sign of increased abdominal pressure, usually from ascites or a large mass. Glistening or taut appearance is associated with ascites. Note prominent venous patterns or engorgement of the veins around the umbilicus. In patients with portal hypertension, the veins are dilated and appear to radiate from the umbilicus. This is caused by the back flow through the collateral veins.[2]

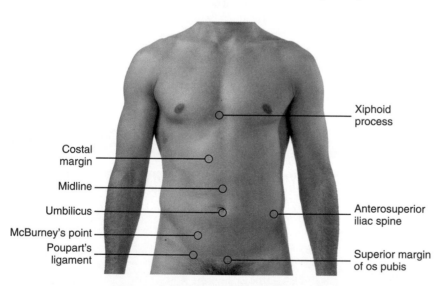

Costal margin

Midline

Umbilicus

McBurney's point

Poupart's ligament

Xiphoid process

Anterosuperior iliac spine

Superior margin of os pubis

FIG. 13-4 Landmarks of the abdomen.

Contour may be sunken, although it may protrude slightly, especially in overweight and obese patients. Adjusting the light source to form shadows may highlight small changes in the contour. Evaluate symmetry by viewing the abdomen from two additional angles: standing behind the patient's head and squatting at the side to view the abdomen at eye level. Ask the patient to take a deep breath and hold it. The contour of the abdomen should remain smooth and symmetric.

Check for marked concavity, which is associated with general wasting signs or anteroposterior rib expansion.

With the patient lying supine, ask him or her to cough to increase intraabdominal pressure while you inspect for a sudden bulge, which is not expected.

Bulges during coughing indicate an abdominal hernia: ventral, umbilical, inguinal, or femoral.[2]

PROCEDURES AND TECHNIQUES WITH EXPECTED FINDINGS	**ABNORMAL FINDINGS**

When abdominal distention is noted, place a measuring tape around the abdomen at the level of the superior iliac crests to measure the abdominal girth (circumference). This provides an objective measure to assess the increase or decrease in abdominal distention.

Inspect the surface for movements. Peristalsis is usually not visible, but an upper midline pulsation may be visible in thin individuals. The abdomen should move smoothly and evenly with respirations. Generally females exhibit thoracic movements during inhalation, whereas males exhibit abdominal movements. Ask the patient to raise his or her head without using the arms for support. The rectus abdominis muscles become prominent, and a midline bulge may appear. Areas of bulges considered expected variations are pregnancy and marked obesity.

AUSCULTATE the abdomen for bowel sounds.

Auscultate *before* palpating and percussing the abdomen so the presence or absence of bowel sounds or pain is not altered. A quiet environment may be necessary. Box 13-1 lists the anatomic correlates of the quarters of the abdomen (Fig. 13-5).

Procedure: Use the diaphragm of the stethoscope and press lightly. Listen in a systematic progression, such as from right upper quadrant (RUQ) to left upper quadrant (LUQ) to left lower quadrant (LLQ) and finally to right lower quadrant (RLQ).

ABNORMAL FINDINGS

Abdominal distention may result from the "seven *F*'s": fat (obesity), fetus (pregnancy), fluid (ascites), flatulence (gas), feces (constipation), fibroid tumor, or fatal tumor. Note any bulges or masses, particularly of the liver or spleen. Abdominal or incisional hernias can also create bulges of the abdomen.

Note visible peristalsis or marked pulsations. The area of pulsation observed is not palpated because it may indicate an abdominal aneurysm (i.e., a weakening in the wall of the abdominal aorta). Grunting or labored movements or restricted abdominal movements with respirations should be recorded.

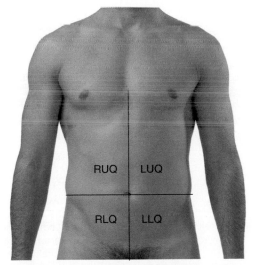

FIG. 13-5 Quadrants of the abdomen.

BOX 13-1	**ANATOMIC CORRELATES OF THE QUADRANTS OF THE ABDOMEN**

Right Upper Quadrant	**Left Upper Quadrant**
Liver and gallbladder	Left lobe of liver
Pylorus	Spleen
Duodenum	Stomach
Head of pancreas	Body of pancreas
Right adrenal gland	Left adrenal gland
Portion of right kidney	Portion of left kidney
Portions of ascending and transverse colon	Portions of transverse and descending colon

Right Lower Quadrant	**Left Lower Quadrant**
Lower pole of right kidney	Lower pole of left kidney
Cecum and appendix	Sigmoid colon
Portion of ascending colon	Portion of descending colon
Bladder (if distended)	Bladder (if distended)
Right ureter	Left ureter
Right ovary and salpinx	Left ovary and salpinx
Uterus (if enlarged)	Uterus (if enlarged)
Right spermatic cord	Left spermatic cord

PROCEDURES AND TECHNIQUES WITH EXPECTED FINDINGS

Findings: Bowel sounds should be noted every 5 to 15 seconds. The duration of a single bowel sound may range from 1 second to several seconds. The sounds are high-pitched gurgles or clicks, although this varies greatly.

AUSCULTATE the abdomen for arterial and venous vascular sounds.

Procedure: Listen with the bell of the stethoscope. Listen over aorta and renal, iliac, and femoral arteries for bruits. They make "swishing" sounds, occur during systole, and are continuous, regardless of the patient's position (Fig. 13-6). Also listen with the bell over the epigastric region and around the umbilicus for a venous hum (i.e., a soft, low-pitched, and continuous sound).

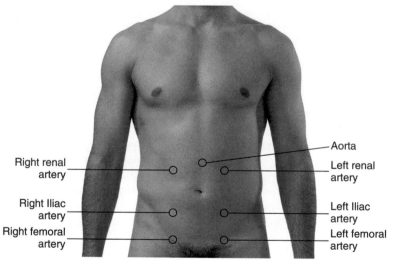

Right renal artery
Right Iliac artery
Right femoral artery
Aorta
Left renal artery
Left Iliac artery
Left femoral artery

FIG. 13-6 Sites to auscultate for bruits: renal arteries, iliac arteries, aorta, and femoral arteries.

Findings: Normally vascular sounds are not heard.

ABNORMAL FINDINGS

Report any absence of sound after listening for several minutes in each quadrant. Decreased or absent bowel sounds occur with mechanical obstruction or paralytic ileus and with peritonitis and bowel obstruction. Audible sounds produced by hyperactive peristalsis are termed *borborygmi* and create rumbling, gurgling, and high-pitched tinkling sounds. Although increased peristalsis is associated with diarrhea, laxative use, and gastroenteritis, true borborygmi are more intense and episodic sounds associated with intestinal obstruction.

A bruit indicates a turbulent blood flow caused by narrowing of a blood vessel. Bruits over the aorta suggest an aneurysm. Two sound patterns may indicate renal arterial stenosis: soft, medium- to low-pitched murmurs heard over the upper midline or toward the flank or epigastric bruits that radiate laterally. Venous hums are rare and are associated with portal hypertension and cirrhosis.

PROCEDURES AND TECHNIQUES WITH EXPECTED FINDINGS	**ABNORMAL FINDINGS**

PALPATE the abdomen lightly for tenderness and muscle tone.

Procedure: Before palpation some nurses ask patients to bend their knees to relax the abdominal muscles. Palpate all quadrants of the abdomen. Use the pads of the fingertips to depress the abdomen 1 to 2 cm (0.4 to 0.8 inches) (Fig. 13-7). When the patient has reported abdominal pain, palpate over the area of pain last. Some nurses reduce ticklishness by sliding their hands into each palpation position to maintain contact with the patient's skin. Another approach is to have the patient place his or her hand atop the nurse's hand as all quadrants are palpated.

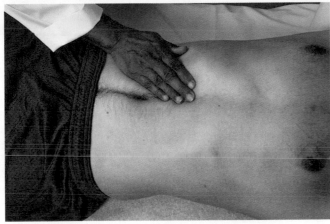

FIG. 13-7 Light palpation of the abdomen.

Findings: No tenderness should be present, and the abdominal muscles should be relaxed, although anxious patients may have some muscle resistance on palpation. Note consistent tension as you move across the smooth surface.

Note any cutaneous tenderness or hypersensitivity. Note superficial masses or localized areas of rigidity or increased tension. Rigidity is associated with peritoneal irritation and may be diffuse or localized.

PALPATE the abdomen deeply for tenderness, masses, and aortic pulsation.

Procedure: Palpate all quadrants. Use either the distal flat portions of the finger pads (Fig. 13-8) and press gradually and deeply 4 to 6 cm (1.6 to 2.4 inches) into the palpation area, or use a bimanual technique with the lower hand resting lightly on the surface and the upper hand exerting pressure for deep palpation (Fig. 13-9). When the patient has abdominal pain, palpate over the area of pain last. Observe for facial grimaces during palpation that may indicate areas of tenderness. Ask the patient to breathe slowly through the mouth to facilitate muscle relaxation.

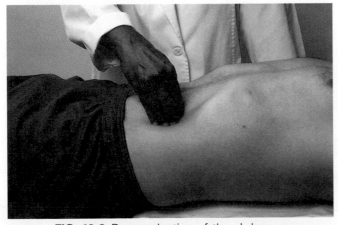

FIG. 13-8 Deep palpation of the abdomen.

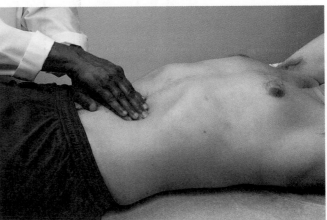

FIG. 13-9 Deep bimanual palpation.

PROCEDURES AND TECHNIQUES WITH EXPECTED FINDINGS

Findings: No tenderness or masses are expected during deep palpation. The aorta is often palpable at the epigastrium and above and slightly to the left of the umbilicus (Fig. 13-10). The borders of the rectus abdominis muscles can be felt, as can the sacral promontory and feces in the ascending or descending colon.

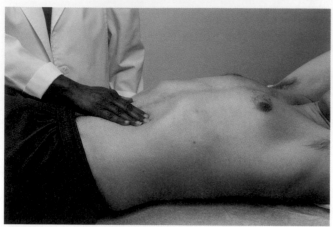

FIG. 13-10 Palpating the aorta.

SPECIAL CIRCUMSTANCES OR ADVANCED PRACTICE: ABDOMEN

★ PERCUSS the abdomen for tones.

Percuss the abdomen when you suspect distention, fluid, or solid masses.

Procedure: See Chapter 3 for the procedures for percussion. Percuss all quadrants for tones, using indirect percussion to assess density of abdominal contents. (Develop a routine for the percussion process to ensure that all areas are covered [Fig. 13-11].) Percuss in each quadrant for tympany and dullness.

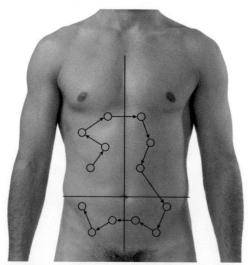

FIG. 13-11 Systematic route for abdominal percussion.

Findings: Tympany is the most common percussion tone heard and is caused by the presence of gas. The suprapubic area may be dull when the urinary bladder is distended.

ABNORMAL FINDINGS

Note any pain that is present in local or generalized areas. The patient may respond to pain by muscle guarding, facial grimaces, or pulling away from the nurse. Abnormal findings include masses that descend during inspiration, lateral pulsatile masses (abdominal aortic aneurysm), laterally mobile masses, and fixed masses.

Note any marked dullness in a localized area that may indicate distention, fluid, or an abdominal mass.

★ Advanced practice

PROCEDURES AND TECHNIQUES WITH EXPECTED FINDINGS

★ PERCUSS the liver to determine span and descent.

Percuss the liver when you suspect enlargement.

Procedure:

1. Beginning below the level of the umbilicus at the right midclavicular line (RMCL), percuss upward until the tone changes from a tympany to a dull percussion tone, indicating the liver border. Mark the border with a pen. The lower border is usually at the costal margin or slightly below it (Fig. 13-12, *A*) (see also Fig. 13-4).
2. Beginning over the lung in the RMCL, percuss the intercostal spaces downward until the tone changes from resonant to dull, indicating the upper liver border. Mark the location with a pen. The upper border usually begins in the fifth to seventh intercostal space (see Fig. 13-12, *B*).
3. Measure the span between the two lines using a ruler or tape measure to estimate the midclavicular liver span.
4. To assess the liver descent, ask the patient to take a deep breath and hold it; then percuss upward from the stomach to the RMCL.

ABNORMAL FINDINGS

★ Advanced practice

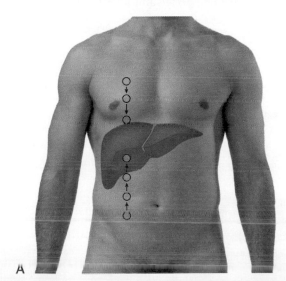

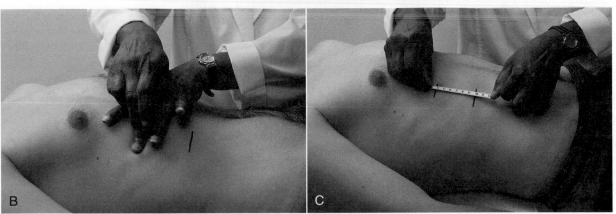

FIG. 13-12 A, Liver percussion route. **B,** Percussion method of estimating size of liver in the midclavicular line. **C,** Distance between the two marks measured in estimating the liver span in midclavicular line is usually 6 to 12 cm.

PROCEDURES AND TECHNIQUES WITH EXPECTED FINDINGS

Findings: The midclavicular liver span is expected to be 6 to 12 cm (about 2.5 to 5 inches) (see Fig. 13-12, *C*). Liver span correlates with body size and gender; large people and men tend to have larger spans. The lower border of the liver is expected to descend downward 2 to 3 cm (0.4 to 0.8 inch).

Note when the lower border of the liver exceeds 2 to 3 cm below the costal margin. This indicates an enlarged liver (hepatomegaly), which is associated with cirrhosis and hepatitis. In addition, patients with chronic obstructive pulmonary disease may have a flat diaphragm, which makes percussion of the upper border of the liver difficult. Obesity can make percussion difficult. Note if the liver fails to move with inspiration or if movement is less than 2 cm.

★ PERCUSS the spleen for size.

Percuss the spleen when you suspect enlargement.

Procedure: With the patient lying supine, percuss in the lowest intercostal space just posterior to the left midaxillary line (LMAL) (Fig. 13-13). Try to outline the spleen by percussing in several directions from dullness to resonance or tympany. Percuss the lowest intercostal space in the left anterior axillary line before and after the patient takes a deep breath.

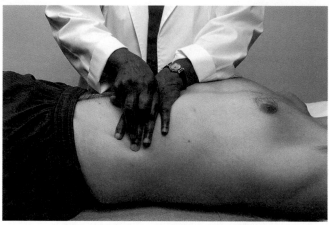

FIG. 13-13 Percussion of the spleen.

Findings: Normally the spleen cannot be percussed, or you may hear a small area of splenic dullness at the sixth to the tenth intercostal spaces. A full stomach or feces in the transverse or descending colon may mimic dullness of splenic enlargement. The area is usually tympanic during inspiration and expiration.

Splenic enlargement may indicate infection or trauma. Note whether the tympany changes to dullness on inspiration. An enlarged spleen is brought forward on inspiration to produce a dull percussion note.

★ PALPATE the liver for lower border and tenderness.

Palpate the liver when you suspect an enlarged liver.

Procedure: Two techniques may be used to palpate the liver.
1. Begin by placing the left hand under the eleventh and twelfth ribs to lift the liver closer to the abdominal wall. Place your right hand parallel to the right costal margin and press down and under the costal margin (Fig. 13-14, *A* and *B*) (see also Fig. 13-4). Ask the patient to take some deep breaths. The border and contour of the liver often are not palpable. The liver may "bump" against the right fingers during inspiration, especially in thin patients.
2. Another technique is called the *hooking technique.* Stand on the patient's right side facing the feet. Place your hands side by side at the right costal margin and curve your fingers to "hook" them under the costal margin (see Fig. 13-14, *C*).

★ Advanced practice

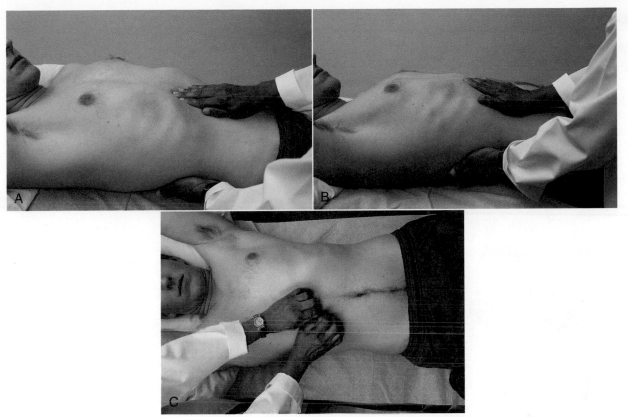

FIG. 13-14 Methods of palpating the liver. **A,** Fingers are extended, with tips on right midclavicular line below the level of liver tenderness and pointing toward the head. **B,** Fingers parallel to the costal margin. **C,** Fingers hooked over the costal margin.

PROCEDURES AND TECHNIQUES WITH EXPECTED FINDINGS	ABNORMAL FINDINGS

Findings: Ask the patient to take a deep breath, and you may feel the liver "bump" against your fingers during inspiration. The border of the liver should feel smooth. No tenderness should be present.

A very enlarged liver may lie under the nurse's hand as it extends downward into the abdominal cavity. Note any irregular surfaces or edges and any tenderness. The patient may complain of pain when taking a deep breath during this assessment.

★ PALPATE the gallbladder for tenderness.

Palpate the gallbladder when you suspect RUQ pain or enlargement.

Procedure: Palpate below the liver margin at the right lateral border of the rectus abdominis muscle for the gallbladder.

Findings: A healthy gallbladder is not palpable.

A palpable, tender gallbladder may indicate cholecystitis. Test for cholecystitis by asking the patient to take a deep breath during deep palpation. Cholecystitis is suspected if the patient experiences pain and abruptly stops inhaling during palpation (Murphy's sign). A nontender, enlarged gallbladder suggests common bile duct obstruction.

★ Advanced practice

| PROCEDURES AND TECHNIQUES WITH EXPECTED FINDINGS | ABNORMAL FINDINGS |

★ PALPATE the spleen for border and tenderness.

Palpate the spleen when you suspect pain or enlargement.

Procedure: Standing at the patient's right side, reach across the patient to place the palm surface of your left hand under his or her left flank at the costovertebral angle and exert pressure upward to elevate the left rib cage and move the spleen anteriorly. Press the palm surface of your right hand gently under the left anterior costal margin (Fig. 13-15). Press your fingertips inward toward the spleen as the patient takes a deep breath. Try to feel the tip of the spleen as it descends during inspiration The spleen is normally not palpable.

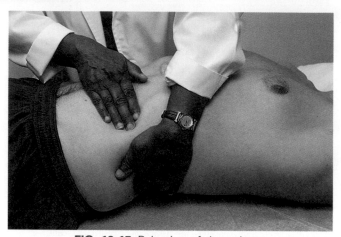

FIG. 13-15 Palpation of the spleen.

An alternative strategy for spleen palpation is to perform the procedure with the patient lying on the right side with the legs and knees flexed. Stand on the patient's right and place your left hand over his or her left costovertebral angle while pressing your right hand under the left anterior costal margin.

Findings: The spleen is normally not palpable.

A palpable spleen feels like a firm mass that bumps against the nurse's fingers. Spleen tenderness may indicate infection or trauma.

★ PALPATE the kidneys for presence, contour, and tenderness.

Palpate the kidney when the patient reports pain in back (flank pain).

Procedure:

Left kidney: Stand to the patient's right side with the patient in a supine position. Place the left hand at the left posterior costal angle (left flank) and the right hand at the patient's left anterior costal margin (see Fig. 13-4). Ask the patient to take a deep breath, elevate his or her left flank with your left hand, and palpate deeply with your right hand (Fig. 13-16).

Right kidney: Repeat the same maneuver on the right side, which is easier to palpate because it lies lower than the left kidney.

Findings: Normally the kidney is not palpable. Occasionally the lower pole of the kidney can be felt during inhalation in thin patients but rarely in the average patient. The contour should be smooth with no tenderness.

Tenderness is associated with kidney trauma or infection (e.g., pyelonephritis or glomerulonephritis).

★ Advanced practice

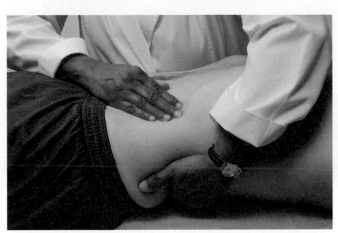

FIG. 13-16 Palpation of the left kidney.

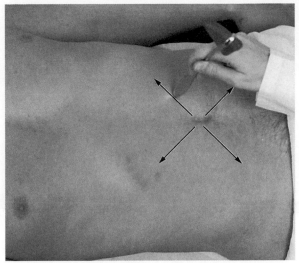

FIG. 13-17 Eliciting superficial abdominal reflexes. Stroke the upper abdominal area upward, away from the umbilicus, and the lower umbilicus area downward, away from the umbilicus. (From Seidel et al., 2003.)

PROCEDURES AND TECHNIQUES WITH EXPECTED FINDINGS	ABNORMAL FINDINGS

★ ELICIT abdominal reflexes for presence.

These reflexes are included here for completeness but are not commonly tested.[2]

Procedure: Elicit the abdominal reflexes by stroking each quadrant with the end of a reflex hammer or tongue blade (Fig. 13-17). For upper abdominal reflexes stroke upward and away from the umbilicus; for lower abdominal reflexes stroke downward and away from the umbilicus.

Findings: The expected response to each stroke is contraction of the rectus abdominis muscle and movement of the umbilicus toward the side stroked.

Diminished reflexes may be found in patients who are obese or have been pregnant. An absence of reflexes is associated with disease of the motor tracts of the spinal cord.

PERCUSS the kidneys for costovertebral angle tenderness.

Percuss kidney when the patient reports pain in back (flank pain).

Procedure: Approach the patient from behind as he or she is seated. One method for percussion is the direct approach. Use direct percussion to tap each costovertebral angle (CVA) with the ulnar surface of the dominant fist (Fig. 13-18, *A*). An alternative method is to use indirect percussion. Place the palmar surface of the nondominant hand over the CVA and tap the dorsum of that hand with the dominant fist (see Fig. 13-18, *B*).

Fig. 13-19 shows the underlying anatomy of the kidney in relation to the CVA or the flank.

Findings: The patient should perceive a thud but no pain.

CVA tenderness or severe pain may indicate pyelonephritis, glomerulonephritis, or nephrolithiasis (kidney stones).

★ Advanced practice

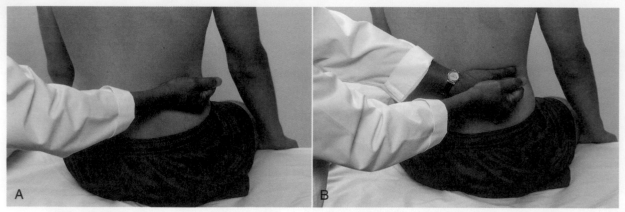

FIG. 13-18 Fist percussion of costovertebral angle for kidney tenderness. **A,** Direct percussion. **B,** Indirect percussion.

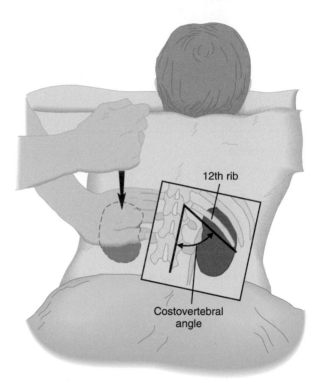

FIG. 13-19 Anatomic drawing showing landmarks for indirect percussion of the costovertebral angle. (From Black and Hawks, 2005.)

PROCEDURES AND TECHNIQUES WITH EXPECTED FINDINGS	ABNORMAL FINDINGS

★ ASSESS the abdomen for fluid.

If fluid is suspected within the abdomen, perform the following tests:

Shifting Dullness

Procedure: Ask the patient to lie supine so any fluid pools in the lateral (flank) area. Percuss the abdomen. Draw lines on the abdomen to indicate the midline tympany (the expected tone) in contrast to lateral dullness (tone created by fluid). Then have the patient turn to the right side and repeat percussion. Listen for the tympanic tone to shift to the upper (left) side and the area of dullness rises toward the midline (Fig. 13-20). Finally have the patient turn to the left lateral position and percuss. Listen as the dullness rises toward the midline.

★ Advanced practice

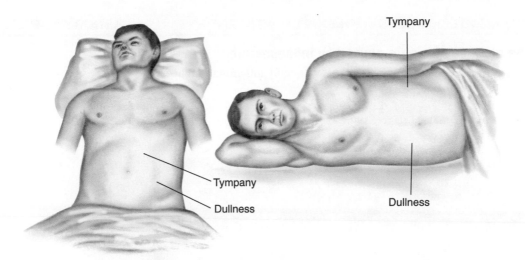

FIG. 13-20 Testing for shifting dullness. Dullness shifts to the dependent side. (From Seidel et al., 2011.)

PROCEDURES AND TECHNIQUES WITH EXPECTED FINDINGS

Findings: Normally tympany is heard throughout the abdomen, except over the bladder when it is distended.

Fluid Wave

Procedure: The patient lies supine. You need the hand of another nurse or the patient to be placed sideways in the middle of the patient's abdomen to stop the transmission of a tap across the skin (Fig. 13-21). Place your hands on either side of the abdomen. Use your fingertips to sharply strike one side of the abdomen. Feel for the fluid wave with the other hand on the opposite side of the abdomen.

Findings: The expected finding is no fluid wave.

ABNORMAL FINDINGS

Movement of the area of dullness as the patient shifts position reflects the shift of fluid in the peritoneal cavity (ascites).

If ascites is present, the tap causes a fluid wave through the abdomen (Fig. 13-22). The wave looks like fluid moving within the abdomen from the side that is tapped to the other side.

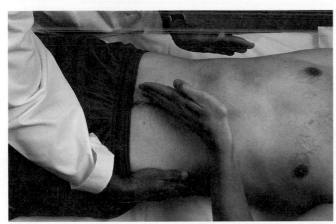

FIG. 13-21 Testing for fluid wave. Strike one side of the abdomen sharply with the fingertips. Feel for the impulse of a fluid wave with the other hand.

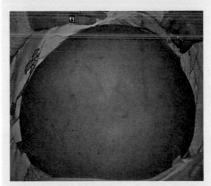

FIG. 13-22 Massive ascites in an individual with cirrhosis. Distended abdomen, dilated upper abdominal veins, and inverted umbilicus are classic manifestations. (From Butcher, 2004.)

PROCEDURES AND TECHNIQUES WITH EXPECTED FINDINGS	ABNORMAL FINDINGS

★ ASSESS the abdomen for pain caused by inflammation.

If the patient has abdominal pain that you suspect is caused by inflammation, test for *rebound tenderness.*

Procedure: Press down firmly at a 90-degree angle to the abdomen in an area away from the point of pain. Press inward deeply (Fig. 13-23) and release your fingers quickly.

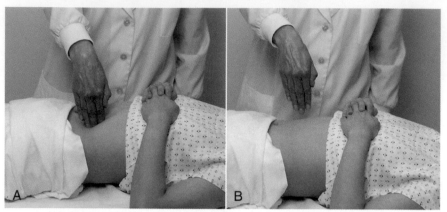

FIG. 13-23 Testing for rebound tenderness. **A,** Press deeply and gently into the abdomen. **B,** Rapidly withdraw the hands and fingers.

Findings: If the patient reports less pain when the pressure is released than when the pressure is exerted, then no pain from inflammation is indicated.

Rebound tenderness is present if the patient experiences more pain when pressure is released than when pressure is exerted and indicates peritoneal inflammation (see Table 13-1).

McBurney's Sign

Testing for *McBurney's sign* is a test for appendicitis.

Procedure: Palpate McBurney's point, which is located halfway between the umbilicus and the right anterior iliac crest (see Fig 13-4). Press firmly into the abdomen and release pressure quickly.

Findings: Absence of pain is a negative McBurney's sign, indicating no appendicitis.

Pain over McBurney's point indicates appendicitis.

Iliopsoas Muscle Test

When acute appendicitis is suspected, perform the *iliopsoas muscle test.*

Procedure: With the patient supine, place your hand over the lower right thigh. Ask the patient to raise the right leg, flexing at the hip. Push down to resist the raising of the leg (Fig. 13-24).

Findings: When the patient reports no pain from the pressure on the iliopsoas muscle, the test is negative.

An inflamed appendix may irritate the lateral iliopsoas muscle. When the patient reports RLQ pain to pressure against the raised leg, the iliopsoas muscle test is positive.

Obturator Muscle Test

When a ruptured appendix or pelvic abscess is suspected, perform the *obturator muscle test.*

Procedure: The patient lies supine and flexes the right hip and knee to 90 degrees. Holding the leg just above the knee and at the ankle, the nurse rotates the leg medially and laterally (Fig. 13-25).

★ Advanced practice

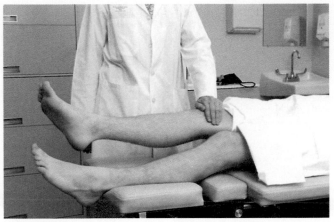

FIG. 13-24 Iliopsoas muscle test. (From Doughty and Jackson, 1993.)

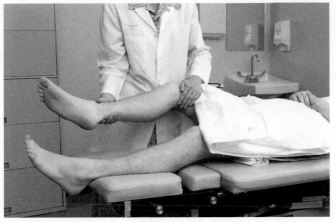

FIG. 13-25 Obturator muscle test. (From Doughty and Jackson, 1993.)

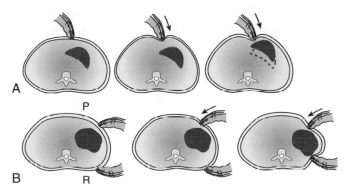

FIG. 13-26 Ballottement technique. **A,** Single-handed ballottement. Push inward at a 90-degree angle; if the object is freely movable, it floats upward to touch the fingertips **B,** Bimanual ballottement. *P,* pushing hand; *R,* receiving hand. (From Seidel et al., 2011.)

PROCEDURES AND TECHNIQUES WITH EXPECTED FINDINGS	ABNORMAL FINDINGS

Findings: If the patient has no pain, the test is negative.

Pain in the hypogastric region is a positive sign indicating irritation of the obturator muscle, which may be caused by a ruptured appendix or pelvic abscess.

★ ASSESS the abdomen for floating mass.

Ballottement is a palpation technique used to determine a floating mass.

Procedure: Use one or two hands to perform ballottement.

Place one hand perpendicular to the abdomen and push in toward the mass with fingertips at a 90-degree angle (Fig. 13-26, *A*). A freely movable mass floats upward and touches the fingertips as fluids and other structures are displaced.

When using the bimanual method, place one hand on the anterior abdomen to push down. Place the other hand against the flank to push up and palpate the mass to determine presence and size (see Fig. 13-26, *B*).

Findings: The normal finding is no palpable mass.

A floating mass may be an abnormal growth or a fetal head.

★ Advanced practice.

DOCUMENTING EXPECTED FINDINGS

Abdomen smooth, flat, and lighter color than extremities, with smooth, symmetric contour and no visible peristalsis. Umbilicus midline and rectus abdominis muscles prominent when head raised. Bowel sounds present in all quadrants with no vascular sounds. No tenderness, masses, or aortic pulsations to light or deep abdominal palpation. Umbilical ring feels round with no irregularities or bulges. Tympany over abdomen and spleen and dullness over suprapubic area. Liver spans 3 inches (7.6 cm) at the midclavicular line, lower border descends downward 1 inch (2.5 cm). Liver border smooth without tenderness. Gallbladder, spleen, and kidneys not palpable. Abdominal reflexes present in each quadrant. No CVA tenderness.

CLINICAL REASONING: THINKING LIKE A NURSE

Gastrointestinal system

A 46-year-old female with a long-standing history of alcoholism presents to the emergency department with severe abdominal pain that has been constant for the last 12 hours. She is screaming in pain and demanding morphine. Her other symptoms include nausea and vomiting.

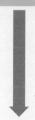

Interpreting

Early in the encounter the nurse considers two possible causes for this patient's abdominal pain and presenting findings: gastritis with gastrointestinal (GI) bleeding or pancreatitis. To determine if either has any probability of being correct, the nurse gathers additional data.

- What are the color and character of the emesis and stool? The woman tells the nurse that her vomit is yellowish green; sometimes she just has "dry heaves." The woman describes the stool from her last bowel movement as "light brown."
- Are there aggravating and alleviating factors? The woman indicates that nothing relieves the pain but any movement makes it worse.

The experienced nurse not only recognizes pancreatitis by the clinical signs (severe, unrelieved, knifelike pain that radiates to the back) and symptoms (nausea, vomiting) but also interprets this information in the context of an adult with a history of alcohol abuse.

Nurse's Background, Experience, Perspective

The experienced nurse immediately has a perceptual grasp of the situation at hand. Extensive practical knowledge about what to expect with this age-group and diagnoses allows the nurse to recognize risk factors given her situation: age and long-standing alcohol abuse.

Noticing

The experienced nurse recognizes that patients with a long history of alcoholism are at risk for GI inflammation and bleeding and liver disorders such as cirrhosis. The nurse also knows that two inflammatory disorders can cause extreme pain like this: pancreatitis and gastritis. The pain is described as knifelike, and it radiates to her back. The patient's bowel sounds are hypoactive; the abdomen is distended, firm, and tender with palpation. The nurse obtains a set of vital signs that include blood pressure 102/58, pulse 120 beats/min, temperature 100° F (37.7° C), respiratory rate 24 breaths/min, oxygen saturation 96%. Her skin is warm and slightly diaphoretic.

Responding

The nurse initiates appropriate initial interventions (oxygen, intravenous access, pain control) and notifies the emergency department provider of the situation, ensuring that the patient receives appropriate immediate and follow-up care.

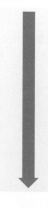

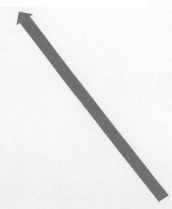

Reflecting

The nurse evaluates the presentation and outcomes of interventions (reflection-in-action); this experience contributes to and deepens the expertise on which to draw (refection-on-action) when encountering a similar situation.

AGE-RELATED VARIATIONS

Little adaptation is needed in techniques and procedures to examine the abdomen and gastrointestinal systems of patients at any age.

INFANTS, CHILDREN, AND ADOLESCENTS

Assessment techniques are the same for infants, children, and adolescents. There are several differences in the assessment findings in infants based on anatomical differences. Children and adolescents may resist abdominal palpation because they

are ticklish. Chapter 19 presents further information for assessing the GI and renal systems of infants, children, and adolescents.

OLDER ADULTS

Procedures and techniques for assessing an older adult are the same as for the younger adult. Chapter 21 presents further information regarding the assessments of these systems for this age-group.

COMMON PROBLEMS AND CONDITIONS

RISK FACTORS

Gastrointestinal Cancers

Esophageal Cancer
- *Age:* Risk increases with age. Less than 15% of cases are found in people younger than 55 years, with the peak between ages 70 and 80.
- *Gender:* Men have a rate three times that of women.
- *Tobacco:* The longer a person smokes, the greater the risk. (M)
- *Alcohol:* Long-term alcohol intake increases risk. Alcohol and smoking together raise a person's risk more than using either alone. (M)
- *Barrett's esophagus:* This condition is associated with long-term gastroesophageal reflux. (M)
- *Overweight:* The risk of this cancer is higher in people who are overweight or obese because obesity increases the risk of esophageal reflux. (M)
- *Diet:* Deficits in fruits and vegetables increase risk. (M)

Stomach Cancer
- *Age:* There is a sharp increase after age 50. Most people are diagnosed between their late 60s and 80s.
- *Gender:* Disease is twice as common in men.
- *Race:* Highest rates are seen in Asians/Pacific Islanders. Rates are higher in Hispanics and African Americans than in non-Hispanic Caucasians.
- *Blood type:* For unknown reasons people with blood type A have a greater risk.
- *Family history:* Risk is higher in those with a first-degree family member with stomach cancer.
- *Previous stomach surgery:* Risk is higher in those who have had surgery to treat noncancerous disease such as peptic ulcer disease.
- *Infection: Helicobacter pylori* infection is a major cause of this cancer.
- *Diet:* Eating large amounts of smoked foods, salted fish and meat, and pickled vegetables increases risk. (M)
- *Tobacco:* The rate of proximal stomach cancer is approximately double in smokers. (M)

Colon Cancer
- *Age:* 90% of people with this cancer are over 50 years old.

- *Family history:* Having a first-degree relative with colorectal cancer increases one's risk.
- *Preexisting gastrointestinal disorder:* Personal history of chronic inflammatory bowel disease (Crohn's disease or ulcerative colitis) increases risk.
- *Diabetes mellitus:* This increases risk. (M)
- *Tobacco:* Smoking for three to four decades causes this cancer. The association is stronger for rectal cancer than for colon cancer. (M)
- *Alcohol:* Moderate alcohol use increases risk. (M)
- *Obesity:* Obesity increases risk, with a stronger association observed in men than in women. (M)
- *Diet:* Diet high in red and/or processed meats increases risk. (M)
- *Physical activity:* Lack of regular physical exercise increases risk. (M)

Liver Cancer
- *Gender:* Men develop this cancer several times more often than women.
- *Race:* In the United States Asian Americans and Pacific Islanders have the highest rate of this cancer.
- *Liver disease:* Hepatitis B and C infections or cirrhosis increase the risk. (M)
- *Obesity:* Risk of developing this cancer is probably increased because obesity can result in fatty liver disease and cirrhosis. (M)

Pancreatic Cancer
- *Age:* The average age of diagnosis is 72 years.
- *Gender:* Men are more likely to develop this cancer.
- *Race:* African Americans are more likely to develop this cancer than Caucasians partly because of higher rates of smoking and diabetes.
- *Family history:* In about 5% to 10% of cases there is an inherited tendency for this cancer.
- *Tobacco:* Risk is 2 to 3 times higher among cigarette smokers. (M)
- *Diet:* A high consumption of red meats and fats increases risk. (M)

Continued

RISK FACTORS
Gastrointestinal Cancers—cont'd

Bladder Cancer
- *Tobacco:* The greatest risk factor for this cancer is smoking. (M)
- *Age:* The average age at diagnosis is 68 years.
- *Gender:* Men get this cancer more often than women.

- *Race:* Caucasians are 2 times more likely to develop this cancer than are African Americans and Hispanic Americans.
- *Chronic bladder inflammation:* Urinary tract infections, kidney stones, and bladder stones are linked to this cancer.

Data from www.cancer.org 2010, accessed October 7, 2011.
M, Modifiable risk factor.

ALIMENTARY TRACT

Gastroesophageal Reflux Disease

Flow of gastric secretions into the esophagus is termed *gastroesophageal reflux disease* (GERD). It is caused by weakening of the lower esophageal sphincter or increased intraabdominal pressure. **Clinical Findings:** Patients complain of heartburn, regurgitation, and dysphagia (difficulty swallowing), which are aggravated by lying down and relieved by sitting up, antacids, and eating.

Hiatal Hernia

A protrusion of the stomach through the esophageal hiatus of the diaphragm into the mediastinal cavity is termed *hiatal hernia* (Fig. 13-27, *A* and *B*). Muscle weakness is a primary factor in developing this type of hernia. **Clinical Findings:** Clinical manifestations are the same as those of GERD: heartburn, regurgitation, and dysphagia.

Peptic Ulcer Disease

An ulcer occurring in the lower end of the esophagus, in the stomach, or in the duodenum is termed *peptic ulcer.* Duodenal ulcer is the most common form, caused by a break in the duodenal mucosa that scars with healing (Fig. 13-28). Gastric and duodenal ulcers may result from infection with *Helicobacter pylori.* Gastric ulcers also are caused by stress and medications such as corticosteroids, aspirin, and nonsteroidal antiinflammatory drugs (NSAIDs). **Clinical Findings:** Patients with gastric ulcers complain of burning pain in the left epigastrium and back 1 to 2 hours after eating. Patients with duodenal ulcers complain of burning pain 2 to 4 hours after eating and at midmorning, at midafternoon, and in the middle of the night, with pain relief after taking antacids or eating.

Crohn's Disease

This chronic inflammatory bowel disease (IBD) is also called *regional enteritis* or *regional ileitis* (Fig. 13-29). Inflammation may occur from mouth to anus, but it commonly affects the terminal ileum and colon. Affected mucosa is ulcerated, with presence of fistulas, fissures, and abscesses that may form adjacent to healthy bowel segments. **Clinical Findings:** Patients complain of severe abdominal pain, cramping, diarrhea, nausea, fever, chills, weakness, anorexia, and weight loss.

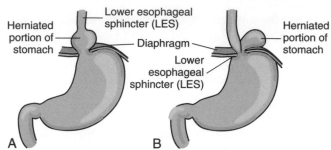

FIG. 13-27 Hiatal hernia. **A,** Sliding hernia. **B,** Paraesophageal. (From Monahan, 2007.)

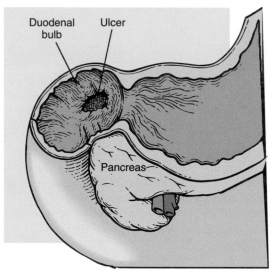

FIG. 13-28 Duodenal peptic ulcer. (From Lewis et al., 2007.)

Ulcerative Colitis

This chronic IBD starts in the rectum and progresses through the large intestine (Fig. 13-30). The submucosa becomes engorged, and mucosa becomes ulcerated and denuded with granulation tissue; it may progress to colon cancer. **Clinical Findings:** Patients complain of severe abdominal pain, fever, chills, anemia, and weight loss. The patient experiences profuse watery diarrhea of blood, mucus, and pus.

Diverticulitis

Inflammation of diverticula is termed *diverticulitis.* Diverticula are herniations through the muscular wall in the colon

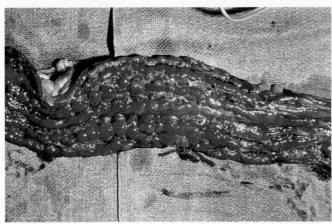

FIG. 13-29 Crohn's disease showing deep ulcers and fissures, creating "cobblestone" effect. (From Doughty and Jackson, 1993.)

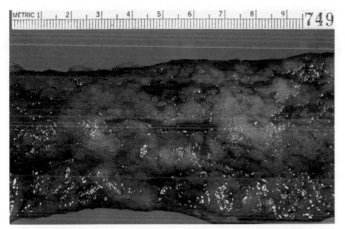

FIG. 13-30 Ulcerative colitis showing severe mucosal edema and inflammation with ulcerations and bleeding. (From Doughty and Jackson, 1993.)

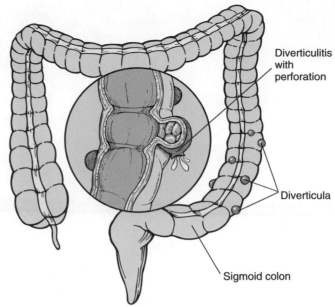

FIG. 13-31 Diverticulosis (diverticulitis). (From Frazier and Drzymkowoki, 2008.)

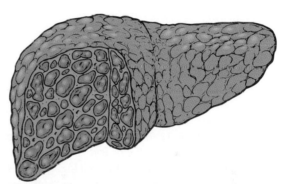

FIG. 13-32 Cirrhosis of the liver. (From Salvo, 2009.)

(Fig. 13-31). Presence of fecal material through the thin-walled diverticula causes inflammation and abscesses. **Clinical Findings:** Patients complain of cramping pain in the left lower quadrant; nausea; vomiting; and altered bowel habits, usually constipation. The abdomen may be distended and tympanic, with decreased bowel sounds and localized tenderness.

HEPATOBILIARY SYSTEM

Viral Hepatitis

This inflammation of the liver results from different viruses. **Clinical Findings:** Common symptoms are anorexia, vague abdominal pain, nausea, vomiting, malaise, and fever. An enlarged liver and spleen are classic findings. Jaundice, tan-colored stools, and dark urine may also be reported or observed.

Cirrhosis

This condition is a chronic degenerative disease of the liver in which diffuse destruction and regeneration of hepatic parenchymal cells occur. Fig. 13-32 illustrates the cobblestone appearance of the cirrhotic liver that results in impaired liver function and blood flow. Causes of cirrhosis include viral hepatitis, biliary obstruction, and alcohol abuse. **Clinical Findings:** The liver becomes palpable and hard. Associated signs include ascites, jaundice, cutaneous spider angiomas, dark urine, tan-colored stools, and spleen enlargement. End-stage cirrhosis is characterized by portal hypertension, esophageal varies, hepatic encephalopathy, and coma.

Cholecystitis with Cholelithiasis

Inflammation of the gallbladder is termed *cholecystitis;* when gallstones are present, the condition is termed *cholelithiasis* (Fig. 13-33). The bile duct becomes obstructed by either edema from inflammation or gallstones. **Clinical Findings:** The primary symptom is right upper quadrant colicky pain that may radiate to midtorso or right scapula. Other indications include indigestion and mild transient jaundice.

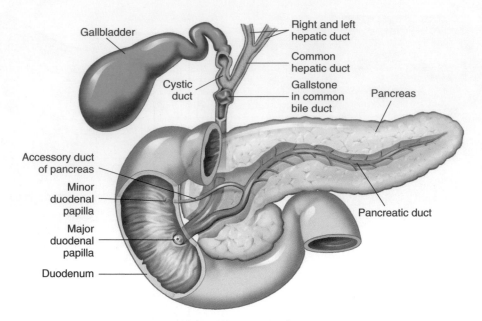

FIG. 13-33 The gallstone in the common bile duct causes biliary colic and may cause jaundice when the bile cannot flow from the liver and gallbladder to the duodenum. (Courtesy Kissane, 1990. From Thibodeau and Patton, 2003.)

PANCREAS

Pancreatitis

Acute or chronic inflammation of the pancreas resulting from autodigestion of the organ is called *pancreatitis*. It can be caused by alcoholism or obstruction of the sphincter of Oddi by gallstones. Fig. 13-33 shows how the location of gallstones could move to obstruct the flow of digestive enzymes from the pancreas. **Clinical Findings:** Patients complain of pain, described as steady, boring, dull, or sharp, that radiates from the epigastrium to the back. Patients prefer the fetal position with knees to the chest. Other manifestations include nausea and vomiting, weight loss, steatorrhea (greater than expected fat in the stool), and glucose intolerance.

URINARY SYSTEM

Urinary Tract Infections

These infections may involve the urethra (urethritis), urinary bladder (cystitis), or renal pelvis (pyelonephritis). Most urinary tract infections result from gram-negative organisms such as *Escherichia coli, Klebsiella, Proteus,* or *Pseudomonas* that originate from the patient's own intestinal tract and ascend through the urethra to the bladder. **Clinical Findings:** Symptoms of urethritis include frequency, urgency, and dysuria. Symptoms of cystitis are the same as those of urethritis plus signs of bacteriuria and perhaps fever. Patients with pyelonephritis complain of flank pain, dysuria, nocturia, and frequency. Manifestations in older adults include confusion or delirium with or without fever.

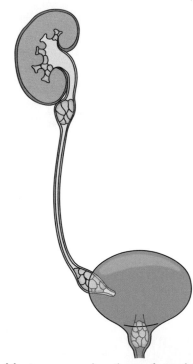

FIG. 13-34 Most common locations of renal calculi formation. (From Monahan et al., 2007.)

Nephrolithiasis

The formation of stones in the kidney pelvis is termed *nephrolithiasis* (Fig. 13-34). Factors contributing to stone formation may be metabolic, dietary, genetic, or climatic. Urinary stasis and infection are important variables in the development of stones. **Clinical Findings:** Signs include fever and hematuria. A symptom is flank pain that may radiate to the groin and genitals.

CLINICAL APPLICATION AND CLINICAL REASONING

See Appendix D for answers to exercises in this section.

REVIEW QUESTIONS

1. What question does a nurse ask a patient with a history of pancreatitis who is complaining of abdominal pain?
   1. Which foods aggravate the pain?
   2. Have you recently traveled outside the United States?
   3. Have you noticed a change in your bowel habits?
   4. How severe is the pain on a scale of 0 to 10?

2. The nurse is interviewing a patient with a history of flank pain, fever, chills, and pain radiating to the groin. Which examination technique is most appropriate for this patient?
   1. Percussion of the costovertebral angle
   2. Deep palpation of the abdomen
   3. Testing for rebound tenderness
   4. Auscultation of all quadrants of the abdomen

3. A patient reports a gnawing, burning pain in the mid-epigastric area that is aggravated by bending over or lying down. Which additional question does the nurse ask for the symptom analysis?
   1. "Do you have a family history of this type of pain?"
   2. "How long ago did you eat?"
   3. "Do you have any symptoms such as nausea with this pain?"
   4. "Have you noticed any yellow coloring in your eyes or on your skin?"

4. The nurse palpates the abdomen to gather data about which organs located in the right upper quadrant?
   1. Liver and gallbladder
   2. Stomach and spleen
   3. Uterus, if enlarged, and right ovary
   4. Right ureter and ascending colon

5. A nurse performing an abdominal examination on a 37-year-old woman would document which finding as abnormal?
   1. Nonpalpable spleen or kidneys
   2. Bowel sounds every 15 seconds in the lower quadrants
   3. Bulges observed when coughing
   4. Silver-white striae and a faint vascular network

6. A 50-year-old patient asks how he can reduce his risk of colon cancer. What is the most appropriate response by the nurse?

   1. "A diet high in animal protein reduces the risk."
   2. "Regular exercise to reduce body fat helps prevent colon cancer."
   3. "Taking antacids for heartburn can help prevent colon cancer."
   4. "Taking vitamin C daily helps reduce the risk."

7. Which is an expected finding of an abdominal examination of an adult?
   1. Dull percussion tones over the bladder
   2. Venus hum over the epigastrium on auscultation
   3. High-pitched gurgles every 5 to 15 seconds on auscultation
   4. Swishing sounds over the abdominal aorta on auscultation

8. Which technique does the nurse use to palpate a patient's abdomen?
   1. Asks the patient to breath slowly though the mouth
   2. Uses the heel of the hand to perform deep palpation
   3. Uses the left hand to lift the rib cage away from the abdominal organs
   4. Depresses the abdomen 1 to 2 inches for light palpation

9. When assessing a patient's abdomen, the nurse uses assessment techniques in which order?
   1. Inspection, palpation, percussion, and auscultation
   2. Inspection, auscultation, palpation, and percussion
   3. Auscultation, inspection, percussion, and palpation
   4. Palpation, auscultation, inspection, and percussion

10. The nurse suspects that the patient has appendicitis. Which assessment techniques can the nurse use to confirm his or her suspicion?
    1. Gently perform fist percussion over the right costovertebral angle
    2. Ask the patient to place her hand on the abdomen while the nurse taps one side of the abdomen and palpates the other side
    3. Palpate the left lower quadrant at a 90-degree angle and quickly release his or her hand
    4. With the patient lying supine and flexing her right knee and hip, tap on the sole of the patient's right foot

CASE STUDY

Fatima Khan is a 22-year-old woman complaining of abdominal pain. The following data are collected by the nurse during an interview and examination.

Interview Data

Ms. Khan tells the nurse that the pain started yesterday evening and has gotten progressively worse. She describes the pain as "really bad." It is constant and located in her right lower abdomen, toward her umbilicus. She says that it feels a little better if she stays curled up and does not move. She tells the nurse that she is in good health and that she has never had a problem with her stomach. Ms. Khan indicates that normally she has a good appetite and can eat anything—except for now. She says that she ate breakfast and lunch yesterday but by dinnertime she was nauseated and had no appetite. She has not eaten anything since. She has had no recent weight changes, but she would like to weigh about 5 lbs (2.5 kg) less than she currently does. Ms. Khan smokes a half pack of cigarettes daily. She does not drink alcoholic beverages, and she takes no medication. She denies discomfort or problems with urination, describing her urine as "usual looking."

Examination Data

* *General survey:* Alert and anxious female in moderate distress lying in a fetal position on the examination table, with her eyes closed. Appears well nourished. Her skin is hot.
* *Inspection:* Abdomen is flat and symmetric. No lesions or scars are noted. No surface movements are seen except for breathing.
* *Auscultation:* Bowel sounds are absent.
* *Palpation:* Tympany is noted over most of abdominal surface; dullness over liver. Midclavicular liver span is 4 inches (10 cm).
* *Light palpation:* Demonstrates pain and guarding in right lower quadrant. Unable to palpate deep structures because of excessive abdominal discomfort. Demonstrates positive rebound tenderness in right lower quadrant.

Clinical Reasoning

1. Which data deviate from normal findings, suggesting a need for further investigation?
2. For which additional information should the nurse ask or assess?
3. Based on the data, which risk factors for cancers in the abdomen does Ms. Khan have?
4. With which team members can the nurse collaborate to meet this patient's needs?

Musculoskeletal System

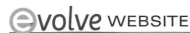
CONCEPT OVERVIEW

The feature concept for this chapter is *Motion*. This concept represents mechanisms that facilitate and impair mobility. Several concepts are interrelated, including oxygenation, perfusion, intracranial regulation, tactile perception, pain, nutrition, tissue integrity, and elimination. These interrelationships are depicted in the following model.

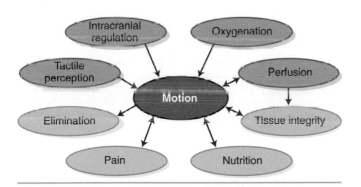

Motion depends on the delivery of oxygenated blood to tissues and coordination of movement regulated by the brain, spinal cord, and peripheral nerves. It can cause pain and thus limit movement. Adequate nutrition is needed for motion, and motion is needed for the procurement and preparation of food. Elimination is impacted by motion, as is the maintenance of tissue integrity. The model shows the interrelationship of concepts associated with motion. As an example, over time excessive body weight damages the joints, causing pain with movement. This pain may limit the walking the person does, which may limit such activities as shopping for food and exercise. Others who have limited mobility may develop constipation and possible skin breakdown because of extended pressure on tissue. An understanding of the relationship of these concepts helps the nurse recognize risk factors and thus increases awareness when conducting a health assessment. The following case provides a clinical example featuring several of these interrelated concepts.

Mrs. Wilcox is a 92-year-old widow who lives alone. One afternoon she fell in her driveway and suffered a hip fracture requiring a surgical repair. After the surgical procedure Ms. Wilcox experienced significant pain and delirium, and she was unable to actively participate in physical therapy. Her lack of mobility contributed to her poor nutritional intake, constipation, and skin breakdown on her sacrum.

ANATOMY AND PHYSIOLOGY

The musculoskeletal system provides both support and mobility for the body and protection for internal organs. This system also produces blood cells and stores minerals such as calcium and phosphorus.

SKELETON

Functions of bones include support for soft tissues and organs, protection of organs such as the brain and spinal cord, body movement, and hematopoiesis. Bones are continually remodeling and changing the collagen and mineral composition to accommodate stress placed on them. The function of each bone dictates its shape and surface features. For example, long bones act as levers; they have a flat surface for the attachment of muscles, with grooves at the end for passage of tendons or nerves. Examples of long bones are the humerus, femur, fibula, and phalanges. Short bones such as carpal and tarsal bones are cube shaped. Flat bones make up the cranium, ribs, and scapula. The vertebrae are irregularly shaped bones.

The human skeleton has two major divisions: the axial and appendicular skeletons. The axial skeleton includes the facial bones, auditory ossicles, vertebrae, ribs, sternum, and hyoid bone; the appendicular skeleton includes the scapula, clavicle, bones of the shoulders and arms, and bones of the pelvis and legs. The subsequent discussion of bones is organized by these divisions.

SKELETAL MUSCLES

Skeletal muscles are composed of muscle fibers that attach to bones to facilitate movement. Although some skeletal muscles move by reflex, all are controlled voluntarily. Skeletal muscle fibers are arranged parallel to the long axis of bones to which they attach, or they are attached obliquely. Muscles attach to a bone, ligament, tendon, or fascia.

JOINTS

Joints are articulations where two or more bones come together. They help hold the bones firmly while allowing movement between them.

Joints are classified in two ways: by the type of material between them (fibrous, cartilaginous, or synovial) and by their degree of movement. Immovable joints are synarthrodial (e.g., the suture of the skull); slightly movable joints are amphiarthrodial (e.g., the symphysis pubis); and freely movable joints are diarthrodial (e.g., the knee and the distal interphalangeal [DIP] joint of the distal fingers).

Diarthrodial joints are further classified by their type of movement. Only the diarthrodial joints have one or more ranges of motion. See Table 14-1 in the examination section of this chapter for types of movement of each diarthrodial joint. Hinge joints (e.g., the knee, elbow, and fingers) permit extension and flexion. Some hinge joints allow hyperextension; however, there is variability among individuals—not all hinge joints are able to hyperextend. Pivot joints permit movement of one bone articulating with a ring or notch of another bone such as the head of the radius, which articulates with the radial notch of the ulna. The ends of saddle-shaped bones articulate with one another: the base of the thumb is the only example. Condyloid or ellipsoidal joints consist of the condyle of one bone that fits into the elliptically shaped portion of its articulating bone (e.g., the distal end of the radius articulates with three wrist bones). Ball-and-socket joints are made of a ball-shaped bone that fits

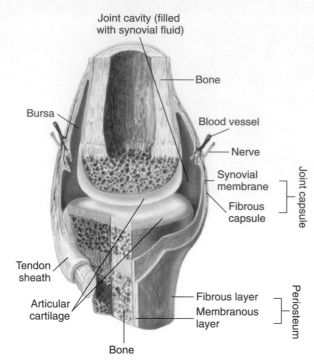

FIG. 14-1 Structures of a synovial joint (the knee). (From Mourad, 1991.)

into a concave area of its articulating bone (e.g., the head of the femur fits into the acetabulum within the pelvis). Gliding joints permit movement along various axes through relatively flat articulating surfaces such as joints between two vertebrae.

Diarthrodial joints are synovial joints because they are lined with synovial fluid (Fig. 14-1). Synovial fluid lubricates the joint to facilitate its movement in various directions. Some synovial joints such as the knee also have a disk called the *meniscus*, which is a pad of cartilage that cushions the joint. These joints have a covering surrounding them called the *joint capsule*, which is an extension of the periosteum of the articulating bone. Ligaments also encase the capsule to add strength.

LIGAMENTS AND TENDONS

The difference between ligaments and tendons is more functional than structural. Ligaments are strong, dense, flexible bands of connective tissue that hold bones to bones (Fig. 14-2). They can provide support in several ways: by encircling the joint, gripping it obliquely, or lying parallel to the bone ends across the joint. They can simultaneously allow some movements while restricting others.

Conversely, tendons are strong, nonelastic cords of collagen located at the ends of muscles to attach them to bones (see Fig. 14-1). Tendons support bone movement in response to skeletal muscle contractions, transmitting remarkable force at times from the contracting muscles to the bone without sustaining injury themselves.

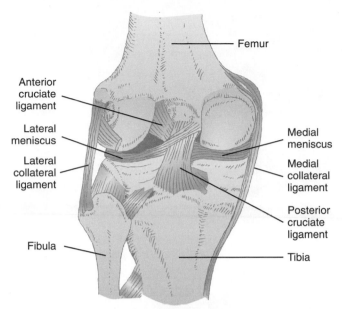

FIG. 14-2 Posterior view of the left knee. The medial collateral ligament prevents the knee from going into too much valgus during stress (inward). The lateral collateral ligament prevents the knee from going into too much varus during stress (outward). (From Black and Hawks, 2009.)

CARTILAGE AND BURSAE

Cartilage is a semismooth, gellike supporting tissue that is strong and able to support weight. The upper seven pairs of ribs are connected directly to the sternum by costal cartilage. The flexibility of the cartilage allows the thorax to move when the lungs expand and contract. Cartilage also reinforces respiratory passages such as the nose, larynx, trachea, and bronchi. It forms a cap over the ends of long bones, providing a smooth surface for articulation (see Fig. 14-1). Because it contains no blood vessels, it receives nutrition from the synovial fluid forced into it during movement and weight-bearing activities. For this reason, weight-bearing activity and joint movement are essential to maintaining cartilage health.

Bursae are small sacs in the connective tissues adjacent to selected joints such as the shoulders (the glenohumeral joint) and knees. Each bursa is lined with synovial membrane containing synovial fluid, which acts as a lubricant to reduce friction when a muscle or tendon rubs against another muscle, tendon, or bone (see Fig. 14-1).

AXIAL SKELETON AND SUPPORTING STRUCTURES

Skull and Neck

The six bones of the cranium (one frontal, two parietal, two temporal, and one occipital) are fused together. The face consists of 14 bones that protect facial structures. Like the skull, these bones are immobile and are fused at sutures, with the exception of the mandible. The mandible articulates with the temporal bone of the skull at the temporomandibular joint,

allowing for movement of the jaw up, down, in, out, and from side to side (see Fig. 10-1). The neck is supported by the cervical vertebrae, ligaments, and the sternocleidomastoid and trapezius muscles, with its greatest mobility at the level of C4-5 or C5-6. The type of movement permitted includes flexion, extension, hyperflexion, lateral movement, flexion, and rotation. The sternocleidomastoid muscle stretches from the upper sternum and anterior clavicle to the mastoid process; the trapezius links the scapula, the lateral third of the clavicle, and the vertebrae, extending to the occipital prominence.

Trunk and Pelvis

The trunk is formed by the vertebrae, ribs, and sternum of the axial skeleton and the scapula and clavicle of the appendicular skeleton. The pelvis is part of the appendicular skeleton. Fig. 14-3 shows the bones of the trunk and pelvis, and Fig. 14-4 shows the muscles. The spine is composed of 7 cervical, 12 thoracic, 5 lumbar, and 5 sacral vertebrae (see Fig. 15-6). The cervical, thoracic, and lumbar vertebrae are separated from each other by fibrocartilaginous disks, whereas the sacral vertebrae are fused. The vertebral joints, separated by disks, glide slightly over the surfaces of one another, permitting flexion, hyperextension, lateral bending, and rotation.

APPENDICULAR SKELETON AND SUPPORTING STRUCTURES

Upper Extremities

The bones of the upper extremities are shown in Fig. 14-5, and the muscles are shown in Fig. 14-6.

Shoulder and Upper Arm

The shoulder joint, also called the *glenohumeral joint*, consists of the point where the humerus and the glenoid fossa of the scapula articulate (Fig. 14-7). The acromial and coracoid processes (see Fig. 14-3) and surrounding ligaments protect this ball-and-socket joint and permit flexion, extension, and hyperextension, abduction and adduction, and internal and external rotation. Besides the glenohumeral joint, two other joints contribute to shoulder movement: the acromioclavicular joint (between the acromial process and the clavicle) and the sternoclavicular joint (between the sternal manubrium and the clavicle).

Elbow, Forearm, and Wrist

The elbow joint consists of the humerus, radius, and ulna enclosed in a single synovial cavity protected by ligaments and a bursa between the olecranon and the skin (see Fig. 14-5). The elbow is a hinge joint; it permits extension, flexion, and sometimes hyperextension. Pronation and supination of the forearm are also provided. The wrist joins the radius and the carpal bones with articular disks of the wrist, ligaments, and a fibrous capsule to form a condyloid joint. This joint permits flexion; extension; hyperextension; and radial and ulnar flexion, also called *radial and ulnar deviation*.

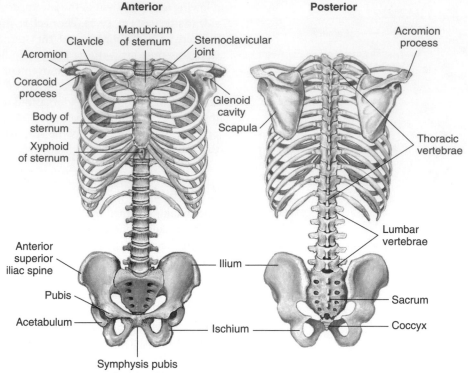

FIG. 14-3 Bones of the trunk and pelvis. (From Mourad, 1991.)

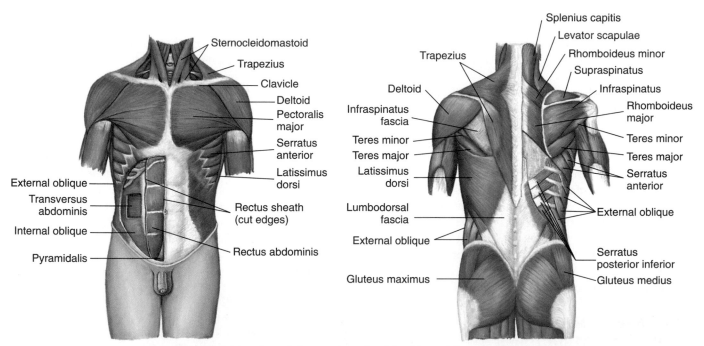

FIG. 14-4 Muscles of the trunk and pelvis. (From Mourad, 1991.)

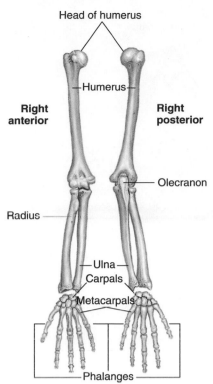

FIG. 14-5 Bones of the upper extremities. (From Mourad, 1991.)

Hand

There are small, subtle movements or articulations within the hand between the carpals and metacarpals, between the metacarpals and proximal phalanges, and between the middle and distal phalanges (see Fig. 14-5). Ligaments protect the diarthrotic joints, which allow flexion, extension, and hyperextension. The fingers are able to flex and extend and abduct and adduct. The names of joints in the hands describe their location. For example, the distal joint of the fingers is called the *distal interphalangeal (DIP) joint*; the middle joint of each finger is called the *proximal interphalangeal (PIP) joint*; and the joint that attaches the metacarpal to the carpal is called the *metacarpophalangeal (MCP) joint*.

Lower Extremities

The bones of the lower extremities are shown in Fig. 14-8, and the muscles are shown in Fig. 14-9.

Hip and Thigh

The acetabulum and femur form the hip joint, protected by a fibrous capsule and three bursae. Three ligaments help stabilize the head of the femur in the joint capsule (Fig. 14-10). Like the shoulder, this is a ball-and-socket joint that provides flexion, extension and hyperextension, abduction and adduction, internal and external rotation, and circumduction.

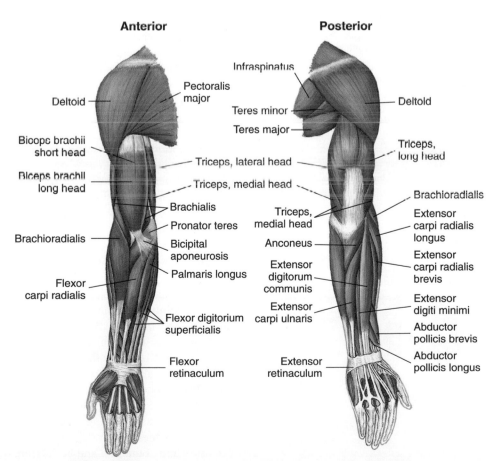

FIG. 14-6 Muscles of the upper extremities. (From Mourad, 1991.)

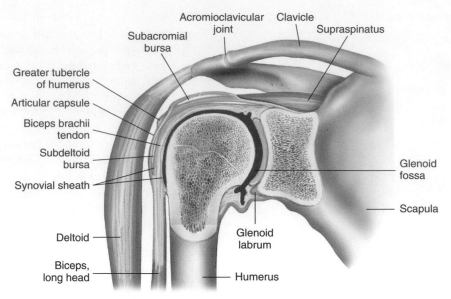

FIG. 14-7 Structures of the glenohumeral and acromioclavicular joint of the shoulder. (From Seidel et al., 2011.)

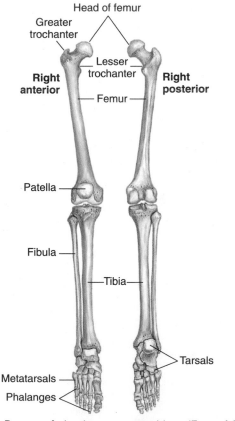

FIG. 14-8 Bones of the lower extremities. (From Mourad, 1991.)

Knee and Lower Leg

The knee is a hinge joint that serves as the point of articulation between the femur, the tibia, and the patella (see Fig. 14-1). The knee has medial and lateral menisci (disk-shaped fibrous cartilage) that cushion the tibia and the femur and connect to the articulated capsule. Ligaments provide stability; the bursae reduce friction on movement between the femur and the tibia. Movements of this joint include flexion, extension, and sometimes hyperextension.

Ankle and Foot

The ankle joint, or tibiotalar joint, forms a hinge joint, permitting flexion, called *dorsiflexion,* and extension in one plane, called *plantar flexion.* Protective medial and lateral ligaments join the tibia, fibula, and talus to form the tibiotalar joint. Smaller joints within the ankle permit a pivot or rotation movement, producing inversion and eversion and adduction and abduction. These joints are the subtalar (talocalcaneal) and the talonavicular (transverse tarsal) joints (Fig. 14-11).

Five metatarsal bones form the sole of the foot. Like the names of joints in the hands, the names of joints in the feet describe their location. For example, the joint between the distal and proximal phalanges is called the *interphalangeal joint;* the joint between the proximal phalanx and the first metatarsal is called the *metatarsophalangeal joint;* and the joint that attaches the first metatarsal to the tarsals is called the *tarsometatarsal joint* (see Fig 14-11).

Each foot has a gliding joint that allows inversion and eversion. The toes are condyloid joints that allow flexion and extension and abduction and adduction.

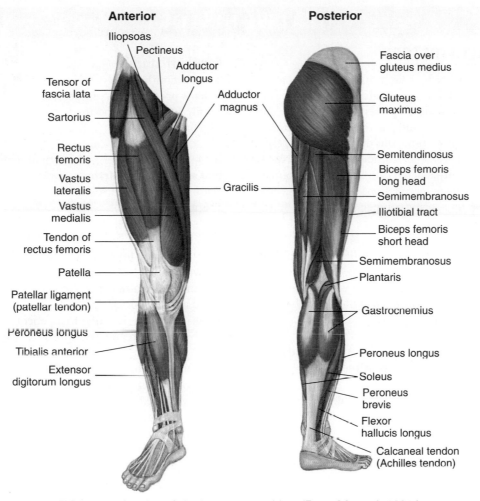

Anterior

Iliopsoas
Pectineus
Adductor longus
Adductor magnus
Tensor of fascia lata
Sartorius
Rectus femoris
Vastus lateralis
Vastus medialis
Tendon of rectus femoris
Patella
Patellar ligament (patellar tendon)
Peroneus longus
Tibialis anterior
Extensor digitorum longus
Gracilis

Posterior

Fascia over gluteus medius
Gluteus maximus
Semitendinosus
Biceps femoris long head
Semimembranosus
Iliotibial tract
Biceps femoris short head
Semimembranosus
Plantaris
Gastrocnemius
Peroneus longus
Soleus
Peroneus brevis
Flexor hallucis longus
Calcaneal tendon (Achilles tendon)

FIG. 14-9 Muscles of the lower extremities. (From Mourad, 1991.)

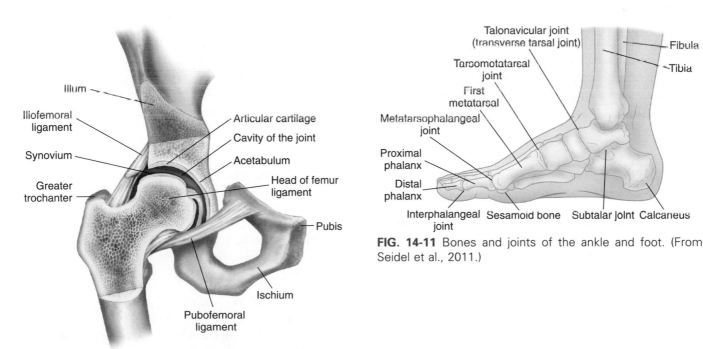

Illum
Iliofemoral ligament
Synovium
Greater trochanter
Articular cartilage
Cavity of the joint
Acetabulum
Head of femur ligament
Pubis
Ischium
Pubofemoral ligament

FIG. 14-10 Structures of the hip. (Modified from Thompson et al., 2002.)

Talonavicular joint (transverse tarsal joint)
Tarsomotatarsal joint
First metatarsal
Metatarsophalangeal joint
Proximal phalanx
Distal phalanx
Interphalangeal joint
Sesamoid bone
Subtalar joint
Calcaneus
Fibula
Tibia

FIG. 14-11 Bones and joints of the ankle and foot. (From Seidel et al., 2011.)

HEALTH HISTORY

GENERAL HEALTH HISTORY

Nurses interview patients to collect subjective data about their present health and any past medical experiences. They ask questions about the patient's present health status, past health history, family history, and personal and psychosocial history, which may affect the functions of the musculoskeletal system. Quality Improvement Competencies for Nurses include providing patient-centered care and interdisciplinary teamwork with physical and occupational therapists. Refer to Table 11-1 on p. 196 for specific competencies.

Present Health Status

Do you have any chronic diseases? Loss of bone density or osteoporosis?
Chronic diseases may affect mobility and activities of daily living. Reduction in weight-bearing activities contributes to loss of bone density and osteoporosis.

Do you take any medications? If yes, what do you take and how often? Are you taking medications as they were prescribed?
Both prescription and over-the-counter medications should be documented. Patients may not report musculoskeletal problems if they are being treated successfully with medications. Many medications for musculoskeletal problems (e.g., aspirin, nonsteroidal antiinflammatory drugs, narcotics, tranquilizers, or sleep aids) can cause adverse effects and may increase risk of injury.

Have you noticed any changes in your ability to move around or participate in your usual activities? Have you noticed any changes in your muscle strength? What do you do to adapt to these changes?
If there are changes, they can be diagnosed and treated at an early stage, or they can generate a discussion about how to prevent further changes. The health care provider needs to determine how the patient is adapting to these changes to determine their impact on his or her quality of life.

Past Health History

Have you ever had any accidents or trauma that affected the bones or joints, including fractures, strains of the joints, sprains, and dislocations? If yes, when? Have you noticed any continuing problems or difficulties that seem related to this previous incident?
Previous injury can leave residual problems such as muscle weakness, decreased range of motion, or impaired mobility.

Have you ever had surgery on any bones, joints, or muscles? If yes, describe the procedure(s), when it (they) occurred, and what the outcome was.
The incidence of surgery may provide additional information about possible musculoskeletal problems and the findings to anticipate during assessment.

Family History

In your family is there a history of curvature of the spine or back problems? If yes, describe.
Family history may be used to determine patient's risk for vertebral disorders.

In your family is there a history of arthritis (i.e., rheumatoid arthritis, osteoarthritis, or gout)?
Family history may be used to determine the patient's risk for a form of arthritis.

Personal and Psychosocial History

What do you do for exercise? How often do you exercise and for what period of time? Do you smoke cigarettes? If yes, how many and how often? Do you drink alcohol? If yes, how much and how often?
These questions identify the patient's learning needs for health promotion and assess for risk factors for osteoporosis.

Do you play sports? If yes, which ones and how often? How do you protect yourself from injury while exercising or playing sports?
These questions assess for risk for injury. Adults should protect themselves from injury (e.g., stretching before running, wearing a bike helmet, and wearing elbow pads and wrist guards for in-line skating).

Do you lift, push, or pull items or bend or stoop frequently as a part of your daily routine either at home or at work? How do you protect yourself from muscle strain or injury?
Many musculoskeletal injuries are caused by heavy lifting and repetitive and forceful motions that may be prevented with proper body mechanics, appropriate help when lifting, and use of protective equipment.

PROBLEM-BASED HISTORY

Commonly reported problems related to the musculoskeletal system are pain, problems with movement, and problems with daily activities. As with symptoms in all areas of health assessment, a symptom analysis is completed using the mnemonic OLD CARTS, which includes the Onset, Location, Duration, Characteristics, Aggravating factors, Related symptoms, Treatment, and Severity (see Box 2-3).

Pain

Where do you feel the pain? When did you first notice it? Is it related to movement? Describe how it feels. How severe is the pain on a scale of 0 to 10, with 10 being the worst pain possible?
Joint pain is the most common musculoskeletal symptom for which patients seek help. Pain is felt in and around the joint and may be accompanied by edema and erythema, indicating

inflammation. Bone pain typically is described as "deep," "dull," "boring," or "intense." Bone pain frequently is not related to movement unless the bone is fractured, in which case the pain is described as "sharp." Muscle pain is described as "cramping." Muscle pain associated with weakness suggests a primary muscular disorder.

Did the pain occur suddenly? When during the day do you feel it?

Sudden onset of pain and erythema in the great toe, ankle, and lower leg suggests gout (also called *gouty arthritis*). Pain from rheumatoid arthritis and tendonitis may awaken the patient, especially when he or she is lying on the affected limb. Patients with rheumatoid arthritis often have morning stiffness lasting 1 to 2 hours. By contrast, patients with osteoarthritis experience pain with weight bearing that is relieved by rest.

Does the pain move from one joint to another? Has there been any injury, overuse, or strain of muscles or joints? Were you ill before the onset of pain?

Some disorders cause migratory arthritis, in which pain moves among joints (e.g., acute rheumatic fever, leukemia, or juvenile arthritis). Viral illnesses can cause muscle aches and pain (myalgia).

What makes the pain worse? Does it change according to the weather?

Learning what makes the pain worse may help to diagnose the disorder. Arthritis pain may become worse with changes in the barometric pressure. Movement usually makes joint pain worse except in rheumatoid arthritis, in which movement may reduce pain.

What have you done to relieve the pain? How effective has it been?

Knowing what relieves pain may help selection of pain relief strategies.

Problems with Movement

How long have you had problems with movement? Are your joints swollen, red, or hot to the touch? Is the movement in your joints limited?

Acute inflammation such as arthritis or gout produces edema, erythema, and warmth. Decreased range of motion occurs with injury to the cartilage or capsule or with muscle contracture or edema.

Have you had a recent sore throat?

Joint pain that occurs 10 to 14 days after a sore throat may be associated with rheumatic fever.

Do you feel any weakness in your muscles? If yes, which muscles? How long have you had this weakness? Does it become worse as the day progresses?

Muscle weakness may be caused by altered nerve innervation or muscle contraction disorder. Atrophied muscles may be the result of prolonged lack of use (e.g., atrophy occurs from disuse when an extremity is casted). Proximal muscle weakness is usually a myopathy, whereas distal weakness is usually a neuropathy.

Have you noticed your knees or ankles giving way when you put pressure on them? If yes, when does it occur? How often does it occur?

This may indicate joint instability that may occur from chronic inflammation or joint trauma. Safety must be a concern of the patient when a joint gives way.

Have your joints felt as if they are locked and will not move? If yes, when does it occur? How often does it occur? What relieves the locking? What makes it worse?

This may indicate joint instability that may occur from chronic inflammation or joint trauma. Data from the symptom analysis helps determine the cause of the movement disorder. Safety must be a concern of the patient when a joint gives way.

Problems with Daily Activities

Which activities are limited? To what extent are your daily activities limited? How do you compensate for this limitation?

- Bathing (getting in and out of the tub, turning faucets on or off)?
- Toileting (urinating, defecating, ability to raise or lower yourself onto or off of the toilet)?
- Dressing (buttoning, zipping, fastening openings behind your neck, hooking your brassiere, pulling a dress or shirt over your head, pulling up your pants, tying shoes, having shoes fit your feet)?
- Grooming (shaving, brushing teeth, brushing or combing hair, washing and drying hair, applying makeup)?
- Eating (preparing meals, pouring, holding utensils, cutting food, bringing food to your mouth, drinking)?
- Moving around (walking, going up or down stairs, getting in or out of bed, getting out of the house)? Sleeping?
- Communicating (writing, talking, using the telephone)?

Any impaired mobility or function may interfere with the person's ability to perform self-care activities. The nurse asks the patient to identify which activities are impaired, to what extent, and how he or she compensates. For example, a patient who reports hip pain when putting on shoes may have degenerative disease, which is aggravated by externally rotating the hip.[1]

For patients who have chronic disability or a crippling disease: How has your illness affected your interactions with your family? How has it affected your relationships with friends?

Assess for disturbance of self-esteem, body image, or role performance; loss of independence; or social isolation. Maintaining social relationships is an important aspect of therapy.

HEALTH PROMOTION FOR EVIDENCE-BASED PRACTICE

Arthritis, Osteoporosis, and Chronic Back Conditions

Arthritis, osteoporosis, and chronic back conditions all have major effects on quality of life, the ability to work, and basic activities of daily living.

There are more than 100 types of arthritis. It commonly occurs with other chronic conditions such as diabetes, heart disease, and obesity. Interventions to treat the pain and reduce the functional limitations from arthritis are important and may also enable people with these other chronic conditions to be more physically active.

Osteoporosis is defined as a bone mineral density (BMD) more than 2.5 standard deviations below the mean for young healthy adult women. Approximately half of all postmenopausal women will have an osteoporosis-related fracture during their lives. The risk for fracture increases as bone density decreases.

Chronic back pain is common, costly, and potentially disabling. The related objective for 2020 tracks activity limitation resulting from chronic back conditions.

Goals and Objectives—*Healthy People 2020*

The *Healthy People 2020* goal is to prevent illness and disability related to arthritis and other rheumatic conditions, osteoporosis, and chronic back conditions.

Recommendations to Reduce Risk (Primary Prevention)

National Osteoporosis Foundation

- Counsel patients to eat a balanced diet rich in calcium and vitamin D. Calcium intake should be between 1000 and 1300 mg per day; vitamin D intake should be between 400 and 800 IU per day.
- Encourage patients to engage in weight-bearing exercise.
- Encourage patients to avoid smoking and excessive alcohol use.

Screening Recommendations (Secondary Prevention)

U.S. Preventive Services Task Force

- Routine screening for osteoporosis for women age 65 and older is recommended.
- For women at increased risk of osteoporotic fracture, routine screening should begin at age 60. Increased risk factors include low body weight (less than 70 kg) and no current use of estrogen therapy.
- Optimal intervals for repeated screening are not established. A minimum of 2 years may be needed to reliably measure a change in BMD.
- Measurement of BMD is considered accurate as a screening method for osteoporosis and the risk for fractures.
- There are no screening recommendations for people with low back pain or arthritis.

Data from US Department of Health and Human Services: *Healthy People 2020,* available at www.healthypeople.gov; US Preventive Services Task Force: *Guide to clinical preventive services*, ed 3, available at www.ahrq.gov.

EXAMINATION

ROUTINE TECHNIQUES

- INSPECT axial skeleton and extremities.
- INSPECT muscles.
- PALPATE bones.
- OBSERVE each major joint and adjacent muscles.
- TEST muscle strength and compare sides.

SPECIAL CIRCUMSTANCES OR ADVANCED PRACTICE

- PERFORM Phalen's test and TEST for Tinel's sign. ★
- PERFORM the drop arm test. ★
- ASSESS for knee effusion. ★
- ASSESS for knee stability. ★
- ASSESS for hip flexion contracture. ★
- ASSESS for nerve root compression.

EQUIPMENT NEEDED

Tape measure • Goniometer

★ Advanced practice.

PROCEDURES AND TECHNIQUES WITH EXPECTED FINDINGS	ABNORMAL FINDINGS

In each specific musculoskeletal region the nurse performs the same skills: inspects the skeleton and muscles; palpates bones, joints, and muscles; observes range of motion; and tests muscle strength.

ROUTINE TECHNIQUES: MUSCULOSKELETAL SYSTEM

CLEAN hands.

INSPECT axial skeleton and extremities for alignment and symmetry.

Observe the patient standing upright and straight from the front, back, and sides (Fig. 14-12, *A* to *C*). He or she should stand erect. The body appears relatively symmetric when one side is compared with the other. The spine should be straight with expected curvatures (cervical concave, thoracic convex, lumbar concave) (see Fig. 14-12, *C*). The knees should be in a straight line between the hips and ankles, and the feet should be flat on the floor and pointing directly forward.

Irregular posture or any asymmetry or misalignment warrants further assessment.

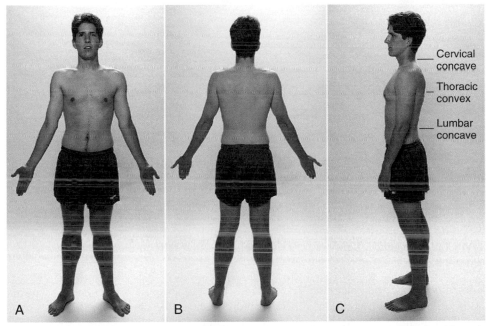

Cervical concave

Thoracic convex

Lumbar concave

A   B   C

FIG. 14-12 Inspection of overall body posture. Note the even contour of the shoulders, level scapulae and iliac crests, alignment of the head over the gluteal folds, and symmetry and alignment of extremities. **A,** Anterior view. **B,** Posterior view. **C,** Lateral view showing normal cervical concave, thoracic convex, and lumbar concave curves of the spine.

| PROCEDURES AND TECHNIQUES WITH EXPECTED FINDINGS | ABNORMAL FINDINGS |

INSPECT muscles for size and symmetry.

Muscle size should appear relatively symmetric bilaterally. (No person has exact side-to-side symmetry.) Muscle circumference can be measured with a cloth or paper tape measure to provide a baseline for future comparisons and make side-to-side comparisons. The dominant side usually is slightly larger than the nondominant side. To ensure consistency of measurement, record the number of centimeters above or below the joint where the muscle was measured or include a diagram such as the one shown in Fig. 14-13. Measurement differences less than 1 cm usually are not significant.

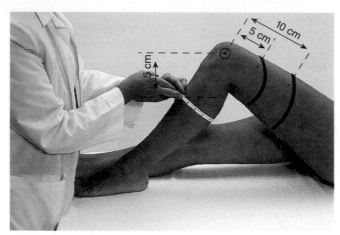

FIG. 14-13 Measurement of the lower leg at 5 cm below the patella and the upper leg at 5 and 10 cm above the patella. Exact location of measurement should be noted for future comparison.

PALPATE bones for tenderness; joints for tenderness, heat, and edema; and muscles for tenderness, heat, edema, and tone.

Procedure: Using the pads of the thumbs and fingers of both hands, palpate both of the patient's shoulders simultaneously. Compare one side with the other. Systematically move distally, palpating the muscles and bones of the arms, elbows, and hands. Use the dorsum of your hands to detect temperature. Use the same technique for palpating the legs from the hips to the toes.

Findings: Bones should be nontender on palpation. No tenderness or edema should be detected on palpation of joints or muscles. The joints and muscles should be the same temperature as the surrounding tissue. Muscles should feel firm, not hard or soft.

OBSERVE range of motion for major joints and adjacent muscles for tenderness on movement, joint stability, and deformity.

Procedure: Ask the patient to perform range of motion actively. Table 14-1 shows range of motion for diarthrodial joints. You may need to demonstrate active range of motion for the patient. When you move the patient's joints passively through the full range of motion, do not force movement of a joint when it is painful or spastic.

ABNORMAL FINDINGS

Atrophy of muscle mass bilaterally may indicate lack of nerve stimulation such as a spinal cord injury or malnutrition. Unilateral muscle atrophy may be from disuse, from pain on movement, or after removal of a cast. Fasciculations (muscle twitching of a single muscle group) may be caused by adverse effects of drugs. Fasciculations are localized, whereas spasms (involuntary muscle contractions) tend to be more generalized.

Tenderness, heat, or edema over bones, joints, or muscles may indicate tumor, inflammation, or trauma. Muscle atrophy may be evident by a decrease in muscle tone.

TABLE 14-1 RANGE OF MOTION FOR DIARTHRODIAL JOINTS

BODY PART	TYPE OF JOINT	TYPE OF MOVEMENT	BODY PART	TYPE OF JOINT	TYPE OF MOVEMENT
Neck and Cervical Spine	Pivotal	Flexion: Bring chin to rest on chest. Extension: Return head to erect position. Hyperextension: Bend head back as far as possible.			Internal rotation: With elbow flexed, rotate shoulder by moving arm until thumb is turned inward and toward back. External rotation: With elbow flexed, move arm until thumb is upward and lateral to head.
		Lateral flexion: Tilt head as far as possible toward each shoulder.			Circumduction: Move arm in full circle. Circumduction is combination of all movements of ball-and-socket joint.
		Rotation: Turn head as far as possible to right and left.			
			Elbow	Hinge	Flexion: Bend elbow so lower arm moves toward its shoulder joint and hand is level with shoulder. Extension: Straighten elbow by lowering hand. Hyperextension: Bend lower arm back as far as possible. Not all elbows hyperextend.
Shoulder	Ball and socket	Flexion: Raise arm from side position forward to position above head. Extension: Return arm to position at side of the body. Hyperextension: Move arm behind body, keeping elbow straight.	**Forearm**	Pivotal	Supination: Turn lower arm and hand so palm is up. Pronation: Turn lower arm so palm is down.
		Abduction: Raise arm to side to position above head with palm away from head. Adduction: Lower arm sideways and across body as far as possible.	**Wrist**	Condyloid	Flexion: Move palm toward inner aspect of the forearm. Extension: Move fingers so fingers, hands, and forearm are in same plane. Hyperextension: Bring dorsal surface to hand back as far as possible.

Continued

TABLE 14-1 RANGE OF MOTION FOR DIARTHRODIAL JOINTS—cont'd

BODY PART	TYPE OF JOINT	TYPE OF MOVEMENT	BODY PART	TYPE OF JOINT	TYPE OF MOVEMENT
		Hyperextension: Bring dorsal surface to hand back as far as possible. Radial flexion: Bend wrist medially toward thumb. Ulnar flexion: Bend wrist laterally toward fifth finger; referred to as radial/ulnar deviation.			Hyperextension: Move leg behind body.
Fingers	Condyloid hinge	Flexion: Make fist. Extension: Straighten fingers. Hyperextension: Bend fingers back as far as possible.			Abduction: Move leg laterally away from body. Adduction: Move leg back toward medial position and beyond if possible.
		Abduction: Spread fingers apart. Adduction: Bring fingers together.			Internal rotation: Turn knee toward the inside. External rotation: Turn knee toward the outside.
Thumb	Saddle	Flexion: Move thumb across palmar surface of hand. Extension: Move thumb straight away from hand. Abduction: Extend thumb laterally (usually done when placing fingers in abduction and adduction).			Circumduction: Move leg in circle.
		Adduction: Move thumb back toward hand. Opposition: Touch thumb to each finger of same hand.	**Knee**	Hinge	Flexion: Bring heel back toward back of thigh. Extension: Return heel to floor.
Hip	Ball and socket	Flexion: Move leg forward and up. Extension: Move leg back beside other leg.			

TABLE 14-1 **RANGE OF MOTION FOR DIARTHRODIAL JOINTS—cont'd**

BODY PART	TYPE OF JOINT	TYPE OF MOVEMENT	BODY PART	TYPE OF JOINT	TYPE OF MOVEMENT
Ankle	Hinge	Dorsiflexion: Move foot so toes are pointed upward. Plantar flexion: Move foot so toes are pointed downward.	**Toes**	Condyloid	Flexion: Curl toes downward. Extension: Straighten toes. Abduction: Spread toes apart. Adduction: Bring toes together.
Foot	Gliding	Inversion: Turn sole of foot medially. Eversion: Turn sole of foot laterally.			

From Potter PA, et al: *Fundamentals of nursing,* ed 7, St Louis, 2009, Mosby.

PROCEDURES AND TECHNIQUES WITH EXPECTED FINDINGS

Findings: There should be full range of motion actively and passively with joint stability but without tenderness, heat, edema, crepitus, deformity, or contracture.

When a joint seems to have increased or decreased range of motion, use a goniometer to measure the angle (Fig. 14-14 and Box 14-1). With the joint in neutral position or fully extended, flex it as far as possible and measure the angles of greatest flexion and extension.

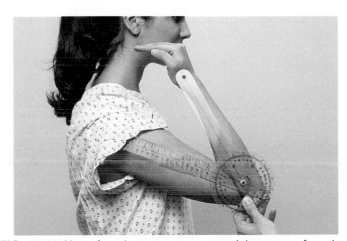

FIG. 14-14 Use of goniometer to measure joint range of motion.

BOX 14-1 **HOW TO USE A GONIOMETER**

A goniometer looks like a protractor with two long arms (see Fig. 14-14). Place the 0 setting of the goniometer over the middle of a joint that is in neutral position. The middle of one arm of the goniometer is aligned with the extremity proximal to that joint, and the other arm is aligned with the middle of the distal joint. Keeping the 0 at the middle of the joint, move the distal joint through its range of motion and notice the degrees of flexion, extension, or hyperextension on the goniometer.

ABNORMAL FINDINGS

Differences found between active and passive range of motion may indicate an actual muscle weakness or a joint disorder (e.g., arthritis or joint effusion). Limited range of motion may indicate inflammation such as arthritis; fluid in the joint; or contracture of muscle, ligament, or capsule. By contrast, increased mobility of a joint may indicate connective tissue disruption, tear of a ligament, or a fracture. *Crepitus* is a crackling sound produced by bone fragments or articular surfaces rubbing together (e.g., osteoarthritis). Crepitus is also heard in chondromalacia patellae, which occurs after knee injury. Joint instability or deformity may indicate a number of disorders, including muscle weakness, fracture, inflammation, strained ligaments, or meniscus tear.

PROCEDURES AND TECHNIQUES WITH EXPECTED FINDINGS	ABNORMAL FINDINGS

TEST muscle strength and compare sides.

Procedure: Testing muscle strength may be performed as part of the musculoskeletal or neurologic system examination. Ask the patient to flex the muscle being evaluated and then to resist when you apply opposing force against it. Screening tests for strength are listed in Table 14-2. Three scales are used to determine the functional level (or "measure") of muscles (i.e., the Lovett scale, grading, and percent of normal), and each requires a subjective assessment of muscle strength. Grading is commonly used. Criteria for grading and recording muscle strength using these scales are described in Table 14-3.

TABLE 14-2 SCREENING TESTS FOR MUSCLE STRENGTH

MUSCLES TESTED	PATIENT ACTIVITY	NURSE ACTIVITY
Ocular musculature		
Lids	Close eyes tightly.	Attempt to resist closure.
Eye muscles	Track object in six cardinal positions.	
Facial musculature	Blow out cheeks.	Assess pressure in cheeks with fingertips.
	Place tongue in cheek.	Assess pressure in cheek with fingertips.
	Stick out tongue; move it to right and left.	Observe strength and coordination of thrust and extension.
Neck muscles	Extend head backward.	Push head forward.
	Flex head forward.	Push head backward.
	Rotate head from side to side.	Observe mobility and coordination.
	Touch shoulders with head.	Observe range of motion.
Deltoid	Hold arms upward.	Push down on arms.
Biceps	Flex arm.	Pull to extend arm.
Triceps	Extend arm.	Push to flex arm.
Wrist musculature	Extend elbow.	Push to flex.
	Flex elbow.	Push to extend.
Finger muscles	Extend fingers.	Push dorsal surface of fingers.
	Flex fingers.	Push ventral surface of fingers.
	Spread fingers.	Hold fingers together.
Hip musculature	In supine position raise extended leg.	Push down on leg above knee.
Hamstring, gluteal, abductor, and adductor muscles of leg	Sit and perform alternate leg crossing.	Push in opposite direction of crossing limb.
Quadriceps	Extend leg.	Push to flex leg.
Hamstring	Bend knees to flex leg.	Push to extend leg.
Ankle and foot muscles	Bend foot up (dorsiflexion).	Push to plantar flexion.
	Bend foot down (plantar flexion).	Push to dorsiflexion.
Antigravity muscles	Walk on toes.	
	Walk on heels.	

From Barkauskas VH et al: *Health and physical assessment,* ed 2, St Louis, 2002, Mosby.

TABLE 14-3 CRITERIA FOR GRADING AND RECORDING MUSCLE STRENGTH

FUNCTIONAL LEVEL	LOVETT SCALE	GRADE	PERCENT OF NORMAL
No evidence of contractility	Zero (0)	0	0
Evidence of slight contractility	Trace (T)	1	10
Complete range of motion with gravity eliminated	Poor (P)	2	25
Complete range of motion with gravity	Fair (F)	3	50
Complete range of motion against gravity with some resistance	Good (G)	4	75
Complete range of motion against gravity with full resistance	Normal (N)	5	100

From Barkauskas VH et al: *Health and physical assessment,* ed 2, St Louis, 2002, Mosby.

| **PROCEDURES AND TECHNIQUES WITH EXPECTED FINDINGS** | **ABNORMAL FINDINGS** |

Findings: Expect muscle strength to be 5, bilaterally symmetric, with full resistance to opposition. The patient's muscle strength is documented as 5/5 (or normal on the Lovett scale), with the patient's value in the numerator and the expected value in the denominator.

Muscle weakness may indicate a muscular or joint disease or atrophy from disuse. A muscle strength of 1/5 means that the patient has slight muscle contraction, with 1 representing the patient's value and 5 representing the expected value.

EXAMINATION OF SPECIFIC MUSCULOSKELETAL REGIONS

OBSERVE gait for conformity, symmetry, and rhythm.

Ask the patient to walk across the room and back. Expected findings are conformity (ability to follow gait sequencing of both stance and swing); regular smooth rhythm; symmetry in length of leg swing; smooth swaying; and smooth, symmetric arm swing.

An unstable or exaggerated gait, limp, irregular stride length, arm swing that is unrelated to gait, or any other inability to maintain straight posture or asymmetry of body parts requires further assessment. When unequal leg length is suspected, measure the leg from the anterior superior iliac spine to the medial malleolus (Fig. 14-15). See Fig. 14-3 for location of the anterior superior iliac spine. The medial malleolus is a rounded bony process on the inside of the ankle bone.

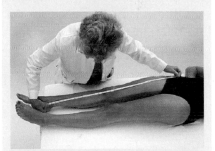

FIG. 14-15 Measure limb length from the anterior superior iliac spine to the medial malleolus.

INSPECT musculature of the face and neck for symmetry.

Patient is in a sitting position. Inspection of the patient's facial symmetry began during the interview. Ask patient to open and close his or her mouth and smile. Muscles of the face should appear symmetric without any facial expressions and during facial expressions. Muscles of the neck should be symmetric.

Asymmetric facial or neck musculature may indicate previous or current facial fractures or previous facial surgery. Facial asymmetry occurs with Bell's palsy (facial cranial nerve palsy) or after cerebrovascular accidents in certain areas of the brain.

PALPATE each temporomandibular joint for movement, sounds, and tenderness.

Use the pads of the first two fingers in front of the tragus of each ear to palpate the temporomandibular joint (TMJ) with the mouth closed and open. The mandible should move smoothly and painlessly. An audible or palpable snapping or clicking in the absence of other symptoms is not unusual (Fig. 14-16, *A*).

Pain or crepitus of the TMJ with locking or popping may indicate a TMJ disorder.

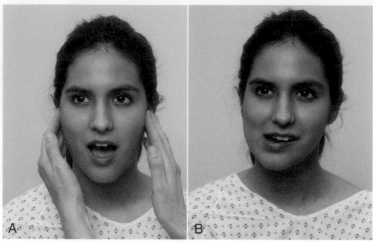

FIG. 14-16 A, Palpation of temporomandibular joint. **B,** Lateral range of motion in the temporomandibular joint.

PROCEDURES AND TECHNIQUES WITH EXPECTED FINDINGS	ABNORMAL FINDINGS

OBSERVE jaw for range of motion.

Ask the patient to open and close the mouth. It should open between 3 and 6 cm between upper and lower teeth. Ask the patient to move the jaw side to side; the mandible should move 1 to 2 cm in each direction (see Fig. 14-16, *B*). Motion should be smooth and without pain. Finally the patient should be able to protrude and retract the chin without difficulty or pain.

> Difficulty opening the mouth or limited range of motion may result from injury or arthritic changes. Pain in the TMJ may indicate malocclusion of teeth or arthritic changes.

PALPATE the neck for pain.

Use the pads of thumbs and fingers to palpate the neck muscles and lymph nodes. The neck is soft and firm, without masses, pain, or spasms.

> Pain on palpation may indicate inflammation of the muscle (myositis). Masses may be enlarged lymph nodes, indicating inflammation or neoplasm. Neck spasm may indicate nerve compression or stress.

OBSERVE the neck for range of motion.

Ask the patient to flex the chin to the chest. It should move to a point 45 degrees from midline. Ask him or her to hyperextend the head if possible; it should reach 55 degrees from midline (Fig. 14-17, *A*). Have the patient laterally bend his or her head to the right and the left. Range should be 40 degrees from midline in each direction (see Fig. 14-17, *B*). Have the patient rotate the chin to the shoulders, first to the right and then to the left. It should reach 70 degrees from midline (see Fig. 14-17, *C*).

> Range of motion may be impaired by pain or muscle spasms. Hyperextension and flexion may be limited because of cervical vertebral disk herniation, degeneration, or osteoarthritic changes. Pain, numbness, or tingling reported during range of motion may indicate compression of cervical spinal root nerves.

TEST the neck muscles for strength.

Ask the patient to rotate the head against resistance of your hand to test strength of the sternocleidomastoid muscles (Fig. 14-18, *A*). (See Fig. 14-4 for location of sternocleidomastoid muscles.) The patient should be able to rotate the neck to withstand your resistance.

> If you can prevent the patient's muscular rotation before the anticipated point, the patient has muscle weakness.

Ask the patient to flex the chin to the chest and maintain the position while you palpate the sternocleidomastoid muscles and try to manually force the head upright (Fig. 14-18, *B*). The sternocleidomastoid muscle should contract, and the patient should be able to flex the neck to withstand your resistance.

> If you can prevent the patient's muscular flexion before the anticipated point, the patient has muscle weakness.

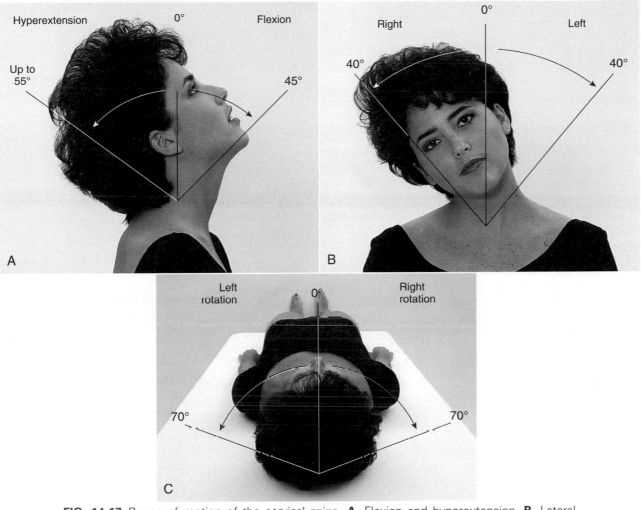

FIG. 14-17 Range of motion of the cervical spine. **A,** Flexion and hyperextension. **B,** Lateral bending. **C,** Rotation.

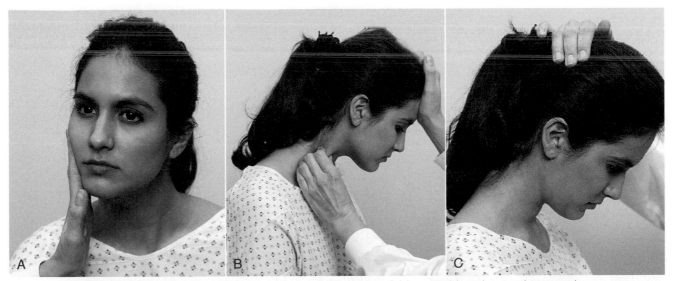

FIG. 14-18 Examination of the strength of the sternocleidomastoid and trapezius muscles. **A,** Rotation against resistance. **B,** Flexion with palpation of the sternocleidomastoid muscle. **C,** Extension against resistance.

PROCEDURES AND TECHNIQUES WITH EXPECTED FINDINGS

Have the patient extend the head and maintain position while you try to manually force the head upright to assess the trapezius muscle strength (Fig. 14-18, *C*). (See Fig. 14-4 for location of trapezius muscles.) The patient should be able to extend the head to withstand your resistance.

If you can prevent the patient's muscular extension before the anticipated point, the patient has muscle weakness.

INSPECT the shoulders and cervical, thoracic, and lumbar spine for alignment and symmetry.

Procedure: Ask the patient to stand; while you stand to his or her side, observe the cervical concave, the thoracic convex, and the lumbar concave (see Fig. 14-12, *C*; Fig. 14-20, *A*). Note the landmarks on the back: spinous processes protruding slightly at C7 and T1, paravertebral muscles, and the alignment across the iliac crests at L4 and the posterior superior iliac spine at S2 (Fig. 14-19). Ask the patient to touch the toes. Move behind the patient to inspect the spine.

Findings: Expected concave and convex curves should be present. Vertebrae should be aligned, indicating a straight spine. Shoulders should be level or at equal heights, indicating symmetry.

Deviation of the spine or asymmetry of shoulder or iliac height is an abnormal finding. *Kyphosis* is a posterior curvature (convexity) of the thoracic spine (see Fig. 14-20, *B*), *lordosis* is an anterior curvature (concavity) of the spine (see Fig. 14-20, *C*), and *scoliosis* is a lateral curvature of the spine (see Fig. 14-20, *E* and *F*). Curvature of the spine may create asymmetry of the shoulders.

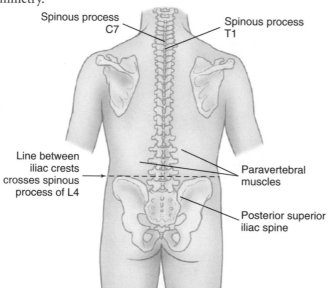

FIG.14-19 Landmarks of the back. (From Seidel et al., 2011.)

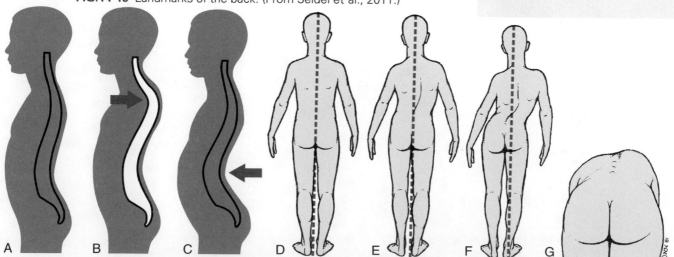

FIG. 14-20 Defects of the spinal column. **A,** Normal spine. **B,** Kyphosis. **C,** Lordosis. **D,** Normal spine in balance. **E,** Mild scoliosis. **F,** Severe scoliosis, not in balance. **G,** Rib hump and flank asymmetry seen in flexion. (Modified from Hilt and Schmitt, 1975. In Hockenberry et al., 2011.)

PROCEDURES AND TECHNIQUES WITH EXPECTED FINDINGS	ABNORMAL FINDINGS

OBSERVE range of motion of the thoracic and lumbar spine.

Ask the patient to bend forward and touch the toes. The patient should be able to reach 75 degrees of flexion while touching his or her toes (Fig. 14-21, *A*). Document how close the patient gets to the floor by measuring from fingertips to the floor (e.g., 6 inches [15 cm] from the floor). Some patients are unable to touch the floor because of tight hamstrings and leg muscles or obesity. These are considered expected variations.

Observe for range of motion as the patient hyperextends the spine; it should reach 30 degrees back from the neutral position (extension) (see Fig. 14-21, *B*).

Ask the patient to bend laterally right and left. (NOTE: You may need to stabilize the patient's hips.) He or she should be able to reach 35 degrees of flexion both ways from midline (see Fig. 14-21, *C*).

Have the patient rotate the upper trunk (you may need to stabilize the pelvis) to the right and left; he or she should achieve 30 degrees of rotation in both directions from a directly forward position (see Fig. 14-21, *D*).

PALPATE the posterior neck, spinal processes, and paravertebral muscles for alignment and tenderness.

Stand behind the patient. Use the pads of the thumbs and fingers for palpation. The posterior neck and spine should be straight and nontender. (NOTE: Having the patient hunch his or her shoulders forward and slightly flex the neck may help your palpation [Fig. 14-22].)

PERCUSS the spinal processes for tenderness.

First tap each process with one finger and then lightly tap each side of the spine with the ulnar surface of your fist. No muscle spasm or tenderness should be noted on palpation or percussion.

ABNORMAL FINDINGS

Flexion less than 75 degrees with pain or muscle spasm is abnormal.

Impaired range of motion during hyperextension or lateral flexion may be caused by pain from muscle strain or spasms or a herniated vertebral disk.

Impaired range of motion during rotation may be caused by pain from muscle strain or spasms.

Misalignment may be caused by muscle weakness. Tenderness may be caused by inflammation such as myositis or herniated vertebral disk.

Tenderness may be caused by inflammation such as myositis or herniated vertebral disk. Muscle spasm may be caused by muscle strain.

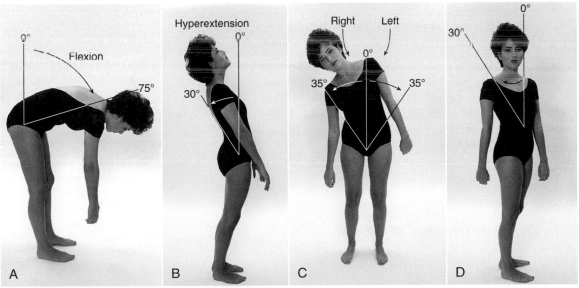

FIG. 14-21 Range of motion of the thoracic and lumbar spine. **A,** Flexion. **B,** Hyperextension. **C,** Lateral bending. **D,** Rotation of the upper trunk.

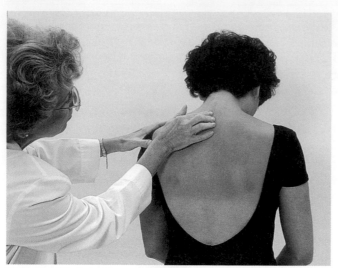

FIG. **14-22** Palpation of the spinal processes of the vertebrae.

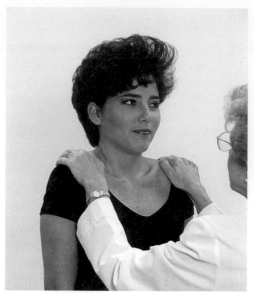

FIG. **14-23** Test strength of the trapezius muscle with the shrugged shoulder movement.

PROCEDURES AND TECHNIQUES WITH EXPECTED FINDINGS

ABNORMAL FINDINGS

INSPECT the shoulders and shoulder girdle for equality of height, symmetry, and contour.

Procedure: Facing the patient, who is in a seated position, inspect scapulae, clavicles, and the acromioclavicular junctions for equality of height and symmetry. (See Fig. 14-7 for review of location of the acromioclavicular joint.) Observe the trapezius muscles for symmetry.

Findings: All structures should be smooth and bilaterally symmetric. Right and left shoulders should be level, rounded, and firm, with smooth contour and no bony prominences. Each shoulder should be equidistant from the vertebral column.

Shoulder joints may have some deformity from trauma, arthritic changes, or scoliosis.

PALPATE the shoulders for firmness, fullness, tenderness, symmetry, and masses.

Use the pads of the thumbs and fingers to palpate the acromioclavicular joint; humerus; and trapezius, biceps, triceps, and deltoid muscles. Compare one side to the other side. These areas should be nontender, smooth, firm and full without masses, and bilaterally symmetric. The muscles of the dominant arm may be slightly larger.

Tenderness may be caused by inflammation of the muscles, overwork of unconditioned muscles, or sports injuries.

TEST the trapezius muscles for strength.

Ask the patient to shrug the shoulders while you attempt to push them down (Fig. 14-23). This also tests function of cranial nerve XI (CN XI; spinal accessory).

Weakness of the trapezius muscles may indicate compressed spinal nerve root or compression of spinal accessory CN XI.

OBSERVE the shoulders for range of motion.

Extension and Hyperextension

Ask the patient to extend the arms straight up beside the ears. The arms should reach 180 degrees from resting neutral position, be bilaterally equal, and cause no discomfort (Fig. 14-24, *A*). Ask the patient to hyperextend the arms backward. They should reach 50 degrees, be bilaterally equal, and cause no discomfort.

Limited range of motion, pain with movement, crepitation, and asymmetry are abnormal findings. Degenerative joint changes or sports injuries may impair range of motion.

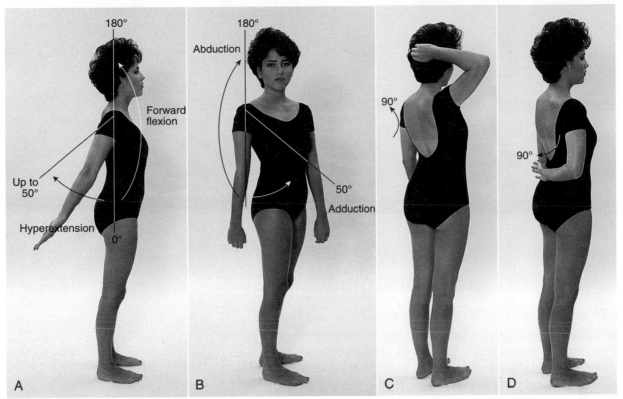

FIG. 14-24 Range of motion of the shoulders. **A,** Forward flexion and hyperextension. **B,** Abduction and adduction. **C,** External rotation and abduction. **D,** Internal rotation and adduction.

PROCEDURES AND TECHNIQUES WITH EXPECTED FINDINGS

Abduction and Adduction

Ask the patient to lift both arms laterally over his or her head. Expected shoulder abduction is 180 degrees. Then ask the patient to swing each arm across the front of the body. Expected adduction is 50 degrees (see Fig. 14-24, *B*).

External Rotation

To test external rotation, have the patient place the hands behind the head with elbows out. A range of 90 degrees is expected; movement should be bilaterally equal and without discomfort (see Fig. 14-24, *C*).

Internal Rotation

To test internal rotation, ask the patient to place the hands at the small of the back. Range should be 90 degrees, with movements bilaterally equal and without discomfort (see Fig. 14-24, *D*).

TEST the arms for muscle strength.

Have the patient hold the arms up while you try to push them down. Remember to compare one side with the other. They should be strong bilaterally, preventing you from moving them out of position. Use criteria in Table 14-3 for grading.

To test triceps muscle strength, ask the patient to extend the arm while you resist by pushing it to a flexed position (Fig. 14-25, *A*). Expected muscle strength is recorded as 5/5 (see Table 14-3).

To test biceps strength, have the patient try to flex the arm while you try to extend his or her forearm. You should be unable to move the arm out of position, and strength should be equal bilaterally, documented as 5/5 (see Fig. 14-25, *B*).

ABNORMAL FINDINGS

Abnormal findings include unequal response, weak response, muscular spasm, and pain. These findings may be caused by joint or muscle inflammation, trauma, or sports injuries.

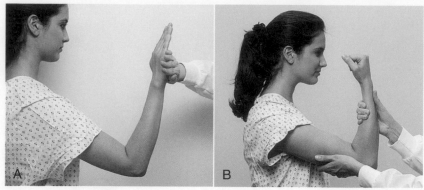

FIG. 14-25 Testing muscle strength of arms. **A,** Testing triceps muscle strength. **B,** Testing biceps muscle strength.

PROCEDURES AND TECHNIQUES WITH EXPECTED FINDINGS	ABNORMAL FINDINGS

PALPATE the elbows for tenderness, edema, and nodules.

Hold the patient's lower arm in your nondominant hand while using the pads of the thumb and fingers of the dominant hand to palpate the olecranon process and lateral epicondyle (Fig. 14-26). Repeat the procedure on the other side. The elbows should be smooth, without discomfort, edema, or nodules.

Abnormal findings include edema, subcutaneous nodules, point tenderness, and palpable nodes. Subcutaneous nodules at pressure points of the ulnar surface may indicate rheumatoid arthritis.

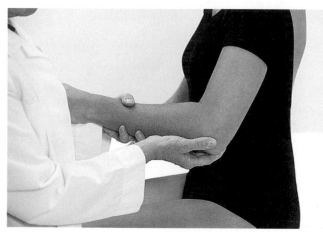

FIG. 14-26 Palpation of the olecranon process grooves.

OBSERVE the elbows for range of motion.

Ask the patient to flex and extend the elbow; 160 degrees of full movement should be present bilaterally without discomfort (Fig. 14-27, *A*). Assess pronation and supination of the elbow by having the patient rotate the hands palms up and palms down (pronate and supinate); 90 degrees should be achieved in each direction, and the movements should be bilaterally equal and without discomfort (see Fig. 14-27, *B*). The patient should demonstrate pronation and supination while keeping the lower arm flexed 90 degrees at the elbow.

Note any limitation of motion, asymmetry of movement, or pain at the elbow. Subcutaneous nodules just inferior to the olecranon process (elbow joint) may indicate rheumatoid arthritis. Tenderness or pain with pronation and supination of the elbow and point tenderness on the lateral epicondyle may indicate lateral tendonitis or epicondylitis (tennis elbow), whereas point tenderness on the medial epicondyle may indicate medial tendonitis (golfer's elbow).

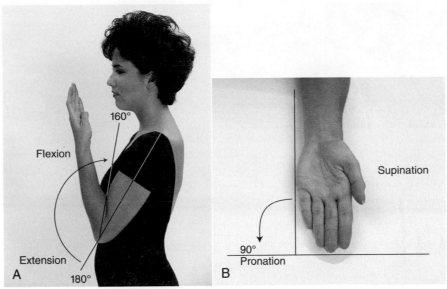

FIG. 14-27 Range of motion of the elbow. **A,** Flexion and extension. **B,** Palm up, supination; palm down, pronation.

PROCEDURES AND TECHNIQUES WITH EXPECTED FINDINGS

INSPECT the joints of the wrists and hands for symmetry, number of digits, and alignment.

Compare the right wrist and hand with the left. They should be symmetric, with no edema or deformities. The hand with five digits is aligned with the wrist, and fingers are aligned with wrist and forearm (Fig. 14-28, *A* and *B*).

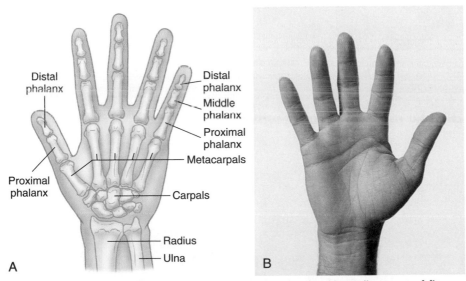

FIG. 14-28 A, Bony structures of the right hand and wrist. Note alignment of fingers with the radius. **B,** Palmar aspect of right hand. (**A** from Seidel et al., 2011.)

ABNORMAL FINDINGS

Missing fingers are recorded. Osteo arthritis may cause Bouchard's nodes in the proximal interphalangeal (PIP) joints, whereas Heberden's nodes form in the distal interphalangeal (DIP) joints (Fig. 14-29). Swan-neck and boutonniere deformities of inter-phalangeal joints may be related to rheumatoid arthritis (Fig. 14-30).

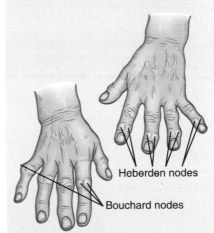

FIG. 14-29 Osteoarthritis. (From Huether and McCance, 2008.)

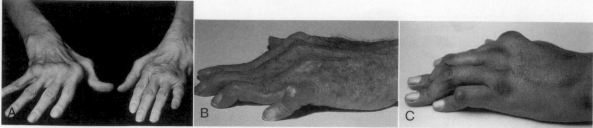

FIG. 14-30 **A,** Ulnar deviation and subluxation of metacarpophalangeal joints. **B,** Swan-neck deformity. **C,** Boutonniere deformity. (**A** and **B** reprinted from the Clinical slide collection of the rheumatic diseases, copyright 1991, 1995, 1997. Used with permission of the American College of Rheumatology. **C** from Seidel et al., 2011.)

PROCEDURES AND TECHNIQUES WITH EXPECTED FINDINGS	ABNORMAL FINDINGS

PALPATE each joint of the hand and wrist for surface characteristics and tenderness.

Palpate the interphalangeal joints with your thumb and index finger. Palpate the metacarpophalangeal joints with both thumbs. Palpate the wrist and radiocarpal groove with your thumbs on the dorsal surface and your fingers on the palmar surface. (See Fig. 14-5 for a review of the hand anatomy.) Joint surfaces should be smooth, without nodules, edema, or tenderness (Fig. 14-31).

Painful, edematous DIP or PIP joints are found in osteoarthritis. A firm mass over the dorsum of the wrist may be a ganglion. Rheumatoid arthritis may cause wrists and PIP joints to appear hot, tender, painful, deformed, and edematous.

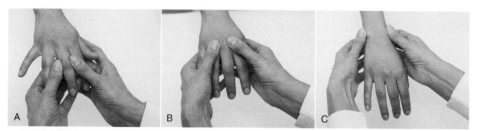

FIG. 14-31 Palpation of joints of the hand and wrist. **A,** Interphalangeal joints. **B,** Metacarpophalangeal joints. **C,** Radiocarpal groove.

TEST for muscle strength and OBSERVE for range of motion of wrists and fingers.

TEST muscle strength.

First ask the patient to extend and spread the fingers (both hands) while you attempt to push them together (Fig. 14-32, *A*). The response should be symmetric, to full flexion and extension, without discomfort and with sufficient muscle strength to overcome the resistance you apply.

Weak muscle strength and impaired range of motion may accompany rheumatoid arthritis and osteoarthritis. Fractures of metatarsals or phalanges may weaken the muscle strength.

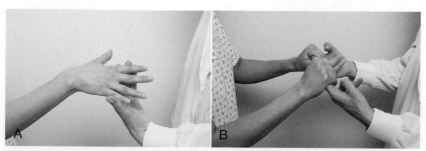

FIG. 14-32 **A,** Assessment of finger strength. **B,** Assessment of grip strength.

PROCEDURES AND TECHNIQUES WITH EXPECTED FINDINGS

Next have the patient grip your first two fingers on each hand. The response should be bilaterally equal, and the grip tight and full flexion (see Fig. 14-32, *B*). Some nurses cross their hands for the patient to grip the fingers so the patient's right hand is gripping the nurse's right hand. This maneuver helps the nurse remember on which side the patient may have deficits.

OBSERVE range of motion.

Procedure: Observe the range of motion of wrists and hands. Ask the patient to:
- Bend the hand up at the wrist (hyperextension to 70 degrees) and down at the wrist (palmar flexion of 90 degrees) (Fig. 14-33, *A*).
- Flex the fingers up and down at the metacarpophalangeal joints (flexion of 90 degrees, hyperextension of 30 degrees) (see Fig. 14-33, *B*).
- Place palms flat on the table and turn them outward and inward (ulnar deviation of 50 to 60 degrees, radial deviation of 20 degrees) (see Fig. 14-33, *C*); spread the fingers apart (see Fig. 14-33, *D*).
- Make a fist (abduction of 20 degrees, fist tight) (see Fig. 14-33, *E*).
- Touch the thumb to each finger (opposition) and to the base of the fifth finger (able to perform all motions) (see Fig. 14-33, *F*).

Findings: Wrists should have flexion, hyperextension, and ulnar and radial deviation. Fingers should have abduction, flexion, extension, and opposition as described above.

ABNORMAL FINDINGS

Abnormal findings include unequal response, weak response, muscular spasm, and pain. The findings may be caused by joint or muscle inflammation.

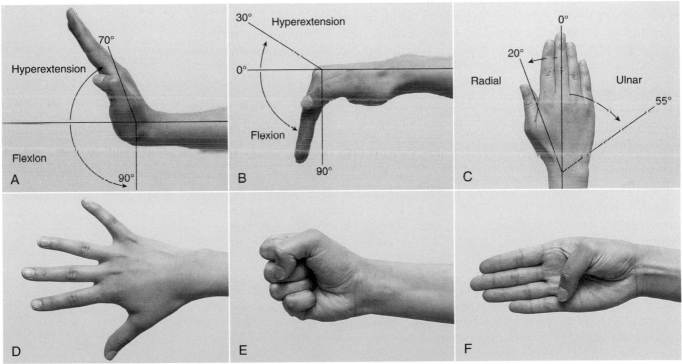

FIG. 14-33 Range of motion of hand and wrist. **A,** Wrist flexion and hyperextension. **B,** Metacarpophalangeal flexion and hyperextension. **C,** Wrist radial and ulnar deviation. **D,** Finger abduction. **E,** Finger flexion: fist formation. **F,** Finger extension: thumb to each fingertip and to base of little finger.

PROCEDURES AND TECHNIQUES WITH EXPECTED FINDINGS	ABNORMAL FINDINGS

INSPECT the hips for symmetry.

Ask the patient to stand. Look at the symmetry of the hips anteriorly and posteriorly. The hips should be the same height and symmetric. You may need to move the patient's clothing aside to visualize the hips.

Asymmetric hips may occur from curvature of the spine.

PALPATE the hips for stability and tenderness.

Assist the patient to a supine position. Use the iliac crests and greater trochanter of the femur as landmarks (see Fig. 14-19). Palpate iliac crests to determine if they are symmetric. Findings should be bilaterally symmetric hips that are stable and painless.

Osteoarthritis or hip dislocation may cause pain and hip instability.

OBSERVE the hips for range of motion.

Hip Flexion with Knee Flexed

Ask the patient to alternately pull each knee up to the chest. The patient should achieve 120-degree flexion from the straight, extended position (Fig. 14-34, *A*).

Osteoarthritis and hip dislocation impair hip range of motion. Vertebral compression of spinal nerves may cause back or leg pain during hip flexion with leg extension.

Hip Flexion with Leg Extended

Next have the patient raise the leg to flex the hip as far as possible without bending the knee. Repeat the procedure with the other leg. Results should be 90 degrees from the straight extended position (see Fig. 14-34, *B*).

External Rotation

To test external hip rotation (Patrick text), ask the patient to place the heel of one foot on the opposite patella. Apply gentle pressure to the medial aspect of the flexed knee as the patient externally rotates the hip until the knee or lateral thigh touches the examination table. Repeat the procedure with the other hip. Rotation should reach 45 degrees from the straight midline position (see Fig. 14-34, *C*).

Internal Rotation

Ask the patient to flex the knee and turn medially (inward) as you pull the heel laterally (outward). Repeat the procedure with the other hip. Rotation should reach 40 degrees from the straight midline position (see Fig. 14-34, *D*).

Abduction and Adduction

Ask the patient to move one leg laterally with the knee straight to test abduction and medially to test adduction. Repeat the procedure with the other leg. The expected range for abduction is up to 45 degrees; the expected range for adduction is up to 30 degrees (see Fig. 14-34, *E*).

Hyperextension

Assist the patient to a prone position. Test hyperextension of the hip by raising the leg upward with the knee straight. Repeat the procedure with the other leg. This assessment can also be performed with the patient in the standing position.
The expected range of movement is up to 30 degrees (see Fig. 14-34, *F*).

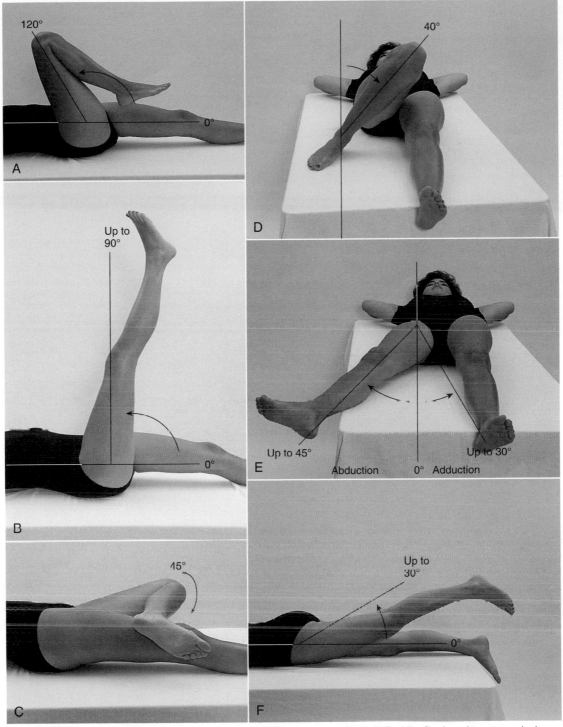

FIG. 14-34 Range of motion of hips. **A,** Hip flexion, knee flexed. **B,** Hip flexion, leg extended. **C,** External rotation of hip. **D,** Internal rotation of hip. **E,** Abduction and adduction of hip. **F,** Hyperextension of hip, leg extended.

PROCEDURES AND TECHNIQUES WITH EXPECTED FINDINGS

TEST the hips for muscle strength.

Assist the patient to a supine position. Ask him or her to attempt to raise the legs while you try to hold them down. Evaluate one leg at a time, noting if the response is bilaterally strong and if you are unable to interfere with the movement. Use the criteria from Table 14-3 for grading muscle strength. It should be 5/5 or normal bilaterally.

Abnormal findings include unequal response, weak response, muscular spasm, and pain. These findings may be caused by joint or muscle inflammation, trauma, or sports injuries.

TEST the leg muscles for strength.

Procedure: To test the quadriceps with the patient sitting, have the patient extend the legs at the knee while you attempt to flex the knee. To evaluate the hamstrings with the patient sitting, have the patient attempt to bend his or her knee while you attempt to straighten it.

Findings: For quadriceps and hamstring, strength should be bilaterally equal, and you should be unable to flex the knee (Fig. 14-35). Use criteria from Table 14-3 for grading muscle strength. It should be 5/5 or normal bilaterally.

Abnormal findings include unequal response, weak response, muscular spasm, and pain. These findings may be caused by joint or muscle inflammation, trauma, or sports injuries.

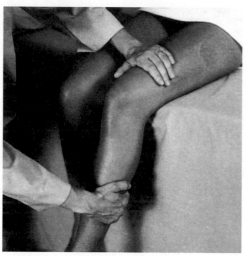

FIG. 14-35 Assessment of hamstring muscle strength. Patient flexes knee while examiner tries to straighten it. (From Barkauskas et al., 2002.)

INSPECT the knees for symmetry and alignment.

The knees should be lined up with the tibia and ankle and symmetric without medial or lateral deviation.

Knees that appear edematous and warm, bowlegged (genu varum), knock-kneed (genu valgum), thick, boggy (spongy), or inflamed are abnormal findings.

PROCEDURES AND TECHNIQUES WITH EXPECTED FINDINGS	**ABNORMAL FINDINGS**

PALPATE the knees for contour, tenderness, and edema.

First palpate the suprapatellar pouch on each side of the quadriceps with the thumb and fingers of one or both hands. Compare one side with the other. The knees should feel smooth, nonedematous, and nontender.

Next, with the knee flexed to 90 degrees, palpate over the medial and lateral aspects of the tibiofemoral joint space. These areas should be nonedematous and nontender. Palpate the popliteal space for contour, tenderness, and edema. It should be smooth and nontender and nonedematous.

Abnormal findings include bogginess, thickening, tenderness, or pain that may occur from rheumatoid arthritis, osteoarthritis, or bursitis. Edema of the suprapatellar pouch may indicate synovitis.

OBSERVE the knees for range of motion.

Evaluate the range of motion by having the patient flex the knees (Fig. 14-36). Flexion should reach 130 degrees from the straight extended position without discomfort or difficulty. If the knee is able to hyperextend, it should reach 15 degrees from the extended position (midline).

A decrease in the range of motion may occur as a result of arthritis, trauma, or ligament, tendon, or meniscus injury.

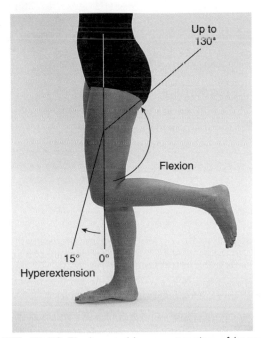

FIG. 14-36 Flexion and hyperextension of knee.

PROCEDURES AND TECHNIQUES WITH EXPECTED FINDINGS	ABNORMAL FINDINGS

INSPECT the ankles and feet for contour, alignment, and number of toes.

The ankles should be smooth, with no deformity. The feet are in straight position aligned with the long axis of the lower leg with five toes that are extended and straight on each foot.

Abnormal findings include misalignment of the feet with the ankle or leg or amputation or deformity of toes. Medial deviation of the toes, hallux valgus (Fig. 14-37), claw toes, hammer toes, and calluses are abnormal findings as well.

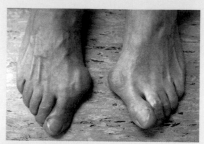

FIG. 14-37 Hallux valgus. (From Jachmann-Jahn, 2009.)

PALPATE the ankles and feet for contour, edema, and tenderness.

Use the pads of the thumbs and fingers to palpate the ankle, heel, and joints; use both hands to palpate one foot at a time. These structures should be smooth, nonedematous, and nontender.

Abnormal findings include tenderness (diffuse versus pinpoint), inflammation, ulcerations, and nodules. Localized pain in one heel may indicate a bone spur. Pain in both feet that is worse on arising may indicate plantar fasciitis.

OBSERVE the ankles and feet for range of motion.

To evaluate the range of motion of both feet and ankles, ask the patient to:

- Dorsiflex the ankle by pointing the toes toward the face. Dorsiflexion should reach 20 degrees from midline.
- Plantar flex the ankle by pointing the toes toward the floor. Plantar flexion should reach 45 degrees from midline (Fig. 14-38, *A*).
- Evert the foot by rotating it inward so the little toe is not touching the floor. (NOTE: You may need to stabilize the heel during these maneuvers.) Eversion should be 20 degrees.
- Invert the foot by rotating it outward so the great toe is not touching the floor. Inversion should be 30 degrees from midline position (see Fig. 14-38, *B*).
- Abduct the foot by turning it away from midline. Expected abduction is 10 degrees.
- Adduct the foot by turning it inward toward midline. Expected adduction is 20 degrees (see Fig. 14-38, *C*).
- Flex and extend the toes. These should be active movements.

All movements should be bilaterally equal and performed without discomfort.

Limitations in range of motion, pain, crepitation, and asymmetry are abnormal findings. Tightening or trauma to the Achilles tendon may cause plantar flexion.

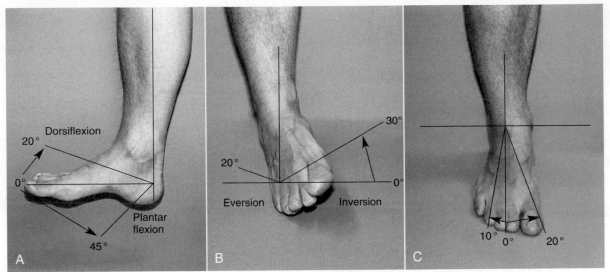

FIG. 14-38 Range of motion of the ankle. **A,** Dorsiflexion and plantar flexion. **B,** Inversion and eversion. **C,** Abduction and adduction. (From Seidel et al., 2011.)

PROCEDURES AND TECHNIQUES WITH EXPECTED FINDINGS

TEST the ankle and feet muscles for strength.

Ask the patient to walk on his or her toes, then heels, followed by walking on the inside of the feet (eversion) and finally walking on the outside of the feet (inversion).

SPECIAL CIRCUMSTANCES OR ADVANCED PRACTICE: MUSCULOSKELETAL SYSTEM

★ ASSESS for carpal tunnel syndrome.

The test for *Phalen's sign* is performed by asking the patient to flex both wrists and press the dorsum of the hands against each other for 1 minute (Fig. 14-39). No report of numbness, tingling, or pain is a negative test.

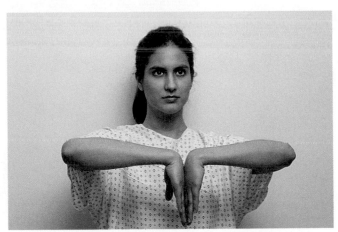

FIG. 14-39 Phalen's test for carpal tunnel syndrome.

ABNORMAL FINDINGS

Abnormal findings include unequal response, weak response, muscular spasm, and pain. These findings may be caused by joint or muscle inflammation, trauma, or sports injuries.

A positive Phalen's sign occurs if the patient complains of numbness, pain, or paresthesia over the palmar surface of the hand and the first three fingers and part of the fourth. This positive finding may indicate carpal tunnel syndrome.

★ Advanced practice

PROCEDURES AND TECHNIQUES WITH EXPECTED FINDINGS

The test for *Tinel's sign* is performed by tapping on the median nerve where it passes through the carpal tunnel under the flexor retinaculum (carpal ligament) and volar carpal ligament. No report of tingling sensation is a negative Tinel's sign (Fig. 14-40).

★ ASSESS for rotator cuff damage.

Rotator cuff damage can be determined with the drop arm test. Abduct the patient's affected arm and ask the patient to lower the arm slowly. The expected response is a slow, controlled adduction of the arm.

★ ASSESS for knee effusion.

Two tests evaluate the presence of fluid in the knee joint. The *bulge sign* tests for small effusions of the knee. Assist the patient to a supine position. Elicit the bulge sign by extending the knee and milking the medial aspect upward two or three times. Then tap on the lateral side of the patella. No fluid waves or bulging should be seen on the opposite side of the joint (Fig. 14-41, *A* and *B*).

ABNORMAL FINDINGS

A positive Tinel's sign occurs when the patient reports a tingling sensation or pain radiating from the wrist to the hand along the median nerve. This positive finding may indicate carpal tunnel syndrome.

Inability to lower the arm slowly and smoothly or severe shoulder pain while adducting the arm may indicate rotator cuff damage.

If fluid is present, fluid waves are palpable on the opposite side of the joint. Fluid in a joint (effusion) is an accumulation of serous exudate as part of an inflammatory process such as osteoarthritis.

★ Advanced practice

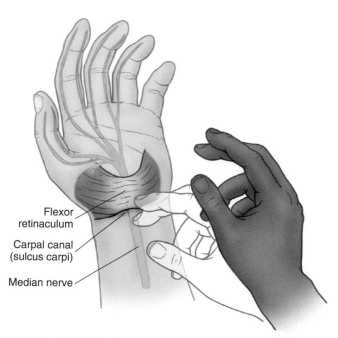

Flexor retinaculum

Carpal canal (sulcus carpi)

Median nerve

FIG. 14-40 Tinel's sign for carpal tunnel syndrome. (From Seidel et al., 2011.)

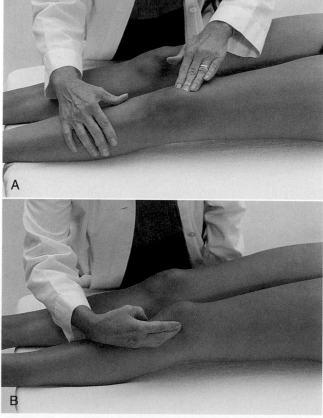

FIG. 14-41 Bulge sign to detect small effusion in knee joint. **A,** Milk the medial aspect of the knee two or three times. **B,** Tap the lateral side of the patella.

PROCEDURES AND TECHNIQUES WITH EXPECTED FINDINGS	ABNORMAL FINDINGS

The second test, *ballottement,* is used for larger effusions. With the knee extended, apply downward pressure on the suprapatellar pouch with the thumb and fingers of one hand, and with the other hand push the patella firmly against the femur. Release the pressure from the patella, but leave your fingers in contact with the knee to detect any fluid wave (Fig. 14-42).

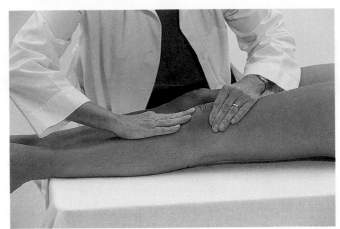

FIG. 14-42 Ballottement procedure to detect large effusion in knee joint.

★ ASSESS for knee stability.

With the patient in supine position, assess knee stability provided by *collateral and cruciate ligaments* (see Fig. 14-2).

Collateral and Cruciate Ligaments

Procedure: Assess the lateral collateral ligament by placing one hand against the medial aspect of the knee joint to keep it from moving and using your other hand to grasp the ankle. Adduct the lower leg (Fig. 14-43, *A*). To test the medial collateral ligament, place your hand on the lateral aspect of the knee, grasp the ankle, and abduct the lower leg. Repeat the procedure on the other knee if indicated.

Findings: Normally there is little motion at the knee.

Movement of the knee medially or laterally suggests collateral ligament damage, which often results from trauma to the knee.

Anterior and Posterior Cruciate Ligaments

Assess the *anterior* and *posterior cruciate ligaments* using the drawer test.

Procedure: The patient remains in supine position with the hip flexed 45 degrees and the knee flexed with the foot flat on the examination table. Sit on the patient's foot to stabilize it. Instruct the patient to relax the muscles in the flexed leg. Palpate the hamstrings at the back of the knee to ensure that they are relaxed. Using both hands, jerk the head of the tibia forward (open drawer) to assess the anterior cruciate ligament and push backward (closed drawer) to assess the posterior cruciate ligament (see Fig. 14-43, *B*). Repeat the procedure on the other knee if indicated.

Findings: You should not be able to displace the knee from its position.

When the tibia can be pulled anteriorly more than 2 cm from the femur, injury to the anterior cruciate ligament may be indicated. When the tibia can be pushed posteriorly from the femur, injury to the posterior cruciate ligament may be indicated.

★ Advanced practice

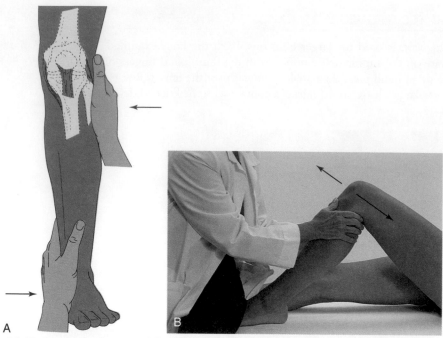

FIG. 14-43 Assessing knee stability. **A,** Assessing collateral ligaments. **B,** Drawer test for assessing anterior and posterior cruciate ligaments. (**A** from Greenberger and Hinthorn, 1993.)

PROCEDURES AND TECHNIQUES WITH EXPECTED FINDINGS	ABNORMAL FINDINGS

Meniscal Damage

Perform *McMurray's test* to evaluate the presence of a damaged medial or lateral meniscus.

Procedure: Ask the patient to lie supine with one foot flat on the table to the knee. Place the thumb and index finger of one hand on either side of the joint space to maintain flexion and stabilize the knee. With the other hand, grasp the patient's heel, raise the lower leg parallel with the table (knee will be flexed 90 degrees), and rotate the knee. External rotation tests the lateral meniscus, and internal rotation tests the medial meniscus (Fig. 14-44).

Findings: The knee should rotate without pain, clicking, or locking.

A positive McMurray's test in the presence of meniscal damage is pain on the medial or lateral surfaces of the knee, audible clicking or locking of the knee on movement, or pain reproduced along the joint lines.

Meniscal Tear

When the patient complains of knee locking, perform the *Apley test* to detect meniscal tear.

Procedure: With the patient in prone position, flex the knee 90 degrees. Press down on the patient's foot so the tibia is firmly against the femur; then rotate the knee externally.

Findings: No pain or locking is a negative test (Fig. 14-45).

If meniscal tear is present, the patient is unable to bear weight or flex the knee. Medial meniscus tear is more common than lateral meniscus tear. A meniscal tear frequently occurs with twisting of the knee playing sports.

Pain, locking of the knee, or clicking during rotation of the knee is a positive Apley test, indicating meniscal tear.

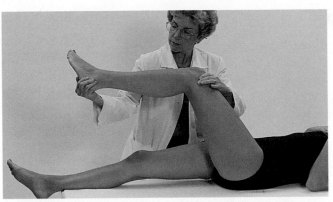

FIG. 14-44 Examination of the knee with McMurray's test. Knee is flexed, stabilized with thumb and index finger; with the other hand rotate and extend the lower leg.

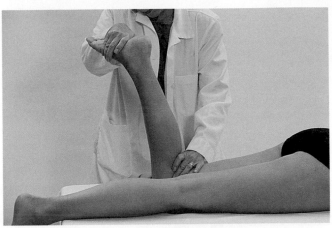

FIG. 14-45 Examination of the knee with the Apley test.

PROCEDURES AND TECHNIQUES WITH EXPECTED FINDINGS

★ ASSESS for hip flexion contractures.

Perform the *Thomas test* to evaluate flexion contractures of the hip.

Have the patient lie supine and ask him or her to fully extend one leg on the table and flex the other knee up to the chest as far as possible. Observe if the extended leg remains flat on the table when the other leg is flexed, which indicates a negative Thomas test (Fig. 14-46).

ASSESS for nerve root compression.

To evaluate for nerve root irritation or lumbar disk herniation, perform *straight leg raises.* With the patient supine, raise one leg, keeping the knee straight.

Tightness of the hamstring may be reported, but no pain should be felt (Fig. 14-47).

ABNORMAL FINDINGS

Lifting of the extended leg off the table in response to flexion of the other leg indicates a hip flexion contracture. Record the degree of flexion.

Pain in the back of the leg with 30 to 60 degrees of elevation indicates pressure on a peripheral nerve by an intervertebral disk.

★ Advanced practice.

DOCUMENTING EXPECTED FINDINGS

Coordinated smooth gait, complete range of motion against gravity with full resistance (5/5) in all joints without pain, muscle size symmetric bilaterally, shoulders aligned, and vertebral column straight.

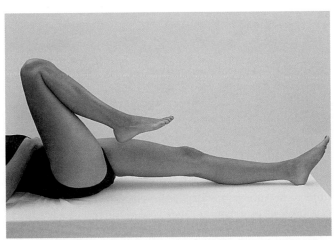

FIG. 14-46 Examination of the hip with the Thomas test. Response is negative in this patient because the extended leg remains flat on the table.

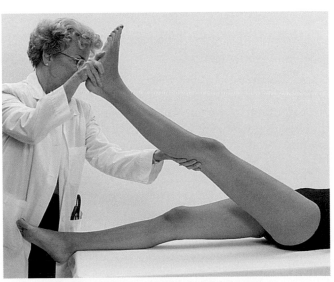

FIG. 14-47 Straight leg–raising test.

⚡ CLINICAL REASONING: THINKING LIKE A NURSE

Musculoskeletal System

A 61-year-old woman presents to the emergency department complaining of severe pain to her right wrist following a 2-foot (61 cm) fall off of a chair. She states that she is unable to move her arm.

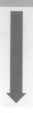

Interpreting

Early in the encounter the nurse considers several possible causes of the pain: hematoma, muscle sprain, fracture, or a combination of these. To determine the probability of being correct, the nurse gathers additional data.

- What is the appearance of the joint? There is moderate edema to the wrist and forearm.
- Is there evidence of joint stability? The nurse notes crepitus and increased pain to the wrist with palpation.

The experienced nurse not only recognizes a fracture by the clinical signs (edema and crepitus) and symptoms (pain, loss of motion) but also interprets this information in the context of an older adult with osteoporosis who has fallen.

Nurse's Background, Experience, Perspective

The experienced nurse immediately has a perceptual grasp of the situation at hand. Extensive practical knowledge about what to expect with this age-group considering the history allows the nurse to recognize risk factors.

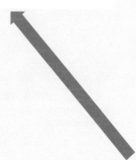

Noticing

The nurse immediately recognizes that a fall from a chair can potentially result in significant injury—particularly with an older adult. The nurse observes the woman holding her arm against her abdomen under a pillow and recognizes that this is a common protective posture with upper-extremity trauma. The nurse learns from the woman that she is in good health but has a history of osteoporosis for which she takes alendronate (Fosamax). Her age and osteoporosis increase her risk for musculoskeletal injury.

Responding

The nurse initiates appropriate initial interventions (protection of the joint, ice, pain relief, monitoring distal perfusion) and notifies the emergency department provider of the situation, ensuring that the patient receives appropriate immediate and follow-up care.

Reflecting

The nurse evaluates the presentation and outcomes of interventions (reflection-in-action); this experience contributes to and deepens the expertise on which to draw (reflection-on-action) when encountering a similar situation.

AGE-RELATED VARIATIONS

Nurses adapt their examinations of the musculoskeletal system when assessing patients at either end of the life span. Neonates and infants are encouraged to make voluntary movements to provide assessment data. The pace of the examination is individualized to accommodate the mobility of the other adult.

▌INFANTS AND CHILDREN

There are several differences in the assessment of the system for infants and young children. Infants' movement is assessed during voluntary movement, and hip joints and feet are assessed for abnormalities. Children's motor development is compared with standardized tables of normal age and sequences described in Chapter 19. Further information regarding musculoskeletal assessment of infants, children, and adolescents is presented in Chapter 19.

▌OLDER ADULTS

Assessing the musculoskeletal system of an older adult usually follows the same procedures as for an adult. Older adults may be slower at performing range of motion, and their muscle strength may be less than that of a younger adult. Chapter 21 presents further information regarding the musculoskeletal assessment of older adults.

COMMON PROBLEMS AND CONDITIONS

RISK FACTORS

Musculoskeletal Conditions

Gout

- *Gender:* Men have a higher uric acid level than women until women reach menopause.*
- *Family history:* Approximately 25% of patients with gout have a positive family history.*[†]
- *Alcohol:* Excessive alcohol use (more than two drinks a day for men and more than one for women) increase risk.* (M)
- *Obesity:* An obese person is four times more likely to develop gout than someone with normal body weight.[†] (M)
- *Hypertension:* Untreated hypertension increases risk.* (M)
- *Diabetes mellitus:* Insulin resistance contributes to the development of gout, and high uric acid levels contribute to insulin resistance.[†]
- *Hyperlipidemia* and atherosclerosis increase risk.* (M)
- *Medications* such as thiazide diuretics used to treat hypertension, low-dose aspirin, and immunosuppressive therapy such as cyclosporine can increase uric acid levels."

Osteoarthritis

- *Age:* Risk increases with age. By age 85 a person has a one-in-two chance of developing osteoarthritis (OA).[‡§]
- *Gender:* OA occurs in women over age 45 years more than in men, but it occurs in men under 45 years more than in women.[‡]
- *Weight:* Being overweight or obese puts stress on joints. An obese person has a two-in-three chance of developing OA.[‡§] (M)

- *Repeated cartilage damage:* Overuse of joints increases risk.[‡] (M)
- *Joint injury:* Injury to the knee or hip increases risk.[‡] (M)

Osteoporosis[¶]

- *Age:* Bone density decreases beginning at age 35 years.
- *Gender:* Women have less bone tissue and lose it more readily than men.
- *Race:* Caucasians and Asians have increased risk.
- *Bone structures and body weight:* Small-boned and thin women (under 127 lb [58 kg]) are at greater risk.
- *Family history:* A family history of osteoporosis increases risk.
- *Lifestyle:* Cigarette smoking, excessive alcohol intake, consuming inadequate calcium, and performing inadequate weight-bearing exercises increase the risk. (M)
- *Medications to treat chronic diseases:* Some medications have adverse effects that lead to osteoporosis, including glucocorticoids and some anticonvulsants. (M)
- *Sex hormones:* Estrogen deficiency from menopause or surgical removal of ovaries (oophorectomy) increases risk in women. Low levels of testosterone and estrogen increase risk in men. (M)

*From www.mayoclinic.com/health/gout, 2011.
[†]From http://gouteducation.org/medical-professionals/about-gouty-arthritis/risk-factors-triggers/ Gout & Uric acid education society.org, 2009.
[‡]From www.cdc.gov/arthritis/basics/risk_factors.htm, September 1, 2011.
[§]From Kennedy S, Jacobson J: Osteoarthritis: Setting nursing's agenda, *Am J Nurs* 111(10): 19-20. 2011.
[¶]Data from www.nof.org, 2011 (National Osteoporosis Foundation)
M, Modifiable risk factor.

BONES

Fracture

A partial or complete break in the continuity of a bone is a fracture. The skin remains intact in a closed fracture, and it is broken in an open fracture (Fig. 14-48). A pathologic or spontaneous fracture is a break in the continuity of the bone resulting from weakness in the bone such as osteoporosis or a neoplasm. Fractures are a common injury at any age but are more likely to occur in children and older adults. Forearm fractures are common in children, whereas hip fractures are common in older adults. **Clinical Findings:** Pain caused by muscle spasm is a common symptom. Deformity and loss of function are caused by the shortening of tissue around the bone and localized edema.

Osteoporosis

Loss of bone density (osteopenia) and decreased bone strength result in osteoporosis, which is defined as a bone mineral density (BMD) more than 2.5 standard deviations

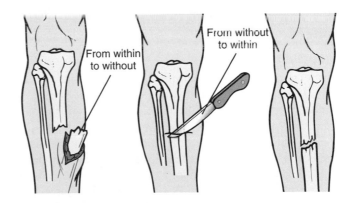

FIG. 14-48 Open and closed fractures. (From Lewis et al., 2007.)

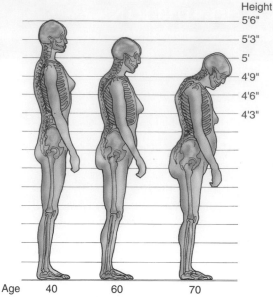

FIG. 14-49 Hallmark of osteoporosis: dowager's hump (kyphosis). (From Ignatavicius and Workman, 2010.)

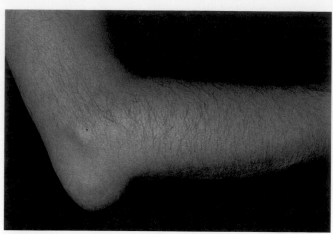

FIG. 14-50 Olecranon bursitis. (Reprinted from the Clinical slide collection of the rheumatic diseases, copyright 1991, 1995, 1997. Used by permission of the American College of Rheumatology.)

below the mean for young healthy adult women. Causes include factors associated with aging such as decline of estrogen and its relationship to calcium deficit and lack of weight-bearing exercise. Use of immunosuppression therapy such as glucocorticoids contributes to osteoporosis. **Clinical Findings:** Osteoporosis is referred to as a *silent disease* because bone loss occurs without signs or symptoms. Patients may not know they have osteoporosis until they discover a loss of height, experience a spontaneous fracture (pathologic fracture) from brittle bones, or develop kyphosis (convex curvature of the thoracic spine) (Fig. 14-49).

JOINTS

Rheumatoid Arthritis

This form of arthritis is a chronic, autoimmune inflammatory disease of the connective tissue. The onset is usually gradual, with fatigue, morning stiffness lasting more than an hour, diffuse muscle ache, and weakness. Eventually the synovial lining of joints becomes inflamed, leading to deterioration of cartilage and erosion of surfaces, causing bone spurs. Ligaments and tendons around inflamed joints become fibrotic and shortened, causing contractures and subluxation (partial dislocation) of joints. **Clinical Findings:** Joint involvement usually is bilateral. Localized symptoms are pain; edema; and stiffness of the fingers, wrists, ankles, feet, and knees. Systemic symptoms caused by the autoimmune response include low-grade fever and fatigue. As the disease process continues, ulnar deviation, swan-neck deformity, and boutonniere deformity may be observed (see Fig. 14-29).

Osteoarthritis

This form of arthritis is caused by degenerative changes of articular cartilage. It affects weight-bearing joints such as vertebrae, hips, knees, and ankles, but it also is noted in fingers. Osteoarthritis also occurs in joints with repetitive movement such as those used when playing sports on a regular basis. As the cartilage wears away, the bones move against one another, causing joint inflammation. Joint involvement may be unilateral or bilateral. **Clinical Findings:** Symptoms include joint edema and aching pain. Joint deformities of fingers develop (Heberden's nodes in DIP joints and Bouchard's nodes in PIP joints) (see Fig. 14-30).

Bursitis

This is an inflammation of a bursa, the connective tissue structure surrounding a joint. Bursa become inflamed by constant friction around joints (Fig. 14-50). Bursitis may be precipitated by arthritis, infection, injury, or excessive exercise. **Clinical Findings:** Painful, limited range of motion; edema; point tenderness; and erythema of the affected joint are common findings. Joints commonly affected include shoulder, elbow, hand, knee, and greater trochanter of the hip.[2]

Gout

This hereditary disorder involves an increase in serum uric acid caused by either increased production or decreased excretion of uric acid and urate salts. The disease is thought to be caused by lack of an enzyme needed to completely metabolize purines for renal excretion. Foods high in purines include poultry, liver, kidney, and legumes. Uric acids commonly accumulate in the great toe but also in other joints such as wrists, hands, ankles, and knees. **Clinical Findings:** Manifestations include erythema and edema of joints that are very painful to move and thus limited in their range of motion. Tophi are a sign of gout; these are round, pealike

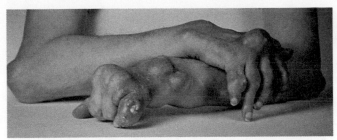

FIG. 14-51 Gout with many tophi present on the hands, on the wrists, and in both olecranon bursae. (Reprinted from the Clinical slide collection of the rheumatic diseases, copyright 1991, 1995, 1997. Used by permission of the American College of Rheumatology.)

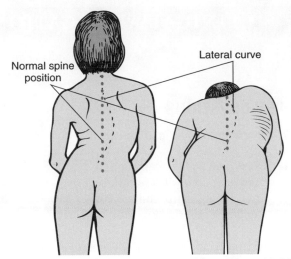

FIG. 14-53 Scoliosis. (From Fraizer and Drzymkowski, 2008.)

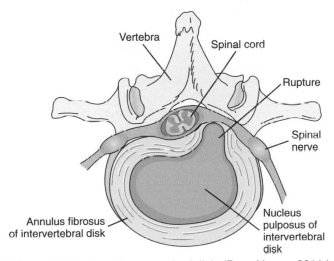

FIG. 14-52 Herniated intervertebral disk. (From Young, 2011.)

deposits of uric acid in ear cartilage or large, irregularly shaped deposits in subcutaneous tissue or other joints (Fig. 14-51). Kidney stones from uric acid crystals can cause manifestations of flank pain and costovertebral angle tenderness.

SPINE

Herniated Nucleus Pulposus

The intervertebral disk provides a cushion between two vertebrae and contains a nucleus pulposus encased in fibrocartilage. When the fibrocartilage surrounding an intervertebral disk ruptures, the nucleus pulposus is displaced and compresses adjacent spinal nerves (Fig. 14-52). *Herniated disk* and *slipped disk* are other names for this disorder. This rupture frequently occurs in the lumbar spine when there is increased strain on the vertebrae such as from lifting heavy objects improperly. **Clinical Findings:** Manifestations depend on the location of the herniated disk. The patient may complain of numbness and radiating pain in the affected extremity from a herniated lumbar disk. Straight leg raises cause pain in the involved leg by putting pressure on the spinal nerve. Cervical

herniated nucleus pulposus causes arm pain and paresthesia. Deep tendon reflexes may be depressed or absent, depending on the spinal nerve root involved.

Scoliosis

An S-shaped deformity of the vertebrae is called *scoliosis*. It is a skeletal deformity of three planes, usually involving lateral curvature, spinal rotation causing rib asymmetry, and thoracic kyphosis (Fig. 14-53). There is evidence that idiopathic scoliosis may be genetic and transmitted as an autosomal-dominant trait with incomplete penetrance, or it may be multifactorial. Causes include congenital malformations of the spine, neuromuscular diseases, traumatic injury, and unequal leg length. **Clinical Findings:** Scoliosis produces uneven shoulders and hip levels. A curvature less than 10% is considered a normal variation, and curves between 10% and 20% are considered mild.[3] Rotation deformity also may cause a rib hump and flank asymmetry on forward flexion. Depending on the severity of the curve, physiologic function of lungs, spine, and pelvis may be compromised.

LIGAMENTS AND MUSCLES

Carpal Tunnel Syndrome

This syndrome occurs when the median nerve is compressed between the flexor retinaculum (carpal ligament) and other structures within the carpal tunnel (see Fig. 14-40). It may be caused by repetitive movements of the hands and arms; injury to the wrist; and systemic disorders such as rheumatoid arthritis, gout, and hypothyroidism. It may also occur with fluid retention that occurs with pregnancy and menopause. **Clinical Findings:** Manifestations include burning, numbness, and tingling in the hands, often at night. Patients report numbness, pain, and paresthesia during the Phalen's sign or Tinel's sign used to assess for this disorder (see Figs. 14-39 and 14-40).

CLINICAL APPLICATION AND CLINICAL REASONING

See Appendix D for answers to exercises in this section.

REVIEW QUESTIONS

1. Which patient's description of pain is consistent with injury to a bone?
   1. "Deep, dull, and boring"
   2. "Cramping even when not moving"
   3. "Intermittent, sharp, and radiating"
   4. "Numbness and tingling with movement"

2. How are expected findings for the musculoskeletal system determined during an examination?
   1. Compare the patient's function with others in the same age-group.
   2. Compare the patient's function with others of the same gender.
   3. Compare the patient's function with others in the same racial group.
   4. Compare the patient's left side with the right side.

3. While testing a patient's bicep muscle strength, the nurse applies resistance and asks the patient to perform which motion?
   1. Extension of the arm
   2. Flexion of the arm
   3. Adduction of the arm
   4. Abduction of the arm

4. The nurse testing the patient's muscle strength finds that the patient has complete range of motion with gravity. Using Table 14-3, how would this finding be documented?
   1. Poor or 2/5
   2. Fair or 3/5
   3. Good or 4/5
   4. Normal or 5/5

5. While assessing the range of motion of the patient's knee, the nurse expects the patient to be able to perform which movements?
   1. Flexion, extension, and hyperextension
   2. Circumduction, internal rotation, and external rotation
   3. Adduction, abduction, and rotation
   4. Flexion, pronation, and supination

6. During an assessment of a young adult, the nurse notes that the patient's shoulders are uneven. Which further examination would the nurse perform for further data?
   1. Ask the patient to rotate each shoulder to assess for shoulder range of motion.
   2. Ask the patient to push against the nurse's hands with his or her forearm to test muscle strength.
   3. Ask the patient to shrug his or her shoulders while the nurse pushes them down to test the muscle strength.
   4. Ask the patient to bend forward at the waist while the nurse checks the alignment of the patient's vertebrae.

7. The nurse is comparing the right and left legs of a patient and notices that they are asymmetric. Which additional data does the nurse collect at this time?
   1. Passively moves each leg through range of motion and compares the findings
   2. Observes the patient's gait and legs as he or she walks across the room
   3. Measures the length of each leg and compares the findings
   4. Palpates the joints and muscles of each leg and compares the findings

8. A patient complains of her jaw popping when chewing. Which examination techniques are appropriate for the nurse to use with this patient?
   1. Inspecting the musculature of the face and neck for symmetry
   2. Observing the range of motion of and palpating each temporomandibular joint for movement, sounds, and tenderness
   3. Asking the patient to move her chin to her chest, hyperextend her head, and move her head from the right side to the left side
   4. Asking the patient to open her mouth as widely as possible and inspecting the lower jaw for redness, edema, or broken teeth

CASE STUDY

Mrs. Soto is a 46-year-old Asian woman with rheumatoid arthritis (RA). The following data are collected by the nurse during an interview and examination.

Interview Data

Mrs. Soto was diagnosed with RA at age 30. Her mother and grandmother had osteoporosis. She has been taking infliximab (Remicade) to treat her RA. She complains of a great deal of pain in her joints, particularly in her hands, and says that she has "just learned to live with the pain because it will always be there." She states that the stiffness and pain in her joints are always worse in the morning or if she sits for too long. She denies muscle weakness other than the fact that her stiffness and soreness prevent her from doing much. Mrs. Soto reports that the RA is progressing to the point at which she is having difficulty doing things requiring fine-motor dexterity such as changing clothes, holding eating utensils, and cutting up her food. She had different faucet handles placed in her home so she could turn the water on and off. Mrs. Soto says that she rarely goes out because she feels ugly.

Examination Data

Patient is able to stand, but standing erect is not possible. Gait is slow and purposeful. Significant edema and tenderness are noted on palpation of wrists, hands, knees, and ankles bilaterally. Hand grips are weak bilaterally. Subcutaneous nodules are noted at ulnar surface of elbows bilaterally.

Clinical Reasoning:

1. Which data deviate from normal findings, suggesting a need for further investigation?
2. For which additional information should the nurse ask or assess?
3. Based on the data, which risk factors for osteoporosis does Mrs. Soto have?
4. With which team members would the nurse collaborate to meet this patient's needs?

CHAPTER

15

Neurologic System

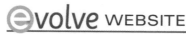

CONCEPT OVERVIEW

The feature concept for this chapter is *Intracranial Regulation.* This concept represents mechanisms that facilitate or impair neurologic function. Because brain function requires perfusion of oxygenated blood and because the respiratory and cardiovascular systems are impacted by neurologic control, strong interrelationships among these concepts exist. Both sensory and tactile perception and motion are extensions of neurologic function that impact other interrelated concepts such as nutrition, development, pain, and elimination. These concepts are represented in the figure below.

This model shows the interrelationships of concepts associated with intracranial regulation. As an example, a stroke results from a lack of oxygenated blood to the brain. Following a stroke an individual may experience problems with sensory and tactile perception and motion, thus impacting elimination, nutrition, pain perception, and independence. Understanding the interrelationship of these concepts helps

the nurse recognize risk factors and thus increases awareness when conducting a health assessment.

The following case provides a clinical example featuring several of these interrelated concepts.

Rose Montya is a 77-year-old female who suffered a stroke in the right hemisphere of the brain 2 months ago. The stroke has resulted in left hemiplegia (meaning that she has no sensation or movement on the left side of her body). She is no longer able to walk and is now confined to a wheelchair or bed. Mrs. Montya has developed a pressure ulcer on her left foot because of a loss of tactile sensation. She can chew and swallow but with difficulty; thus she has experienced weight loss. She is unable to meet basic care needs (dressing, bathing, and toileting), making her fully dependent on others. This previously independent woman is now experiencing depression as a result of her current health status.

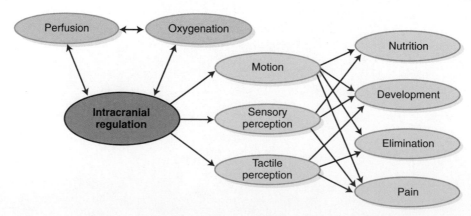

ANATOMY AND PHYSIOLOGY

The nervous system controls body functions through voluntary and autonomic responses to external and internal stimuli. Structural divisions of the nervous system are the central nervous system (CNS), which consists of the brain and spinal cord; the peripheral nervous system; and the autonomic nervous system (ANS).

CENTRAL NERVOUS SYSTEM

Protective Structures

The skull protects the brain. At the base of the skull in the occipital bone is a large oval opening termed the *foramen magnum*, through which the spinal cord extends from the medulla oblongata. There are other openings (foramina) at this base for the entrance and exit of paired cranial nerves and cerebral blood vessels.

Between the skull and the brain lie three layers termed *meninges*. The outer layer is a fibrous layer termed the *dura mater*. The middle meningeal layer, the *arachnoid*, is a two-layer, fibrous, elastic membrane that covers the folds and fissures of the brain. The inner meningeal layer, the *pia mater*, contains small vessels that supply blood to the brain. Between the arachnoid and the pia mater is the subarachnoid space, where the cerebrospinal fluid (CSF) circulates. A fold of dura mater termed the *falx cerebri* separates the two cerebral hemispheres. Another fold of dura mater, the *tentorium cerebelli*, supports the temporal and occipital lobes and separates the cerebral hemispheres from the cerebellum. Structures above the tentorium cerebelli are referred to as *supratentorial*, and those below it as *infratentorial* (Fig. 15-1).

Cerebrospinal Fluid and Cerebral Ventricular System

Cerebrospinal fluid (CSF) is a colorless, odorless fluid containing glucose, electrolytes, oxygen, water, carbon dioxide, protein, and leukocytes. It circulates around the brain and spinal cord to provide a cushion, maintain normal intracranial pressure, provide nutrition, and remove metabolic wastes.

The cerebral ventricular system consists of four interconnecting chambers or ventricles that produce and circulate CSF (see Fig. 15-1). There is one lateral ventricle in each hemisphere, with a third ventricle adjacent to the thalamus and a fourth adjacent to the brainstem. The CSF circulates from the lateral ventricles through the interventricular foramen to the third ventricle and through the aqueduct of Sylvius to the fourth ventricle and into the cisterna magna, which is a small reservoir for CSF. From the cisterna magna the CSF flows within the subarachnoid space up around the brain and down around the spinal cord. The CSF is absorbed through arachnoid villi that extend into the subarachnoid space and is returned to the venous system.

Brain

The brain, consisting of the cerebrum, diencephalon, cerebellum, and brainstem, is made up of gray matter (cell bodies) and white matter (myelinated nerve fibers). The carotid arteries supply most of the blood to the brain and branch off into the posterior cerebral, middle cerebral, and anterior cerebral arteries (see Figs. 12-12 and 12-14). The remaining blood flows through two vertebral arteries and into the posterior and anterior communicating arteries that supply blood through the circle of Willis. Blood leaves the brain through venous sinuses that empty into the jugular veins.

Cerebrum

The cerebrum is the largest part of the brain and is composed of two hemispheres. Each hemisphere is divided into four lobes: frontal, parietal, temporal, and occipital (Fig. 15-2).

The frontal lobe contains the primary motor cortex and is responsible for functions related to voluntary motor activity. The distribution of the nerves that provide movement to specific parts of the body is shown in Fig. 15-3, *A*. The left frontal lobe contains Broca's area (see Fig. 15-2), which is involved in formulation of words. The frontal lobe also controls intellectual function, awareness of self, personality, and autonomic responses related to emotion.

The parietal lobe contains the primary somesthetic (sensory) cortex. One of its major functions is to receive sensory input such as position sense, touch, shape, and texture of objects. The distribution of the nerves that receive sensations from specific parts of the body is adjacent to the motor cortex and is shown in Fig. 15-3, *B*.

The temporal lobe contains the primary auditory cortex. Wernicke's area (see Fig. 15-2), located in the left temporal lobe, is responsible for comprehension of spoken and written language. The temporal lobe also interprets auditory, visual, and somatic sensory inputs that are stored in thought and memory.

The occipital lobe contains the primary visual cortex and is responsible for receiving and interpreting visual information.

Diencephalon

The thalamus, hypothalamus, epithalamus, and subthalamus make up the diencephalon. The thalamus is a relay and integration station from the spinal cord to the cerebral cortex and other parts of the brain. The hypothalamus has several important functions in maintaining homeostasis. Some of these functions include regulation of body temperature, hunger, and thirst; formation of ANS responses; and storage and secretion of hormones from the pituitary gland. The epithalamus contains the pineal gland, which causes sleepiness and helps regulate some endocrine function. The subthalamus is part of the basal ganglia.

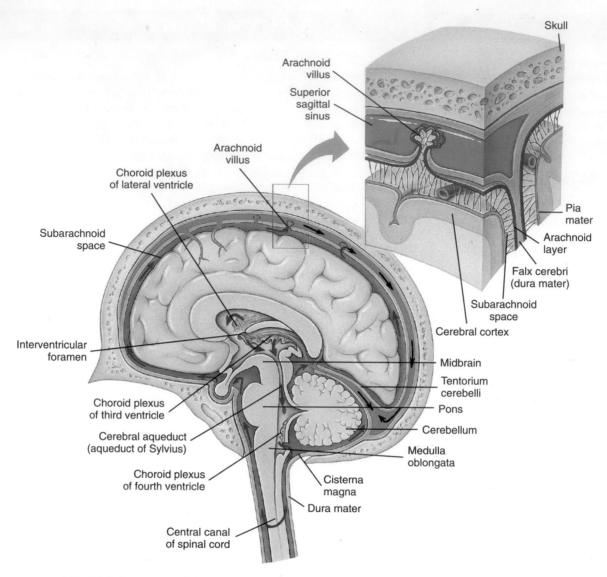

FIG. 15-1 Structures of the brainstem and cerebrospinal fluid (CSF) circulation. *Red arrows* represent the route of the CSF. *Black arrows* represent the route of blood flow. Cerebrospinal fluid is produced in the ventricles, exits the fourth ventricle, and returns to the venous circulation in the superior sagittal sinus. The *inset* depicts the arachnoid granulations in the superior sagittal sinus, where the CSF enters the circulation. (Modified from Thibodeau and Patton, 1999.)

Basal Ganglia

Between the cerebral cortex and midbrain and adjacent to the diencephalon lie the structures that form the basal ganglia (Fig. 15-4). The six ganglia that comprise the basal ganglia are the putamen, caudate nucleus, globus pallidus, thalamus, red nucleus, and substantia nigra. The function of the basal ganglia is to create smooth, coordinated voluntary movement by balancing the production of two neurotransmitters: acetylcholine and dopamine.

Brainstem

The midbrain, pons, and medulla oblongata make up the brainstem (see Fig. 15-1). Ten of the twelve cranial nerves originate from the brainstem (Fig. 15-5). The major function of the midbrain is to relay stimuli concerning muscle

movement to other brain structures. It contains part of the motor tract pathways that control reflex motor movements in response to visual and auditory stimuli. The oculomotor nerve (CN III) and trochlear nerve (CN IV) originate in the midbrain.

The pons relays impulses to the brain centers and lower spinal nerves. The cranial nerves that originate in the pons are trigeminal (CN V), abducens (CN VI), facial (CN VII), and acoustic (CN VIII).

The medulla oblongata contains reflex centers for controlling involuntary functions such as breathing, sneezing, swallowing, coughing, vomiting, and vasoconstriction. Motor and sensory tracts from the frontal and parietal lobes cross from one side to the other in the medulla, so lesions on the right side of the brain create abnormal movement and sensation

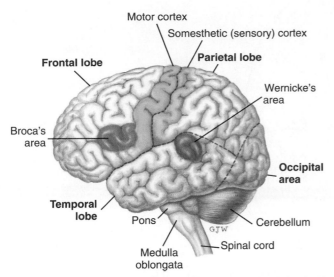

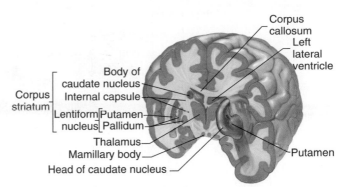

FIG. 15-2 Cerebral hemispheres. Lateral view of the brain. The motor cortex in the frontal lobe is depicted in pink, and the somesthetic cortex in the parietal lobe is depicted in blue. (Modified from Chipps, Clanin, and Campbell, 1992.)

FIG. 15-4 Frontal section of the brain shows nuclei that make up the basal ganglia. (From Patton and Thibodeau, 2010.)

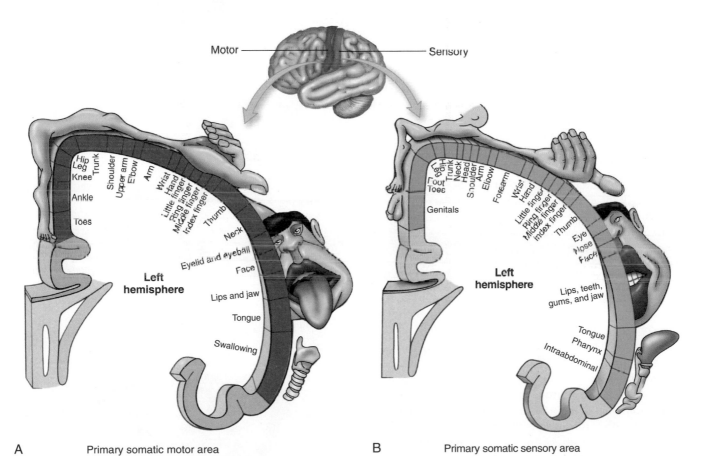

A   Primary somatic motor area

B   Primary somatic sensory area

FIG. 15-3 Topography of the somesthetic and motor cortex. Cerebral cortex is seen in coronal section on the left side of the brain. The figure of the body (homunculus) depicts the relative nerve distributions; the size indicates the relative number of nerves in the distribution. Each cortex occurs on both sides of the brain but appears only on one side in this illustration. The inset shows the motor and somesthetic regions of the left hemisphere. **A,** Primary somatic motor area. **B,** Primary somatic sensory area. (From Patton and Thibodeau, 2010.)

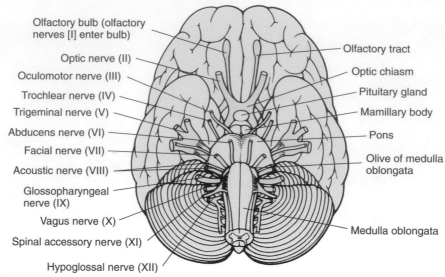

Olfactory bulb (olfactory nerves [I] enter bulb)
Optic nerve (II)
Oculomotor nerve (III)
Trochlear nerve (IV)
Trigeminal nerve (V)
Abducens nerve (VI)
Facial nerve (VII)
Acoustic nerve (VIII)
Glossopharyngeal nerve (IX)
Vagus nerve (X)
Spinal accessory nerve (XI)
Hypoglossal nerve (XII)

Olfactory tract
Optic chiasm
Pituitary gland
Mamillary body
Pons
Olive of medulla oblongata
Medulla oblongata

FIG. 15-5 Inferior surface of the brain showing the origin of the cranial nerves. (From Seeley, Stephens, and Tate, 1995.)

on the left side and vice versa. The cranial nerves that originate in the medulla are glossopharyngeal (CN IX), vagus (CN X), spinal accessory (CN XI), and hypoglossal (CN XII).

Cerebellum

The cerebellum is separated from the cerebral cortex by the tentorium cerebelli (see Fig. 15-1). Functions of the cerebellum include coordinating movement, equilibrium, muscle tone, and proprioception. Each of the cerebellar hemispheres controls movement for the same (ipsilateral) side of the body.

Spinal Cord

The spinal cord is a continuation of the medulla oblongata that begins at the foramen magnum and ends at the first and second lumbar (L1 and L2) vertebrae. At L1 and L2 the spinal cord branches into lumbar and sacral nerve roots termed the *cauda equina.* The spinal cord consists of 31 segments, each giving rise to a pair of spinal nerves (Fig. 15-6). Nerve fibers, grouped into tracts, run through the spinal cord transmitting sensory, motor, and autonomic impulses between the brain and the body. Myelinated nerves form the white matter of the spinal cord and contain ascending and descending tracts of nerve fibers. The descending, or motor, tracts (e.g., anterior and lateral corticospinal or pyramidal tracts) carry impulses from the frontal lobe to muscles for voluntary movement. They also play a role in muscle tone and posture.

The ascending, or sensory, tracts carry sensory information from the body through the thalamus to the parietal lobe. The fasciculus gracilis track travels in the posterior (dorsal) column carrying sensations of touch, deep pressure, vibration, position of joints, stereognosis, and two-point discrimination. The lateral spinothalamic tract carries fibers for sensations of light touch, pressure, temperature, and pain. The gray matter, which contains the nerve cell bodies, is arranged in a butterfly shape with anterior and posterior horns.

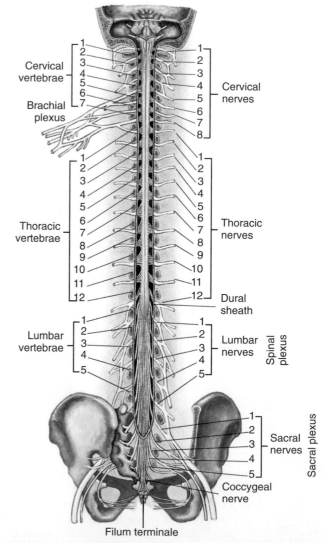

Cervical vertebrae
Brachial plexus
Thoracic vertebrae
Lumbar vertebrae

Cervical nerves
Thoracic nerves
Dural sheath
Lumbar nerves
Spinal plexus
Sacral nerves
Sacral plexus
Coccygeal nerve
Filum terminale

FIG. 15-6 View of the spinal column showing vertebrae, spinal cord, and spinal nerves exiting. (From Chipps, Clanin, and Campbell, 1992.)

PERIPHERAL NERVOUS SYSTEM

Cranial Nerves

Of the 12 pairs of cranial nerves, some have only motor fibers (five pairs) or only sensory fibers (three pairs); whereas others have both motor and sensory fibers (four pairs). Table 15-1 lists the 12 cranial nerves and their functions. Box 15-1 describes ways to remember the names and functions of the cranial nerves. Fig. 15-5 shows the location of the cranial nerves on the inferior surface of the brain.

Spinal Nerves

The 31 pairs of spinal nerves emerge from different segments of the spinal cord: 8 pairs of cervical, 12 pairs of thoracic,

TABLE 15-1	THE CRANIAL NERVES AND THEIR FUNCTIONS
CRANIAL NERVE	**FUNCTION**
Olfactory (I)	Sensory: Smell reception and interpretation
Optic (II)	Sensory: Visual acuity and visual fields
Oculomotor (III)	Motor: Raise eyelids, most extraocular movements Parasympathetic: Pupillary constriction, change lens shape
Trochlear (IV)	Motor: Downward, inward eye movement
Trigeminal (V)	Motor: Jaw opening and clenching, chewing and mastication Sensory: Sensation to cornea, iris, lacrimal glands, conjunctiva, eyelids, forehead, nose, nasal and mouth mucosa, teeth, tongue, ear, facial skin
Abducens (VI)	Motor: Lateral eye movement
Facial (VII)	Motor: Movement of facial expression muscles except jaw, close eyes, labial speech sounds (b, m, w, and rounded vowels) Sensory: Taste—anterior two thirds of tongue, sensation to pharynx Parasympathetic: Secretion of saliva and tears
Acoustic or vestibulocochlear (VIII)	Sensory: Hearing and equilibrium
Glossopharyngeal (IX)	Motor: Voluntary muscles for swallowing and phonation Sensory: Sensation of nasopharynx, gag reflex, taste—posterior one third of tongue Parasympathetic: Secretion of salivary glands, carotid reflex
Vagus (X)	Motor: Voluntary muscles of phonation (guttural speech sounds) and swallowing Sensory: Sensation behind ear and part of external ear canal Parasympathetic: Secretion of digestive enzymes; peristalsis; carotid reflex; involuntary action of heart, lungs, and digestive tract
Spinal accessory (XI)	Motor: Turn head, shrug shoulders, some actions for phonation
Hypoglossal (XII)	Motor: Tongue movement for speech sound articulation (l, t, n) and swallowing

From Seidel HM et al: *Mosby's guide to physical examination*, ed 7, St Louis, 2011, Mosby.

BOX 15-1	HOW TO REMEMBER NAMES AND NERVE TYPE OF CRANIAL NERVES

Read the words in the column on the left from top to bottom. The first letter of each word is the same as the first letter in the name of the cranial nerve (CN). The fourth column gives the type of impulses carried by the nerves (i.e., sensory, motor, or both sensory and motor). The last column is a phrase to remember the type of nerve for each cranial nerve.

MEMORY WORD	CN NUMBER	CN NAME	TYPE	MEMORY WORD
On	CN I	Olfactory	Sensory	Some
Old	CN II	Optic	Sensory	Say
Olympus	CN III	Oculomotor	Motor	Marry
Towering	CN IV	Trochlear	Motor	Money
Top	CN V	Trigeminal	Both	But
A	CN VI	Abducens	Motor	My
Fin	CN VII	Facial	Both	Brother
And	CN VIII	Acoustic (vestibulocochlear)	Sensory	Says
German	CN IX	Glossopharyngeal	Both	Bad
Viewed	CN X	Vagus	Both	Business to
Some	CN XI	Spinal accessory	Motor	Marry
Hops	CN XII	Hypoglossal	Motor	Money

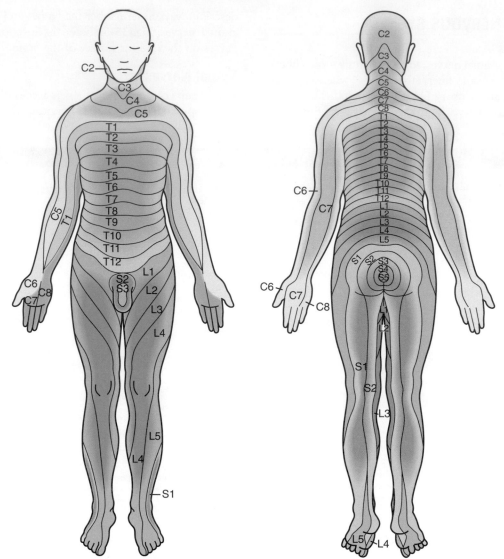

FIG. 15-7 Dermatome map. Letters and numbers indicate the spinal nerves innervating a given region of skin. (From Marx, Hockberger, and Walls, 2010.)

5 pairs of lumbar, 5 pairs of sacral, and 1 pair of coccygeal nerves. The first seven cervical nerves exit above their corresponding vertebrae. There are eight cervical nerves but seven cervical vertebrae. The remaining spinal nerves exit below the corresponding vertebrae (see Fig. 15-6).

Each pair of spinal nerves is formed by the union of an efferent, or motor (ventral), root and an afferent, or sensory (dorsal), root. The motor fibers carry impulses from the brain (frontal lobe) through the spinal cord to muscles and glands, whereas sensory fibers carry impulses from the sensory receptors of the body through the spinal cord to the brain (parietal lobe). Each pair of spinal nerves and its corresponding part of the spinal cord make up a spinal segment and innervate specific body segments. The dorsal root of each spinal nerve supplies the sensory innervation to a segment of the skin known as a dermatome. Refer to the dermatome map to determine the spinal nerve that

corresponds to the area where the patient reports sensory alteration (Fig. 15-7). For example, if the patient complains of pain with numbness and tingling across the right knee, the nurse knows that the fourth lumbar spinal segment is involved, perhaps compressed.

Reflex Arc

Reflex arcs are tested by observing muscle movement in response to sensory stimuli. Deep tendon reflexes are responses to stimulation of a tendon that stretches the neuromuscular spindles of a muscle group. Striking a deep tendon stimulates a sensory neuron that travels to the spinal cord, where it stimulates an interneuron that stimulates a motor neuron to create movement (Fig. 15-8). Superficial reflexes are tested in the same manner. Each reflex corresponds to a specific spinal segment. Table 15-2 shows the

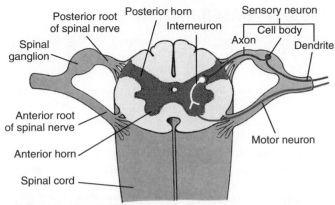

FIG. 15-8 Cross-section of the spinal cord showing three-neuron reflex arc. (From Chipps, Clanin, and Campbell, 1992.)

TABLE 15-2	SUPERFICIAL AND DEEP TENDON REFLEXES
REFLEX	**SPINAL LEVEL**
Superficial	
Upper abdominal	T8, T9, and T10
Lower abdominal	T10, T11, and T12
Cremasteric	T12, L1, and L2
Plantar	L5, S1, and S2
Deep	
Biceps	C5 and C6
Brachioradial	C5 and C6
Triceps	C6, C7, and C8
Patellar	L2, L3, and L4
Achilles	S1 and S2

Modified from Seidel HM et al: *Mosby's guide to physical examination,* ed 7, St Louis, 2011, Mosby.

deep tendon and superficial reflexes and the segments of the spinal cord that innervate each reflex.

AUTONOMIC NERVOUS SYSTEM

The ANS regulates the internal environment of the body in conjunction with the endocrine system. It has two components: the sympathetic nervous system (SNS) and the parasympathetic nervous system (PNS). The SNS arises from the thoracolumbar segments of the spinal cord and is activated during stress (the fight-or-flight response). The SNS actions include increasing blood pressure and heart rate, vasoconstricting peripheral blood vessels, inhibiting gastrointestinal peristalsis, and dilating bronchi. By contrast, the PNS arises from craniosacral segments of the spinal cord and controls vegetative functions (breed and feed). The PNS actions are involved in functions associated with conserving energy such as decreasing heart rate and force of myocardial contraction, decreasing blood pressure and respiration, and stimulating gastrointestinal peristalsis.

HEALTH HISTORY

Nurses interview patients to collect subjective data about their present health and any past medical experiences. They ask questions about the patient's present health status, past health history, family history, and personal and psychosocial history, which may affect the functions of the nervous system. Quality Improvement Competencies for Nurses include providing patient-centered care and interdisciplinary teamwork with physical and occupational therapists and vocational counselors. See Table 11-1 on p. 196 for examples of competencies.

GENERAL HEALTH HISTORY

Present Health Status

Have you noticed any changes in your ability to move around or participate in your usual activities?
The patient's perception of his or her functioning is the primary source of data. Difficulty moving because of weakness or spasticity may indicate a neuromuscular problem.

Often patients can identify that they are having difficulty in performing their usual activities, but they may not associate it with a neurologic disorder.

Do you have any chronic diseases? If yes, describe. In what ways does this chronic disease keep you from maintaining a healthy lifestyle?
Chronic diseases may affect mobility and daily living. These questions may help identify risks for injury, opportunities for teaching, and needs for additional resources.

Which medications do you take? Are you taking medications as prescribed?
Both prescription and over-the-counter medications should be documented. Adverse effects of medications may influence the nervous system. Drugs (prescription or street drugs) or alcohol may interfere with the functioning of the nervous system. Note any anticonvulsant medications, antitremor drugs, antivertigo agents, or pain medications that could alter a patient's neurologic examination.

Past Health History

Have you ever had injury to your head or spinal cord? If yes, describe when this happened. What residual changes have you experienced since the injury?

Previous injury to the central nervous system may leave residual deficits such as weakness or spasticity that you can anticipate during the examination. Injury to the frontal lobe can cause changes in memory and cognition.

Have you ever had surgery on your brain, spinal cord, or any of your nerves? If yes, describe. What was the outcome of the surgery?

A history of surgery may provide additional information about possible neurologic problems and the findings to anticipate during the examination.

Have you ever had a stroke? If yes, describe when and what residual changes you have as a result of the stroke.

Previous stroke (cerebrovascular accident [CVA]) may leave residual deficits such as aphasia that affect your subjective data collection or hemiparesis, which you will assess further during the examination.

Do you have a seizure disorder? If yes, describe the kind of seizure, how often you have them, and what you do to prevent the seizures.

Although seizure is probably not evident during the examination, you need to determine how the patient is caring for this disorder to maintain safety and prevent recurrence of seizures.

Family History

In your family has anyone ever had a stroke, seizures, or tumor of the brain or spinal cord?

Family history may be used to determine the patient's risk for these conditions.

Personal and Psychosocial History

Have you had any changes in your ability to perform your personal care or daily activities?

Disorders of the neurologic system such as Parkinson's disease or myasthenia gravis may interfere with the patient's completion of functional abilities.

How much alcohol do you drink per week? Do you use or have you ever used substances such as marijuana, cocaine, barbiturates, tranquilizers, or any other mood-altering drugs?

Documentation of these substances is necessary because they may alter the patient's cognitive or neuromuscular function. In addition, the actions of these substances may interfere with medications that may be prescribed.

Do you use the seat belts when riding in a car? If you ride a bicycle, motorcycle, or all-terrain vehicle, do you wear a helmet?

Brain injury can be prevented by using seat belts and wearing helmets when indicated.

PROBLEM-BASED HISTORY

Commonly reported problems related to the neurologic system are headache, dizziness, seizures, loss of consciousness, changes in movement (tremors, weakness, or incoordination), changes in sensations (numbness or tingling), difficulty swallowing, or difficulty communicating such as inability to understand speech or inability to speak. As with symptoms in all areas of health assessment, a symptom analysis mnemonic OLD CARTS, which includes the *O*nset, *L*ocation, *D*uration, *C*haracteristics, *A*ggravating factors, *R*elated symptoms, *T*reatment, and *S*everity (see Box 2-3).

Headache

Describe your headaches. What do they feel like? Where do you feel the pain? How long do they last? How often do you have them?

These questions analyze the symptoms of headaches to help determine the cause. Headaches may be related to compression from tumors or increased intracranial pressure or ischemia from impaired circulation within the brain. (Also see Chapter 10 for history of migraine, cluster, and tension headaches.)

Have you had any recent surgeries or medical procedures such as spinal anesthesia or lumbar puncture?

A transient headache can occur after some diagnostic tests, such as a lumbar puncture. When the patient is in an upright position, the loss of CSF creates tension on the meninges, causing a headache.

Dizziness

What does it feel like when you are dizzy or light-headed? Do you feel as if you may faint? How often do you experience this dizziness? What makes it worse?

The word "dizziness" means different things to different people. It can be used by patients to refer to different sensations such as light-headedness, vertigo, or ataxia. Distinguish among these disorders by asking the patient what he or she experienced because these symptoms have different causes. Dizziness may be a sensation of light-headedness or fainting with an inability to maintain balance caused by decreased cerebral blood flow. To others dizziness means vertigo, a sensation of instability described in the following paragraphs. Dizziness may refer to ataxia, which is an inability to coordinate movement or a staggering gait caused by a cerebellar disorder.

Have you ever experienced a perception that feels like the room is spinning (objective vertigo) or a sensation that you are spinning (subjective vertigo)? Does this happen suddenly or gradually? What makes the vertigo worse? What relieves it?

Vertigo may occur as a perception or a sensation. It may be caused by a neurologic dysfunction (usually with a gradual onset) or a problem with the vestibule such as an inner ear infection (labyrinthitis) or Meniere's disease (usually with a sudden onset). Vertigo suggests a balance problem that may be related to equilibrium involving the cerebellum or inner ear.[1] Chapter 10 has additional questions about vertigo related to inner ear problems.

Seizures

Have you had a seizure? How often are you having seizures or convulsions? When was your last seizure? What are they like? Do you become unconscious?

Seizures may be caused by idiopathic epilepsy, a pathologic process, endogenous or exogenous poison, metabolic disturbances, or fever (see Common Problems and Conditions later in this chapter).

Do you have any warning signs before the seizure starts? Describe what happens.

An aura can precede a seizure; it can involve auditory, gustatory, olfactory, visual, or motor sensations. The area in the brain that corresponds to the aura provides information about seizure origin.

When the patient loses consciousness during the seizure, refer the following questions to people who observed the seizure. Describe the seizure movements that you observed. Did you notice any other signs such as a change in color of the face or lips; loss of consciousness (note how long)? Did the patient urinate or have a bowel movement during the seizure? After the seizure, how long did it take him or her to return to the preseizure level of consciousness?

Responses to these questions help identify the areas of the brain involved in the seizure activity. Fig. 15-3, *A,* is helpful in understanding the path that a seizure may follow. For example, if the seizure begins in the wrist and travels to the head, neck, and trunk, you can follow the path of the excessive nervous discharge of the seizure along the motor cortex. This is an example of a simple seizure in which the patient maintains consciousness.

How do you feel after the seizure? Are you confused? Have a headache or aching muscles? Do you sleep more than usual?

Affirmative answers to these questions may indicate the expected recovery phase of a generalized seizure. Patients may be weak, confused, or sleepy after a seizure because the glucose supply of the brain was used during the seizure and it takes time to replace it.

Do any factors such as stress, fatigue, activity, or discontinuing medication seem to start these seizures? Do you take any actions to prevent hurting yourself during seizures?

Answers to these questions help plan prevention strategies for seizures or any injury experienced during the seizure.

How have the seizures affected your life? Your occupation? Do you wear any identification that indicates that you have seizures?

Because seizures may be a chronic disease that affects patients' driving, personal relationships, and employment, the nurse needs to learn how seizures have affected the patient's life and if he or she has adapted to the seizure condition. Carrying identification about seizures helps those who may assist a patient who is seizing.

Loss of Consciousness

When did you lose consciousness, have a blackout or faint, or feel that you were not aware of your surroundings? Did the change occur suddenly? Can you describe what happened to you just before you lost consciousness? Were there other symptoms associated with the change of consciousness?

Loss of consciousness may be caused by cardiovascular disorders, which tend to cause symptoms more rapidly, or neurologic disorders. It is also associated with drugs; psychiatric illness; or metabolic diseases such as hypoxia, liver or kidney failure, or diabetes mellitus.

Changes in Movement

How long have you had a change in your mobility? Describe the change. Is it continuous or intermittent?

The patient's description helps guide subsequent questions for the symptom analysis.

Have you noticed any tremors or shaking of the hands or face? When did they start? Do they seem worse when you are anxious or at rest? When you focus on doing something (intention)? What relieves the tremors—rest, activity, or alcohol? Do they affect your performance of daily activities?

Answers to these questions may help identify the cause of the altered mobility. For example, Parkinson's disease causes tremor at rest, whereas cerebellar disorders cause tremor with intentional movement.

Have you felt any sense of weakness in or difficulty moving parts of your body? Is this confined to one area or generalized? Is it associated with anything in particular (e.g., activity)? How does the weakness affect your daily activities?

Decreased circulation to the brain can cause these symptoms. Some type of transient ischemic attack (TIA) or CVA may have occurred.

Do you have problems with coordination? Do you have difficulty keeping your balance when you walk? Do you lean to one side or fall? Which direction? Do your legs suddenly give way?

A CVA may be the cause, but dysfunction of the cerebellum or inner ear should be considered when balance is impaired. Multiple sclerosis, Parkinson's disease, or brain tumor may also be causes. If a patient reports falls in one direction such as to the right, this may indicate that muscle weakness is caused by impaired nerve function on the left side of the brain.

Changes in Sensation

Where are you experiencing numbness or tingling? How does it feel? Is it associated with any activity?

These questions relate to some types of central nervous system disorder (e.g., multiple sclerosis or CVA), peripheral nerve disorder (e.g., diabetes mellitus may cause peripheral neuropathy), peripheral vascular disease, or anemia (vitamin B_{12} deficiency anemia causes paresthesia). Paresthesias often fluctuate with posture, activity, rest, edema, or underlying disease. Hypoesthesia is decreased sensation that may indicate a sensory problem from impaired circulation or nerve compression. Identifying the location of the abnormal sensation may help identify its cause.

Difficulty Swallowing (Dysphagia)

How long have you had problems swallowing? Do these problems involve liquids or solids? Both? Do you have excessive saliva or drooling? Do you cough or choke when trying to swallow?

These may be caused by dysfunction of CN IX (glossopharyngeal), CN X (vagus), or CN XII (hypoglossal).

Parkinsonism and myasthenia gravis may cause excessive salivation that may increase the need to swallow. A CVA may cause weakness of muscles involved in swallowing.

Difficulty Communicating (Dysphasia/Aphasia)

How long have you had problems speaking? Are you having difficulty forming words or finding the right words? Have you had difficulty understanding things that are said to you? When did this begin?

Aphasia is the term for defective or absent language function, whereas *dysphasia* is an impairment of speech not as severe as aphasia. Inability to comprehend speech of others and of oneself is termed *receptive aphasia* or *fluent aphasia* and is associated with lesions in Wernicke's area in the temporal lobe (see Fig 15-2). Inability to spontaneously communicate or translate ideas into meaningful speech or writing is termed *expressive aphasia* or *nonfluent aphasia* and is associated with lesions in Broca's area in the frontal lobe. Lesions in the frontal or temporal lobe may occur following a brain tumor, head injury, or CVA. Parkinson's disease may create difficulty forming words because of bradykinesia (slow movement) of facial muscles. NOTE: These questions may need to be asked of the person accompanying the patient when the patient is unable to respond.

HEALTH PROMOTION FOR EVIDENCE-BASED PRACTICE

Traumatic Brain Injury

Traumatic brain injury (TBI) results from a blow or sudden jolt to the head. The severity of injury may range from mild to severe. An estimated 1.5 million people sustain TBI in the United States each year. Injuries are the leading cause of death for Americans ages 1 to 44 and a leading cause of disability for all ages, regardless of gender, race/ethnicity, or socioeconomic status. More than 180,000 people die from injuries each year, and approximately 1 in 10 sustains a nonfatal injury serious enough to be treated in a hospital emergency department.

Crashes (involving motor vehicles, bicycles, pedestrians, and recreational vehicles), falls, assaults, and sports-related injuries are common causes. Driving while impaired and failing to take safety precautions are two important risk factors for such injury.

Goals and Objectives—*Healthy People 2020*

Injuries and violence are widespread in society. The *Healthy People 2020* goals for injury and violence involving TBI are to reduce fatal and nonfatal brain injuries. Both unintentional injuries and those caused by acts of violence are among the top 15 killers for Americans of all ages. Most events resulting in injury, disability, or death are predictable and preventable. Increased use of automobile safety belts, use of child restraints,

and increased use of helmets by motorcyclists and bicyclists prevent TBIs.

Recommendations to Reduce Risk (Primary Prevention)
U.S. Preventive Services Task Force

- Counsel individuals to use lap/shoulder belts while in a car. Children should ride in an appropriate-size child safety seat in accordance with the manufacturer's instructions in the middle of the rear seat.
- Advise individuals against riding in the back of pickup trucks or in cargo areas of vehicles unless equipped with seat belts.
- Counsel individuals against driving while under the influence of drugs or alcohol or riding as a passenger with an impaired driver.
- Advise individuals who ride on motorcycles to wear a safety helmet.
- Discuss with individuals and parents of children and adolescents the importance of wearing approved safety helmets and not riding in motor vehicle traffic while riding bicycles and all-terrain vehicles.
- The value of counseling to prevent pedestrian injuries is unknown.

From www.healthypeople.gov/2020/topicsobjectives2020/overview.aspx?topicid=24. Last updated September 23, 2011, accessed October 24, 2011; and www.uspreventiveservicestaskforce.org/uspstf07/mvoi/mvoirs.htm, last updated August, 2007, accessed October 24, 2011.

EXAMINATION

ROUTINE TECHNIQUES	SPECIAL CIRCUMSTANCES OR ADVANCED PRACTICE

• ASSESS mental status and level of consciousness.
• EVALUATE speech.
• NOTICE cranial nerve functions.
• OBSERVE gait.
• EVALUATE extremities for muscle strength.
• TEST deep tendon reflexes.
• TEST for ankle clonus.
	• ASSESS cranial nerves.
	  • TEST nose (CN I).
	  • ASSESS eyes (CN II, CN III, CN IV, and CN VI).
	  • TEST ears (CN VIII).
	  • ASSESS face (CN V and VII).
	  • TEST tongue for taste (CN VII and CN IX).
	  • INSPECT tongue (CN XII).
	  • INSPECT oropharynx (CN IX and CN X).
	  • TEST shoulders and neck muscles (CN XI).
	• ASSESS cerebellum.
	  • TEST cerebellar function.
	• ASSESS peripheral nerves.
	  • TEST extremities for sensation.
	  • TEST for Babinski's reflex.
	  • TEST for superficial reflexes.

EQUIPMENT NEEDED

Aromatic materials • Penlight • Tuning fork (200 to 400 Hz) • Cotton-tipped applicator • Tongue blade • Examination gloves • 4 × 4 gauze • Reshaped paper clip • Cotton ball • Percussion hammer

PROCEDURES AND TECHNIQUES WITH EXPECTED FINDINGS	ABNORMAL FINDINGS

ROUTINE TECHNIQUES: NEUROLOGIC SYSTEM

CLEAN hands.

ASSESS mental status and level of consciousness.

Say the patient's name and note the response. The patient is expected to turn toward you and respond appropriately. While taking the patient's history you gather data about his or her mental status and level of consciousness. More detail is provided on this assessment in Chapter 7. The patient should be oriented to time, place and person.

Patients who do not know their name or location are disoriented. Those who require excessive stimulation or even painful stimuli to respond have a decrease in level of consciousness and require follow-up care and close supervision to maintain safety. A change in level of consciousness is the first sign of impaired cerebral function.

EVALUATE speech for articulation and voice quality and conversation for comprehension of verbal communication.

The patient's voice should have inflection and sufficient volume with clear speech. His or her responses indicate an understanding of what is said.

Errors in choice of words or syllables; difficulty in articulation, which could involve impaired thought processes or dysfunction of the tongue or lips; slurred speech (tone sounds slurred); poorly coordinated or irregular speech; monotone or weak voice; nasal tone, rasping, or hoarseness; whispering voice; and stuttering are abnormal responses.

PROCEDURES AND TECHNIQUES WITH EXPECTED FINDINGS	ABNORMAL FINDINGS

NOTICE cranial nerve functions.

Assessing cranial nerves is not performed ordinarily during a routine examination. They are assessed when you suspect an abnormal finding of one or more of the cranial nerves. However, you collect data about the expected cranial nerve functions during the interview. If you notice the following expected findings, you document "CN II- CN XII grossly intact."

- The olfactory nerve (CN I) is frequently not tested; however, if the patient mentions altered taste, this may indicate a need to test for smell.

Patient reports of absence of smell or lack of taste of food and drink are abnormal.

- When the patient walks around in the room and sees the chair to sit down, the optic nerve (CN II) is intact.

If the patient bumps into furniture, squints, or needs assistance to locate a chair, it may be an indication of a vision problem.

- Observe the patient's eye movements during the interview. When his or her eyes move equally from side to side, up and down, and obliquely, the oculomotor nerve (CN III), trochlear nerve (CN IV), and abducens nerve (CN VI) are intact.

If the patient's eyes do not move or move in opposite directions, it is abnormal.

- When the patient's eyes blink, the ophthalmic branch of the trigeminal nerve (CN V) is intact.

Lack of blinking is abnormal.

- When the patient's face is symmetric when talking, the facial nerve (CN VII) is intact.

Patient's face appears asymmetric.

- When the patient hears you, the acoustic or vestibulocochlear nerve (CN VIII) is intact.

Indications of hearing loss include the patient asking you to repeat yourself; repeatedly misunderstanding questions asked; leaning forward or placing the hands behind his or her ears to screen out environmental noises.

- When you observe the patient swallowing, the glossopharyngeal nerve (CN IX) and vagus nerve (X) are intact.

Inability to swallow saliva is an abnormality.

- Hearing the patient's guttural speech sounds (e.g., k or g) indicates another function of the vagus nerve (CN X).

Absence of guttural sounds or nasal speech may indicate a vagus nerve abnormality.

- When the patient shrugs the shoulders or turns the head during the interview, the spinal accessory nerve (XI) is intact.

Absence or difficulty in turning the head may indicate a CN XI abnormality.

- When the patient enunciates words, the tongue and hypoglossal nerve (CN XII) are intact.

Speech that is not clearly articulated may indicate an abnormality with the tongue.

OBSERVE gait for balance and symmetry.

When the patient walks into the room, notice the gait. The patient should be able to maintain upright posture, walk unaided, maintain balance, and use opposing arm swing. Observing equilibrium is a test of CN VIII (acoustic or vestibulocochlear nerve).

Poor posture, ataxia, unsteady gait, rigid or absent arm movements, wide-based gait, trunk and head held tight, lurching or reeling, scissors gait, or parkinsonian gait (stooped posture; flexion at hips, elbows, and knees) is abnormal.

PROCEDURES AND TECHNIQUES WITH EXPECTED FINDINGS

ABNORMAL FINDINGS

EVALUATE extremities for muscle strength.

Test muscle strength according to the procedures outlined in Chapter 14. Muscle strength may be part of the musculoskeletal or neurologic system assessment. Ask the patient to flex the muscles being evaluated and then resist when you apply opposing force against the muscles. Expect muscle strength to be 5/5, bilaterally symmetric, with full resistance to opposition.

A fasciculation is a localized uncontrollable twitching of a single muscle group innervated by a single motor nerve fiber that may be observed or palpated. Causes of fasciculation include adverse effects of medications, cerebral palsy, neuralgia, and poliomyelitis.

Paralysis is lack of voluntary movement that is spastic or flaccid. Spastic paralysis is the involuntary contraction of muscles and occurs with pyramidal tract injury that occurs after a spinal cord injury or cerebrovascular accident (CVA). Flaccid paralysis is the lack of muscle tone and deep tendon reflexes that occurs after lower motor neuron damage such as injury to the cauda equina from spina bifida.

TEST extremities for deep tendon reflexes.

Test deep tendon reflexes for muscle contraction in response to direct or indirect percussion of a tendon. Box 15-2 outlines the scoring system. Table 15-2 lists the spinal level of each reflex. Hold the reflex hammer between your thumb and index finger and briskly tap the tendon with a flick of the wrist. The patient must be relaxed and sitting or lying down.

- To elicit the *triceps reflex,* ask the patient to let his or her relaxed arm fall onto your arm. Hold the arm, with elbow flexed at a 90-degree angle, in one hand. Palpate and then strike the triceps tendon just above the elbow with either end of the reflex hammer (Fig. 15-9, *A*). (Some nurses prefer the flat end because of the wider striking surface.) An alternative arm position is to grasp the upper arm and allow the lower arm to bend at the elbow and hang freely; then strike the triceps tendon. The expected response is the contraction of the triceps muscle that causes visible or palpable extension of the elbow.
- The biceps reflex is elicited by asking the patient to let his or her relaxed arm fall onto your arm. Hold the arm with elbow flexed at a 90-degree angle and place your thumb over the biceps tendon in the antecubital fossa and your fingers over the biceps muscle. Using the pointed end of the reflex hammer, strike your thumb instead of striking the tendon directly (see Fig. 15-9, *B*). The expected response is the contraction of the biceps muscle that causes visible or palpable flexion of the elbow.

Abnormal response may range from a hyperactive to a diminished response. Observe whether the abnormal reflex response is unilateral or bilateral.

Hyperactive reflexes are found in spinal cord injuries, calcium and magnesium deficits, and hyperthyroidism.[2] Diminished reflexes are found in calcium or magnesium excesses, hypothyroidism, spina bifida, or Guillain-Barré syndrome.

BOX 15-2 SCORING DEEP TENDON REFLEXES

Test the five deep tendon reflexes (triceps, biceps, brachioradial, patellar, and Achilles) using a reflex hammer. Compare the reflexes bilaterally. Reflexes are graded on a scale of 0 to 4, with 2 being the expected findings. Findings are recorded as follows:

0 = No response

1 + = Sluggish or diminished

2 + = Active or expected response

3 + = Slightly hyperactive, more brisk than normal; not necessarily pathologic

4 + = Brisk, hyperactive with intermittent clonus associated with disease

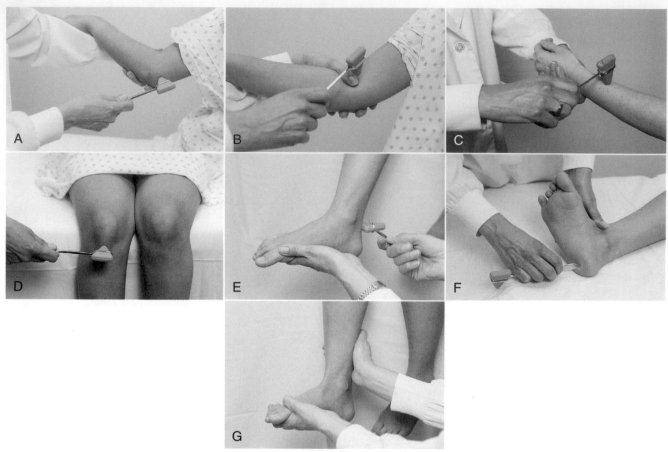

FIG. 15-9 Location of tendons for evaluation of deep tendon reflexes. **A,** Triceps reflex. **B,** Biceps reflex. **C,** Brachioradialis reflex. **D,** Patellar reflex. **E,** Achilles reflex. **F,** Babinski's reflex. **G,** Ankle tonus.

PROCEDURES AND TECHNIQUES WITH EXPECTED FINDINGS

- The *brachioradialis reflex* is elicited by asking the patient to let his or her relaxed arm fall into your hand. Hold the arm with the hand slightly pronated. Using either end of the reflex hammer, strike the brachioradialis tendon directly about 1 to 2 inches (2.5 to 5 cm) above the wrist (see Fig. 15-9, *C*). The expected response is pronation of the forearm and flexion of the elbow.
- The *patellar reflex* is tested with the patient sitting with legs hanging free. Flex his or her knee at a 90-degree angle and strike the patellar tendon just below the patella (see Fig. 15-9, *D*). The expected response is the contraction of the quadriceps muscle, causing extension of the lower leg. When no response is found, divert the patient's attention to another muscular activity by asking him or her to pull the fingers of each hand against the other. While the patient is pulling, strike the patellar tendon.
- The *Achilles tendon* is tested by flexing the patient's knee and dorsiflexing the ankle 90 degrees. Hold the bottom of the patient's foot in one hand while you use the flat end of the reflex hammer to strike the Achilles tendon at the level of the ankle malleolus (see Fig. 15-9, *E*). The expected response is the contraction of the gastrocnemius muscle, causing plantar flexion of the foot.
- Test for ankle clonus if reflexes are hyperactive. Support the patient's knee in a partly flexed position. With the other hand sharply dorsiflex the foot and maintain it in flexion (see Fig. 15-9, *G*). There should be no movement of the foot.

ABNORMAL FINDINGS

Rhythmic oscillations between dorsiflexion and plantar flexion are abnormal responses.

PROCEDURES AND TECHNIQUES WITH EXPECTED FINDINGS	ABNORMAL FINDINGS

SPECIAL CIRCUMSTANCES OR ADVANCED PRACTICE: CRANIAL NERVES

ASSESS cranial nerves.

Test these nerves when you suspect an abnormality.

TEST nose for smell.

Evaluate the olfactory cranial nerve (CN I). Have the patient close his or her eyes and mouth. Occlude one nostril while testing the other. Ask the patient to identify common aromatic substances held under the nose. Examples include coffee, toothpaste, orange, and oil of cloves (Fig. 15-10). The patient should be able to identify aromas.

An inability to smell anything or incorrect identification of odors is abnormal. Nasal allergies can impair ability to smell. Loss of smell may be caused by an olfactory tract lesion. *Anosmia* is the term used for loss of or impaired sense of smell.

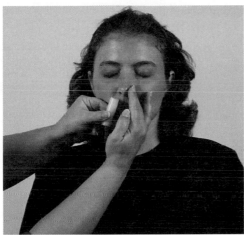

FIG. 15-10 Examination of the olfactory cranial nerve (CN I). (From Chipps, Clanin, and Campbell, 1992.)

TEST eyes for visual acuity.

Test the optic nerve (CN II) for visual acuity using Snellen's chart and an ophthalmoscopic examination of the eye (see Chapter 10).

Refer the patient to an ophthalmologist for further evaluation of vision and eye function when abnormalities are suspected. Chapter 10 provides more details.

TEST eyes for peripheral vision.

See Chapter 10 for the confrontation test. The presence of peripheral vision indicates function of the optic nerve (CN II).

If the patient cannot see the pencil or finger at the same time you see it, peripheral field loss is suggested. Refer the patient for further evaluation. Lesions in the central nervous system (e.g., tumors) may cause peripheral visual defects such as loss of vision in one half or one quarter of the visual field, either medially or laterally.

OBSERVE eyes for extraocular muscle movement.

The oculomotor (CN III), trochlear (CN IV), and abducens (CN VI) nerves are tested together because they control muscles that provide eye movement (see Chapter 10).

Eye movements that are not parallel indicate extraocular muscle weakness or dysfunction of CN III, CN IV, or CN VI. Report nystagmus other than that noted as normal. Report ptosis (eyelid droop) that may occur with ocular myasthenia gravis.

| PROCEDURES AND TECHNIQUES WITH EXPECTED FINDINGS | ABNORMAL FINDINGS |

OBSERVE eyes for pupillary size, shape, equality, constriction, and accommodation.

Pupils should appear equal, round, and reactive to light and accommodation. See Chapter 10 for this assessment technique.

Increased intracranial pressure or trauma to the midbrain may exert pressure on CN III, resulting in diminished-to-absent pupillary constriction. Pupil size can be changed by drug effects (e.g., constricted by heroin or morphine and dilated by cocaine).

EVALUATE face for movement and sensation.

• Evaluate the trigeminal nerve (CN V) for facial movement and sensation. Test motor function by having the patient clench his or her teeth; then palpate the temporal and masseter muscles for muscle mass and strength. There should be bilaterally strong muscle contractions (Fig. 15-11, *A*).

Inequality in muscle contractions, pain, twitching, or asymmetry is abnormal. Disorders of the pons (e.g., a tumor) may cause altered function of CN V or CN VII. A tic or mimic spasm is an involuntary movement of small muscles, usually of the face. Occasional tics may have psychogenic causes aggravated by anxiety or stress.

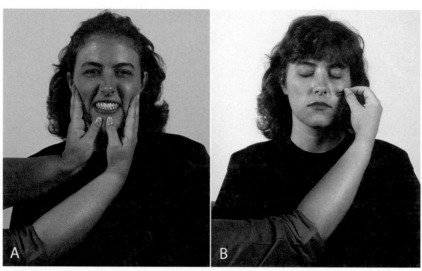

FIG. 15-11 Examination of the trigeminal nerve (CN V) for motor function **(A)** and sensory function **(B)**. (From Chipps, Clanin, and Campbell, 1992.)

• To test sensation of light touch, have the patient close his or her eyes while you wipe cotton lightly over the anterior scalp (ophthalmic branch), paranasal sinuses (maxillary branch), and jaw (mandibular branch). A tickle sensation should be reported equally over the three areas touched. Repeat the procedure on the other side of the face.

Decreased or unequal sensation is abnormal. Record the extent of the involved areas of the face.

• To test deep sensation, use alternating blunt and sharp ends of a paper clip over the patient's forehead, paranasal sinuses, and jaw. The patient should be able to feel pressure and pain equally throughout these areas and differentiate between sharp and dull (see Fig. 15-11, *B*). Repeat the procedure on the other side of the face.

Decreased or unequal sensation is abnormal. Trigeminal neuralgia is characterized by stablike pain radiating along the trigeminal nerve, caused by degeneration of or pressure on the nerve.

• Test the ophthalmic branch (sensory) of CN V and motor function of CN VII by testing for the corneal reflex. *This test may be omitted when the patient is alert and blinking naturally.* Ask the patient to remove contact lenses if applicable and to look up and away from you. Approach him or her from the side and lightly touch the cornea with a wisp of cotton. There should be a bilateral blink to corneal touch. Patients who wear contact lenses regularly may have diminished or absent reflex.

Absence of a blink is abnormal. Be sure to check that this abnormal response is not caused by the presence of contact lenses.

PROCEDURES AND TECHNIQUES WITH EXPECTED FINDINGS

- Evaluate the facial cranial nerve (CN VII) for movement. Inspect the face at rest and during conversation. Have the patient raise the eyebrows, purse the lips, close the eyes tightly, show the teeth, smile, and puff out the cheeks. He or she should be able to correctly perform each request, and the movements should be smooth and symmetric (Fig 15-12, *A* to *F*).

TEST ears for hearing.

Evaluate the acoustic or vestibulocochlear nerve (CN VIII) for hearing. Assessment of sensorineural hearing loss using the Rinne and Weber's test is described in Chapter 10. Tests for the vestibular function of CN VIII usually are not performed.[2]

ABNORMAL FINDINGS

Asymmetry, facial weakness, drooping of one side of the face or mouth, or inability to maintain position until instructed to relax is abnormal. Unilateral paralysis of the facial nerve occurs in Bell's palsy.

Sensorineural hearing loss may be indicated using Weber's test by lateralization of sound to the unaffected ear or the Rinne test when air conduction is longer than bone conduction in the affected ear but by a less than 2:1 ratio.

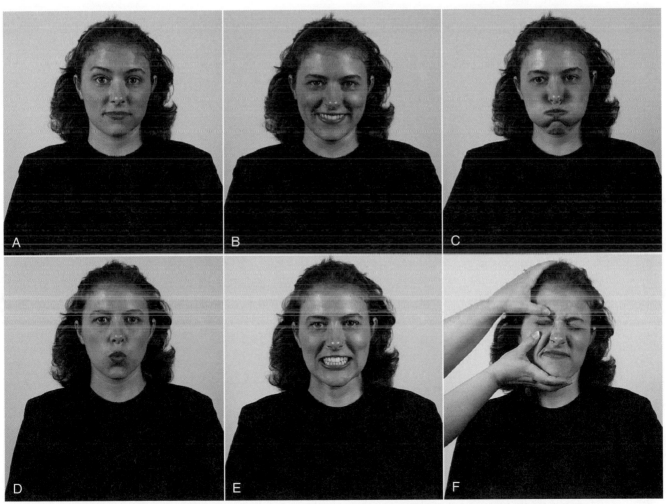

FIG. 15-12 Examination of the facial nerve (CN VII). Ask the patient to make the following movements: **A,** Raise eyebrows and wrinkle forehead. **B,** Smile. **C,** Puff out cheeks. **D,** Purse lips and blow out. **E,** Show teeth. **F,** Squeeze eyes shut while you try to open them. (From Chipps, Clanin, and Campbell, 1992.)

PROCEDURES AND TECHNIQUES WITH EXPECTED FINDINGS

TEST tongue for taste.

Evaluate taste over the anterior and posterior tongue. For the anterior two thirds of the tongue (CN VII), instruct the patient to stick out the tongue and leave it out during the testing process. Use a cotton applicator to place on the patient's anterior tongue small quantities of salt, sugar, and lemon one at a time. The patient should be able to correctly identify salty and sweet tastes (Fig. 15-13). Test the glossopharyngeal nerve for taste of the posterior one third of the tongue or pharynx (CN IX). The patient should be able to taste bitter and sour tastes. Taste, the sensory component of CN VII and CN IX, usually is not tested unless the patient reports a problem.

Inability to identify tastes or consistently identifying a substance incorrectly is abnormal. Loss of smell and taste may occur together. Patients who are chronic smokers may have decreased taste.

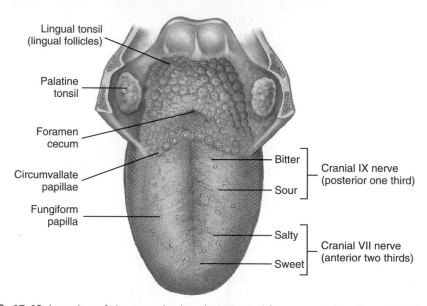

FIG. 15-13 Location of the taste bud regions tested for sensory function of the facial and glossopharyngeal cranial nerves. (From Seidel et al., 2011.)

INSPECT oropharynx for gag reflex and movement of soft palate.

Evaluate the glossopharyngeal nerve (CN IX) and the vagus nerve (CN X) together for movement of the soft palate and gag reflex. Instruct the patient to say "ah" to test CN X. There should be equal upward movement of the soft palate and uvula bilaterally. To test the gag reflex, touch the posterior pharynx with the end of a tongue blade; the patient should gag momentarily. Movement of the posterior pharynx and gag reflex test CN IX. See Chapter 10 for more detail.

Asymmetry of the soft palate or tonsillar pillar movement, any lateral deviation of the uvula, or absence of the gag reflex may indicate disorders of the medulla oblongata. For example, tumors in the medulla oblongata may cause pressure on CN IX or CN X.

TEST the tongue for movement, symmetry, strength, and absence of lesions.

Evaluate the hypoglossal nerve (CN XII) for movement and symmetry. Ask the patient to protrude his or her tongue. Note symmetry. Then ask him or her to move the tongue toward the nose, the chin, and side to side (Fig. 15-14).

Wearing gloves, grasp the tongue with a 4 × 4 gauze pad and palpate all sides (see Fig. 10-50). Test the muscle strength of the tongue by asking the patient to press the tip of the tongue inside the check while you resist the pressure from outside of the patient's cheek with your fingers. Repeat the procedure on the other side. The tongue should be moist, pink, and symmetric without lumps, nodules, or ulcers. Tongue strength should be evident by resistance to outside pressure.

Asymmetric movement or weakness of the tongue may indicate impairment of the hypoglossal cranial nerve (CN XII). The tongue deviates toward the impaired side. Tumors of the tongue may develop from alcohol, tobacco, or chronic irritation.

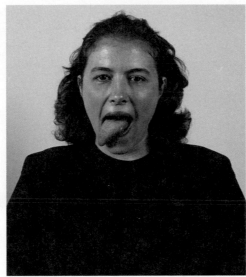

FIG. 15-14 Examination of the hypoglossal nerve (CN XII). (From Chipps, Clanin, and Campbell, 1992.)

PROCEDURES AND TECHNIQUES WITH EXPECTED FINDINGS	ABNORMAL FINDINGS

TEST shoulders and neck muscles for strength and movement.

Have the patient turn his or her head to the side against your hand; repeat with the other side (see Fig 14-18, A). Observe the contraction of the opposite sternocleido-mastoid muscle and note the force of movement against your hand. Movement should be smooth, and muscle strength should be strong and symmetric.

Weakness or pain when pushing against your hand or asymmetry is abnormal.

Evaluate the spinal accessory nerve (CN XI) for movement. Ask the patient to shrug his or her shoulders upward against your hands (see Fig 14-23). Contraction of the trapezius muscles should be strong and symmetric.

Unilateral or bilateral muscle weakness or any pain or discomfort is abnormal.

TEST cerebellar function for balance and coordination.

When patient reports or you observe impaired balance, test cerebellar function. Use at least two techniques for each area assessed (e.g., balance and coordination of upper and lower extremities). Choose these techniques based on the patient's age and overall physical ability. For example, not every patient should have to perform deep knee bends.

TEST for balance.

• Perform the Romberg test. Have the patient stand with feet together, arms resting at sides, eyes open, and then eyes closed. Stand close to the patient with arms ready to "catch" him or her if he or she begins to fall off balance. There will be slight swaying, but the upright posture and foot position should be maintained.

If the patient sways with eyes closed but not open, the problem is probably proprioceptive. If the patient sways with eyes open and closed, the problem is probably a cerebellar or vesticular disorder and is documented as a positive Romberg sign.[3]

• Have the patient close his or her eyes and stand on one foot and then the other. He or she should be able to maintain position for at least 5 seconds.

Inability to maintain single-foot balance for 5 seconds is abnormal.

• Have the patient walk in tandem, placing the heel of one foot directly against the toes of the other foot. The patient should be able to maintain this heel-toe walking pattern along a straight line (Fig. 15-15).

Inability to walk heel-to-toe or using a wide-based gait to maintain the upright posture is abnormal.

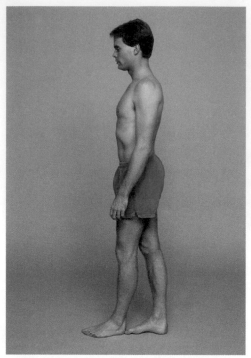

FIG. 15-15 Evaluation of balance with heel-toe walking on a straight line. (From Seidel et al., 2006.)

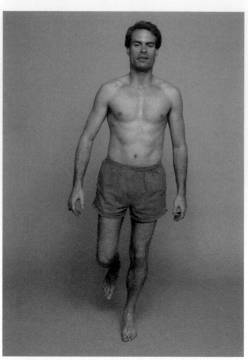

FIG. 15-16 Evaluation of balance with the patient hopping in place on one foot. (From Seidel et al., 2006.)

PROCEDURES AND TECHNIQUES WITH EXPECTED FINDINGS

- Have the patient hop first on one foot and then on the other. He or she should be able to follow directions successfully and have enough muscle strength to accomplish the task (Fig. 15-16).

- Have the patient hold one hand outward and perform several shallow or deep knee bends. He or she should be able to follow directions successfully, with muscle strength adequate to accomplish the task.

- Have the patient walk on toes, then heels. He or she should be able to follow directions, walking several steps on the toes and then on the heels. The patient may need to use the hands to maintain balance, but should be able to walk several steps.

Upper Extremity Coordination

- Have the patient alternately tap thighs with hands using rapid pronation and supination movements. Timing should be equal bilaterally, and movement purposeful; the patient should be able to maintain a rapid pace (Fig. 15-17).

ABNORMAL FINDINGS

Inability to hop or maintain single-leg balance is abnormal.

Inability to perform activity because of difficulty with balance or lack of muscle strength is abnormal.

Inability to retain balance, poor muscle strength, or inability to complete the activity is abnormal.

Inability to maintain rapid pace is abnormal. An intention tremor (i.e., an involuntary muscle contraction during a purposeful movement of an extremity that disappears when the extremity is not moving) may indicate cerebellar dysfunction.

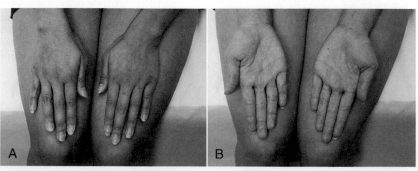

FIG. 15-17 Examination of coordination with rapid alternating movements. Ask patient to tap top of thighs with both hands, alternately with palms down **(A)** and palms up **(B)**.

PROCEDURES AND TECHNIQUES WITH EXPECTED FINDINGS	ABNORMAL FINDINGS

PROCEDURES AND TECHNIQUES WITH EXPECTED FINDINGS

- Have the patient close eyes and stretch arms outward. Use index fingers to alternately touch the nose rapidly. The patient should be able to touch the nose repeatedly in a rhythmic pattern.

- Evaluate the patient's ability to perform rapid, rhythmic, alternating movement of fingers by having him or her touch each finger to the thumb in rapid sequence. Test each hand separately. The patient should be able to perform movement rapidly and purposefully, touching each finger to thumb (Fig. 15-18).

- Have the patient rapidly move his or her index finger back and forth between his or her nose and your finger 46 cm (18 in) apart. Test one hand at a time. The patient should be able to maintain the activity with a conscious, coordinated effort (Fig. 15-19).

Lower Extremity Coordination

With the patient lying supine, ask him or her to place the heel of one foot to the knee of the other leg, sliding it all the way down the shin (Fig. 15-20). Repeat on the other leg. The patient should be able to run the heel down the opposite shin purposefully, with equal coordination.

ABNORMAL FINDINGS

Cerebellar dysfunction may cause the patient to miss touching his or her nose several times or cause the arms to drift downward.

Inability to coordinate fine, discrete, rapid movement is abnormal. An intention tremor may be observed during the movement, indicating a cerebellar dysfunction.

Inability to maintain continuous touch both with the patient's own nose and your finger, inability to maintain the rapid movement, or obvious difficulty coordinating is abnormal.

Patients with cerebellar disease may overshoot the knee and oscillate back and forth. With loss of position sense, the patient may lift the heel too high and have to look to ensure that it is moving down the shin.

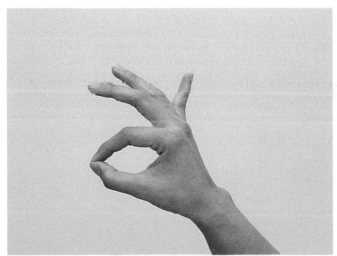

FIG. 15-18 Examination of finger coordination. Ask patient to touch each finger to thumb in rapid sequence.

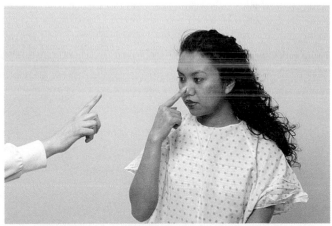

FIG. 15-19 Examination of fine-motor function. Ask patient to alternately touch own nose and the nurse's index finger with the index finger of one hand.

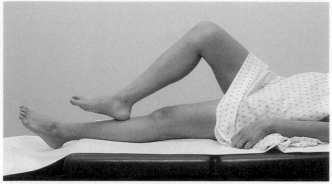

FIG. 15-20 Examination of lower-extremity coordination. Ask patient to run heel of one foot down shin of other leg. Repeat with opposite leg.

| **PROCEDURES AND TECHNIQUES WITH EXPECTED FINDINGS** | **ABNORMAL FINDINGS** |

ASSESS peripheral nerves.

ASSESS for sensation.

Ask the patient to close his or her eyes during the tests of sensory function. Areas routinely assessed are the hands, lower arms, abdomen, lower legs, and feet. If sensation is intact, no further evaluation is needed; if impaired, assess sensation systemically from digits up or from shoulder or hip down to identify the area that is without sensation. Compare bilateral responses in each sensory testing area. Try to map out the area involved using the dermatome map (see Fig. 15-7) to identify the spinal nerve providing sensation to that area of the body.

Impaired or absent sensation is abnormal. Absence of sensation may be caused by compression of the nerve, whereas inflammation of the nerve may cause abnormal sensation. Diabetes mellitus may cause absent or abnormal sensation.

- To test sensation to light touch (superficial touch), use a cotton wisp and the lightest touch possible to test each designated area (patient's eyes are closed) (Fig. 15-21, *A*). The patient should perceive light sensation and be able to correctly point to or name the spot touched.

Abnormal findings include the patient reporting that he or she does not feel the light touch, incorrectly identifying the area touched, not feeling the vibration, or reporting an asymmetric response.

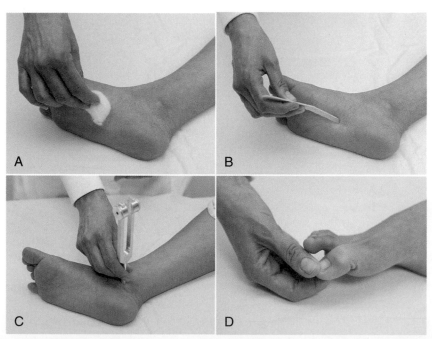

FIG. 15-21 Evaluation of peripheral nerve sensory function. **A,** Superficial tactile sensation. **B,** Superficial pain sensation. **C,** Vibratory sensation. **D,** Position sense of joints.

PROCEDURES AND TECHNIQUES WITH EXPECTED FINDINGS

- ★ A monofilament is used to test peripheral sensation (see Fig. 3-27).

- Test sharp and dull sensation by using the pointed tip of a paper clip (or broken tongue blade) to lightly prick each designated area (patient's eyes are closed) (see Fig. 15-21, *B*). Alternate sharp and dull sensations to more accurately evaluate the patient's response. The patient should be able to distinguish sharp from dull and identify the area touched.

- Ask the patient to close his or her eyes for the test of vibratory sense. Place a vibrating tuning fork on a bony area such as the styloid process of the radius (wrist), medial or lateral malleolus (ankle), and sternum (chest) and ask the patient to describe the sensation (see Fig. 15-21, *C*). He or she should feel a sense of vibration. Also ask the patient to report when he or she no longer feels vibration; then stop vibration of the tuning fork by touching it with your fingers without moving it from its location on the bony prominence.

- Test kinesthetic sensation by grasping the patient's finger or toe and moving its position 1 cm up or down (patient's eyes are closed) (see Fig. 15-21, *D*). The patient should be able to describe how the position has changed.

- ★ Test stereognosis by asking the patient to close his or her eyes. Place a small, familiar object in the patient's hand and ask him or her to identify it (Fig. 15-22, *A*). The object should be properly identified.

ABNORMAL FINDINGS

Inability to feel monofilament indicates reduced peripheral sensation. This abnormal finding may occur in patients with diabetes mellitus who have peripheral neuropathy.

Abnormal findings include the patient reporting that he or she does not feel the sharp or dull touch, being unable to distinguish between sharp and dull, or reporting an asymmetric response.

Unequal or decreased vibratory sensation is abnormal. The patient may not be able to distinguish the change in sensation from vibration to nonvibration or may not feel the vibration in one or more locations. Referring to the dermatome drawing (see Fig. 15-7) helps to identify the spinal nerve supplying this area. This may be found in patients with diabetes mellitus and those who have had a CVA or spinal cord injury.

Inability to distinguish the change in position may indicate impairment of sensory (afferent nerves) or parietal lobe.

Altered stereognosis may indicate a parietal lobe or sensory nerve tract dysfunction and is documented as tactile agnosia[3].

★ Advanced practice

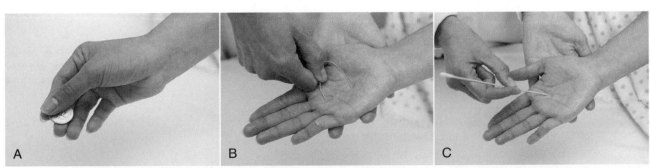

FIG. 15-22 Evaluation of cortical sensory function. **A,** Stereognosis: identification of a familiar object by touch. **B,** Two-point discrimination. **C,** Graphesthesia: draw letter or number on palm and ask patient to identify by touch.

BOX 15-3	MINIMAL DISTANCES FOR DISTINGUISHING TWO POINTS
LOCATION	**MINIMAL DISTANCE**
Tongue	1 mm or $\frac{1}{32}$ inch*
Fingertips	2-8 mm or $\frac{2}{32}$* to $\frac{5}{16}$ inch
Toes	3-8 mm or $\frac{3}{32}$* to $\frac{5}{16}$ inch
Palm of hand	8 to 12 mm or $\frac{5}{16}$ to $\frac{1}{2}$ inch
Chest and forearms	40 mm or $1\frac{1}{2}$ inches
Back	40-70 mm or $1\frac{1}{2}$ to $2\frac{3}{4}$ inches
Upper arms and thighs	75 mm or 3 inches

*Too small to measure with conventional ruler.

PROCEDURES AND TECHNIQUES WITH EXPECTED FINDINGS

ABNORMAL FINDINGS

- ★ Test two-point discrimination by touching selected parts of the body simultaneously while the patient's eyes are closed (see Fig. 15-22, *B*). Use the points of two cotton-tipped applicators or reshape a paper clip so two prongs can be pressed lightly against the patient's skin simultaneously. Ask the patient how many points he or she detects. The expected values for two-point discrimination are listed in Box 15-3.

Inability to distinguish two-point discrimination is abnormal. Report the anatomic location of the sensory alteration.

- Evaluate graphesthesia using a blunt instrument to draw a number or letter on the patient's hand, back, or other area (patient has eyes closed) (see Fig. 15-22, *C*). He or she should be able to recognize the number or letter drawn.

If the patient cannot distinguish the number or letter, he or she may have a parietal lobe lesion.

- ★ Check for the plantar reflex (Babinski reflex). Using the end of the handle on the reflex hammer, stroke the lateral aspect of the sole of the foot from heel to ball, curving medially across the ball of the foot (see Fig. 15-9, *F*). The expected findings should be plantar flexion of all toes.

Dorsiflexion of the great toe with fanning of the other toes is an abnormal response termed a *positive Babinski's sign* and may indicate pyramidal (motor) tract disease.

EVALUATE for superficial reflexes.

Testing abdominal reflexes is described in Chapter 13 (see Fig. 13-17). In assessing the neurologic system, you correlate the expected response with the spinal level involved. See Table 15-2 for the spinal level of these reflexes. The testing of superficial reflexes is included here for completeness; however, there is little clinical significance to their presence or absence.[2]

Diminished-to-absent response is found on the side of a corticospinal tract (motor tract) lesion.[2]

For male patients: Check the cremasteric reflex. Lightly stroke the upper, inner aspect of the thigh with the reflex hammer or tongue blade. The ipsilateral testicle should rise slightly.

Absence of the cremasteric reflex is seen in disorders of the pyramidal (motor) tract above the level of the first lumbar vertebrae.

DOCUMENTING EXPECTED FINDINGS

Oriented to person, place, and time. Speech understandable and of sufficient volume. Cranial nerves II to XII grossly intact. Balanced gait with upright posture. Muscle strength 5/5 and movement coordinated bilaterally; negative Romberg sign. Peripheral sensation intact. Deep tendon reflexes 2+ bilaterally. No clonus present.

★ Advanced practice.

❓ CLINICAL REASONING: THINKING LIKE A NURSE

Neurologic System

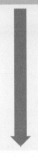

A 19-year-old male college student is brought to the student health services with a chief complaint of headache. He is accompanied by his roommate, who explains that the patient was playing a game of football with friends and struck the right side of his head when he collided with another player.

Interpreting

Early in the encounter the nurse considers two possible causes of the headache: scalp trauma (hematoma, laceration), closed head injury (CHI), or both. The nurse also knows that CHI can present in many ways, depending on the type of injury. The nurse gathers additional data.

- Is there evidence of external trauma? The nurse palpates a lump over the right temporal region of the scalp. The skin is intact.
- Was there a loss of consciousness? The patient was "knocked out" for a few minutes.
- Are there any neurologic changes? The patient does not recall playing football or sustaining the injury. The roommate reports that he keeps asking the same questions. The nurse notes an unsteady gait with ambulation; pupils equal, round, react to light and accommodation (PERRLA).

The experienced nurse not only recognizes abnormal clinical findings (loss of consciousness, headache, memory impairment, unsteady gait) but also interprets this information in the context of an individual who has had a recent blow to the head.

Nurse's Background, Experience, Perspective

The experienced nurse knows that this type of injury can result in mild or significant brain injury and that neurologic changes may be overt or subtle.

Noticing

This background knowledge sets up the possibility of noticing signs of a prevalent complication in an individual presenting with these data. The patient is alert and oriented to time, place, and person; his vital signs are within expected parameters. The nurse learns that the incident took place 4 hours ago. The patient has a headache that is getting worse. Given the nature of his injury and symptoms, the nurse recognizes the possibility of closed head injury (CHI); this background knowledge sets up the possibility of noticing signs of brain swelling in an individual presenting with these manifestations.

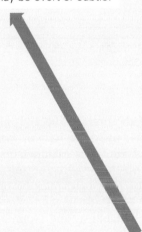

Responding

The nurse initiates appropriate initial interventions and notifies the primary care provider of the situation, ensuring that the patient receives appropriate immediate and follow-up care.

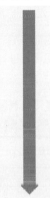

Reflecting

The nurse evaluates the presentation and outcomes of interventions (reflection-in-action); this experience contributes to and deepens the expertise on which to draw (reflection-on-action) when encountering a similar situation.

AGE-RELATED VARIATIONS

Nurses adapt their examinations of the neurologic system when assessing patients at either end of the life span. Neonates and infants have age-dependent reflexes to assess, whereas the development of children is compared with standardized norms. Older adults are assessed for falls.

▌INFANTS AND CHILDREN

There are several differences in the assessment of the system for infants and young children. Infants' sensation and cranial nerves are assessed by observation. Unique reflexes are assessed in infants. Children's motor development is compared with standardized tables of normal age and sequences of motor development. Assessment of the older child and adolescent follows the same procedures as for adults and reveals similar expected findings. Chapter 19 presents further information regarding neurologic assessment of infants, children, and adolescents.

OLDER ADULTS

Assessing the neurologic system of an older adult usually follows the same procedures as for the younger adult. Tests for balance and gait of older adults are often assessed to identify those at risk for falls. Chapter 21 presents further information regarding the neurologic assessment of older adults.

COMMON PROBLEMS AND CONDITIONS

RISK FACTORS

Cerebrovascular Accident (Stroke)

- *Age:* Older adults are at greater risk.
- *Gender:* Men have a greater risk than women. However, women account for more than half of the deaths from cerebrovascular accidents (CVAs). Women who are pregnant have a higher risk than nonpregnant women as do women who take birth control pills or hormone replacement therapy and smoke or have hypertension. Women who have migraine headaches with an aura are at greater risk.
- *Family history:* Risk is greater if parent, grandparent, or sibling had a CVA.
- *Race:* African Americans have a higher risk of death from CVA than Caucasians. Stroke is the fourth leading cause of death among Hispanics.
- Previous CVA or heart attack increases risk of a CVA.
- High blood pressure (greater than 120/80 mm Hg) puts undue pressure on arteries. (M)

- *Smoking:* Nicotine constricts blood vessels, and carbon monoxide reduces the oxygen in the blood. (M)
- Diabetes mellitus contributes to hypertension, hypercholesterolemia, and thrombus formation. (M)
- Atherosclerosis narrows the carotid vessels, reducing the blood flow to the brain. (M)
- High serum cholesterol forms plaques in the vessels that impair blood flow to the brain. (M)
- Obesity increases workload on the heart and risk of high cholesterol and physical inactivity. (M)
- Excessive alcohol intake increases blood pressure. (M)
- Transient ischemic attacks (TIAs) are warning signs that there is inadequate blood flow to the brain. (M)
- Atrial fibrillation may form blood clots in the atrium that can travel to the brain. (M)
- Cocaine use increases risk of CVAs. (M)

Data from http://www.strokeassociation.org/STROKEORG/LifeAfterStroke/HealthyLivingAfterStroke/UnderstandingRiskyConditions/Understanding-Risky-Conditions_UCM_310897_Article.jsp, updated January, 2011, accessed October 24, 2011.
M, Modifiable risk factor.

DISORDERS OF THE CENTRAL NERVOUS SYSTEM

Multiple Sclerosis

Progressive demyelination of nerve fibers of the brain and spinal cord results in multiple sclerosis. It is an autoimmune disorder initiated by a virus that attacks the myelin at various sites of the central nervous system. **Clinical Findings:** Manifestations vary, depending on the areas of the central nervous system that are affected by the demyelination. Common symptoms are fatigue, depression, and paresthesias. Other manifestations are focal muscle weakness; ocular changes (diplopia, nystagmus); bowel, bladder, and sexual dysfunction; gait instability; and spasticity.

Meningitis

Inflammation of the meninges that surround the brain and spinal cord is termed *meningitis*. It may result from invasion of bacteria, viruses, fungi, parasites, or other toxins. **Clinical Findings:** Meningitis produces severe headache, fever, and malaise. A sign of meningeal irritation is nuchal rigidity or a stiff neck. Level of consciousness may decrease with drowsiness and reduced attention span, which may progress to stupor and coma. Confusion, agitation, and irritability may occur.

Encephalitis

Inflammation of the brain tissue and meninges is termed *encephalitis.* It is caused by bacteria, viruses, fungi, and parasites. **Clinical Findings:** Manifestations of encephalitis vary, depending on the invading organism and the part of the brain involved. The onset may be gradual or sudden, with symptoms of headache and nausea and signs of fever, lethargy, irritability, and vomiting. Over several days the patient may develop decreased consciousness, motor weakness, tremors, seizures, aphasia, and positive Babinski's sign.[4]

Spinal Cord Injury

Any traumatic disruption of the spinal cord can result in a spinal cord injury. Common causes of spinal cord injuries are vertebral fractures and dislocations such as those suffered by individuals involved in car accidents, sports injuries, and other violent impacts. Injury to the cervical spinal cord may result in quadriplegia, whereas injury to the thoracic and lumbar spinal cord may result in paraplegia. **Clinical Findings:** Manifestations of complete spinal cord transection include paresthesia or anesthesia, and signs are paralysis below the level of injury with loss of bowel and bladder control. Spinal cord injuries damage the upper motor neurons, causing a spastic paralysis. When the injury to the spinal cord is incomplete, manifestations are variable and correlate to the location and extent of injury.

Craniocerebral Injury (Head Injury)

Any injury to the scalp, skull, or brain that is sufficient to alter normal function can result in craniocerebral injury. Open head injuries result from fractures or penetrating wounds; closed head injuries result from blunt head injury producing cerebral concussion or contusion. **Clinical Findings:** Manifestations of head injury vary, depending on the severity of the trauma and the areas of the brain involved. Residual deficits in memory, cognition, and motor and sensory abilities depend on the extent of injury to the brain.

Parkinson's Disease

Parkinson's disease develops slowly due to degeneration of the dopamine-producing neurons in the substantia nigra of the basal ganglia. **Clinical Findings:** The disease is characterized by resting tremor, bradykinesia, and rigidity. Other manifestations include masklike facies, trunk-forward flexion, muscle weakness, shuffling gait, and finger pill-rolling tremor (Fig. 15-23).

Cerebrovascular Accident (Stroke)

When cerebral blood vessels become occluded by a thrombus or embolus or when intracranial hemorrhage occurs, the brain tissues become ischemic, resulting in a CVA or stroke. Hemorrhage can be caused by hypertension or a cerebral aneurysm (a weakened area in an artery that balloons out as a result of the high pressure of blood). **Clinical Findings:** Manifestations are directly related to the area of the brain involved and the extent of ischemic area. For example, ischemia to the left frontal lobe may result in paralysis of the right arm or leg. There may be sudden unilateral numbness or weakness of the face, arm, or leg. The patient may complain of trouble walking, dizziness, or loss of balance or coordination. A sudden, severe headache with no known cause may be a symptom. There may be sudden confusion, difficulty swallowing (dysphagia), difficulty speaking or understanding speech (aphasia), or partial loss of vision. See the problem-based history for additional information on assessing patients with aphasia or dysphagia.

Alzheimer's Disease

This is an incurable, degenerative neurologic disorder that begins with a decline in memory. It is the most common cause of dementia in western countries. The exact cause is unknown; however, theories suggest genetic tendency, altered function of neurotransmitters, or a mutation for encoding certain precursor proteins as contributing factors. **Clinical Findings:** Three stages of Alzheimer's disease have been described. The early stage lasts 2 to 4 years when the patient's memory (e.g., forgetting names and misplacing items) begins to fail. The second stage lasts from 2 to 12 years when the patient experiences progressive memory loss and has difficulty with activities of daily living. Language skills deteriorate, and the patient becomes disoriented and confused with poor concentration. During the final stage the patient requires total care and is unable to communicate.[4]

DISORDERS OF CRANIAL NERVES

Trigeminal Neuralgia

An intense paroxysmal pain along one or all three of the branches of the trigeminal nerve (CN V) is termed *trigeminal neuralgia* or *tic douloureux*. Although the etiology is unknown, trauma to the face or head and infection of the teeth or jaw are contributing factors. Many patients can identify trigger points in small areas on the cheek, lip, gum, or forehead that initiate pain when stimulated. **Clinical Findings:** Patients report an abrupt, intense unilateral pain along the tissue innervated by the trigeminal nerve that lasts a few seconds.[4]

Bell's Palsy

This is an acute unilateral paralysis of the facial nerve. About 80% of patients recover fully after a few weeks to months. **Clinical Findings:** Patients report a history of pain behind the ear or on the face a few hours or days before the onset of paralysis. On the affected side the eye does not close, the forehead does not wrinkle, and the patient is unable to whistle or smile.[4]

DISORDERS OF PERIPHERAL NERVES

Myasthenia Gravis

This neuromuscular disease is characterized by weakness of voluntary muscles that improves with rest and administration of anticholinesterase drugs. In myasthenia gravis acetylcholine receptor sites are destroyed by autoantibodies, causing muscle weakness. In some cases it is associated with tumors

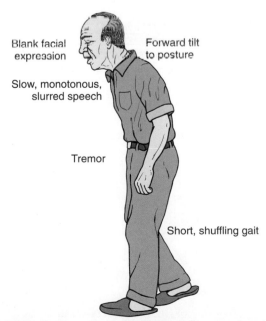

Blank facial expression

Forward tilt to posture

Slow, monotonous, slurred speech

Tremor

Short, shuffling gait

Fig. 15-23 Posture and shuffling gait associated with Parkinson's disease. (From Christensen and Kockrow, 2011.)

of the thymus gland. There are three types of myasthenia: (1) ocular, which affects only the eyes; (2) bulbar, which involves the nerves that innervate the muscles needed for swallowing (CN IX, CN X, CN XI, and CN XII); and (3) generalized, which affects skeletal muscles of the arms, legs, and trunk. **Clinical Findings:** Manifestations vary with the type of myasthenia. Ocular myasthenia produces muscle weakness confined to the muscles of the eye, causing ptosis and diplopia. Patients with bulbar myasthenia often aspirate saliva and other fluids because of impaired swallowing. Generalized myasthenia produces weakness of the face, limbs, and trunk, including the muscles of breathing.

Guillain-Barré Syndrome

This acute syndrome is characterized by widespread demyelinization of nerves of the peripheral nervous system. Guillain-Barré syndrome affects the motor component of peripheral nerves and is believed to be caused by a cell-mediated autoimmune response to a viral infection. Patients usually have a respiratory or gastrointestinal viral infection weeks before the onset. Between 80% and 90% of patients recover from this syndrome with few or no residual deficits; however, patients may die when respiratory depression develops rapidly. **Clinical Findings:** The usual manifestation is an ascending paralysis that begins with weakness and paresthesia in the lower extremities and ascends to the upper extremities and face. If ascending paralysis reaches the thorax, respiratory depression may result. There is a descending variation of Guillain-Barré syndrome that begins with the facial, glossopharyngeal, vagus, and hypoglossal cranial nerves and moves downward more commonly to the hand, but it can reach the feet. Deep tendon reflexes are absent.[4]

CLINICAL APPLICATION AND CLINICAL REASONING

See Appendix D for answers to exercises in this section.

REVIEW QUESTIONS

1. The nurse gives a key to a patient with a tumor in the cerebrum and asks the patient to close her eyes and identify the object. The patient manipulates the key, but she cannot identify what it is. From this finding the nurse suspects that the patient's tumor is located in which lobe of the cerebrum?
   1. Frontal lobe
   2. Parietal lobe
   3. Temporal lobe
   4. Occipital lobe

2. During a symptom analysis the patient reports a pain that radiates from the right lateral thigh, over the knee, and around to the right medial ankle. The nurse refers to the dermatome map (see Fig. 15-7) to determine that the patient's description of pain is consistent with dysfunction of which spinal nerve?
   1. Second lumbar (L2)
   2. Third lumbar (L3)
   3. Fourth lumbar (L4)
   4. Fifth lumbar (L5)

3. The nurse is checking the deep tendon reflexes of a patient who has compression of the fifth and sixth cervical nerves on the right. Which deep tendon reflex is diminished?
   1. Right biceps reflex
   2. Left brachioradialis reflex
   3. Right triceps reflex
   4. Left patellar reflex

4. When assessing a patient with a tumor within the medulla oblongata, the nurse notes which abnormal finding?
   1. Absent gag reflex
   2. Inability to smile and raise eyebrows
   3. Loss of sensation to the face
   4. Hearing deficit with unsteady gait

5. Which techniques does the nurse use to test the triceps reflex?
   1. Holds the knee in a slightly flexed position while he or she strokes the end of the foot with a dull object
   2. Holds the patient's relaxed forearm with the hand slightly pronated while striking the appropriate tendon with a reflex hammer
   3. Hold the patient's relaxed arm with elbow flexed at a 90-degree angle, places a thumb over the appropriate tendon, and strikes the thumb with the pointed end of the reflex hammer
   4. Holds the patient's relaxed arm with elbow flexed at a 90-degree angle in one hand and strikes the appropriate tendon just above the elbow with either end of the reflex hammer

6. Which technique is used to assess the cerebellum?
   1. Application of a pointed tip of a paper clip to lightly prick various areas of the upper and lower extremities to test for sensation
   2. Having the patient walk on the heels and then on the toes to test for balance
   3. With the patient's eyes closed, grasping his or her finger or toe and moving its position 1 cm up or down to determine if the patient perceives that the digit has moved
   4. Having the patient lie supine and flex the hips and knees to test for mobility and range of motion.

CASE STUDY

Leo Thompson is a 54-year-old African American man admitted to the hospital with a diagnosis of acute CVA. The following data are collected by the nurse during an interview and examination.

Interview Data

Mr. Thompson's wife tells the nurse that he was fine until this morning, when he suddenly had a headache, fell to the floor, and could not get up. Mrs. Thompson adds that her husband made only mumbling noises and she could not understand him. He has type 2 diabetes mellitus and hypertension. He stopped smoking last year.

Examination Data

- *Neurologic examination:* Awake, alert man. Unable to talk but able to follow commands. Cries and avoids eye contact with his wife and nurse.
- Cranial nerves III, IV, V, VI, and VIII are intact bilaterally. Patient has asymmetry and unequal movements of face, with a drooping of the left side of face. He has asymmetry of shoulder shrug, with weakness noted on left side. He has supination and pronation of right hand and is unable to perform with left hand. Light touch with sharp and dull sensation is present on right arm and leg; there is no sensation on left arm or leg. Right arm and leg muscle strength is 5, left arm muscle tone 0, left leg 1. He is unable to move around in bed unassisted at this time. Assessment of balance is deferred.

Clinical Reasoning

1. Which data deviate from expected findings, suggesting a need for further investigation?
2. For which additional information should the nurse ask or assess?
3. Based on the data, which risk factors for CVA does Mr. Thompson have?
4. With which team member would the nurse collaborate to meet this patient's needs?

CHAPTER

16

Breasts and Axillae

evolve WEBSITE

http://evolve.elsevier.com/Wilson/assessment

ANATOMY AND PHYSIOLOGY

The breasts are paired mammary glands located within the superficial fascia of the anterior chest wall. Breasts are a feature of all mammals, evolving as milk-producing organs to provide nourishment for offspring. During embryologic development these glands develop along paired "milk lines," an embryonic ridge that extends between the limb buds of what will become the axillae and the inguinal regions. Normally only one gland develops on each side in the pectoral region. After birth the glands undergo little additional development in the male. However, in the female the breasts undergo considerable development during adolescence under the influence of estrogen and progesterone.

FEMALE BREAST

The breast of the mature female has a distinctive shape; however, the "normal" breast size varies greatly. The breasts extend vertically from the second to the sixth ribs and laterally from the sternal margin to the midaxillary line. To facilitate description (or location of lesions), breasts are divided into quadrants by imaginary vertical and horizontal lines intersecting at the nipple (Fig. 16-1).

The female breast is composed of three types of tissue: glandular, fibrous, and subcutaneous and retromammary fat. The glandular tissue is arranged into 15 to 20 lobes per breast, radiating around the nipple in a spokelike pattern (Fig. 16-2). Each lobe is composed of 20 to 40 lobules, or alveoli, containing the milk-producing acini cells. During lactation, milk produced by acini cells empties into the lactiferous ducts. These ducts drain milk from the lobes to the surface of the nipple. The largest amount of glandular tissue lies in the upper outer quadrant of each breast. From this quadrant the breast tissue extends into the axilla, forming the axillary tail of Spence.

The breast is supported by a layer of subcutaneous fibrous tissue and by multiple fibrous bands termed *Cooper's ligaments.* These suspensory ligaments extend from the connective tissue layer and run through the breast, attaching to the underlying muscle fascia. Subcutaneous and retromammary fat surrounds the glandular tissue and composes most of the breast.

Centrally located on the breast, the nipple is surrounded by the pigmented areola. The nipples are composed of epithelium intertwined with circular and longitudinal smooth muscle fibers. These muscles contract in response to sensory, tactile, or autonomic stimuli, producing erection of the nipple and causing the lactiferous ducts to empty. A number of sebaceous glands, termed *Montgomery's glands,* are located within the areolar surface, aiding in lubrication of the nipple during lactation.

Throughout the reproductive years the breasts undergo a cyclic pattern of size change, nodularity, and tenderness during the menstrual cycle. The breasts are smallest during days 4 through 7 of the menstrual cycle. Three to four days before the onset of menses, many women experience breast fullness, tenderness, and pain because of hormonal changes and fluid retention.

The breasts undergo a dramatic change during pregnancy and lactation in response to luteal and placental hormones. These changes include an increase in the number of lactiferous ducts and the size and number of alveoli. See Chapter 20 for further information.

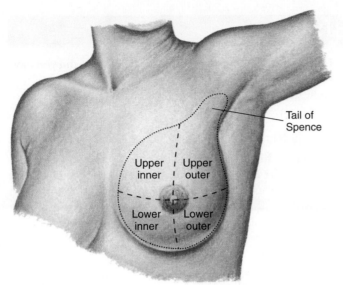

FIG. 16-1 Quadrants of the left breast and axillary tail of Spence. (From Seidel et al., 2011.)

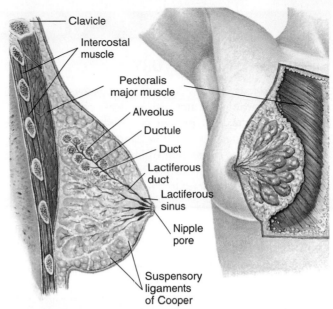

Fig. 16-2 Anatomy of the breast, showing position and major structures. (From Seidel et al., 2011.)

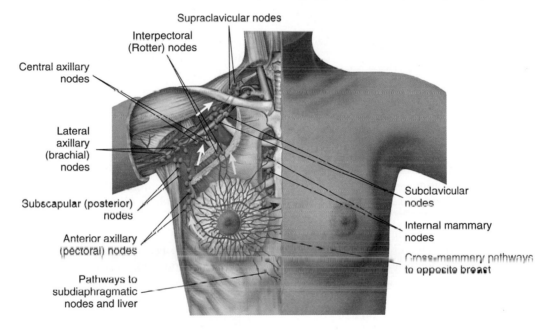

FIG. 16-3 Lymphatic drainage of the breast. (From Seidel et al., 2011.)

Lymphatic Network

Each breast contains an extensive lymphatic network, which drains into lymph nodes in several areas. As blood flows through the capillary bed, fluid is forced out into the interstitial space and into the cells. Most of the fluid is immediately resorbed into the capillaries; however, fluid left in the interstitial spaces is eventually absorbed by the lymph system and carried through the lymph nodes. More than 75% of lymph drainage from the breast flows outward toward the axillary lymph node groups and then upward to the subclavicular and supraclavicular nodes. Other routes for lymph drainage include flow through the anterior axillae (pectoral) nodes (above the breast), internal mammary nodes (in the thorax), and subdiaphragmatic nodes (toward the abdomen)

and through cross-mammary pathways to the opposite breast (Fig. 16-3).[1]

MALE BREAST

The male breast undergoes very little additional development after birth, and the gland remains rudimentary. It consists of a thin layer of undeveloped tissue beneath the nipple. The areola of the nipple is small when compared with that of the female. During puberty the male breast may become slightly enlarged, producing a temporary condition termed *gynecomastia*. Although gynecomastia is usually unilateral, it may occur bilaterally. The older male may also have gynecomastia secondary to a decrease in testosterone.

HEALTH HISTORY

GENERAL HEALTH HISTORY

Nurses interview patients to collect subjective data about their present health and any past medical experiences. They ask patients about their present health status, past medical history, family history, and personal and psychosocial history as they relate to the assessment of breasts and axilla. Quality Improvement Competencies for Nurses include providing patient-centered care. Refer to Table 11-1 on p. 196 for specific competencies.

Present Health Status

Do you take any medications? If so, what do you take and how often? Why do you take them?

Some medications such as oral contraceptives can cause cyclic breast discomfort or nipple discharge. Some individuals take a vitamin E supplement to reduce symptoms of breast edema and tenderness.

How much chocolate and caffeine do you consume each day or each week?

A diet high in methylxanthines (found in foods containing caffeine) may cause benign breast disease such as fibrocystic changes.[2]

Past Health History

Have you ever had a breast problem such as fibrocystic changes to the breast, fibroadenoma, or breast cancer? If so, describe. When did it occur? How was it diagnosed? How was it treated?

A history of breast cancer increases the risk of recurrence.[3] Fibrocystic changes to the breast and fibroadenoma complicate the evaluation of the breasts because the presence of cysts makes it difficult to detect new masses or lumps. Determination of the time frame and previous treatment is included in the history as baseline information for the present visit.

Do you have a past medical history involving ovarian cancer, endometrial cancer, or colon cancer?

A personal history of ovarian, endometrial, or colon cancer increases the risk of breast cancer.

Have you ever had surgery on a breast (e.g., biopsy, mastectomy, lumpectomy, or breast reduction or augmentation)? If so, when was it and why did you have it?

This is helpful background information; it may affect findings noted with examination.

How old were you when you began menstruating? How old were you at menopause (if appropriate)?

Menarche before age 12 or menopause after age 50 increases the risk for breast cancer.

Have you ever been pregnant? If so, at what age did you have your children?

Nulliparous or first child born after age 30 is a risk factor for breast cancer.

Family History

Is there a history of breast cancer or breast disease in your family? If so, in whom? At what age did this relative have breast cancer or disease? Did it affect one or both breasts?

Family history is a risk factor for breast cancer, particularly if it involves first-degree relatives (mother, sister, or daughter). Having one first-degree relative with breast cancer approximately doubles a woman's risk; two first-degree relatives with breast cancer triples the risk.[3]

Personal and Psychosocial History

Do you perform breast self-examination (BSE)? If so, how often?

Evaluating self-care behaviors helps guide further education and encourages health-enhancing behaviors. Women should know how their breasts normally feel and be encouraged to report any breast change promptly to their health care providers.

Do you have regular examination of your breasts by a health care professional? If so, how often? Have you ever had a mammogram? If so, when was your last mammogram? How frequently do you have a mammogram?

Clinical breast examination (CBE) is performed as part of an examination, and documenting the last CBE is important for baseline information. Because mammography is considered an effective method for breast cancer screening in women over 40 years of age,[4] the nurse asks these patients if and when the last mammography was performed.

PROBLEM-BASED HISTORY

The most commonly reported problems related to the breasts are pain or tenderness, breast lump, nipple discharge, pain or lumps in the axillae, and breast swelling or enlargement in men. As with symptoms in all areas of health assessment, a symptom analysis is completed using the mnemonic OLD CARTS, which includes the Onset, Location, Duration, Characteristics, Aggravating factors, Related symptoms, Treatments, and Severity (see Box 2-3).

Breast Pain or Tenderness

Where does it hurt? Is the pain in one breast or both? Is there a specific location or is the pain generalized? When did the pain in your breasts first begin?

Along with breast mass, breast pain is among the most common breast-related symptoms.[5] Determine the onset and location of the breast pain. Pain occurring bilaterally is more likely attributed to hormonal effects; pain in one breast could suggest a pathologic condition.

Describe the pain. Rate the severity of the pain on a scale from 0 to 10. Does the pain or tenderness prevent you from carrying out routine activities?
Determine the characteristics of the pain. Some women with breast cancer report a burning or pulling sensation in addition to a vague pain. Rapidly growing cysts may be very painful. Limitations in activity may also help the nurse understand how the pain affects the patient.

Have you noticed any specific activities that bring on the pain? For example, do you experience it during sexual activity? When you exercise? When wearing a certain bra or when not wearing a bra?
Determine any aggravating factors for the pain. Strenuous activity can bring on pain, as can the other specific causes noted.

Have you noted any recent changes in your breasts such as changes in size, shape, tenderness, lumps, or discharge?
Question the patient for associated symptoms with the breast pain.

Is the breast tenderness associated with a swollen feeling to the breasts? If yes, when do you notice the swelling? Is it related to your menstrual cycle?
Cyclic bilateral breast edema or fullness is a normal occurrence caused by hormonal fluctuations associated with the menstrual cycle. Significant edema should be further evaluated, especially if it is unilateral, has other associated findings, or influences the woman's ability to participate in usual activities.

Breast Lump

Where is the breast lump? When did you first notice it?
Establish the onset and location of all breast lumps. Some lumps may be present over a period of several years. If they do not undergo change, they may be insignificant but still should be examined. Any new lumps or changes in a previously identified and documented lump should be of particular concern.

Is the lump always present or does it seem to come and go? Is there a relationship between the lumps and your menstrual cycle?
Lumps that change in size in relation to the menstrual cycle may be influenced by hormonal fluctuations.

Is the lump tender to the touch? If yes, does the severity of the tenderness change related to menstruation?
Determine the characteristics of the lump. Some lumps are tender, whereas others are painless. The degree of pain or tenderness may be affected by hormonal fluctuations.

Have you recently experienced injury to the breasts? If yes, did the lump develop after the injury?
Lumps resulting from an injury may be associated with a hematoma. Typically these resolve in a short period of time.

Have you noticed other symptoms such as redness, swelling, or dimpling associated with this lump?
Determine associated changes to the breast (i.e., redness, edema, localized heat, rash, and dimpling), which are all symptoms requiring further evaluation.

Nipple Discharge

When did you first notice the discharge from your nipple? Have you ever noticed it before? Does it affect one or both nipples?
Determine onset, location, and duration of nipple discharge. Unilateral nipple discharge is concerning because it is more commonly associated with a pathologic condition than is bilateral nipple discharge.[6]

Describe the discharge. Color? Is it thick or thin? Is there an odor associated with the discharge? Does the discharge occur at specific times such as always before your menstrual period or with breast manipulation?
Nipple discharge may indicate a pathologic condition. A bloody or blood-tinged discharge is alarming and must be investigated.

Does the discharge occur spontaneously or only when expressed?
If the discharge is spontaneous, it is helpful to know if it occurs intermittently or constantly. Spontaneous discharge is considered an abnormal finding. Discharge that is not spontaneous may result from medications or endocrine disorders.

Have you noticed other symptoms such as breast pain or a breast lump?
Determine if there are any other associated breast symptoms or onset of other symptoms. Headaches or changes in vision along with nipple discharge may suggest a pituitary tumor or mass.[6]

Axillary Lumps or Tenderness

When did you first notice the lumps or tenderness under your arms?
Because the tail of Spence extends up into the axilla and most lymphatic drainage flows toward the axillary nodes, a symptom analysis for lumps and tenderness is needed. Determine the onset of symptoms.

Where is the lump or tenderness located? Under one arm or both arms? Do the symptoms come and go or are they always present? Has the tenderness or lump gotten worse?
Determine the location and characteristics of the lump or tenderness.

Do you shave your underarms? If so, how often? Do you notice a relationship to shaving your arms and the tenderness? Do you use deodorant or antiperspirant?

Shaving and use of deodorants and antiperspirants can cause discomfort and a mild inflammation to the axilla.

What have you done to treat this, if anything?

Explore self-care practices; this may be helpful to guide future treatment strategies.

Breast Swelling or Enlargement (Men)

Describe the change you have been experiencing to your breast. When did you first notice it? Have the changes occurred on one or both sides? Have they been associated with weight gain?

Gynecomastia is the enlargement of one or both breasts in the male. Although it may occur at any time, it is most prevalent during puberty, among older adult men, or among men who are overweight. Although breast cancer in men is rare, the most common initial symptom is a breast mass.

Have you experienced any other symptoms such as pain or discharge?

Although a painless palpable mass is the most common initial finding with male breast cancer, nipple discharge may be the only symptom.[7]

HEALTH PROMOTION FOR EVIDENCE-BASED PRACTICE

Breast Cancer

An estimated 226,870 women were diagnosed with breast cancer in 2012, making it the most frequently diagnosed non-skin cancer in women. In addition, breast cancer is the second leading cancer-related cause of death in women; an estimated 39,510 women were expected to die from breast cancer in 2012.

Goals and Objectives—*Healthy People 2020*

The overall *Healthy People 2020* goal related to cancer is to reduce the number of new cancer cases and illness, disability, and death caused by cancer. Three specific objectives relate to breast cancer: (1) reduce the breast cancer death rate, (2) reduce late-stage female breast cancer, and (3) increase the proportion of women who receive a breast cancer screening based on the most recent guidelines.

Screening Recommendations (Secondary Prevention)
U.S. Preventive Services Task Force
- Women whose family history is associated with increased risk for genetic mutation of the breast cancer 1 or 2 genes

(BRCA 1 or BRCA 2) should be referred for genetic counseling and evaluation for BRCA testing.
- Biennial screening mammography should be done for women ages 50 to 74. Women should have the opportunity to become informed about the benefits, limitations, and potential harm associated with regular screening.
- Clinical breast examination (CBE) is recommended as part of a periodic health examination at least every 3 years for average-risk, asymptomatic women in their twenties and thirties and annually for asymptomatic women age 40 and over.
- Breast self-examination (BSE) is optional for women after age 20. Women should be informed about the benefits and limitations of BSE. They may choose not to perform BSE or to perform it on an irregular basis. The U.S. Preventive Services Task Force recommends against teaching BSE.

From *Healthy People 2020, Cancer.* Available at: http://www.healthypeople.gov/2020/topicsobjectives2020/overview.aspx?topicid=5; American Cancer Society: *Cancer facts and figures, 2012,* Atlanta, 2012, American Cancer Society; *American Cancer Society Guidelines for the early detection of cancer,* available at http://www.cancer.org/Healthy/FindCancerEarly/CancerScreeningGuidelines/american-cancer-society-guidelines-for-the-early-detection-of-cancer.

EXAMINATION

ROUTINE TECHNIQUES
- INSPECT both breasts.
- INSPECT the skin of the breasts.
- INSPECT the areolae.
- INSPECT the nipples.
- INSPECT the axillae.

SPECIAL CIRCUMSTANCES OR ADVANCED PRACTICE
- INSPECT the breasts in various postures.
- PALPATE the breasts and axillae.
- PALPATE the nipples.

EQUIPMENT NEEDED
Gloves in presence of nipple drainage or open lesions

PROCEDURES AND TECHNIQUES WITH EXPECTED FINDINGS	ABNORMAL FINDINGS

ROUTINE TECHNIQUES: FEMALE BREAST EXAMINATION

Always explain the procedure to the patient before you begin. Let her know that you will be touching her breasts and be sure to obtain her permission before you begin the examination. Initially position the patient so she is sitting on the examination table facing you. She should be sitting erect with her gown dropped to the waist.

CLEAN hands.

INSPECT the breasts, noting size, symmetry, and shape.

Start by inspecting the breasts with the patient sitting with her arms at her sides. Breasts may be slightly unequal in size. Breast size may vary significantly, but symmetry or only slight asymmetry should be considered normal. The breast shape should be smooth, convex, and even (Fig. 16-4). Gently lift each breast with your fingers and inspect the lower and outer aspects for dimpling, retraction, or bulging.

Note evidence of marked asymmetry of breast size or shape. Significant and rapid changes in the size of one breast could indicate an inflammatory process or a growth. Dimpling, retraction, or bulging could indicate a malignancy.

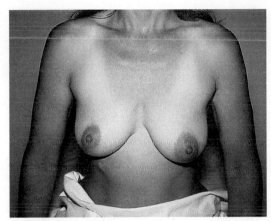

FIG. 16-4 Breasts should appear bilaterally symmetric.

INSPECT the skin of the breasts for color, venous patterns, surface characteristics, and lesions.

The skin of the breast should appear smooth, with an even color. The skin color should be similar to skin on the rest of the body, although it may be lighter in color compared with sun-exposed skin surfaces. The venous patterns (visible veins under the skin) should be bilaterally similar. The venous pattern may be pronounced in obese or pregnant females.

Note any localized or generalized areas of discoloration. Inflammation (e.g., cellulitis or breast abscess) in the breast tissue may cause surface erythema and heat (Fig. 16-5).

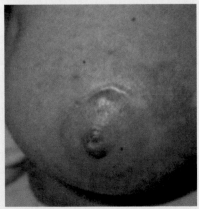

FIG. 16-5 Erythema of the breast. (From Swartz, 2010.)

PROCEDURES AND TECHNIQUES WITH EXPECTED FINDINGS

A rash on both breasts is likely caused by dermatitis; unilateral breast rash, especially surrounding the areola, could be associated with Paget's disease of the breast (a rare type of breast cancer).

Unilateral hyperpigmentation is also considered an abnormal finding. Obese women or women with large breasts may have a red rash with demarcated borders from candidiasis caused by excessive moisture.

Unilateral venous patterns on the breast may occur secondary to dilated superficial veins from an increased blood flow to a malignancy. Roughened, tough, or thickened skin is considered abnormal. Edema may give the skin an orangelike texture and appearance termed *peau d'orange* (Fig. 16-6). Note any lesions.

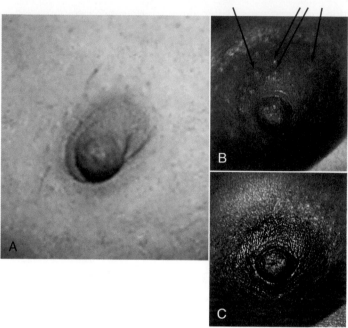

FIG. 16-7 Variations in color of areola. **A,** Pink. **B,** Brown. **C,** Black. Note presence of Montgomery's tubercles in **B.** (**B** and **C** from Seidel et al., 2011.)

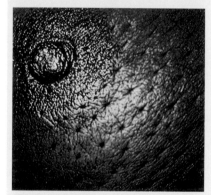

FIG. 16-6 Peau d'orange appearance caused by edema. (From Gallager et al., 1978.)

INSPECT the areolae for color, shape, and surface characteristics.

The color of the areola may vary, depending on the patient's skin color. Fig. 16-7, *A* to *C* shows the variations of areola color, ranging from pink to black. The areola should be round or oval and appear bilaterally similar. Montgomery's tubercles (see Fig. 16-7, *B*) may appear as slightly raised bumps on the areola tissue. Hairs on the nipple may also be seen. These are all expected variations.

Abnormal findings include areolae that are unequal bilaterally, have an irregular shape, or have lesions or changes in color.

INSPECT the nipples for position, symmetry, surface characteristics, lesions, bleeding, and discharge.

Most women's nipples protrude, although some may appear to be flat or actually inverted. All should be considered normal if they have remained unchanged throughout adult life and the nipples are symmetric bilaterally. Nipple *inversion* (a nipple that is recessed as opposed to protruding) can be a normal or an abnormal finding (Fig. 16-8). Consider it normal if it is not a new finding and if it can be everted with manipulation. Inspect nipples for lesions, bleeding, and discharge. Lesions, bleeding, and discharge are not expected.

Nipples that point in different directions or those that are not symmetric should be considered abnormal. Recent nipple inversion or nipple *retraction* (a nipple that is pointing or pulled in a different direction) suggests malignancy, and the patient should be referred for further evaluation (Fig. 16-9).

PROCEDURES AND TECHNIQUES WITH EXPECTED FINDINGS

ABNORMAL FINDINGS

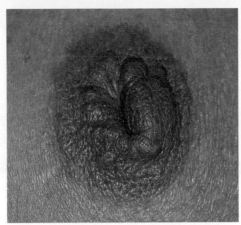

FIG. 16-8 Nipple inversion. (Courtesy Lemmi and Lemmi, 2013.)

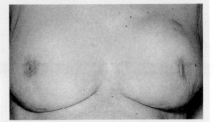

FIG. 16-9 Nipple retraction. (From Mansel and Bundred, 1995.)

Nipples are normally smooth and intact without evidence of crusting, lesions, bleeding, or discharge. Note presence of supernumerary nipples. Supernumerary nipples are considered a normal variation, although they are uncommon. These nipples look similar to pink or brown moles and generally appear along the embryonic "milk line" (Fig. 16-10).

Deviations from normal include nipple edema, redness, pigment changes, ulceration or crusting, erosion or scaling, and wrinkling or cracking. A red, scaly nipple with discharge and crusting that lasts more than a few weeks could indicate *Paget's disease* (Fig. 16-11). Nipple discharge is usually considered an abnormal finding. If a patient has nipple discharge, a specimen should be collected for possible cytologic examination for malignancy (see Box 16-1 on p. 378). Table 16-1 presents various types of discharge and possible causes

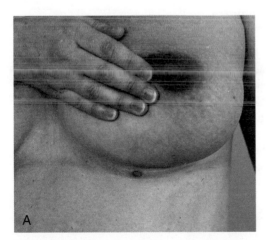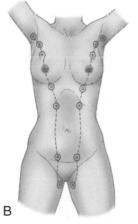

FIG. 16-10 A, Supernumerary nipple. **B,** Supernumerary nipples may arise along the "milk line." (**A** from Mansel and Bundred, 1995. **B** from Seidel et al., 2011.)

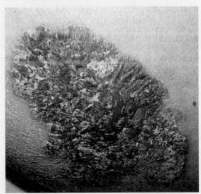

FIG. 16-11 Paget's disease. (From Habif, 1996.)

FREQUENTLY ASKED QUESTIONS

I am embarrassed to think about performing a breast examination on a patient. What can be done to get over this?

This is not an uncommon feeling for a beginner to have. Probably the most important thing to consider first is your own feelings about breast examination in general. Are you uncomfortable about the thought of touching someone else's breasts? Is the discomfort associated with your own perceived inability or lack of experience?

Another key point is to consider the therapeutic purpose for the examination; remember that this is simply a process of data collection and an opportunity for patient teaching. Like most other skills, you will become less nervous with experience. As you gain experience, you will also gain confidence. You will also feel more confident about performing a breast examination if you have established a rapport with your patient. Typically you will perform less invasive examination procedures first; thus, by the time you get to the breast examination, you and the patient will feel more at ease with one another.

TABLE 16-1 NIPPLE DISCHARGE

COLOR OF DISCHARGE	POSSIBLE CAUSE
Serous (yellow)	Usually normal
Serosanguineous (straw colored)	Carcinoma Ductal ectasia
Sanguineous (bloody)	Carcinoma Intraductal papilloma Ductal ectasia Prepartum women from vascular engorgement
Clear (watery)	Pharmacologic causes Carcinoma
Milky	Pituitary adenoma Pharmacologic causes Galactorrhea
Purulent	Infectious process Ductal ectasia
Multicolored (green, gray, brown)	Fibrocystic changes Carcinoma Infectious process Ductal ectasia

---

PROCEDURES AND TECHNIQUES WITH EXPECTED FINDINGS

ABNORMAL FINDINGS

SPECIAL CIRCUMSTANCES OR ADVANCED PRACTICE: FEMALE BREAST EXAMINATION

These techniques are usually performed by an advanced practice or specialty nurse as part of an annual clinical breast examination.

INSPECT the breasts in various positions for bilateral pull, symmetry, and contour.

Procedure: Ask the patient to remain seated and raise her arms over her head (Fig. 16-12, *A*). This position adds tension to the suspensory ligaments and accentuates dimpling or retractions. Observe and compare the breasts, areolae, and nipples. The breasts should appear equal on both sides (bilaterally symmetric).

With her arms still raised, have the patient lean forward (see Fig. 16-12, *B*). The nurse may hold onto the patient's hands to provide balance.

Inspect the breasts for symmetry as previously described. The breasts should hang equally with a smooth contour, and pull should be symmetric. Having the patient lean forward is an especially useful technique if she has large and pendulous breasts because the breasts fall away from the chest wall and hang freely.

Next inspect the breasts while the seated patient pushes her hands onto her hips or pushes her palms together, thus contracting the pectoral muscles (see Fig. 16-12, *C*).

Findings: There should be no deviations in contour and symmetry of the breasts.

Asymmetry or appearance of attachment (fixation), bulging, or retraction of either breast is abnormal.

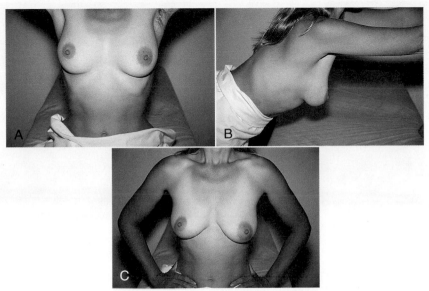

FIG. 16-12 A, Patient with arms extended overhead. **B,** Patient with arms raised and leaning forward. **C,** Patient sitting and pressing her hands on hips.

| PROCEDURES AND TECHNIQUES WITH EXPECTED FINDINGS | ABNORMAL FINDINGS |

INSPECT and PALPATE the axillae for evidence of enlarged lymph nodes, rash, lesions, or masses.

Procedure: (If the patient has a rash or an open lesion in the axilla, wear examination gloves.) You must have short fingernails to prevent injury to the patient.

Instruct the patient to relax both arms at her sides. Using your left hand (if you are right-handed), lift one of the patient's arms and support it so her muscles are loose and relaxed (Fig. 16-13). While in this position, use your right hand to palpate that axilla.

Reach your fingers deep into the axilla and slowly and firmly slide your fingers along the patient's chest wall, first down the middle of the axilla, then along the anterior border of the axilla, and finally along the posterior border. Then turn your hand over and examine the inner aspect of the patient's upper arm. Repeat the same palpation in the opposite axilla. During all maneuvers position the patient's arm with your other hand to maximize the examining area. In all positions palpate for areas of enlargement, masses, or lymph nodes or isolated areas of tenderness. Palpation of lymph nodes in the axilla is included with clinical breast examination because lymph nodes are accessible and may provide clues regarding the presence of inflammation or lesions.

Findings: Lymph nodes or masses should not be palpable in the axillae. There should be no evidence of lesions or rashes.

Infections in the breast, arm, and even the hand may cause lymphatic drainage into the axillary area. Enlargement and tenderness of lymph nodes in the axilla may indicate such an infection. Hard, fixed nodules or masses may suggest metastatic carcinoma or lymphoma.

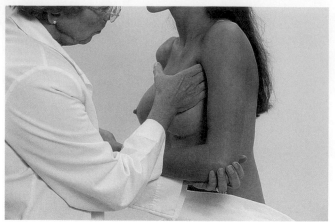

FIG. 16-13 Raise and support patient's arm while palpating axilla.

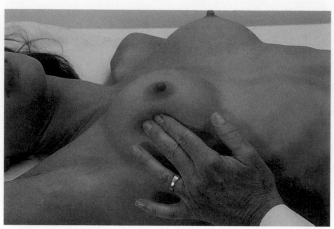

FIG. 16-14 Palpate the breasts using your finger pads.

PROCEDURES AND TECHNIQUES WITH EXPECTED FINDINGS

PALPATE the breasts for tissue characteristics.

Position: The preferred position for breast palpation is supine with a small pillow or towel placed under the shoulder of the breast to be examined. Instruct the patient to place her arm over her head. The combination of the slight shoulder elevation and the arm positioning flattens the breast tissue evenly over the chest wall. A sitting position may be used if the patient has difficulty lying down, if she is young and has very small breasts, or if she has very large breasts, making palpation difficult in a supine position.

Procedure: Using the finger pads of the first two or three fingers of your examining hand, gently, firmly, and systematically palpate all quadrants of the breast and the tail of Spence (Fig. 16-14). Use a systematic approach to breast palpation that begins and ends at a designated point. This ensures that all areas of the breast are palpated.

Several motions may be used for breast palpation (Table 16-2). Press firmly enough to feel the underlying tissue but not so firmly that the tissue is compressed against the rib cage. Do not lift your fingers from the chest wall during the palpation because this breaks the continuity of the palpation. Instead gently slide your fingers over the breast tissue, moving along the designated pattern of palpation.

If the sitting position is used for a woman with very large breasts, ask the patient to lean forward slightly and position your hands between the breasts as shown in Fig. 16-15. While supporting the inferior side of the breast with one hand, palpate the breast with the other hand, starting at the top of the breast, and slowly slide the finger pads down the breast. Repeat the technique until all breast tissues of both breasts are examined. If a mass is identified, specifically palpate the mass for characteristics, including its location, size, shape, consistency, tenderness, mobility, delineation of borders, and retraction (Fig. 16-16). Characteristics that should be included when assessing a mass are presented in Box 16-2. Transillumination may be used to confirm the presence of fluid in superficial masses.

Findings: The breast should feel firm, smooth, and elastic, without the presence of lumps or nodules. Typically it should be nontender on palpation. After pregnancy or menopause the breast tissue may feel softer and looser. During the premenstrual period the patient's breasts may be engorged, be slightly tender, and have generalized nodularity. Most women have a firm transverse ridge along the lower edge of the breast termed the *inframammary ridge*. This firm ridge is normal and should not be mistaken for a breast mass.

ABNORMAL FINDINGS

Abnormal findings during the breast palpation include masses or isolated areas of tenderness or pain. Conditions that may cause lumps or masses include breast cancer, fibroadenoma, and fibrocystic changes to the breast. These are discussed in greater detail in the common problems and conditions later in this chapter. Breast engorgement (in patients who are not pregnant or premenstrual) is also an abnormal finding.

TABLE 16-2	METHODS FOR BREAST PALPATION

CIRCULAR METHOD

This is the most common palpation technique. Place the finger pads of your middle three fingers against the outer edge of the breast. Press gently in small circles around the breast until you reach the nipple. Try not to lift your fingers off the breast as you move from one point to another.

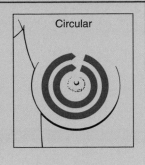

Circular

WEDGE METHOD

Place the finger pads of your middle three fingers on the areola and palpate from the center of the breast outward. Return your fingers to the areola and again palpate from the center outward, covering another section of the breast (in a spokelike fashion). Repeat this until the entire breast has been covered.

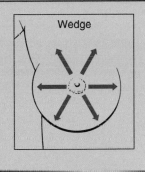

Wedge

VERTICAL STRIP METHOD

Place the finger pads of your middle three fingers against the top outer edge of the breast. Palpate downward and then upward, working your way across the entire breast.

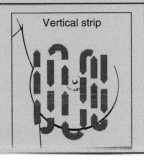

Vertical strip

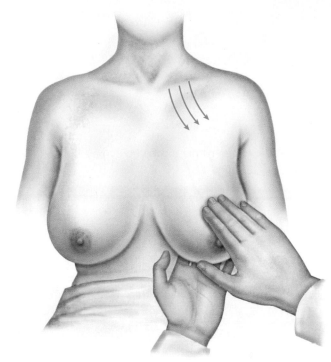

FIG. 16-15 Manual palpation of large breasts. (From Seidel et al., 2003.)

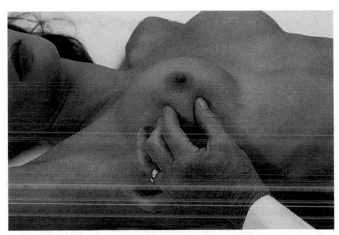

FIG. 16-16 Palpate the borders and mobility of a breast mass.

PROCEDURES AND TECHNIQUES WITH EXPECTED FINDINGS

PALPATE the nipples for surface characteristics and discharge.

NOTE: Wear examination gloves if there is a history of nipple discharge or if discharge is observed. With the patient in the supine position, palpate the nipples. They should be soft and pliable with no masses or discharge. If a discharge is present, note the color, consistency, quantity, and odor. Try to determine the origin of the discharge by gently palpating the areola completely around the nipple with your index finger (Fig. 16-17). Observe for the appearance of discharge through one of the duct openings.

ABNORMAL FINDINGS

Thickening of the nipple tissue, a mass, and loss of elasticity are signs consistent with malignancy. Nipple discharge is considered an abnormal finding except during pregnancy or lactation (see Table 16-1). Discharge may occur secondary to fluid retention of the ducts, infection, hormonal flux, or carcinoma. If a nipple discharge is present, a specimen should be collected for possible cytologic evaluation (Box 16-1).

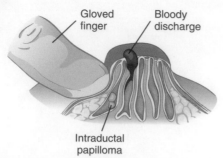

FIG. 16-17 Express nipple discharge by palpating on the areola.

Gloved finger Bloody discharge Intraductal papilloma

FREQUENTLY ASKED QUESTIONS

What is the difference between a clinical breast examination and a breast self-examination?

A *clinical breast examination* (CBE) is performed by a health care professional, usually as part of an annual examination. It involves inspection and palpation of the breasts and axillae. Although this examination can be performed by any nurse, most often it is performed by nurse practitioners. The primary goal of the CBE is to detect breast cancer. A *breast self-examination* (BSE) is performed by women on themselves. Until recently it was strongly recommended that all women perform BSE; it is now considered optional. Women who choose to do this are taught to inspect their breasts in the mirror and palpate their breasts and axillae on a monthly basis. The primary goal of BSE is to increase women's self-awareness regarding how their breasts normally feel so that any changes will be detected.

BOX 16-1 COLLECTING A SPECIMEN FOR CYTOLOGIC EXAMINATION

Cytologic examination of nipple discharge requires proper specimen collection and management. Wearing gloves, express a small amount of nipple discharge. Use a cotton-tipped applicator to collect a small sample of the discharge. Using a rolling technique, smear the discharge from the cotton-tipped applicator on a clear microscopic slide and spray with cytologic fixative. Be sure to label the specimen with the patient's name, the date, and the source (right or left breast).

BOX 16-2 BREAST MASS CHARACTERISTICS

Note and record the following:
- *Location:* Which breast is being examined; which quadrant (may describe as position on the clock or draw on chart to show location)?
- *Size:* Measure the width, length, and thickness in centimeters.
- *Shape:* Is the mass oval, round, lobed, irregularly shaped, or indistinct?
- *Consistency:* Is the mass hard, soft, firm, or rubbery?
- *Tenderness:* Is the mass tender during palpation?
- *Mobility:* Does the lump move during palpation or is it fixed to the overlying skin or the underlying chest wall?
- *Borders:* Are the edges of the mass discrete or poorly defined?
- *Retractions:* Is there any dimpling of the tissue around the mass?

Modified from Seidel HM et al: *Mosby's guide to physical examination,* ed 6, St Louis, 2006, Mosby.

PROCEDURES AND TECHNIQUES WITH EXPECTED FINDINGS

ABNORMAL FINDINGS

ROUTINE TECHNIQUES: MALE BREAST EXAMINATION

As part of a comprehensive examination, nurses examine a male patient's breasts. Inspect the male breast while the patient is seated with his arms at his sides.

CLEAN hands.

INSPECT the breasts and nipples for symmetry, color, size, shape, rashes, and lesions.

With the patient in a seated position, inspect both breasts, looking for breast symmetry, color, size, rashes, and skin lesions. The breasts should be flat and without rashes or lesions. Men who are overweight often have a thicker fatty layer of tissue on the chest, giving the appearance of breast enlargement. If this is noted, determine if he has a history of weight gain. If the patient reports that his breasts became full as he gained weight, the condition is most likely within expected limits. The nipple and areolar areas should be intact; smooth; and of equal color, size, and shape bilaterally.

Note any asymmetry or distinct differences between the two sides. Note any ulcerations, masses, or swelling. If the patient reports a sudden bilateral or unilateral breast enlargement with associated tenderness, the nurse should consider the situation abnormal and refer the patient for further evaluation.

PROCEDURES AND TECHNIQUES WITH EXPECTED FINDINGS

ABNORMAL FINDINGS

PALPATE the breasts and nipples for surface characteristics, tenderness, size, and masses.

With the patient in the same position, palpate the breasts and areolar areas. The tissue should feel smooth, intact, and nontender. Note evidence of tenderness, unilateral enlargement, or masses.

Unilateral or bilateral breast enlargement in men is termed *gynecomastia*. Breast cancer can occur in men, usually manifesting as a hard, painless, irregular nodule often fixed to the area under the nipple. These conditions are discussed in greater detail later in this chapter.

PALPATE the axilla for lymph nodes.

The procedure for palpation of axillary lymph nodes in men is the same as previously described for women. Lymph nodes should not be palpable; or they should be small, soft, mobile, and nontender.

The presence of a lump is considered abnormal. See abnormal findings of axillae previously described in the female examination.

DOCUMENTING EXPECTED FINDINGS

Female Breast Examination
Breasts moderate size, even color, bilaterally symmetric, and hang equally with smooth contour. Venous patterns bilaterally similar. Breasts firm; smooth; elastic; without tenderness, lumps, or nodules. Areolae round, nipples protruding, symmetric, soft, pliable, smooth, and intact without discharge. Axillary lymph nodes not palpated.

Male Breast Examination
Nipples and areolae intact; smooth; evenly pigmented; and of equal color, size and shape bilaterally. Tissue smooth, intact, and nontender. Axillary lymph nodes not palpated.

AGE-RELATED VARIATIONS

This chapter discusses conducting an examination of the breasts with adult patients. These data are important to assess for individuals of all ages, but the approach and techniques used to collect the information may vary depending on the patient's age.

INFANTS AND CHILDREN

The breast assessment among infants and children requires only inspection. Neonates of both genders may have slightly enlarged breasts secondary to the mother's estrogen. Maternal hormones are also responsible for a small, watery, whitish discharge referred to as "witch's milk" seen in a small percentage of newborns during the first few weeks of life. Chapter 19 presents further information regarding the assessment of the breasts in these age-groups.

ADOLESCENTS

Breast development (known as *thelarche*) initially begins in preadolescence and continues through adolescence. Girls are often sensitive about having their breasts exposed for examination; thus the nurse must take the time to reassure them and ensure privacy. Males may experience an unexpected enlargement of the breasts (known as gynecomastia) as a result of obesity or body change transition during early puberty. Chapter 19 presents further information regarding breast assessment among adolescent patients.

OLDER ADULTS

Atrophic changes to the female breast begin by age 40 and continue through menopause. As the glandular tissue atrophies, the breast tissue is gradually replaced with fat and connective tissue. Postmenopausal women should continue to have regular breast examinations because of the increased risk of breast cancer with age. Chapter 21 presents further information regarding breast assessment among older adults.

SITUATIONAL VARIATIONS

PATIENTS WITH A MASTECTOMY

Women who have had a mastectomy require the same breast assessment as all other women. Many women experience anxiety or fear as they worry about the recurrence of cancer or metastasis. Some women may also have personal issues regarding body image and feel self-conscious about exposing the chest. The nurse should be sensitive to this but also reassure the patient that it is necessary to perform a comprehensive examination. In addition to examining the remaining breast in the usual manner, the nurse should assess the mastectomy site and the scar because malignancy recurrence is possible at the scar site (Fig. 16-18, *A*). The mastectomy site and axilla should be inspected for color changes; redness; rash; irritation; and visible signs of edema, thickening, or lumps. Note areas that may have had muscle resection. Also note any signs of lymphedema in the affected upper extremity. Lymphedema is a localized accumulation of lymph fluid in the interstitial spaces caused by removal of the lymph nodes.

Using the finger pads of your examining hand, palpate the side with the mastectomy, especially around the area of the scar. Use a small circular motion, assessing for thickening, lumps, edema, or tenderness; then use a sweeping motion to palpate the entire chest area on the affected side to ensure that no abnormalities have been missed. Finally palpate the axillary and supraclavicular areas for lymph nodes. If the patient has had breast reconstruction or augmentation, perform the breast examination in the usual manner, paying particular attention to scars (see Fig. 16-18, *B* and *C*).

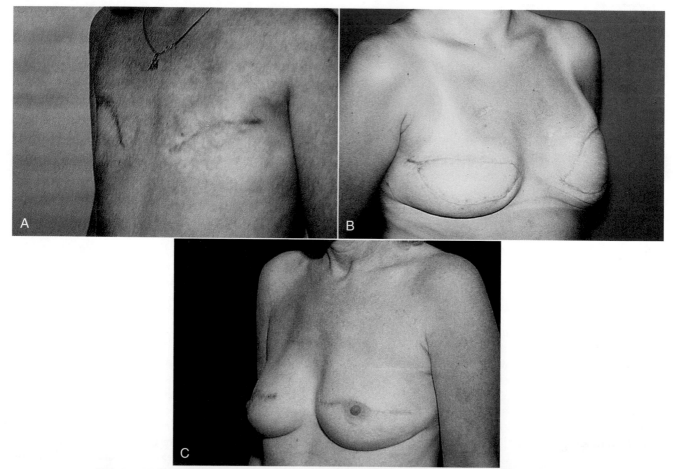

FIG. 16-18 A, Appearance of chest following bilateral mastectomy. Postoperative breast reconstruction before **(B)** and after **(C)** nipple-areolar reconstruction. (Courtesy Brian W. Davies. From Fortunato and McCullough, 1998.)

COMMON PROBLEMS AND CONDITIONS

RISK FACTORS

Breast Cancer

- *Gender:* Females account for 99% of breast cancer cases.
- *Age:* Risk increases with age; 18% of cases are diagnosed in women between ages 40 and 50, and 77% are older than age 50.
- *Race/ethnicity:* White women have the highest incidence of breast cancer.
- *Genetic:* 10% of breast cancer cases are associated with a genetic mutation of breast cancer 1 or 2 genes (BRCA-1 or BRCA-2).
- *Family history:* Breast cancer in a first-degree family relative (on either maternal or paternal side) especially before age 50 increases risk; risk is highest if relative is mother or sister.
- *Personal medical history:*
  - Those with a history of breast cancer have increased risk of subsequent episodes.
  - Those with a history of proliferative breast disease with a biopsy-confirmed atypical hyperplasia have increased risk.
- Exposure to ionizing radiation to chest area as child or young adult (for treatment of other cancer such as Hodgkin's disease) increases risk.
- *Reproductive history:*
  - Long menstrual history (menarche before age 12; menopause after age 50) increases risk.
  - Nulliparity increases risk.
  - First full-term pregnancy after age 30 increases risk.
- *Breast density:* Increased breast density is associated with higher risk of breast cancer.
- *Estrogen replacement:* Hormone replacement therapy for more than 5 years after menopause increases risk. (M)
- *Physical inactivity* (M)
- *Alcohol intake:* Increased alcohol intake (two to five drinks a day) is associated with increased risk. (M)
- *Obesity:* Obesity, especially after age 50, or increased weight gain as an adult increases breast cancer risk. (M)

From American Cancer Society: *Cancer facts and figures, 2012,* Atlanta, 2012, American Cancer Society; Centers for Disease Control and Prevention: *Breast cancer rates by race and ethnicity,* http://www.cdc.gov/cancer/breast/statistics/race.htm. *M,* Modifiable risk factor.

BENIGN BREAST DISEASE

Noncancerous breast conditions account for 90% of clinical breast problems. *Benign breast disease* is a term that represents a number of breast-related symptoms and problems, including breast pain or tenderness, swelling, lumps, discharge, and inflammation.

Fibrocystic Changes to the Breast

The term *fibrocystic changes to the breast* refers to a variety of conditions associated with multiple benign masses within the breast caused by ductal enlargement and the formation of fluid-filled cysts, commonly seen among middle-age women (Fig. 16-19). **Clinical Findings:** Typically cysts manifest as one or more palpable masses that are round, well-delineated, mobile, and tender. The degree of discomfort experienced can range from slightly tender to very painful; the cysts often fluctuate in size and tenderness with the menstrual cycle.[8] Symptoms tend to subside after menopause (Table 16-3).

Fibroadenoma

This is a common benign breast tumor among young women that consists of glandular and fibrous tissue (Fig. 16-20). **Clinical Findings:** Fibroadenoma usually manifests unilaterally as a small, solitary, firm, rubbery, nontender lump. It is generally mobile and well-delineated. This tumor does not change premenstrually.

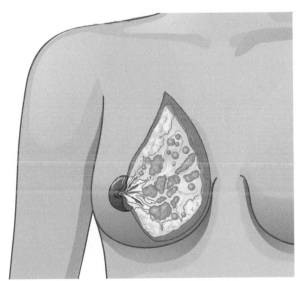

FIG. 16-19 Fibrocystic changes to the breast. The cysts are depicted as green masses.

Ductal Ectasia

Ductal ectasia is a benign breast disease characterized by inflammation and dilation involving one or multiple subareolar ducts. It affects perimenopausal and postmenopausal women. **Clinical Findings:** The initial symptom is a sticky nipple discharge that is commonly dark green or black.[9] As the disease progresses, inflammatory signs and symptoms

TABLE 16-3 DIFFERENTIATION OF BREAST MASSES

	FIBROCYSTIC CHANGES TO BREAST	FIBROADENOMA	CANCER
Age range	20-49	15-55	30-80
Occurrence	Usually bilateral	Usually bilateral	Usually unilateral
Location	Upper outer quadrant	No specific location	48% occur in the upper outer quadrant but may occur in any part of the breast or axillary tail
Nipple discharge	No	No	If present, may be bloody or clear
Pain	Yes	No	Usually none
Number	Multiple or single	Single; may be multiple	Single
Shape	Rounded	Rounded or discoid	Irregular or stellate
Consistency	Soft to firm; tense	Firm, rubbery	Hard, stonelike
Mobility	Mobile	Mobile	Fixed
Retraction signs	Absent	Absent	Often present
Tenderness	Usually tender	Usually nontender	Usually nontender
Borders	Well delineated	Well delineated	Poorly delineated; irregular
Variations with menses	Yes	No	No

Modified from Seidel HM et al: *Mosby's guide to physical examination,* ed 6, St Louis, 2006, Mosby; Fogel CI, Woods NF: *Health care of women: a nursing perspective,* St Louis, 1981, Mosby.

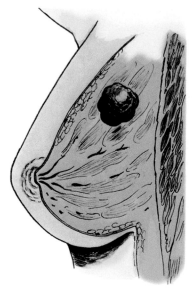

FIG. 16-20 Fibroadenoma.

occur. The woman may experience burning or itching of the nipple and edema in the areolar area. The discharge may become purulent or sanguineous. A complication that can occur is a breast abscess.

Intraductal Papilloma

An intraductal papilloma is a small, benign tumor growth in the major ducts usually within 1 to 2 cm of the areolar edge. One or more ducts may be affected. This commonly occurs in women 40 to 60 years of age. **Clinical Findings:**

The clinical presentation usually associated with intraductal papilloma is a spontaneous bloody discharge from the nipple; occasionally a painful mass is palpated.[10]

BREAST CANCER

Breast cancer is a major health problem for women. It is the most common non–skin-related malignancy in American women.[11]

⊕ ETHNIC, CULTURAL, AND SPIRITUAL VARIATIONS

Breast Cancer Screening

One of the *Healthy People 2020* goals is to achieve health equity, eliminate disparities, and improve the health of all groups. Eliminating racial and ethnic disparities in health requires enhanced efforts at preventing disease, promoting health, and delivering appropriate care. One of the focus areas in which racial and ethnic minorities experience disparity related to health access and outcome is breast cancer screening and management.

- White non-Hispanic women have a higher incidence of breast cancer than nonwhites and Hispanics.
- Hispanic women have the lowest rate of cancer screening of any ethnic group.
- African American women are more likely to die from breast cancer than are women of any other racial or ethnic group.

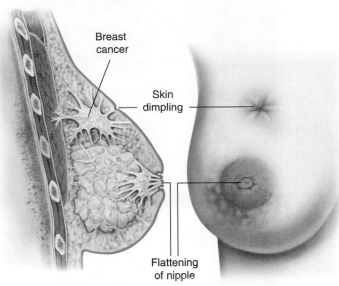

FIG. 16-21 Clinical signs of breast cancer: nipple retraction and dimpling of skin. (From Seidel et al., 2011.)

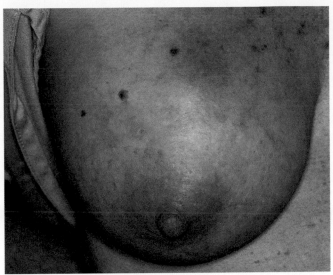

FIG. 16-22 Mastitis 4 weeks after delivery. (Courtesy Lemmi and Lemmi, 2013.)

Invasive Breast Cancer

The most common type of breast cancer is an invasive malignancy arising from the ducts or lobules. Breast cancer is most prevalent in women ages 40 to 60 years (see Table 16-3). **Clinical Findings:** A breast malignancy usually manifests as a solitary, unilateral, nontender lump, thickening, or mass (Fig. 16-21). As the mass grows, there may be breast asymmetry, discoloration (erythema or ecchymosis), unilateral vein prominence, peau d'orange, ulceration, dimpling, puckering, or retraction of the skin. The lesion is sometimes fixed to underlying tissue. Its borders are irregular and poorly delineated. The nipple may be inverted or diverted to one side. A serosanguineous or clear nipple discharge may be present. There may be crusting around the nipple or erosion of the nipple or areola. Lymph nodes may be palpable in the axilla.

Noninvasive Breast Cancer

Two types of cancers categorized as noninvasive are ductal carcinoma in situ (DCIS) and lobular carcinoma in situ (LCIS). The term *in situ* is used to describe an early, noninvasive stage of cancer. DCIS is a true precursor of invasive ductal carcinoma and is considered the more important of the two. LCIS is a risk factor for subsequent development of breast cancer. **Clinical Findings:** The most common manifestation of DCIS or LCIS is an abnormal mammogram. Occasionally DCIS is clinically detected as a lump with well-defined margins or nipple discharge.

OTHER BREAST CONDITIONS

Mastitis

Mastitis is an inflammatory condition of the breast usually caused by a bacterial infection. The condition occurs most

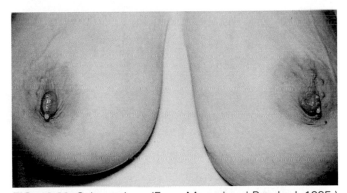

FIG. 16-23 Galactorrhea. (From Mansel and Bundred, 1995.)

frequently in lactating women secondary to milk stasis or a plugged duct. The incidence is highest in the first few weeks after delivery and decreases thereafter.[12] In nonlactating women mastitis may also result from foreign bodies such as nipple rings and breast implants or from trauma. **Clinical Findings:** The infection generally occurs in one area of the breast, which appears as red, edematous, tender, warm to the touch, and hard. Axillary lymph nodes are often enlarged and tender. The patient usually has associated fever and chills and often experiences general malaise (Fig. 16-22).

Galactorrhea

The term *galactorrhea* means inappropriate lactation. Causes include endocrine-related disorders such as a pituitary tumor; systemic diseases such as renal failure; and adverse effects of many medications, especially those that interfere or suppress dopamine (e.g., codeine, morphine, metoclopramide, phenothiazines, and reserpine). **Clinical Findings:** The manifestation is milky-appearing nipple discharge (Fig. 16-23).

There are no other specific symptoms because any additional signs or symptoms are likely based on the underlying cause (e.g., headache or change in vision if caused by a pituitary tumor).

Gynecomastia

Gynecomastia is a noninflammatory enlargement of one or both male breasts representing the most common breast problem in men. It can occur at any age. In neonates the cause is typically associated with maternal hormones. At puberty the condition is idiopathic and transient. Common causes in adult men include adverse effects of medications, adrenal or testicular tumors, liver disease, obesity, or renal disease. **Clinical Findings:** Gynecomastia may be unilateral or bilateral and manifests as enlargement of the male breast (Fig. 16-24).

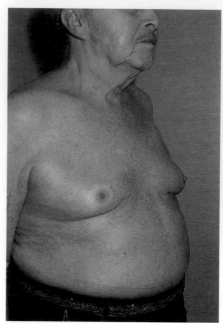

Fig. 16-24 Gynecomastia in an adult male. (From Swartz, 2010.)

CLINICAL APPLICATION AND CLINICAL REASONING

See Appendix D for answers to exercises in this section.

REVIEW QUESTIONS

1. Which finding is considered abnormal when conducting an examination on a 68-year-old woman?
   1. Dark pink areola
   2. Pendulous breasts
   3. Serous nipple drainage
   4. Granular feeling when palpating the breast

2. During a routine health examination a 47-year-old female patient tells the nurse that she performs breast self-examination (BSE) "once in a while." The nurse should base his or her response on which fact?
   1. Those who routinely perform BSE are more likely to survive breast cancer.
   2. Because breast cancer is always found by health care professionals, BSE is no longer indicated.
   3. Performance of BSE is an important indication of a patient's compliance with health care.
   4. BSE is now considered optional; it is a personal choice.

3. A 58-year-old woman has found a small lump in her breast. Which data from her history are risk factors for breast cancer?
   1. Her husband's mother died from breast cancer at age 43.
   2. She drinks a glass of wine each night with dinner.
   3. Menarche occurred at age 14; menopause occurred at age 46.
   4. She underwent radiation treatment for Hodgkin's disease at age 17.

4. What is the reason for palpating axillary lymph nodes during a clinical breast examination?
   1. Axillary nodes fluctuate during the month in response to the menstrual cycle.
   2. Axillary node tenderness is the most common initial symptom of breast cancer.
   3. The lymph network in the breast primarily drains toward the axillary lymph nodes.
   4. This is a matter of convenience because of the close proximity of the axillae to the breasts.

5. A 19-year-old college student comes to the student health center because she discovered a small, nontender, firm, rubbery lump in her right breast. What is the most common cause of breast lumps in women her age?
   1. Breast cancer
   2. Fibroadenoma
   3. Ductal ectasia
   4. Breast abscess

6. A 58-year-old man seeks treatment for "recent breast enlargement." On examination the nurse notes bilateral enlargement of the breasts. Which question asked by the nurse is most appropriate based on this finding?
   1. "What medications are you currently taking?"
   2. "Have you recently been lifting weights?"
   3. "Did your mother have large breasts?"
   4. "Have you ever had cancer?"

CASE STUDY

Julie Fisher is a 46-year-old woman who came to the clinic because she had discovered a lump in her left breast. The following data are collected during an interview and examination.

Interview Data

Ms. Fisher tells the nurse that she first noticed the lump about 9 months ago. Because it seemed small and didn't hurt, she didn't worry about it that much. Recently she noticed that the lump felt bigger and decided that she should have someone look at it. Ms. Fisher tells the nurse, "I just know it's not cancer because I'm much too young and healthy. And if it is, I'm not about to let some doctor mutilate me with a knife. I'd rather die than have my breast cut off." The nurse asks her if she has noticed any redness or dimpling of the breast. Ms. Fisher tells the nurse, "No, not really, but I don't pay attention to those things." She tells the nurse that she started having regular menstrual cycles at age 11 and has not reached menopause. She has never been married and has no children.

Examination Data

- *General survey:* Alert, well-nourished female; hesitant to expose her breast for examination.

- *Breast examination:* Inspection reveals breasts of typical size with right and left breast symmetry. The skin of both breasts is smooth with even pigmentation. The nipples protrude slightly with no drainage noted. The left nipple is slightly retracted. Significant dimpling is noted on left breast in upper outer quadrant when arms are raised over her head. Right breast is firm, smooth, elastic, without lumps or tenderness. Palpation of the left breast reveals a large, hard lump in the upper outer quadrant. No lumps or masses are noted in the right breast. The left nipple produces a serosanguineous discharge when squeezed; the right nipple is unremarkable.

Clinical Reasoning

1. Which data deviate from normal findings, suggesting a need for further investigation?
2. For what additional information should the nurse ask or assess?
3. Which risk factors for breast cancer does Ms. Fisher have?
4. With which additional health care professionals should the nurse consider collaborating to meet her health care needs?

CHAPTER

17

Reproductive System and the Perineum

evolve WEBSITE

http://evolve.elsevier.com/Wilson/assessment

Organization of this chapter begins with anatomy and physiology of the female reproductive system followed by that of the male reproductive system and rectum and anus. The history questions are applicable to both genders, except when noted (e.g., obstetric history). Examination of the female is followed by examination of the male and rectal examination.

Common problems and conditions begin with infections that affect either gender, followed by disorders specific to women and then those specific to men. Conditions of the anus and rectum are described, followed by prolapse or hernia, which affects either gender.

ANATOMY AND PHYSIOLOGY

FEMALE REPRODUCTIVE SYSTEM

The anatomy of the female reproductive system can be categorized into external genitalia and internal structures. Physiologic functions discussed in the chapter are limited to menstrual cycle and menopause. The process of pregnancy is discussed in Chapter 20.

External Genitalia

The external female genitalia are collectively referred to as the *vulva*. The vulva includes the mons pubis, labia majora, labia minora, clitoris, prepuce, vaginal vestibule, ducts of the Skene's and Bartholin's glands, vaginal orifice, urethral meatus, and perineum (Fig. 17-1).

The mons pubis is a layer of adipose tissue that lies over the symphysis pubis. After puberty this surface is covered with coarse hair that extends down over the outer labia to the perineal and anal areas. The labia majora are folds of tissue that extend downward from the mons pubis, surround the vestibule, and come together at the perineum. The outer surfaces are covered with hair, whereas the inner surfaces are hairless and smooth.

Lying inside the labia majora are darker, smooth folds called the *labia minora*. In some women the labia minora are completely enclosed within the labia majora; in others the labia minora protrude between the labia majora. Each of the labia minora divides into a medial and lateral aspect. The medial aspects join superior to the clitoris to form the clitoral hood (prepuce), and the lateral aspects join inferior to the clitoris to form the frenulum. The clitoris is a small, cylindric bud of erectile tissue that is a primary center of sexual stimulation. The fourchette is a tense band or fold of mucous membrane connecting the posterior ends of the labia minora, just behind (posterior to) the vagina.

The vaginal vestibule is the area that lies between the labia minora and contains the urethral (urinary) meatus, the introitus (vaginal opening), hymenal tissue, and Bartholin's and Skene's glands. The urethral meatus is located just below the clitoris and appears as an irregularly shaped slit. The vaginal introitus lies immediately below the urethral meatus and varies in size and shape. The hymen is a fold of mucous membrane at the vaginal opening separating the external genitalia from the vagina and appears as small, fleshy tags of skin (sometimes referred to as *hymenal remnants* or *hymenal tags*).

The ducts of Skene's glands and Bartholin's glands open within the vestibule. The tiny Skene's glands are numerous and are located in the paraurethral area. During sexual

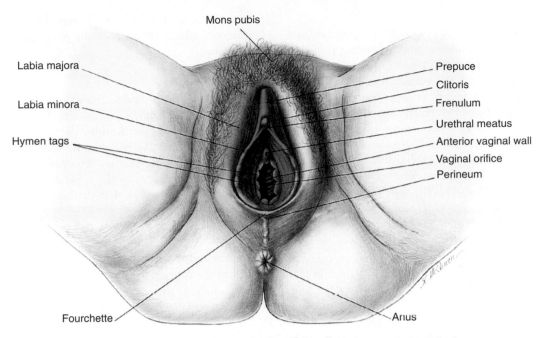

Mons pubis

Labia majora

Labia minora

Hymen tags

Prepuce

Clitoris

Frenulum

Urethral meatus

Anterior vaginal wall

Vaginal orifice

Perineum

Fourchette

Anus

FIG. 17-1 Female external genitalia. (From Stenchever et al., 2001.)

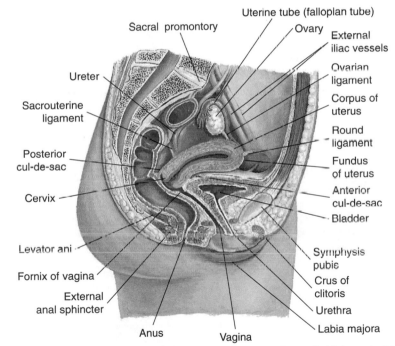

Sacral promontory

Uterine tube (fallopian tube)

Ovary

External iliac vessels

Ureter

Ovarian ligament

Sacrouterine ligament

Corpus of uterus

Round ligament

Posterior cul-de-sac

Fundus of uterus

Cervix

Anterior cul-de-sac

Bladder

Levator ani

Symphysis pubis

Fornix of vagina

Crus of clitoris

External anal sphincter

Urethra

Labia majora

Anus

Vagina

FIG. 17-2 Midsagittal view of female pelvic organs. (From Seidel et al., 2011.)

intercourse they secrete a lubricating fluid. The ducts usually are not visible. Bartholin's glands are small and round, located on either side of the introitus, at approximately the 5 and 7 o'clock positions. The ducts of the Bartholin's glands open onto the sides of the vestibule in the space between the hymen and the labia minora. The ductal openings are usually not visible. During sexual excitement Bartholin's glands secrete a mucoid material into the vaginal orifice for lubrication.

The perineal surface is the triangular-shaped area between the vaginal opening and the anus. The pelvic floor consists of a group of muscles that form a suspended sling supporting the pelvic contents. These muscles attach to various points on the bony pelvis and form functional sphincters for the vagina, rectum, and urethra.

Internal Structures

The internal structures include the vagina, uterus, fallopian tubes, and ovaries (Fig. 17-2). They are supported by four pairs of ligaments: cardinal, uterosacral, round, and broad ligaments.

Vagina

The vagina is a canal composed of smooth muscle and is lined with mucous membrane that extends posteriorly from the vestibule to the uterus. It inclines posteriorly at an angle of approximately 45 degrees to the vertical plane of the body. The canal has transverse ridges of mucous membrane lining the vagina in the reproductive years. The uterine cervix enters superiorly and anteriorly into the vaginal cavity to form a recess, or fornix, around the cervix. The fornix is divided into anterior, posterior, and lateral fornices, through which the internal pelvic walls can be palpated. The vagina carries menstrual flow from the uterus and is the receptive organ for the penis during sexual intercourse. During birth the vagina becomes the terminal portion of the birth canal.

Uterus

The uterus is a hollow, thick, pear-shaped, muscular organ. It is suspended and stabilized in the pelvic cavity by the four pairs of ligaments (listed previously). It is fairly mobile, usually loosely suspended between the bladder and rectum. The cervix is a mucus-producing gland that is the lowest portion of the uterus. It is visible (during a speculum examination) and palpable in the upper vagina. The cervical opening, or the os, is visible on the surface of the cervix. It appears as a small, round opening in a nulliparous woman (never having borne a child) or as an irregular slit in parous women. The outer surface of the cervix (known as the *ectocervix*) is layered with squamous cells, and the cervical canal is layered with columnar cells. In some women the juncture of these two types of cells (the squamocolumnar junction) can be observed as a circumscribed red circle around the os (Fig. 17-3).

The portion of the uterus above the cervix is known as the corpus. The corpus is composed of three sections: the isthmus (the narrow neck from which the cervix extends into the vagina); the main body of the uterus; and the fundus, which is the bulbous top portion of the uterus (Fig. 17-4). The fundus maintains its anterior position by the attached round ligaments, which are occasionally palpable on either side of the uterus.

Fallopian Tube

The fallopian tubes extend from the fundus laterally 3 to 5 inches (7.5 to 12.5 cm) to the ovaries. The fimbriated ends of the fallopian tubes (uterine tube) partially project around the ovary to capture and draw ova into the tube for fertilization (see Fig. 17-4). The ova are transported to the uterus by rhythmic contractions of the tubal musculature. The inner tube is lined with cilia that further assist in transport of the ova.

Ovaries

The almond-shaped ovaries are connected to the uterine body by the ovarian ligaments. The primary functions of the ovaries include ovulation and secretion of reproductive hormones. Ovulation is the release of an ovum (egg), which

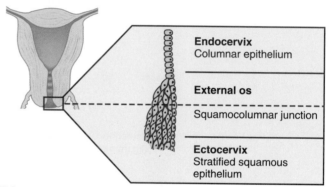

FIG. 17-3 Types of cervical cells: endocervix, external os, and ectocervix. (Used with permission from Mashburn and Scharbo-DeHaan: A clinician's guide to Pap smear interpretation, *Nurse Pract* 22(4):115-118, 124, 126-127, 1997. Springhouse Corporation.)

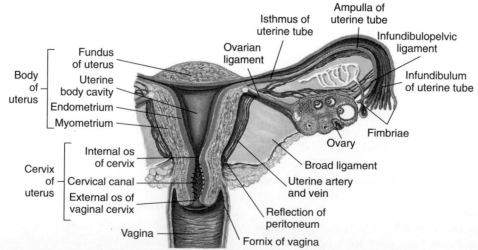

FIG. 17-4 Cross-sectional view of internal female genitalia and pelvic contents. (From Seidel et al., 2011.)

usually occurs monthly as part of the menstrual cycle. The two dominant female sex hormones produced by the ovaries are estrogen and progesterone. These hormones have several functions, including triggering sexual maturation at puberty, development of secondary sex characteristics, and regulation of the menstrual cycle.

Menstrual Cycle

The hypothalamus, the anterior pituitary, and the ovaries together regulate the menstrual cycle. The menstrual cycle follows a predictable 28-day cycle. The five stages are described here and illustrated in Fig. 17-5.

Stage 1: Menstrual Phase (Days 1 to 4). The menstrual cycle begins with the menstrual phase. During this phase estrogen and progesterone levels have decreased, triggering a shedding of the upper layers of endometrium and menstrual bleeding.

Stage 2: Postmenstrual or Preovulatory Phase (Days 5 to 12). The follicle-stimulating hormone (FSH) stimulates follicular growth during this stage. The ovary and maturing follicle produce estrogen, which supports egg development within the follicle.

Stage 3: Ovulation (Days 13 or 14). Ovulation is characterized by a steep rise in estrogen and luteinizing hormone (LH). The egg is expelled from the follicle and drawn into the fallopian tube by the fimbriae and cilia. A subsequent rise in progesterone causes thickening of the uterine wall.

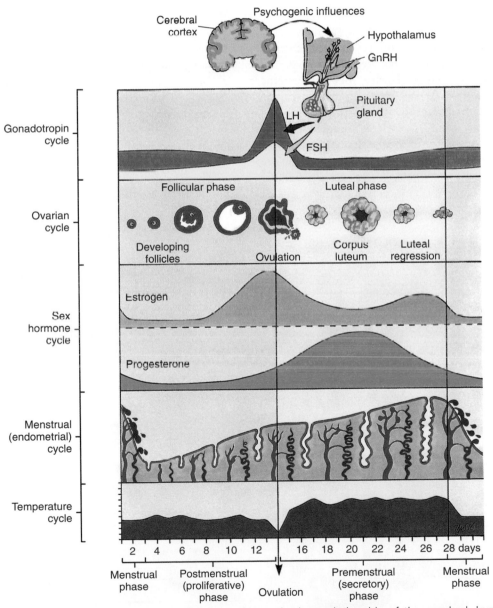

FIG. 17-5 Female menstrual cycle. Diagram shows the interrelationship of the cerebral, hypothalamic, pituitary, and uterine functions throughout a standard 28-day menstrual cycle. The variations in basal body temperature are also shown. (From Thibodeau and Patton, 2007.)

Stage 4: Secretory Phase (Days 15-20). After ovulation the FSH and LH hormones decline. The egg moves into the uterus, and the follicle becomes a corpus luteum. Secretion of progesterone rises and predominates while estrogen declines. The uterine wall continues to thicken in anticipation of receiving a fertilized egg.

Stage 5: Premenstrual Phase (Days 21 to 28). If fertilization of the egg and subsequent implantation do not occur, the corpus luteum degenerates, and progesterone production decreases. Estrogen levels begin to rise again as a new follicle develops. When the thickened uterine wall begins to shed, menstruation starts, which marks the beginning of another menstrual cycle.

Menopause

Women undergo a period of decreased hormonal function starting between ages 35 and 40. This period is termed the *climacteric,* a long transition phase extending many years. It includes endocrine, somatic, and psychologic changes involving a complex relationship between the ovarian and hypothalamic-pituitary factors. During this period the woman undergoes a series of changes associated with aging and estrogen depletion. *Menopause* is defined as the permanent cessation of menses and is considered complete after the woman has experienced an entire year with no menses. Ovulation usually ceases 1 to 2 years before menopause. The age at which women reach menopause varies greatly, but the mean age is 50.

MALE REPRODUCTIVE SYSTEM

The anatomy of the male reproductive system can be categorized into internal structures (testes, ducts, and glands) and external genitalia (penis, scrotum) (Fig. 17-6).

Internal Structures
Testes

The testes are paired sex organs located within the scrotum. They are oval shaped, with a smooth surface and rubbery texture. The primary function of the testes is the production of sperm (spermatogenesis). Each testicle contains a series of coiled ducts (seminiferous tubules) where spermatogenesis occurs. As sperm are produced, they move toward the center of the testis, traveling into the efferent tubules adjacent to the epididymis (see Fig. 17-6).

Ducts

The ducts are responsible for the transportation of sperm. Sperm travel from the epididymides to the vas deferens, to the ejaculatory duct, and out the urethra.

Once formed in the testes, sperm move into the comma-shaped *epididymis*—a long and elaborately coiled duct that lies on the posterolateral surface of each testis (Fig. 17-7). As sperm move through the epididymis, they receive nutrients and mature. Eventually they exit the epididymis through the vas deferens.

The *vas deferens* (also known as the *ductus deferens*) transport sperm from the epididymis to the ejaculatory duct. It is

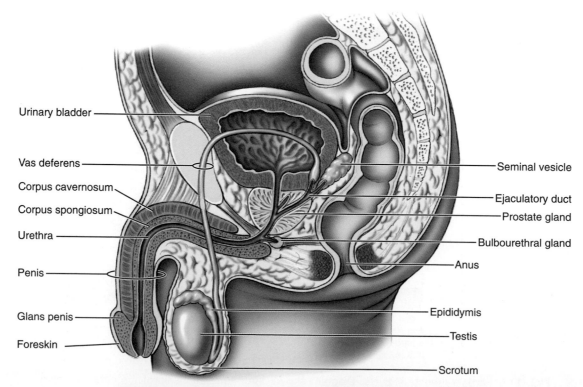

FIG. 17-6 Male reproductive organs. (From Herlihy et al., 2011.)

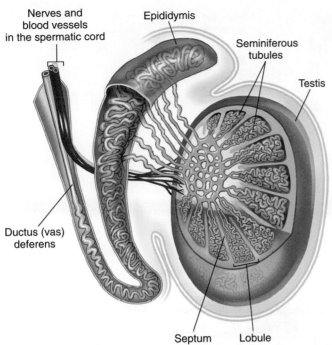

Nerves and blood vessels in the spermatic cord

Epididymis

Seminiferous tubules

Testis

Ductus (vas) deferens

Septum   Lobule

FIG. 17-7 Scrotum and its contents. (From Thibodeau and Patton, 2007.)

enclosed within the spermatic cord (a connective tissue sheath) along with arteries, veins, and nerves as it ascends through the inguinal canal. The cord enters the inguinal canal through the external inguinal ring; this ring is vulnerable to hernias, or protrusion of the abdominal contents. In the abdominal cavity the vas deferens travels up and around to the posterior aspect of the bladder, where it unites with the seminal vesicle. The union of the seminal vesicles with the vas deferens forms the *ejaculatory duct* just before the entrance into the prostate gland. Within the ejaculatory duct sperm are transported downward through the prostate gland and into the prostatic portion of the urethra.

The innermost tube of the penis, the *urethra*, is usually about 18 to 20 cm from bladder to meatus. It extends out of the base of the bladder, traveling through the prostate gland into the pelvic floor and through the penile shaft (see Fig. 17-6). The urethral orifice is a small slit at the tip of the glans. The urethra is the terminal passageway for both urine and sperm. During ejaculation sperm travel from the ejaculatory duct through the urethra and out of the body.

Glands

Three glands (seminal vesicles, prostate gland, and bulbourethral glands) produce and secrete fluid that makes up most of the fluid in the ejaculate (semen). These secretions serve as a medium for the transport of sperm and also provide an alkaline environment that promotes sperm motility and survival.

The *seminal vesicles* (small pouches lying between the rectum and the posterior bladder wall) join the ejaculatory

duct at the base of the prostate (see Fig. 17-6). The *prostate gland* lies beneath the urinary bladder and surrounds the upper portion of the urethra. The posterior surface of the prostate lies adjacent to the anterior rectal wall. Two of the three prostate lobes are palpable through the rectum (right and left lateral lobes). These lobes are divided by a slight groove known as the median sulcus. The third lobe (median lobe) is anterior to the urethra and cannot be palpated. *Bulbourethral glands,* located on either side of the urethra just below the prostate, also secrete fluid that contributes to the semen, providing a medium for transport of the sperm.

External Genitalia
Scrotum

The scrotum is a pouch covered with thin, darkly pigmented, rugous (wrinkled) skin. A septum divides the scrotum into two pendulous compartments, or sacs. Each sac contains a testis, which contains seminiferous tubules arranged within lobules, and an epididymis, which is suspended by the *spermatic cord* (i.e., a network of nerves, blood vessels, and the vas deferens discussed previously) (see Fig. 17-7). Because sperm production requires a temperature slightly below body temperature, the testes are suspended outside the body cavity; the temperature of the scrotum is controlled by a layer of muscle under the scrotal skin that contracts or relaxes in response to the outside temperature. When the temperature is cold, the scrotal sac and its contents move close to the body; conversely, when the temperature rises, the scrotal sac relaxes, and the testes drop downward.

Penis

The penis serves two functions: It is the final excretory organ in urination, and during intercourse it introduces sperm into the vagina. The body of the penis contains two layers of tissue, the corpora cavernosa and the corpus spongiosum, which encase the urethra (see Fig. 17-6). This smooth, spongy tissue becomes firm when engorged with blood, forming an erection. The corpus spongiosum expands at its distal end to form the glans penis.

The glans penis is lighter pink in color than the rest of the penis. It is exposed when the prepuce (the foreskin) is either pulled back or surgically removed (circumcision). The corona is the ridge that separates the glans from the shaft of the penis. The skin covering the penis is thin, hairless, and a little darker than the rest of the body; it adheres loosely to the shaft to allow for expansion with erection.

Erection is a neurovascular reflex that occurs when increased arterial dilation and decreased venous outflow cause the two corpora cavernosa to become engorged with blood. This reflex can be induced by psychogenic and local reflex mechanisms, both under the control of the autonomic nervous system. The psychogenic erection can be initiated by any type of sensory input (auditory, visual, tactile, or imaginative), whereas local reflex mechanisms are initiated by tactile stimuli. Ejaculation (i.e., the emission of semen from

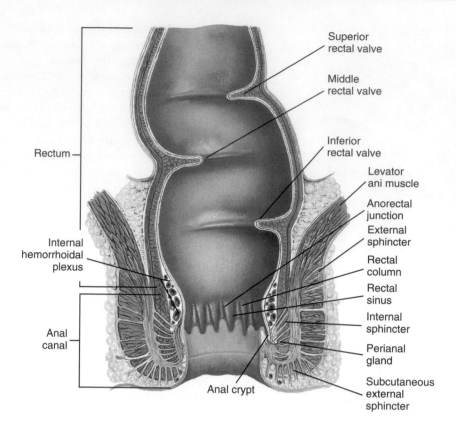

FIG. 17-8 Anatomy of the anus and rectum. (From Seidel et al., 2011.)

the vas deferens, epididymides, prostate, and seminal vesicles) is followed by constriction of the vessels supplying blood to the corpora cavernosa and gradual return of the penis to its relaxed, flaccid state.

RECTUM AND ANUS

The rectum and anus are the terminal structures of the gastrointestinal (GI) tract. They are presented in this chapter because they make up the posterior portion of the perineum in the male and female and because they are usually examined in conjunction with examination of the reproductive system.

Rectum

The proximal end of the rectum lies at the distal end of the sigmoid colon and extends down for approximately 12 cm to the anorectal junction (Fig. 17-8). Three semilunar folds of tissue called *rectal valves* (superior, middle, and inferior rectal valves) lie within the rectal wall and extend across half the circumference of the rectal lumen. The function of these valves is not well understood but is thought to support feces while allowing flatus to pass. The most distal of these valves

(the inferior rectal valve) can be palpated with digital examination.

Anal Canal and Anus

The anal canal extends from the anorectal junction to the anus (see Fig. 17-8). The anal canal is lined with mucous membranes arranged in longitudinal folds called *rectal columns* that contain a network of arteries and veins (frequently referred to as the *internal hemorrhoidal plexus*). Between each of the columns is a recessed area called the *anal crypt* into which the perianal glands empty. Surrounding the anal canal are two concentric rings of muscle, the internal and external sphincters. The internal sphincter consists of smooth muscle and is under involuntary control. The external sphincter, consisting of skeletal muscle, is under voluntary control, allowing for control of defecation. The lower portion of the anal canal is sensitive to painful stimuli, whereas the upper portion is relatively insensitive.

The anus is the terminal portion of the rectum, located on the perineum. It is hairless, moist mucosal tissue surrounded by hyperpigmented perianal skin. Normally the anus is closed, except during defecation.

HEALTH HISTORY

Nurses interview patients to collect subjective data about their present health status, past health history, family history, personal and psychosocial history, and sexual and obstetric history, which may affect the health condition of their reproductive systems. Quality Improvement Competencies for Nurses include providing patient-centered care. See Table 11-1 on p. 196 for examples of competencies.

GENERAL HEALTH HISTORY

Present Health Status

Do you have any chronic illnesses? If so, describe.
Many chronic illnesses may affect the reproductive functioning in women and men. For example, endocrine disorders may impact a woman's menstrual cycle; diabetes mellitus, vascular insufficiency, cardiac, and respiratory disease can contribute to erectile dysfunction.

Do you take any medications? If so, what do you take, and how often?
Both prescription and over-the-counter medications should be noted. Ask if the medications are taken as prescribed. Many medications can affect reproductive system functioning or libido. For example, medications such as oral contraceptives and broad-spectrum antibiotics can alter the balance of the normal vaginal flora in women. In men, some medications such as diuretics and antihypertensive agents can cause impotence.

Past Health History

Have you had any reproductive problems in the past? If so, describe.
Identify previous problems with the reproductive system because this information may be helpful when documenting current problems or risk factors for other medical problems. For example, women with endometriosis have been shown to have an increased risk of ovarian cancer.[1]

Have you ever had surgery on your reproductive organs or rectum? If so, when? How has it affected you?
If a woman reports that she has had a hysterectomy, ask if it was an abdominal or a vaginal approach and if she had a total (uterus, fallopian tubes, and ovaries removed) or a partial (only uterus removed) hysterectomy. In addition, ask the patient why she had the hysterectomy, when it was performed, if she had any accompanying bowel or bladder repairs, and what problems or concerns she has had since the surgery.

Men may have had surgery to treat an enlarged prostate, prostate cancer, hydrocele, varicocele, or testicular cancer.

Both men and women may have had surgical procedures to prevent pregnancy (vasectomy or a tubal ligation) or involving the anus or rectum (such as hemorroidectomy).

Do you have a history of cancer? If so, which type of cancer? How was it treated?
In women, a history of breast cancer or nonpolyposis colon cancer is a risk factor for some types of female reproductive cancers. In men a history of testicular cancer increases risk of recurrence in the other testicle.[2]

Have you received the hepatitis A or B vaccine? Females: Have you received the human papillomavirus (HPV) vaccine?
Assess self-care behaviors. Preexposure vaccination is one of the most effective methods for preventing some sexually transmitted diseases. The hepatitis B vaccination is recommended for all unimmunized individuals at risk for sexually transmitted disease (STD). The hepatitis A vaccine is recommended for unimmunized men who have sex with men. The HPV vaccine is now available and is recommended for females ages 9 to 26.[3]

Family History

Women: Has any woman in your family ever had cancer of the cervix, ovary, uterus, breast, or colon? If so, who? When?
A family history of these cancers (particularly in a first-degree relative) increases risk for certain female reproductive cancers.[2]

Men: Has any man in your family ever had cancer of the prostate or testicle? If so, who? When?
A family history of these cancers (particularly in a first-degree relative) increases risk for certain prostate and testicular cancers.[2]

Personal and Psychosocial History

Do you ever perform self-examination of your genitalia?
Assess the self examination behaviors of all men and women. In one study the majority of adolescent males were aware of testicular cancer, but only 10% performed testicular self-examination regularly.[4] Health care awareness does not necessarily translate to health practice.

How often do you have an examination of your genitalia by a health care professional? What were the results?
Assess self-care behaviors. Ideally women should have a pelvic examination and Papanicolaou (Pap) test at least every 3 years through age 65 if sexually active.[5] Men should have an examination of their genitalia and prostate on a regular basis, depending on their age.

Sexual History

Are you currently in a sexual relationship? If yes, do you prefer relationships with men, women, or both? In which type of sex do you engage (penile-vaginal, penile-rectal, recipient rectal, oral)?

The type of sex in which one participates may provide useful information for risk assessment of sexually transmitted infections. Cross-infections from mouth, anus, and genitalia can occur. Men and women need to feel accepted when discussing their health concerns. If the nurse seems genuinely interested and concerned, the patient may appreciate the opportunity to discuss sexuality issues or problems.

How frequently do you engage in sexual activities? Are you and your partner(s) satisfied with the sexual relationship? Do you communicate comfortably about sexual activity?
Determining the frequency of sexual activity and the patient's satisfaction are important. Questions related to sexual activities and satisfaction are found on health history forms; however, health care practitioners have been found to offer little discussion related to sexuality unless an issue is raised by the patient.[6] For this reason, nurses should engage in this conversation.

Do you or your partner(s) have multiple partners? How many sexual partners have you had in the past 3 months?
This information may be used to determine the patient's risk for STD.

How do you protect yourself from STD? Do you use a protective barrier such as a condom every time you have intercourse?
Determine level of understanding and practice regarding safe sex and STD and prevention. Individuals may not have accurate information. When used correctly and consistently, condoms are highly effective in preventing sexual transmission of human immunodeficiency virus (HIV), chlamydia, gonorrhea, and trichomoniasis. The effectiveness of preventing transmission of herpes simplex virus type 2 is less well established.[3]

Are you currently using any birth control measures? If so, which type(s)? How effective do you think it (they) has (have) been? Do you have any difficulty with the birth control measures? Do you use birth control measures every time you have intercourse?
All women who have the potential to become pregnant or men who have the potential to create a pregnancy should be questioned about contraceptive practices. Information should be gathered about appropriate use of the contraception, length of use, and satisfaction with the product.

How old were you when you first had intercourse? Was it by choice? Have you ever been forced into sexual acts as a child or an adult? If so, how has this impacted you and your partner?
Inquire about current or past sexual abuse. Research has shown that women may wait years before disclosing sexual abuse or assault; delay in disclosure is even more likely when the perpetrator is a family member.[7] Sexual abuse or assault often causes ongoing sexual difficulties for the victims and their partners; male partners of women who are sexually assaulted often feel angry, guilty, and helpless. Men can also be victims of physical and sexual abuse, and often it is very difficult for them to admit to such abuse.

Do you or your partner(s) frequently use drugs or alcohol before you engage in sexual activity?
Drug and alcohol use leads to high-risk sexual behavior.

OBSTETRIC HISTORY

Menstruation

What was the date of the first day of your last menstrual period (LMP)? How often do you have periods? How long do they usually last?
A menstrual history consists of the LMP, usual menstrual interval, and the duration of menses. Women who are menopausal should be asked at what age menopause occurred.

How would you describe your usual amount of flow—light, moderate, heavy? How many pads or tampons do you use over the course of a day? An hour?
Normal flow is difficult to determine, but any change from the "normal" for the patient should be noted.

Have you noted any change in your periods recently?
Change in menstruation could reflect hormone imbalance. Menstruation that is irregular or of frequently long or short intervals may indicate a lack of ovulation.[8]

How old were you when you started having periods?
Menarche typically occurs between ages 12 and 14 years, although the range spans ages 8 to 16. Onset between ages 16 and 17 suggests an endocrine problem. Early onset of menarche (before age 11) is a risk factor for endometrial and ovarian cancer.[2]

Pregnancy

Have you ever been pregnant? If so, how many times? How many babies have you had? Have you had any miscarriages, abortions, or infants who died before they were born? If so, how many?
Gravida refers to the number of pregnancies; *para* refers to the number of pregnancies that reached 20 weeks or longer. See Chapter 20 for more information regarding documentation of obstetric history.

Do you think you may be pregnant now? If so, what symptoms have you noticed?
Symptoms may include missed or abnormal periods, nausea or vomiting, breast changes or tenderness, and fatigue.

Have you ever had difficulty becoming pregnant? If so, have you seen a health care practitioner? What have you tried to do to become pregnant? How do you feel about not being able to become pregnant?
Inquiring about difficulty becoming pregnant is as important as asking about actual pregnancy. When couples trying

unsuccessfully to become pregnant are highly distressed, they may need a nurse to provide a referral for counseling or to encourage them to discuss their feelings.

PROBLEM-BASED HISTORY

The most commonly reported problems related to the reproductive system and perineum for men and women include pain, genital lesions and discharge, problems with urination, and rectal bleeding. Common problems unique to women include problems or changes with menstrual cycle and menopausal symptoms. As with symptoms in all areas of health assessment, a symptom analysis is completed using the mnemonic OLD CARTS, which includes the *Onset, Location, Duration, Characteristics, Aggravating Factors, Related* symptoms, *Treatment,* and *Severity* (see Box 2-3).

Pain

When did the pain begin? Where is it located? Describe its characteristics. On a scale of 0 to 10, how would you rate the intensity of the pain? Is it aggravated by other activity or function (e.g., menstrual cycle)?

Men and women may experience lower abdominal, pelvic, or rectal pain from a number of problems involving the reproductive system, urinary tract (urethra, bladder, ureters), or rectum and anus. Women with unexplained pelvic pain should be screened for chlamydia.[9]

Rectal discomfort may be associated with a number of factors, including poor hygiene, infection, hemorrhoids, and abscess. Symptoms such as burning with urination suggest urinary tract infection (UTI).

Among men, pain in the groin or scrotum may occur from hernia or problems in the spermatic cord, testicles, or prostate gland. Testicular pain can occur secondary to almost any problem of the testis or epididymis, including epididymitis, orchitis, hydrocele, spermatic cord torsion, and testicular cancer.

Do you have associated symptoms such as discharge or bleeding, abdominal distention or tenderness, or pelvic fullness?

Determine if there are any associated symptoms with the pain to help identify the cause. Vaginal and penile discharges are described later in the chapter.

What have you done, if anything, to treat the pain? How effective was the treatment?

Knowledge of previous self-treatment measures may be helpful in identifying appropriate treatment strategies.

Lesion

When did you first become aware of the lesion? Where exactly is it located? What does it look like? Is it tender?

A lesion or sore on the genitalia is often caused by STD or cancer but may also be associated with other problems.

Establish when the lesion was first noticed because this may be important in identifying the cause.

Do you have any other symptoms (e.g., pain, bleeding, discharge, burning pain with urination, pelvic fullness, or abdominal pain)?

These are symptoms commonly associated with STD.

Have you had a sexual relationship with someone who has an STD? If so, when? Have you ever been treated for any of these infections? If so, was the treatment successful?

Sexual contact with a partner with untreated STD increases a person's risk for STD.

Vaginal or Penile Discharge

When did the discharge begin? What color is it? Describe its odor and consistency.

Identify onset of the symptom. Penile discharge suggests infection. Among women, normal discharge is clear or cloudy with minimal odor. A change may suggest a vaginal infection. Specific appearance or odor of the discharge may help identify the causative organism. For example, bacterial vaginosis produces an unpleasant fishy odor with vaginal discharge in some women.

Do you have other symptoms such as pain or itching?

These are associated symptoms. Irritation from the discharge can cause itching, rash, or pain with intercourse. Pelvic, abdominal, or urinary pain associated with discharge suggests infection.

If sexually active, does your partner have a discharge? Have you or your partner had a recent change or addition in sex partners?

A common cause of penile and vaginal discharge is STD.

Problems with Menstruation

What kinds of problems with menstruation are you experiencing? Have you noticed clotted blood during your periods? If so, when did it begin? Is it becoming worse over time?

Menorrhagia is a term for heavy menses. Clotting of blood indicates a heavy flow or vaginal pooling.

Do you have cramps or other pains associated with your period? Do they occur each month? What relieves the discomfort? Do the cramps or pains interfere with your normal activities?

Dysmenorrhea is a term for painful or difficult menses. It is often associated with hormone imbalance or endometriosis.

Do you ever have spotting between periods?

Spotting between periods or midcycle bleeding may indicate hormone imbalance or a need for dose adjustment if the patient is taking hormonal contraceptives or hormone replacement.

Do you have any other problems or symptoms before menses such as headaches, bloated feeling, weight gain, breast tenderness, irritability, or moodiness? Do they seem to be associated with your periods, or do they occur at other times? Do they interfere with your routine activities?

Hormone fluctuation associated with the menstrual cycle may cause the patient to have symptoms that are frequently referred to as premenstrual syndrome (PMS). Asking how routine activities are affected by symptoms helps the nurse gain a better understanding of the significance of the symptoms.

Menopausal Symptoms

When did your menstrual periods slow or stop? Describe the symptoms you are experiencing.

Amenorrhea means absent menses. The perimenopausal period for most women occurs between ages 42 and 58. Common symptoms experienced during menopause include hot flashes, excessive sweating, back pain, palpitations, headaches, vaginal dryness, painful intercourse, changes in sexual desire, or mood swings.[8]

Are you being treated for any symptoms associated with menopause? Are you taking hormone replacement? If so, what are you taking and how much? Have you noted any adverse effects?

Hormone replacement therapy (HRT) includes taking estrogen for women without a uterus or taking estrogen and progesterone for women with a uterus. Adverse effects of estrogen include headache, nausea, fluid retention, breast pain or enlargement, and vaginal bleeding. A link between cardiovascular disease and estrogen replacement therapy has also been found. Adverse effects of progesterone include weight gain and increased appetite, fluctuations in mood (irritability and depression), breast tenderness, and spotting.

Difficulty with Erection

When did you first notice problems with attaining or maintaining an erection? Did this problem develop suddenly or over a period of time? Do you have this problem consistently, or does the problem come and go?

Erectile dysfunction (ED) is a common problem, yet a very delicate topic. It is highly age dependent; 4% of men in their 50s and 17% of men in their 60s are unable to achieve an erection. By age 75 the incidence jumps to 47%.[10]

Do you have an idea about what might be contributing to the problem?

ED may be associated with medications, chronic illness (e.g., diabetes, hypertension, or treatment for prostate cancer), sexual dissatisfaction, or emotional problems. It may also be an indicator for underlying complications among men with diabetes.[11] If the nurse identifies a patient who has difficulty with erection, he or she recommends a referral to a health care professional who specializes in this area.

Problems with Urination

What kind of problem or change with urination are you experiencing? Is it hard to urinate? Do you have to urinate more frequently than normal?

Infection is the most common problem among men and women. A common problem among older men is urinary obstruction caused by an enlarged prostate.

Have you experienced any pain or burning with urination? Is the urine clear or cloudy? Discolored? Bloody? Foul smelling? If so, do you have other symptoms such as frequent urination in small amounts? Feeling that you cannot wait to urinate? Incontinence?

These symptoms may accompany problems such as UTI or acute cystitis among men and women and prostatitis among men. Urethritis in the young, sexually active male may indicate an STD such as chlamydia or gonorrhea.[3]

Do you think you are urinating more frequently than you consider normal? Do you awaken at night because you have to urinate?

Medications, especially those for cardiovascular problems, diuretics, and antihistamines, may cause increased urination. When the patient has a urinary tract disorder or prostate enlargement, nocturia (awakening at night to urinate), urinary frequency, and urgency usually also increase.

Men: Do you have any trouble initiating or maintaining a urine stream? Is the stream narrower or weaker than usual? Afterward do you feel that you still have to urinate?

Hesitancy, straining, loss of force or decreased caliber of the stream, terminal dribbling, sensation of residual urine, and recurrent episodes of acute cystitis may be symptoms of a progressive prostate enlargement. Prostate enlargement, a common condition among older men, gradually obstructs the urethra, impeding urinary flow. Determine onset of the problem. If benign prostatic hyperplasia is suspected, use the symptom index tool (Table 17-1).[12]

🌐 **ETHNIC, CULTURAL, AND SPIRITUAL VARIATIONS**

Menopausal Symptoms

A study involving Israeli women found differences in reporting of menopausal symptoms (i.e., hot flashes, mental and somatic symptoms) between minority (i.e., immigrants and Arab women) and majority (long-term Jewish residents) women. There was a lower report of symptoms by the minority women. Researchers concluded that the differences were culturally based.

Data from Lerner-Geva L et al: The impact of education, cultural background, and lifestyle on symptoms of the menopausal transition: the women's health at midlife study, *J Women's Health* 19(5):975-985, 2010.

Rectal Bleeding

When did the rectal bleeding first start? Is the problem constant or does it come and go? Describe the color and amount of blood.

Determine onset and duration of the problem. Determine characteristics of the bleeding. Bleeding from high in the intestinal tract produces black, tarry stools (melena); whereas bleeding near the rectum is associated with bright red bleeding (hematochezia). Black or dark, nontarry stools may occur when taking certain medications such as iron supplements.

Have you had accompanying abdominal cramping or pain? Have you been constipated? Have you felt fatigued?

Identify associated symptoms. Some conditions such as ulcerative colitis can cause rectal bleeding accompanied by abdominal cramping. The passage of hard, dry stools can contribute to rectal bleeding. Fatigue is a significant finding in patients who develop anemia secondary to rectal bleeding.

TABLE 17-1	**THE AMERICAN UROLOGICAL ASSOCIATION SYMPTOM INDEX FOR BENIGN PROSTATIC HYPERPLASIA**					
QUESTIONS	**NOT AT ALL**	**LESS THAN 1 TIME IN 5**	**LESS THAN HALF THE TIME**	**ABOUT HALF THE TIME**	**MORE THAN HALF THE TIME**	**ALMOST ALWAYS**
1. During the last month or so, how often have you had a sensation of not emptying your bladder completely after you finished urinating?	0	1	2	3	4	5
2. During the last month or so, how often have you had to urinate less than 2 hours after you finished urinating?	0	1	2	3	4	5
3. During the last month or so, how often have you stopped and started again several times when you urinated?	0	1	2	3	4	5
4. During the last month or so, how often have you found it difficult to postpone urination?	0	1	2	3	4	5
5. During the last month or so, how often have you had a weak urinary stream?	0	1	2	3	4	5
6. During the last month or so, how often have you had to push or strain to begin urination?	0	1	2	3	4	5
	NONE	**1 TIME**	**2 TIMES**	**3 TIMES**	**4 TIMES**	**5 OR MORE TIMES**
7. During the last month, how many times did you most typically get up to urinate from the time you went to bed at night until the time you got up in the morning?	0	1	2	3	4	5

From Barry MJ et al: The American Urologic Association symptom index for benign prostatic hyperplasia, *J Urol* 148(11):1549-1557, 1992.
Score: 7 or below = mild symptoms; 8-19 = moderate symptoms; above 20 = severe symptoms.

HEALTH PROMOTION FOR EVIDENCE-BASED PRACTICE

Sexually Transmitted Disease

Background

There are an estimated 19 million new sexually transmitted disease (STD) cases each year in the United States; nearly 50% of these involve young people ages 15 to 24 years. Women tend to suffer more serious consequences of STD than do men; ethnic groups with the highest incidence of STD are African Americans and Hispanics.

Goals and Objectives—Healthy People 2020

The overall Healthy People 2020 goal related to STD is to promote healthy sexual behaviors, strengthen community capacity, and increase access to quality services to prevent STDs and their complications. Ten specific objectives are related to STDs, including increasing screening efforts, reduction of disease, and appropriate treatment.

Recommendations to Reduce Risk (Primary Prevention)
Centers for Disease Control and Prevention (CDC)

- Abstinence and reduction of number of sex partners: Abstain from sexual intercourse or be in a long-term, mutually monogamous relationship with an uninfected partner. Before initiating sexual activity with a new partner, both should be tested for STDs, including human immunodeficiency virus (HIV).
- Preexposure vaccination:
  - Human papillomavirus (HPV) vaccination is recommended for girls ages 11 to 12 and girls and young women ages 13 to 26 who did not receive the vaccination when they were younger.
  - Hepatitis B vaccine is recommended for all adolescents if not given with childhood immunizations; unimmunized adults who have more than one sex partner or men who have sex with men (MSM) should be encouraged to receive vaccination.
  - Hepatitis A vaccine is recommended for all adolescents if not given with childhood immunizations; unimmunized MSM should be encouraged to receive vaccination.

- Barrier protection:
  - A male condom should be used if sexual activity will involve an individual whose infection status is unknown or who is infected with an STD. Use of a spermicide alone is not effective in preventing sexually transmitted infection.
  - Female condoms have also been found to be an effective mechanical barrier to prevent STD. Although the female condom is more expensive than male condoms, it should be used if a male condom cannot be used.

Screening Recommendations (Secondary Prevention)
Centers for Disease Control and Prevention

- *HIV:* HIV screening is recommended for all persons seeking evaluation and treatment for STDs. HIV testing should be offered for all pregnant women at the first prenatal visit or at delivery if they did not receive prenatal care.
- *Chlamydia:* Annual screening should be offered for all sexually active women under age 20; sexually active women ages 20 to 24 who meet *either* of the following criteria: inconsistent use of a barrier contraceptive or more than one sexual partner during the last 3 months; and sexually active women older than age 24 who meet *both* previously stated criteria. Pregnant women should be screened at the first prenatal visit and again during the third trimester if they have high-risk behaviors.
- *Gonorrhea:* Annual screening is recommended for all sexually active women under age 25 and all high-risk sexually active women over age 25. All pregnant women with high-risk behaviors should be screened at the first prenatal visit.
- *Syphilis:* All high-risk individuals should be screened. Screening should be performed on all pregnant women at the first prenatal visit and again during the third trimester or at delivery if they have high-risk behaviors.

From Centers for Disease Control and Prevention: Sexually transmitted diseases treatment guidelines 2010, *MMWR* 59(RR12); *Healthy People 2020* (available at http://www.healthypeople.gov/2020/default.aspx).

HEALTH PROMOTION FOR EVIDENCE-BASED PRACTICE

Reproductive Cancers

Background

Reproductive cancers accounted for an estimated 311,150 new cases and 51,680 deaths in the United States in 2012. The large majority of new cases and deaths involve prostate cancer (241,740 and 28,170, respectively). Among women nearly half of new cancer cases (47,130) were caused by endometrial cancer, and over half of the deaths (15,500) were caused by ovarian cancer. Despite these facts, cancer of the cervix receives the most attention in health promotion literature because effective screening through cytologic testing exists only for cervical cancer.

Goals and Objectives—Healthy People 2020

The overall *Healthy People 2020* goal related to cancer is to reduce the number of new cancer cases and illness, disability, and death caused by cancer.

Recommendations to Reduce Risk (Primary Prevention)
U.S. Preventive Services Task Force

- It is unknown if counseling women about measures for primary prevention of gynecologic cancers is effective in reducing long-term morbidity and mortality rates.

HEALTH PROMOTION FOR EVIDENCE-BASED PRACTICE

Reproductive Cancers—cont'd

- There are no specific recommendations for prevention of prostate or testicular cancers.
- Clinicians are encouraged to promote the practice of certain healthy behaviors (e.g., smoking cessation, safe sex practices, and maintaining healthy body weight) because these may reduce the incidence of certain cancers.

Screening Recommendations (Secondary Prevention)
Cervical Cancer
- The U.S. Preventive Services Task Force (USPSTF) and American Cancer Society (ACS) recommend routine screening for cervical cancer. USPSTF recommends screening in all sexually active women at least every 3 years after onset of sexual activity or age 21 (whichever comes first) through age 65.

Endometrial Cancer
- ACS recommends annual screening with biopsy for women age 35 who have or are at risk for hereditary nonpolyposis colon cancer.

Prostate Cancer
- Because longer-term outcomes are unclear, USPSTF reports that there is insufficient evidence to recommend for or against routine screening for prostate cancer using PSA testing because of no reduction in prostate cancer mortality.
- The ACS recommends that PSA and DRE screening tests be done annually for men starting at age 50 or at age 45 for men with increased risk factors (African American men or men with a first-degree relative who had prostate cancer at a young age).

Ovarian Cancer
- Routine screening for ovarian cancer is not recommended by USPSTF or ACS.
- Women who have a family history of mutations in breast cancer 1 or 2 genes (BRCA-1 or BRCA-2) should be referred for genetic counseling and an evaluation from BRCA testing.

Testicular Cancer
- Routine screening for testicular cancer is not recommended by USPSTF or ACS.

Data from American Cancer Society: *Cancer facts and figures 2012,* Atlanta, 2012, American Cancer Society; US Department of Health and Human Services: Cancer. In *Healthy People 2020,* available at http://www.healthypeople.gov/2020/default.aspx); US Preventive Services Task Force: *Guide to clinical preventive services,* available at http://www.uspreventiveservicestaskforce.org/recommendations.htm).
DRE, Digital rectal examination; *PSA,* prostate-specific antigen.

EXAMINATION

FEMALE EXAMINATION OVERVIEW

ROUTINE TECHNIQUES	SPECIAL CIRCUMSTANCES OR ADVANCED PRACTICE
• INSPECT the pubic hair and skin over the mons pubis and inguinal area. • INSPECT the labia majora, labia minora, and clitoris. • INSPECT the urethral meatus, vaginal introitus, and perineum. • INSPECT the perianal area and anus.	• PALPATE the Skene's and Bartholin's glands. ★ • INSPECT and PALPATE for vaginal wall tone ★ **Speculum Examination** • INSPECT the cervix. ★ • OBTAIN specimens for laboratory testing. ★ • INSPECT the vaginal walls. ★ **Bimanual Examination** • PALPATE the vagina. ★ • PALPATE the cervix and uterus. ★ • PALPATE the adnexa and ovaries. ★ • PALPATE the uterus and ovaries using a rectovaginal approach. ★ **Rectal Examination** • PALPATE the rectal wall. ★ • PALPATE the anal sphincter. ★ • EXAMINE the stool.

EQUIPMENT NEEDED
Examination gloves • Light source • Speculum • Swabs • Lubricating gel

★ Advanced practice.

PREPARING FOR THE FEMALE EXAMINATION

Before you begin this procedure, prepare the room. Assemble the equipment; obtain a sheet, pillow, and gown; and be sure that the room temperature is warm. Clean your hands and don examination gloves.

Women may feel apprehensive about having their genitalia examined, especially if the nurse is male. If necessary, arrange for a female assistant. Before bringing the woman to the examination room, ask her to empty her bladder. Provide for privacy as the woman prepares for the examination. She should be instructed to undress completely and put on a gown. Some women may be more comfortable wearing their socks.

Assist the woman into the lithotomy position, with body supine, feet in the stirrups, and knees apart. Provide adequate draping with a sheet. Position her with her buttocks at the edge of the examination table. Ask her to place her arms at her sides or across her chest but not over her head (this tightens the abdominal muscles). Position the sheet completely over the patient's lower abdomen and upper legs, exposing only the vulva for your examination. Push the sheet down so you can see the woman's face as you proceed. Sit on a stool at the end of the table between the patient's legs.

Help the woman relax. The lithotomy position may make her feel embarrassed and vulnerable. If she seems uncomfortable or embarrassed, you may ask her if she would like her head elevated so she can see you better. Readjusting the stirrups either outward or inward may help reduce the stress on the pelvis and legs. In addition, make sure that the patient is adequately covered and that you are in a private location where others may not walk in during the examination.

As you start the examination, reassure her that you will tell her everything that you are going to do before you actually do it. Assure her that, if she becomes too uncomfortable, you will stop what you are doing and reassess what is happening. Always remember to touch the inner aspect of her thigh before you touch the external genitalia. (Don't be tentative with your touch; once you make physical contact, maintain it throughout the procedure.) Be sure to talk to the woman throughout the examination to tell her what you are doing, what you are seeing or feeling, and how long it will be until you are finished.

PROCEDURES AND TECHNIQUES WITH EXPECTED FINDINGS	ABNORMAL FINDINGS

ROUTINE TECHNIQUES: FEMALE GENITALIA EXAMINATION

CLEAN hands.

INSPECT the pubic hair and skin over the mons pubis and inguinal area for distribution and surface characteristics.

Hair distribution varies but usually covers an inverse triangle with the base over the mons pubis; some hair may extend up midline toward the umbilicus. The skin should be smooth and clear (Fig. 17-9).

Note any male hair distribution (diamond-shaped pattern), patchy loss of hair, or absence of hair in any patient over 16 years of age. Observe for presence of skin lesions or infestations (nits or lice) of skin or pubic hair. *Monilial infections* are red, eroded patches with scaling and pustules and are associated with immobility, systemic antibiotics, and immunologic deficits.

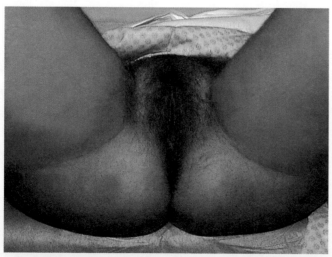

FIG. 17-9 Inspection of the external genitalia.

PROCEDURES AND TECHNIQUES WITH EXPECTED FINDINGS	ABNORMAL FINDINGS

INSPECT and PALPATE the labia majora, labia minora, and clitoris for pigmentation and surface characteristics.

The skin pigmentation of the labia majora should be darker than the patient's general skin tone; and the tissues may appear shriveled or full, gaping or closed, usually symmetric, with a smooth skin surface and a dry or moist texture.

Gently touch the patient on the inner thigh and tell her that you are going to spread the labia apart. Spread the labia majora to view the inner surface of the labia majora, labia minora, and the surface of the vestibule (Fig. 17-10). Pigmentation should be dark pink. The area should appear moist; and the tissue should appear symmetric and without drainage, lesions, or sores.

Observe for signs of inflammation, edema, excoriation, leukoplakia (white patches), ulceration, drainage, lesions, nodules, and marked asymmetry.

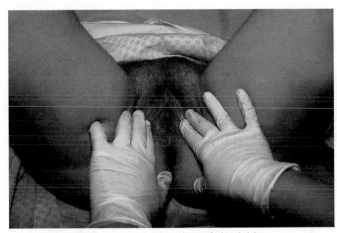

FIG. 17-10 Inspection of the labia.

Palpate the labia minora between your thumb and the second fingers of your other hand. The tissue should feel smooth and soft without nodules or masses, and the palpation should elicit no statements of discomfort from the patient.

Inflammation, irritation, excoriation, vaginal discharge, and pain are abnormal findings. Discoloration or tenderness may be the result of traumatic bruising.

The clitoris is located midline between the labia minora. It is normally a smooth, pink, and moist cylindric structure about the size of an eraser head.

Note any enlargement, atrophy, inflammation, lesions, or discharge.

INSPECT the urethral meatus, vaginal introitus, and perineum for positioning and surface characteristics.

Inspect the urethral meatus and the tissues immediately surrounding it. There should be a midline location of an irregular opening or slit close to or slightly within the vaginal introitus. The vaginal introitus may appear as a thin vertical slit or a large orifice with irregular edges from the hymenal remnants; the tissues should appear moist. The posterior skin surface of the perineum between the vaginal introitus and the anus should appear smooth and without lesions or discoloration. If the patient has had an episiotomy, a scar (midline or mediolateral) may be visible.

Note any discharge from the surrounding (Skene's) glands or the urethral opening, polyps, inflammation, or a lateral position of the meatus. Note any surrounding inflammation, discolored or foul-smelling vaginal discharge, bleeding or blood clots, edema, skin discoloration indicative of tissue bruising, or lesions. Note scars, skin tags, lesions, fissures, lumps, or excoriation.

PROCEDURES AND TECHNIQUES WITH EXPECTED FINDINGS

INSPECT the perianal area and anus for color and surface characteristics.

The anus should exhibit increased pigmentation and coarse skin; no lesions should be present, and the skin should be intact. The anus should be closed tightly. Hemorrhoids may be seen in the adult; differentiate hemorrhoids from other lesions. If a lesion is seen, identify the location of the abnormality in terms of the position of a clock, with the 12 o'clock position being toward the symphysis pubis and the 6 o'clock position toward the sacrococcygeal area.

Ask the patient to bear down. While the patient is straining, observe for the presence of internal hemorrhoids, polyps, tumors, and rectal prolapse. None should be seen.

SPECIAL CIRCUMSTANCES OR ADVANCED PRACTICE: FEMALE GENITALIA EXAMINATION

The procedures that follow are part of the female pelvic examination. This is done by an advanced practice nurse as a routine annual examination or when a patient presents with pelvic pain or discharge.

★PALPATE the Skene's and Bartholin's glands for surface characteristics, discharge, and pain or discomfort.

With the labia still spread apart, insert the index finger of your dominant hand (palm surface up) into the vagina as far as possible. Exert upward pressure on the anterior vaginal wall surface and milk the Skene's glands by moving your finger outward toward the vaginal opening (Fig. 17-11). The glands are located in the paraurethral area and usually are not visible. The gland area should be nontender and without discharge.

Next palpate the lateral tissue of the vagina bilaterally. Use your thumb and index finger to palpate the entire area, paying attention to the posterolateral portion of the labia majora where the Bartholin's glands are located (Fig. 17-12). The glands usually are not visible. There should be no tenderness or discharge.

Note lesions or fissures around the anus. Lesions associated with sexually transmitted disease frequently appear on or around the anus. Lesions that may be seen include external hemorrhoids, ulcerations, warty growths (condylomata acuminata), skin tags, inflammation, fissures, and fistulas. Internal hemorrhoids, polyps, tumors, and rectal prolapse are also abnormal findings.

Note any tenderness or discharge; collect a sample of any discharge that is present for culture. Discharge from the Skene's and Bartholin's glands usually indicates an infection. Edema in the area of the Bartholin's glands that is painful and "hot to the touch" may indicate an abscess of the Bartholin's gland. The abscess is generally pus filled and is gonococcal or staphylococcal in origin. A nontender mass, which is the result of chronic inflammation of the gland, usually indicates a Bartholin's cyst.

★Advanced practice.

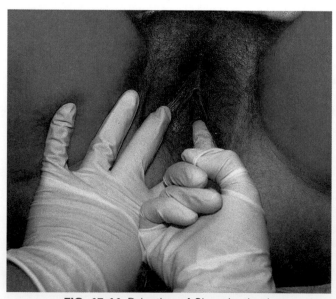

FIG. 17-11 Palpation of Skene's gland.

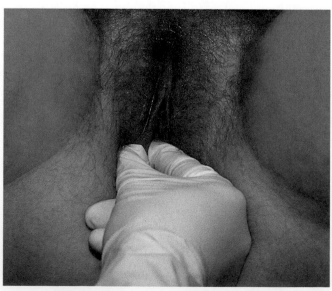

FIG. 17-12 Palpation of Bartholin's gland.

PROCEDURES AND TECHNIQUES WITH EXPECTED FINDINGS	**ABNORMAL FINDINGS**

★PALPATE for vaginal wall tone.

NOTE: Vaginal wall tone is not assessed routinely unless there is a specific indication such as a history of incontinence or discomfort.

With your examining finger still in the vagina, instruct the patient to squeeze the vaginal orifice around your finger. The nulliparous patient is usually able to squeeze tightly so you feel the vaginal wall tissue firmly around your examining finger (Fig. 17-13). If the woman has had children by vaginal delivery, she may not squeeze as tightly.

Note inability of patient to constrict the vaginal orifice around your finger.

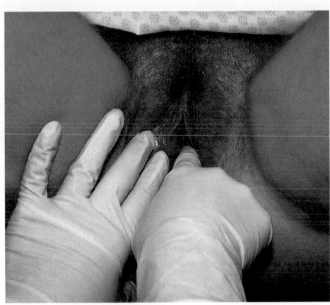

FIG. 17-13 Assessing vaginal tone.

Remove your finger from the vagina. Holding the labia apart, ask the patient to bear down as you inspect for vaginal wall bulging and urinary incontinence. Ask the patient to cough and again inspect for bulging and incontinence.

No bulging or incontinence should be observed.

Bulging of the anterior wall may indicate a cystocele. Bulging of the posterior vaginal wall may indicate a rectocele. If the cervix is visible at the opening of the vagina, it may indicate signs of a uterine prolapse. The presence of urine during either bearing down or coughing may indicate stress incontinence.

★Advanced practice.

PROCEDURES AND TECHNIQUES WITH EXPECTED FINDINGS

ABNORMAL FINDINGS

SPECIAL CIRCUMSTANCES OR ADVANCED PRACTICE: SPECULUM EXAMINATION

The speculum examination is part of the female pelvic examination. This is done by an advanced practice nurse as a routine annual examination or when a patient presents with pelvic pain or discharge.

Tell the patient that you will now use a speculum to do the internal examination (Box 17-1). Using a speculum of appropriate size, follow these steps:

1. Locate the cervix using the middle finger on your nondominant hand; visualize the location in your "mind's eye"; this helps you to locate the cervix with the speculum.
2. Place the index and middle fingers of your nondominant hand inside the vaginal introitus and spread it apart about 2.5 cm. Exert downward pressure against the posterior wall; wait for the vaginal wall muscles to relax (Fig. 17-14).
3. As downward pressure is exerted, simultaneously insert the speculum (with blades closed) over your fingers, holding the speculum at an oblique angle (Fig. 17-15). After the blades pass over your fingers, the speculum must be rotated to a horizontal position as it is inserted.

BOX 17-1   CLINICAL NOTES

- Make sure that you know how to use the speculum before you start, including how to lock the blades open in place and how to release the lock.
- Make sure that the speculum is warm (especially if it is metal). If necessary, run it under warm water to warm it. The speculum may also be kept warm by wrapping it in a heating pad or placing it under a warming light.
- Pick the correct size speculum for the patient. Do not assume that a wide-blade Graves' speculum is comfortable for all women. If the patient is not sexually active, she most likely needs a narrower-blade speculum.
- Lubricate the speculum with warm water. Do not use lubricant because it interferes with cytologic analysis.
- Make sure that you have all of the necessary supplies within reach before you start (e.g., slides, applicators, test tubes with potassium hydroxide [KOH], and saline).

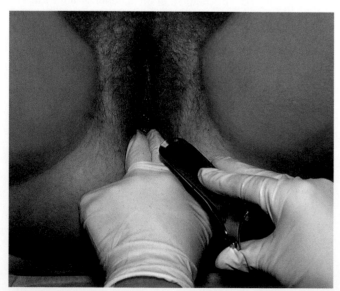

FIG. 17-14 Apply downward pressure on vagina before inserting the speculum.

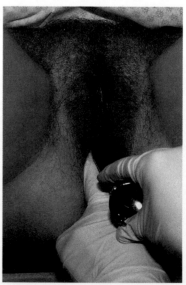

FIG. 17-15 Insertion of closed speculum blades with oblique angle.

PROCEDURES AND TECHNIQUES WITH EXPECTED FINDINGS

4. After the blades have passed the introitus, remove your fingers while exerting downward pressure. Maintain downward and posterior pressure on the blades directed at a 45-degree angle until the speculum is inserted completely (Fig. 17-16, *A* and *B*).

5. With speculum fully inserted and blades horizontal, open the blades of the speculum and look for the cervix. If you see a smooth, shiny wall, you are probably below the cervix; if you see rough or rugated wall, you are probably above the cervix. Reposition the speculum if necessary to visualize the cervix; once visualized, lock the blades in the open position (Fig. 17-17, *A* and *B*).

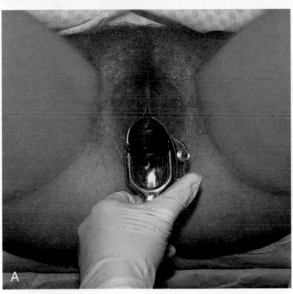
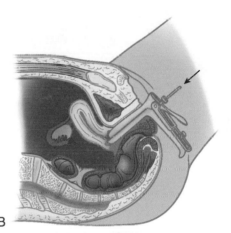

FIG. 17-16 A, Direct the speculum downward at a 45-degree angle. **B,** Cross-sectional view. (**B** from Seidel et al., 2011.)

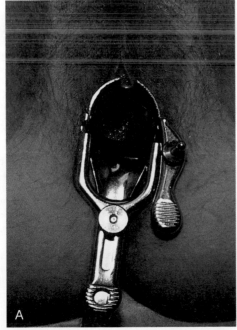
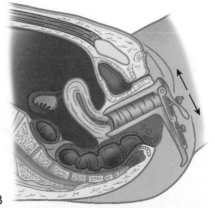

FIG. 17-17 A, Open speculum blades. **B,** Cross-sectional view. (**B** from Seidel et al., 2011.)

PROCEDURES AND TECHNIQUES WITH EXPECTED FINDINGS

★INSPECT the cervix for surface characteristics, color, position, size and shape, and discharge.

The cervix should appear smooth, and it should be an evenly distributed pink color (except during pregnancy, when it is a bluish color secondary to increased vascularity). A symmetric, circumscribed erythema surrounding the os (the opening) may indicate the normal condition of exposed columnar epithelium, known as the *squamocolumnar junction*. You may see nabothian cysts, which appear as smooth, round, small, yellow, raised areas (Fig. 17-18, *F*). Absence of a cervix may be an expected finding for a woman who has had a hysterectomy that included removal of the cervix (Box 17-2).

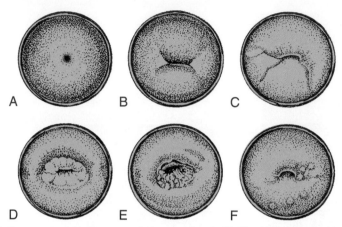

FIG. 17-18 Common appearances of the cervix. **A,** Nulliparous cervix. Note rounded os. **B,** Parous cervix. Note slit appearance of os. **C,** Multigravidous, lacerated. **D,** Everted. **E,** Eroded. **F,** Nabothian cysts. (From Seidel et al., 2011.)

BOX 17-2 CLINICAL NOTE

Performing a speculum examination on a patient who has had a *hysterectomy* is essentially the same as examining any other patient. The most obvious finding during the assessment is the absence of a cervix and uterus. If the patient has had her ovaries removed and is not taking hormone replacement therapy, many findings are consistent with findings present in older, postmenopausal women.

The cervix should be midline and point in a direction related to the position of the uterus. An anterior-pointing cervix indicates a retroverted uterus. A posterior-pointing cervix indicates an anteverted uterus. A midline cervix indicates a midposition uterus (see Table 17-3).

The cervix should be about 2.5 cm in diameter and project into the vagina slightly (2.5 cm or less), forming fornices. The os of a nulliparous patient is small and round. The os of a parous patient is generally slit shaped and may be irregular. An everted cervix (a normal variant) is manifested by a circular, raised erythematous area around the os (see Fig. 17-18). A mucus plug may be present at the os of the cervix.

If discharge is present, determine whether it is coming from the cervix itself or from the vagina and has only pooled near the cervix. Discharge should be odorless; creamy or clear; and thin, thick, or stringy. At the middle of the menstrual cycle or immediately after menstruation, the discharge may be heavier.

ABNORMAL FINDINGS

Note any reddened granular area around the os (especially if asymmetric), friable tissue (tissue that readily bleeds), red patches or lesions, strawberry spots, or white patches. A pale-appearing cervix may be associated with menopause or anemia. Reddened, irregular color or patchy appearance with irregular borders can be an abnormal finding and requires further investigation.

The cervix deviating to either the right or left from a midline position may indicate a pelvic mass, uterine adhesions, or pregnancy and requires further investigation.

Note if the cervix is over 4 cm in diameter. A projection of more than 2.5 cm into the vaginal canal is an abnormal finding and may indicate a pelvic or uterine mass. A lacerated cervix has a torn slit appearance, indicating injury.

A discharge with an odor or a discharge that is colored such as yellow, green, or gray usually indicates a bacterial or fungal infection.

★Advanced practice.

PROCEDURES AND TECHNIQUES WITH EXPECTED FINDINGS	ABNORMAL FINDINGS

★OBTAIN specimens for laboratory testing.

Often during the speculum examination, collection of a specimen for laboratory analysis is indicated. These specimens should be collected while the speculum is still in place but after the cervix and surrounding tissue have been inspected.

Papanicolaou (Pap) test: The Pap test should always be the first specimen collected. It is used as a screening test to detect cervical dysplasia or cancer. Follow the guidelines in Table 17-2 for specimen collection.

★Advanced practice.

TABLE 17-2　PROCEDURE FOR COLLECTING PAP TEST SPECIMEN

	PROCEDURE	RATIONALE
Ectocervical specimen	Insert vertical projection of spatula into os until lateral projection is against cervix. Rotate 360 degrees, maintaining contact with cervix, scraping the entire cervical surface. Remove and spread material from both sides of the spatula thinly on glass slide. Immediately spray slide with cytologic fixative; label slide "ectocervical specimen."	Avoid applying a thick sample on the slide—it makes it difficult to visualize cells. 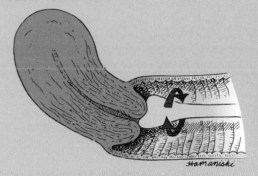
Endocervical specimen	Insert a cytobrush into cervical os. Rotate 360 degrees. Remove and place sample on slide using a rolling or twisting motion on the slide. Immediately spray slide with cytologic fixative; label slide "endocervical specimen."	Use of brush as opposed to cotton-tipped applicator has improved the quality of the sample of endocervical cells. 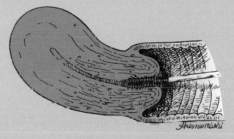
Ectocervical/ endocervical specimen	Use a Cervex-Brush. (It collects both ectocervical and endocervical specimens at the same time.) Insert the central long bristles into the os until the lateral bristles bend against the ectocervix. Apply gentle pressure and rotate the brush 3 to 5 times to the left and right. Withdraw brush and paint the glass slide with two single strokes in the same place on the slide, applying the first stroke with one side to the brush, the second stroke with the other side of the brush. Apply a fixative; label the slide "ectocervical and endocervical specimen."	Use of a Cervex-Brush reportedly causes less spotting after the examination yet provides a quality sample of ectocervical and endocervical cells. 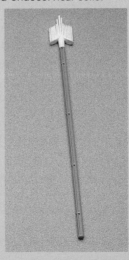

Specimens are not collected while the patient is menstruating or if she took a bath, used a vaginal douche, or inserted topical vaginal inserts or lubrications within the last 48 hours. In addition, do not use lubrication jelly on the speculum if specimens are to be collected. These affect the quality of samples taken and could result in false-negative results. In women who have undergone a hysterectomy in which the cervix was removed, Pap testing is not required unless the hysterectomy was performed because of cervical cancer or its precursors. If a routine Pap test is indicated, the sample should be collected from along the suture line, using the blunt end of a spatula. Label the specimen as vaginal cells taken from the suture line.

Additional screening tests or cultures may be collected at this time; the decision to do this is based on risk factors, the history, or clinical findings.

★INSPECT the vaginal walls for color and surface characteristics.

Procedure: Following the specimen collection, carefully unlock the speculum and, while the blades are still partially open, begin to remove the speculum gently from the vagina. The blades of the speculum tend to close by themselves. As the speculum is being removed, slowly rotate the blades and inspect the walls of the vagina. Apply posterior downward pressure to avoid causing discomfort to the sensitive urethra with blade removal.

Findings: The walls should be pink and moist, with transverse rugae that diminish after vaginal deliveries and with age, and homogeneous in consistency. Note any vaginal secretions. They should be thin, clear or cloudy, odorless, and minimal-to-moderate in amount.

Note if the wall is red or pale; if there are lesions, leukoplakia, cracks, a dried surface, or bleeding; or if it appears nodular or edematous. Report any secretions that are thick, curdy, frothy, gray, green, yellow, foul smelling, or profuse.

SPECIAL CIRCUMSTANCES OR ADVANCED PRACTICE: BIMANUAL EXAMINATION

The bimanual examination is part of the female pelvic examination. This is done by an advanced practice nurse as a routine annual examination or when a patient presents with pelvic pain or discharge.

Tell the patient that you are going to perform an internal examination with your fingers and hand. Move to a standing position at the end of the examination table between the patient's legs. If your gloves have become soiled or contaminated, put on a clean pair of gloves. Lubricate the index and middle fingers of the hand that will be placed internally. Gently insert the middle and index fingers into the vaginal opening. Insert downward pressure on the posterior vaginal wall. Wait a moment for the vaginal opening to relax. Then gradually insert your fingers their full length into the vagina.

★PALPATE the vagina for surface characteristics and discomfort.

Palpate the vaginal wall as you insert your fingers. The wall should feel smooth and be nontender. Once your fingers are fully extended into the vaginal wall, position your thumb (which is outside the vagina and near but not on the urethra and clitoris) out of the way so it is not uncomfortable for the patient.

Abnormalities of the vaginal wall include nodules, cysts, discomfort, and unusual tissue growths.

★PALPATE the cervix and uterus for position, size, surface characteristics, mobility, and discomfort.

Procedure: Locate the cervix with the fingers of your internal hand. Place the palmar surface of the fingers of your other hand on the lower abdomen midway between the umbilicus and the pubis (Fig. 17-19). The hand on the abdomen should gently hold the uterus downward against the internal examination hand so the cervix can be evaluated. Palpate the cervix and vaginal fornices with the palmar surfaces of the fingers of your internal hand.

★Advanced practice.

| **PROCEDURES AND TECHNIQUES WITH EXPECTED FINDINGS** | **ABNORMAL FINDINGS** |

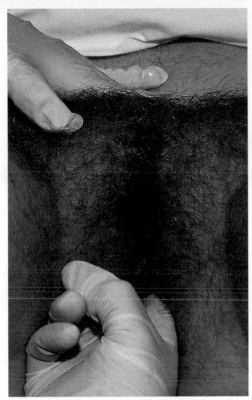

FIG. 17-19 Bimanual palpation.

Findings: The cervix should feel evenly rounded or slightly ovoid, firm (like the tip of a nose), and smooth. It should be slightly mobile in each direction without causing discomfort (documented as no cervical motion tenderness [CMT] noted). It should be located in the midline position; the fornices (pockets surrounding the cervical protrusion) should be pliable and smooth, and there should be no tenderness.

Note if the cervix is enlarged, irregular, soft or nodular, hard, immobile, or associated with discomfort as it moves and if it is laterally displaced (not in the midline). Painful cervical movement suggests an inflammatory process such as acute pelvic inflammatory disease or a ruptured tubal pregnancy.

Procedure: Move the fingers from the cervical os into the anterior fornix of the vagina. Slowly slide the hand that is on the abdomen toward the pubis with the palmar surface of your fingers pressing downward to push the pelvic organs closer for your internal fingers to palpate. It may be helpful to visualize the hands working together to "trap" the uterus between the two hands. The uterus is generally assessed with the *internal fingers*; it is normally not palpable abdominally by the external hand. Determine the uterine size and position.

Findings: The nonpregnant uterus is small and usually lies under the symphysis pubis in the pelvis. In a parous patient the uterus may feel larger. Various uterine positions include anteverted, anteflexed, midposition, retroverted, and retroflexed (Table 17-3). Most women have an anteverted uterus.

An enlarged uterus in a nonpregnant woman is abnormal and requires further evaluation. An enlarged uterus may be caused by fibroid tumor, adenomyosis, or carcinoma.

TABLE 17-3 POSITIONS OF THE UTERUS

Anteverted

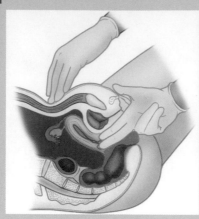

The uterus is palpated at the level of the pubis between the external and internal hands; the uterus points anteriorly; the cervix is aimed posteriorly.

Anteflexed

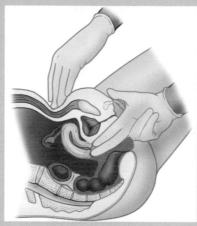

The uterus is palpable at the level of the pubis between the external and internal hands; the uterus points anteriorly, the cervix points along the axis of the vaginal canal.

Midposition

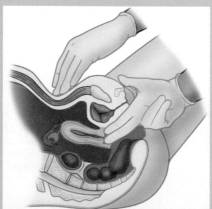

The uterus may not be palpable between the external and internal hands; the uterus points upward, the cervix is pointed along the axis of the vaginal canal.

Retroverted

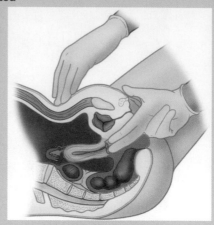

The uterus is positioned posteriorly and is not palpable between the external and internal hands. The cervix is pointed anteriorly.

Retroflexed

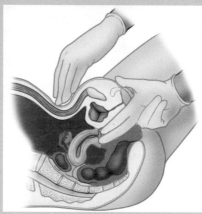

The uterus is positioned posteriorly and is not palpable between the external and internal hands. The cervix is directed along the axis of the vaginal canal.

Illustrations from Seidel et al., 2011.

PROCEDURES AND TECHNIQUES WITH EXPECTED FINDINGS	**ABNORMAL FINDINGS**

Determine surface characteristics by palpating the uterine wall with the internal fingers in the vaginal fornices. Normally it feels smooth and firm. Gently move the uterus between your external hand and internal fingers. It should move freely and be nontender.

Report any irregular contour; soft, nodular consistency; or masses. A uterus that feels irregular or non-smooth is abnormal and requires further evaluation. A soft uterus is usually associated with pregnancy; an irregular surface suggests fibroids. Note if the uterus is fixed or tender during this maneuver. A fixed uterus may indicate adhesions. Tenderness may indicate pelvic inflammation or a ruptured tubal pregnancy.

★PALPATE the adnexa and ovaries for size, shape, and tenderness.

Procedure: Place the abdominal hand on the left lower abdominal quadrant and the intravaginal hand in the left fornix of the vagina. Lift the internal fingers upward as the external fingers press down and inward to "trap" the ovary between the hands (Fig. 17-20). You know that you have located the ovary when you reach a slight bulging area in the lower quadrant and when the patient complains of a "twinge" sensation of slight tenderness.

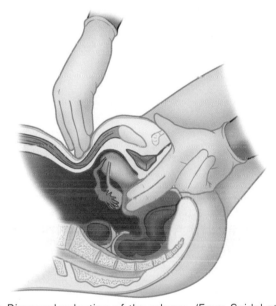

FIG. 17-20 Bimanual palpation of the adnexa. (From Seidel et al., 2011.)

Findings: The ovary may not always be palpable; but, if it is, it should feel smooth, firm, and ovoid. The ovaries are approximately walnut sized and should be mobile. Fallopian tubes have a very small diameter and normally are not palpable or sensitive. Move the hands to the right side and use the same techniques to evaluate the right ovary and adnexa.

An ovary larger than 5 cm is considered abnormal and requires further evaluation. If any masses are noted in the adnexa, evaluate their characteristics: size, shape, location, tenderness, and consistency. Tenderness with palpation is an abnormal finding.

★Advanced practice.

★PALPATE the uterus and ovaries using the rectovaginal approach.

Procedure: The rectovaginal examination allows for a more complete evaluation of the posterior side of the uterus. To prepare for rectovaginal examination, change the intravaginal glove. (This prevents transfer of organisms from the vagina to the rectum.) Tell the patient what you will be doing and that the procedure will be uncomfortable; she may feel the pressure similar to that during a bowel movement. Lubricate the first two fingers of the newly gloved hand. Place your middle finger, palm side up, over the anus. Ask the patient to bear down; while she is doing so, gently insert your middle finger into the rectum. Insert your index finger into the vagina and locate the cervix. Place the external hand on the lower abdomen and apply downward pressure. Repeat the steps as described in the bimanual examination (Fig. 17-21). Keep the index finger of the internal hand under the cervix as a landmark.

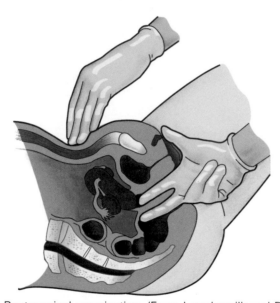

FIG. 17-21 Rectovaginal examination. (From Lowdermilk and Perry, 2007.)

Findings: Normally the uterus feels smooth and firm; the uterus should move freely and be nontender.

Note marked tenderness, nodularity, enlargement, and masses that seem immobile. All of these findings should be considered abnormal. If a mass is detected in the adnexa, evaluate its characteristics, including size, shape, location, tenderness, and consistency.

SPECIAL CIRCUMSTANCES OR ADVANCED PRACTICE: FEMALE RECTAL EXAMINATION

NOTE: The female rectal examination may be done in conjunction with the pelvic examination or independent of a pelvic examination.

This is done by an advanced practice nurse as a routine annual examination or when a patient presents with rectal pain, bleeding, or fullness.

★Advanced practice.

PROCEDURES AND TECHNIQUES WITH EXPECTED FINDINGS	**ABNORMAL FINDINGS**

The female patient should remain in a lithotomy position (if the examination is being done in conjunction with the pelvic examination). If the examination is independent of a pelvic examination, she should assume the left lateral position. Before the examination, tell the patient what you will be doing and that the procedure will be uncomfortable; she may feel the pressure similar to that during a bowel movement.

★PALPATE the rectal wall for surface characteristics.

Procedure: Lubricate the first two fingers of a gloved hand. Place your middle finger, palm side up, over the anus. Ask the patient to bear down; while she is doing so, gently insert your middle finger into the rectum. (If in conjunction with a pelvic exam, simultaneously insert your index finger of the same hand into the vagina and locate the cervix.)

With the index and middle fingers inserted as far as possible, instruct the patient to bear down. This brings more rectal wall into the range of palpation. Gently rotate the finger in the rectum (middle finger) to evaluate the characteristics of the rectal wall.

Findings: The rectal wall should feel smooth and be without any areas of masses, fistulas, fissures, or tenderness.

When this procedure is done in conjunction with the pelvic exam, note the septum (the tissue between the vagina and the rectum); it should be thin, smooth, and intact. Occasionally the cervix may be palpable on the anterior wall; this could be mistaken for a mass.

Note any areas of masses, polyps, nodules, irregularities, and tenderness.

★ASSESS the anal sphincter for muscle tone.

Withdraw your fingers slowly and evaluate the characteristics of the anal tone with the middle finger. The anus should tighten evenly around the examination finger.

Note the presence of rectal stricture. A hypotonic sphincter can occur with neurologic deficits, following rectal surgery, or with anal/rectal trauma (especially trauma associated with frequent anal sex). Hypertonic sphincter may be associated with lesions, inflammation, scarring, or anxiety related to the examination. Extreme pain with anal palpation almost always indicates a local inflammation such as a fissure, fistula, or cyst.

★EXAMINE stool for characteristics and presence of occult blood.

Slowly remove the gloved finger from the patient's rectum. Inspect the gloved finger for color and consistency of stool. It should be brown and soft. Use a guaiac test to evaluate for occult blood (Box 17-3). A negative response is expected.

Note the presence of blood, pus, mucus, or abnormal color of stool (Box 17-4). A positive guaiac test indicates the presence of blood.

★Advanced practice.

BOX 17-3   GUAIAC TESTING

Use the guaiac test to check the stool for occult blood.
1. Obtain a guaiac slide and developer *(A)*.
2. Open the flap of the cardboard guaiac slide.
3. Dab the gloved finger containing stool on the paper in the boxes of the slide *(B)*.
4. Close the flap and remove soiled gloves. Don clean examination gloves.
5. Turn the slide to the reverse side and open the cardboard flap.

6. Apply 2 drops of developing solution on each box of guaiac paper *(C)*.
7. Wait 30 to 60 seconds and note the color of the paper. A bluish discoloration of the paper indicates presence of occult blood and is documented as guaiac positive.

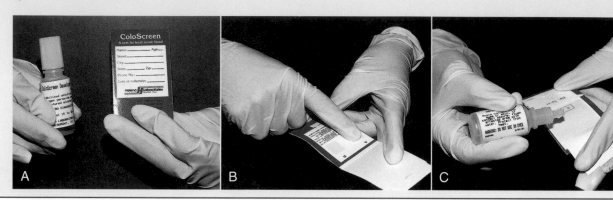

BOX 17-4   STOOL COLORS AND SIGNIFICANCE

COLOR	SIGNIFICANCE
Bright red	Hemorrhoidal or lower rectal bleeding
Tarry black	Upper intestinal tract bleeding or excessive iron or bismuth ingestion
Light tan or gray	Obstruction of the biliary tract (obstructive jaundice)
Pale yellow	Malabsorption syndrome

FREQUENTLY ASKED QUESTIONS

In which situations does a nurse perform a rectal examination? It seems like this is something a health care provider would do.
Remember that a rectal examination includes both an inspection of the anus and an internal examination. Inspection of the anus is done routinely by nurses in a number of situations. For example, when a patient has rectal bleeding or pain, the nurse inspects the anus; he or she also inspects the anus before inserting a suppository or administering an enema. A common indication for a nurse to palpate the rectum is with a patient who is suspected of having a fecal impaction.

DOCUMENTING EXPECTED FINDINGS

Pubic hair inverse triangle pattern with smooth, clear, and intact skin. Labia symmetric, smooth, soft, and moist with pigment darker than general skin tone. Clitoris midline between labia minora with smooth, pink, moist cylindric structure. Urinary meatus midline with an irregular opening. Vaginal introitus moist and appears as a thin vertical slit. No tenderness or discharge noted in the areas of Skene's or Bartholin's glands.

Cervix smooth, pink, midline, posterior pointing, round, about 2.5 cm in diameter, nulliparous, easily movable and without discharge or tenderness. Uterus smooth, firm, anteverted, and freely movable. Ovaries size of walnut, oval, smooth, firm, and mobile bilaterally. Vaginal walls smooth; pink; moist with transverse rugae and minimal thin, clear, and odorless discharge. Skin of perineum intact and smooth. Anus more darkly pigmented; skin is coarse and tightly closed. Rectal wall smooth and intact. Septum between vagina and rectum thin, smooth, and intact. Anal sphincter tone tight, and stool soft and brown.

MALE EXAMINATION OVERVIEW

ROUTINE TECHNIQUES	SPECIAL CIRCUMSTANCES OR ADVANCED PRACTICE
• INSPECT the pubic hair. • INSPECT and PALPATE the penis. • INSPECT the scrotum. • INSPECT the inguinal region and the femoral area. • INSPECT and PALPATE the sacrococcygeal areas. • INSPECT the perianal area and anus.	**Scrotum and Testes** • PALPATE the scrotum. • PALPATE the testes, epididymides, and vas deferens. • TRANSILLUMINATE the scrotum. ★ **Inguinal Region** • PALPATE the inguinal canal. ★ **Rectal Examination** • PALPATE the anus. • PALPATE the anal canal. ★ • PALPATE the prostate. ★ • EXAMINE stool.

EQUIPMENT NEEDED

Examination gloves • Lubricating gel • Light source (if transillumination is needed)

★Advanced practice.

PREPARING FOR THE MALE EXAMINATION

The patient is positioned in one of two ways, either standing or lying down. (He needs to stand to evaluate for a hernia.) If the patient is standing, the nurse should be seated facing him and wearing gloves.

Men may feel apprehensive about having their genitalia examined, especially if the examiner is female. This may be seen as an invasion of privacy rather than accepted as a necessary component of examination. As a nurse you must be aware of these concerns and approach the genitalia examination in a professional, matter-of-fact way, projecting confidence throughout the examination (Box 17-5). Before begining, wash your hands.

BOX 17-5 CLINICAL NOTE

When examining male genitalia, use a firm, deliberate touch. If an erection occurs, reassure the patient that this is a normal physiologic response to touch and that he could not have prevented it. Do not stop the evaluation; stopping focuses further on the erection and reinforces the patient's embarrassment.

PROCEDURES AND TECHNIQUES WITH EXPECTED FINDINGS

ABNORMAL FINDINGS

ROUTINE TECHNIQUES: MALE GENITALIA EXAMINATION

CLEAN hands.

INSPECT pubic hair for distribution and skin for general characteristics.

Hair distribution varies widely but is normally in a diamond-shaped pattern that may extend to the umbilicus. The hair should appear coarser than scalp hair. It should be free of parasites; and the skin should be intact, smooth, and clear.

Note patchy growth, loss, or absence of hair; distribution of hair in a female pattern (triangular, with the base over the pubis); nits or pubic lice; scars; lower abdominal or inguinal lesions; or a rash. *Tinea cruris* ("jock itch") is a common fungal infection found in the groin that appears as large, clearly marginated, red patches that are pruritic. *Monilial infections* are red eroded patches with scaling and pustules and are associated with immobility, systemic antibiotics, and immunologic deficits.

PROCEDURES AND TECHNIQUES WITH EXPECTED FINDINGS

INSPECT and PALPATE the penis for surface characteristics, color, tenderness, and discharge.

The dorsal vein should be apparent on the dorsal surface of the shaft of the penis. The skin is usually dark and hairless, with a wrinkled surface and frequently apparent vascularity. In uncircumcised men the prepuce is present and folded over the glans (Fig. 17-22, *A*); in circumcised men the amount of prepuce varies (see Fig. 17-22, *B*). If the patient has not been circumcised, ask him to retract the foreskin. The foreskin should retract easily and completely over the glans.

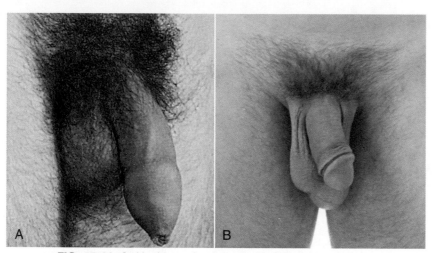

FIG. 17-22 **A,** Uncircumcised penis. **B,** Circumcised penis.

⊕ ETHNIC, CULTURAL, AND SPIRITUAL VARIATIONS
Circumcision

Circumcision has been a common practice of the dominant American culture. Rationales for circumcision include prevention of phimosis and decreased incidence of glans penis inflammation, cancer of the penis, urinary tract infections in infants, and sexually transmitted disease (particularly syphilis, gonorrhea, and warts). However, the decision to circumcise a newborn infant is based largely on cultural practice. Judaism and Islam incorporate circumcision as part of their belief systems. On the other hand, most Native Americans, Alaskan Natives, and Hispanics may be uncircumcised because of their belief system.

ABNORMAL FINDINGS

Failure of the ability to retract the foreskin, discomfort on retraction, or difficulty returning the foreskin to the original position should be considered abnormal. *Phimosis* is a very tight foreskin that cannot be retracted over the glans (Fig. 17-23). *Paraphimosis* is the inability to return the foreskin over the glans (Fig. 17-24).

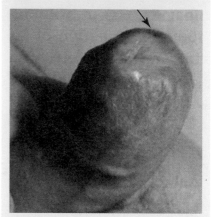

FIG. **17-23** Phimosis. (From 400 Self-assessment picture tests in clinical medicine, 1984. By permission of Mosby International.)

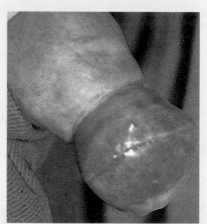

FIG. **17-24** Paraphimosis. (From Lloyd-Davies et al., 1994.)

PROCEDURES AND TECHNIQUES WITH EXPECTED FINDINGS

Inspect the glans and under the fold of the prepuce. The glans should be smooth, pink, and bulbous. Note any erythema, lesions, edema, nodules, or presence of discharge. (If discharge or smegma is present, obtain a specimen on a slide for microscopic examination.) The prepuce fold is wrinkled and loosely attached to the underlying glans; it is darker than the glans. NOTE: Circumcised penises have varying lengths of foreskin remaining; some have multiple folds, and others have none.

Inspect the urethral meatus. It should be located centrally at the distal tip of the glans and should appear as a slit-like opening. No discharge should be present.

ABNORMAL FINDINGS

Erythema, edema, or redness may indicate *balanitis,* an inflammation of the glans that commonly occurs in patients with phimosis (Fig. 17-25).

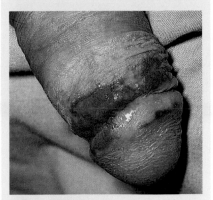

FIG. 17-25 Balanitis. (From Swartz, 2010.)

Note if the meatus is located either on the upper surface of the penis (epispadias) or on the bottom of the penis (hypospadias). Note if a discharge is present. The discharge may be yellow-green or milky white or have a foul odor (Fig. 17-26).

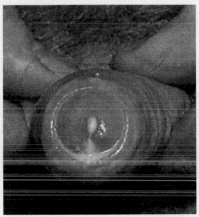

FIG. 17-26 Purulent penile discharge. (From Swartz, 2010.)

PROCEDURES AND TECHNIQUES WITH EXPECTED FINDINGS	ABNORMAL FINDINGS

Palpate the glans anteroposteriorly to open the distal end of the urethra (Fig. 17-27). The surface should be pink and smooth, and no discharge should be present.

Report any erythema, edema, discharge, or crusting.

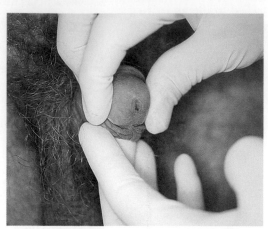

FIG. 17-27 Examination of urethral meatus.

Palpate the entire shaft of the penis between the thumb and first two fingers. The penis shaft should be nontender and smooth with a semifirm consistency.

Note tenderness, edema, nodules, or induration.

INSPECT and PALPATE the sacrococcygeal areas for surface characteristics and tenderness.

The sacrococcygeal area is located betweeen the sacrum and the coccyx. See Fig. 14-3 for landmarks. The skin surface should be smooth, without lesions. There should be no tenderness with palpation.

A dimple with an inflamed tuft of hair or a tender palpable cyst in the sacrococcygeal area suggests a pilonidal cyst or sinus (see Common Problems and Conditions later in this chapter).

INSPECT the perianal area and anus for pigmentation and surface characteristics.

The buttocks are spread with both hands to inspect this area. The anus should exhibit increased pigmentation and coarse, intact skin. The anus should be tightly closed. No lesions or inflammation should be present. Ask the patient to bear down while you inspect the anal area. Again, no lesions should be observed.

Note the presence and location of inflammation and lesions. Identify the location of the abnormality in terms of the position of a clock, with the 12 o'clock position being toward the symphysis pubis and the 6 o'clock position toward the sacrococcygeal area. Lesions that may be seen include external hemorrhoids, ulcerations, warty growths (condylomata acuminata), skin tags, inflammation, fissures, and fistulas. While the patient is straining, note the presence of internal hemorrhoids, polyps, tumors, and rectal prolapse (see Common Problems and Conditions later in this chapter).

PROCEDURES AND TECHNIQUES WITH EXPECTED FINDINGS	**ABNORMAL FINDINGS**

INSPECT the scrotum for color, texture, surface characteristics, and position.

Move the penis out of the way with the back of your hand (or ask the patient to hold the penis out of the way) while you inspect the scrotum (Fig. 17-28). The scrotal sac is divided in half by the septum; the two sides often appear asymmetric; the left side tends to hang lower than the right because of a longer spermatic cord (see Fig. 17-22, *B*). The scrotal skin is usually more deeply pigmented than the body skin, with a coarse-appearing surface. Small bumps on the scrotal skin are known as *sebaceous cysts* or *sebaceous glands*; they are considered a normal finding. The scrotal surface should be a consistent color without lesions. Be sure to lift the scrotum to examine the underside as well. This area is deeply pigmented, hairless, and has a rugous surface.

Temperature affects the appearance of the scrotum. When the environmental temperature is very cold, the testes retract slightly upward, causing the scrotum to become smaller and tighter in appearance. Conversely, when the temperature is hot, the testes extend downward, and the scrotal sac hangs loosely. A patient who has a fever may have a pendulous-appearing scrotum.

Scrotal lesions or scrotal redness (either generalized or isolated) is considered abnormal and may indicate an infection. Excessive differences between the right and left sides are an abnormal finding.

INSPECT the inguinal region and the femoral area for bulges.

The patient should assume a standing position for this part of the examination. Ask him to bear down. While he is straining, inspect the inguinal canal and femoral area (area just above where the femoral artery is palpated) for presence of a bulge. There should be no bulges.

NOTE: If a bulge is seen, palpate the inguinal ring (described in the Special Circumstances or Advanced Practice section that follows).

Note any bulges in the area of the external ring or the femoral area. Presence of bulges suggests a hernia. See Table 17-4 on p. 436 and Common Problems and Conditions later in this chapter.

SPECIAL CIRCUMSTANCES OR ADVANCED PRACTICE: MALE GENITALIA EXAMINATION

PALPATE the scrotum for surface characteristics and tenderness.

This procedure is done to screen for scrotal masses or when the patient reports pain or edema.

Palpate each half of the scrotum (Fig. 17-29). The surface should feel coarse, with the skin intact and loose over a muscle layer. The thickness of the skin of the scrotum changes with temperature and age. In cold or cool temperatures, the scrotal skin feels thickened. As the individual ages, the skin thins. The scrotum should be nontender.

Note any marked tenderness or edema.

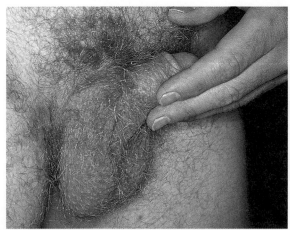

FIG. 17-28 Inspect the scrotum and ventral surface of the penis as the patient positions his penis.

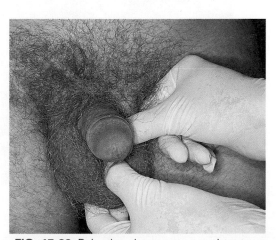

FIG. 17-29 Palpating the scrotum and testes.

PROCEDURES AND TECHNIQUES WITH EXPECTED FINDINGS	ABNORMAL FINDINGS

PALPATE the testes, epididymides, and vas deferens for location, consistency, tenderness, and nodules.

This procedure is done to screen for testicular cancer or when the patient reports pain or edema.

Palpate the testes simultaneously with both hands, using the thumb and the first two fingers. Note that the testes are present in each sac; they should be equal in size, mildly sensitive but nontender to moderate compression, smooth and ovoid, and movable.

Note if the testes have not distended into the sac or are enlarged (unilaterally or bilaterally), atrophied, markedly tender, nodular or irregular, or fixed.

On the posterolateral surface of each testis, palpate the epididymis; it will feel like a tubular, comma-shaped structure that collapses when gently compressed between your fingers and thumb. This area should be smooth and nontender.

If a problem is noted with the epididymis, determine its position in relation to the testes (i.e., proximal or distal); whether it can be moved with your fingers; and if it disappears when the patient lies down. Report any tenderness, irregular placement, enlargement, induration, or nodules.

The vas deferens lies within the spermatic cord. To palpate, grasp both spermatic cords between the thumb and forefinger and palpate, starting at the base of the epididymides, moving upward to the inguinal ring. Because the vas deferens lies within the spermatic cord along with arteries and veins, it is difficult to specifically identify with palpation. The vas deferens feels like a smooth, cordlike structure. It should be nontender and palpable from the epididymis to the external inguinal ring.

Report any tenderness, tortuosity (twisting), thickened or beaded area, or induration.

★TRANSILLUMINATE the scrotum for evidence of fluid and masses.

If a mass, fluid, or irregularity is suspected, transilluminate each scrotal sac. This technique is performed by using a bright penlight or transilluminator and pressing the light source up against the scrotal sac (Fig. 17-30).

There should be no additional contents or fluid. The testes and epididymides do not transilluminate.

Note any mass that is distal or proximal to the testis. It may or may not be tender. Hydroceles and spermatoceles are fluid-filled masses and therefore transilluminate; tumors, hernias, and epididymitis do not.

★Advanced practice.

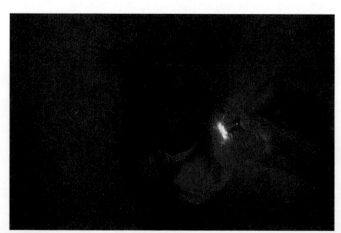

FIG. 17-30 Transillumination of the scrotum. (From Swartz, 2006.)

PROCEDURES AND TECHNIQUES WITH EXPECTED FINDINGS

★PALPATE the inguinal canal for evidence of indirect hernia or direct hernia.

With the patient in a standing position, palpate both the right and left inguinal rings. Use your index or middle finger of the hand corresponding to the patient's side (Fig. 17-31, *A* and *B*) (e.g., right hand for right side). Insert your finger into the lower aspect of the scrotum. The finger should follow the spermatic cord upward through the triangular, slitlike opening of the inguinal ringer into the inguinal canal. Ask the patient to bear down or cough. You should not feel any bulging against your fingertip.

SPECIAL CIRCUMSTANCES OR ADVANCED PRACTICE: MALE RECTAL EXAMINATION

The male patient should assume the left lateral position with the hips and knees flexed, a knee-chest position, or the standing position with the hips flexed and the patient bending over the examination table with feet pointed together (Fig. 17-32, *A* to *D*).

ASSESS the anus for sphincter tone.

Ask the patient to bear down. Place the finger pad surface of a gloved and lubricated index finger at the anal opening; as the sphincter relaxes, slowly insert the finger, pointing toward the patient's umbilicus (Fig. 17-33, *A* and *B*). Ask the patient to tighten the anus around your examining finger. The sphincter should tighten evenly around your finger with minimum discomfort to the patient.

ABNORMAL FINDINGS

Note any palpable mass that touches your fingertip or pushes against the side of your finger.

A hypotonic sphincter can occur with neurologic deficits, following rectal surgery, or with anal/rectal trauma (especially trauma associated with frequent anal sex). Hypertonic sphincter may be associated with lesions, inflammation, scarring, or anxiety related to the examination. Extreme pain with anal palpation almost always indicates a local inflammation such as a fissure, fistula, or cyst.

★Advanced practice.

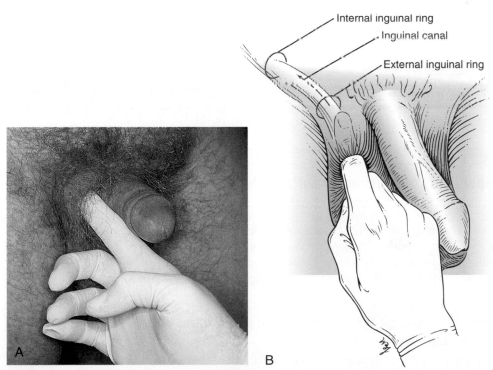

FIG. 17-31 A, Palpating for inguinal hernia. **B,** Position of gloved finger inserted through inguinal canal. (**B** from Swartz, 2011.)

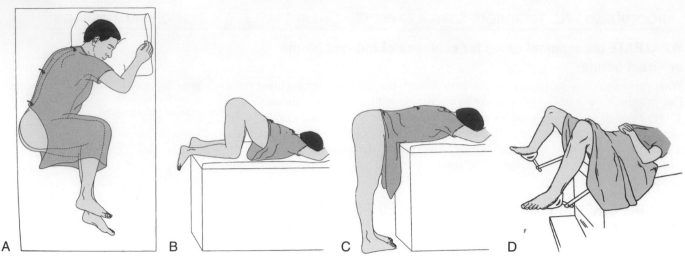

FIG. 17-32 Positions for rectal examination. **A,** Left lateral or Sims' position. **B,** Knee-chest position. **C,** Standing position. **D,** Lithotomy position. (From Barkauskus et al., 2002.)

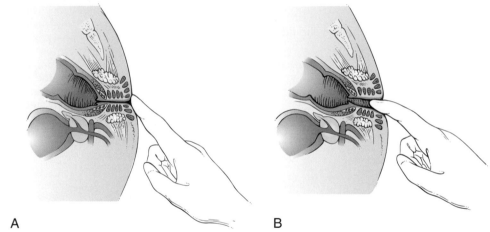

FIG. 17-33 Rectal examination. **A,** Relax sphincter with gentle pressure with the palmar surface of the finger. **B,** Insert the finger into the anal canal. (From Swartz, 2011.)

PROCEDURES AND TECHNIQUES WITH EXPECTED FINDINGS

★PALPATE the anal canal and rectum for surface characteristics.

This procedure is done as part of the rectal examination to detect masses in the rectum.

Rotate the finger around the musculature of the anal ring to palpate the surface characteristics. The area should be smooth, with even pressure on your finger. Insert the finger as far as possible into the rectum to palpate all four rectal walls. There should be a continuous smooth surface, and the patient should experience only minimal discomfort.

★PALPATE the prostate (through the anterior rectal surface) for size, contour, consistency, mobility, and tenderness.

This procedure is done as part of the rectal examination to detect prostate enlargement or to screen for prostate cancer.

ABNORMAL FINDINGS

Note any nodules, irregularities, masses, presence of hard stool, or tenderness.

★Advanced practice.

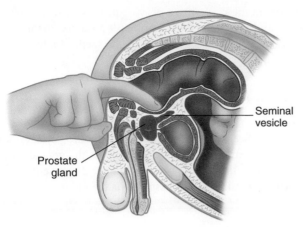

FIG. 17-34 Palpation of the anterior surface of the prostate gland. Feel for the lateral lobes and median sulcus. (From Seidel et al., 2011.)

BOX 17-6	CLASSIFICATIONS OF PROSTATE ENLARGEMENT
GRADE	**PROTRUSION INTO RECTUM**
Grade I	1 to 2 cm
Grade II	2 to 3 cm
Grade III	3 to 4 cm
Grade IV	4 cm

PROCEDURES AND TECHNIQUES WITH EXPECTED FINDINGS

Palpate the posterior surface of the prostate gland by palpating the anterior surface of the rectum (Fig. 17-34). (NOTE: The patient may state that he has the urge to urinate during the prostate examination. Reassure him that this is an expected sensation.) Note the size, contour, consistency, and mobility of the gland. It should be about 3.8 cm in diameter and project less than 1 cm into the rectum. The contour is symmetric and bi-lobed with a palpable vertical groove in the center (referred to as the sulcus). The prostate should feel firm, smooth, and slightly mobile. Palpation should not produce tenderness.

EXAMINE stool for characteristics and presence of occult blood.

Slowly remove the gloved finger from the patient's rectum. Inspect the gloved finger for color and consistency of stool. It should be brown and soft. Use a guaiac test to evaluate for occult blood (see Box 17-3). A negative response is the expected finding.

ABNORMAL FINDINGS

Note if the prostate projects more than 1 cm into the rectum. Estimate classification of prostate enlargement (Box 17-6). Note if there is asymmetry or if the median sulcus is obliterated; also note any tenderness, a boggy feeling, irregularity, or nodules. A rubbery or boggy consistency may indicate benign hyperplasia. A stony-hard or nodular prostate may indicate carcinoma, prostate calculi, or fibrosis.

Note the presence of blood, pus, mucus, or abnormal color of stool (see Box 17-4). A positive guaiac test indicates the presence of blood.

DOCUMENTING EXPECTED FINDINGS

Pubic hair diamond pattern with smooth, clear, and intact skin. Penis uncircumsized, hairless, wrinkled surface and dorsal vein noted. Shaft smooth and nontender. Glans smooth, pink, and bulbous. Urinary meatus slitlike opening in center of glans with pink, smooth urethra without discharge. Sacrococcygeal area smooth, clear, and nontender. Scrotum deeply pigmented, hairless, coarse with rugous surface and intact skin. Testicles smooth, ovoid, and movable bilaterally; epididymis smooth and nontender bilaterally. No bulges or hernia detected in inguinal area.

Skin of perineum intact and smooth. Anus more darkly pigmented with coarse skin; tightly closed. Rectal wall smooth and intact. Prostate symmetric, firm, smooth, slightly mobile. Anal sphincter tone tight, and stool soft and brown.

AGE-RELATED VARIATIONS

This chapter discusses conducting an examination of the reproductive system with adult patients. These data are important to assess for individuals of all ages, but the approach and techniques used to collect the information may vary depending in the patient's age.

INFANTS AND CHILDREN

Infants and children have functionally immature reproductive systems. For this reason examination is usually limited to inspection of external genitalia. Further examination may be warranted if parents, caregivers, or the nurse notice a problem. The nurse should always maintain an awareness of the potential for sexual abuse among infants and children. Chapter 19 presents further information regarding reproductive assessment for this age-group.

ADOLESCENTS

The onset of puberty (pubescence) marks the beginning of sexual development for boys and girls. A focus for this age-group is assessing sexual maturity and the patient's response. Adolescents are often self-conscious about the changes; for this reason the nurse must provide privacy, ensure confidentiality, and be reassuring. Chapter 19 presents further information regarding assessment of the reproductive system among adolescents.

OLDER ADULTS

The history and examination of older adults is similar to that which has been previously described for the younger adult. Sexual response and physical changes to the genitalia occur as a result of the aging process. Chapter 21 presents further information related to assessment of the older adult.

COMMON PROBLEMS AND CONDITIONS

RISK FACTORS

Reproductive Cancer

Female Reproductive Cancers

Cervical Cancer
- The most important risk factor is infection with human papillomavirus (HPV) virus.
- Sexual intercourse at early age and a lifetime history of multiple sex partners or partners with multiple sexual partners increase the risk of HPV infection; thus it is linked to cervical cancer risk. (M)
- Cigarette smoking is a risk factor. (M)

Ovarian Cancer
- Age (increased risk with aging)
- Nulliparity
- Increased body weight (M)
- Estrogen use for postmenopausal hormone replacement therapy (M)
- Personal history of breast cancer
- Genetic condition known as Lynch syndrome (also known as hereditary nonpolyposis colon cancer)
- Strong family history of ovarian and breast cancer
- BRCA-1 and BRCA-2 gene mutations
- Elevated tumor marker CA 125

Endometrial Cancer
- Early menarche and late onset of menopause (increased number of ovulatory cycles)
- Nulliparity
- Obesity (M)

- Estrogen use for postmenopausal hormone replacement therapy (M)
- Infertility
- Genetic condition known as Lynch syndrome (also known as hereditary nonpolyposis colon cancer)
- Family history of endometrial, breast, colon, or ovarian cancer

Male Reproductive Cancers

Testicular Cancer
- Age (highest incidence in young men ages 20 to 34)
- Cryptorchidism (undescended testicle at birth)
- Family history (increased risk if brother has had testicular cancer)
- History of testicular cancer in other testicle
- Ethnicity and culture (highest incidence among white men in the United States and the United Kingdom)

Prostate Cancer
- *Age:* Highest incidence is in older men; 62% of new cases occur in men over age 65; 92% of new cases occur in men age 50 or over.
- *Family history:* First-degree relative with prostate cancer increases risk.
- *Ethnicity:* African American men have the highest incidence of prostate cancer—two times higher than white men. Worldwide the highest prevalence is in North America and northwestern Europe.

Data from American Cancer Society: *Cancer facts and figures 2012,* Atlanta, 2012, American Cancer Society; National Cancer Institute website, available at www.nci.nih.gov.
BRCA-1, BRCA-2, Breast cancer 1 or 2 genes.
M, Modifiable risk factor.

RISK FACTORS
Sexually Transmitted Diseases

Sexually transmitted diseases (STDs) can occur with oral, vaginal, or rectal sex and between heterosexual or homosexual partners.
- Sexual activity with new or multiple sex partners, including prostitutes who trade sex for money or drugs; two or more sex partners in last year (M)
- Sexual activity with individual who has multiple partners (M)
- Sexual activity with individual with history of STD (M)
- Failure to consistently and correctly use protective barrier* (M)
- Not vaccinated against human papillomavirus (HPV) or hepatitis B (M)

M, Modifiable risk factor.
*Latex condoms are effective in preventing infections transmitted via mucosal surfaces (e.g., gonorrhea, chlamydia, human immunodeficiency virus) but may not be as effective in preventing infections transmitted by skin-to-skin contact (e.g., herpes simplex virus, HPV, syphilis).

INFECTIONS

Bacterial Vaginosis

Bacterial vaginosis (BV) is caused by an alteration of the normal vaginal flora with other bacteria; a number of bacteria can cause BV, including *Gardnerella vaginalis*, *Mobiluncus*, and *Mycoplasma hominis*. **Clinical Findings:** The typical signs and symptoms of BV include malodorous vaginal discharge and vulvar itching and irritation.

Candida Vaginitis

Candidiasis is a fungal (yeast) infection usually caused by *Candida albicans*. The Centers for Disease Control and Prevention (CDC) estimates that 75% of all women have at least one fungal infection; 40% to 45% will have two or more infections at some point during their lifetime.[3] *Candida* infections are more prevalent in women who have diabetes mellitus or who are pregnant. **Clinical Findings:** Some women have asymptomatic infections. Those who have symptoms frequently experience vulvar pruritus associated with a thick, cheesy, white vaginal discharge. Vaginal soreness and external dysuria (caused by splash of urine on inflamed tissue) may occur. Erythema and edema to the labia and vulvar skin may be visible.

Sexually Transmitted Disease

Sexually transmitted disease (STD), also commonly referred to as *sexually transmitted infection (STI)*, represents a large number of infections that are transmitted through sexual activity. There are well over 50 different STDs. Listed here are those that the nurse may observe in conjunction with examination of the genitalia.

Chlamydia

Chlamydia is the most common STD in the United States, occurring most frequently among sexually active adolescents and young adults under the age of 25.[3] It is transmitted from genital-genital, oral-genital, and rectal-genital contact. Neonatal exposure during vaginal delivery can cause ophthalmia neonatorum—a purulent conjunctivitis and keratitis. **Clinical Findings, Women:** Chlamydia infection is asymptomatic in up to 75% of women because it often does not cause enough inflammation to produce symptoms.[3] When symptoms occur, the most common are urinary (e.g., dysuria, frequency, or urgency) and vaginal (e.g., spotting or bleeding after sex or purulent cervical discharge). The most important examination findings in a chlamydia infection include purulent or mucopurulent cervical discharge, cervical motion tenderness, or cervical bleeding on introduction of a cotton swab (friability). **Clinical Findings, Men:** This infection usually occurs in the urethra, but it can also affect the rectum. The most common symptoms associated with urethral infection include dysuria, discharge, and urethral itch. If untreated, urethral infection can spread to the epididymis and cause epididymitis.

Gonorrhea

Caused by the aerobic, gram-negative diplococcus *Neisseria gonorrhoeae*, this is currently the second most frequently *reported* STD in the United States. It is transmitted from genital-genital, oral-genital, and rectal-genital contact. Neonatal exposure during vaginal delivery can cause corneal ulceration. **Clinical Findings, Women:** In most women gonorrhea causes a yellow or green vaginal discharge, dysuria, pelvic or abdominal pain, and abnormal menses. Vaginal itching and burning may be severe. **Clinical Findings, Men:** The most common clinical manifestation of gonorrhea is urethritis. Specific clinical findings include mucopurulent or purulent discharge and dysuria.[3] If untreated, gonorrhea can lead to epididymitis.

Syphilis

Syphilis is caused by *Treponema pallidum*, which is transmitted congenitally or by sexual contact. Syphilis infection begins as a local infection in the primary phase and can become systemic. It progresses through four stages if left untreated: primary, secondary, latent, and tertiary. Primary and secondary phases occur within months of exposure; latent and tertiary syphilis occur over a number of years.[8] Fetal exposure (from an infected mother) results in congenital syphilis. **Clinical Findings, Adults:** The clinical manifestations of syphilis vary, depending on the phase of infection. Primary syphilis produces a single, firm, painless open sore or chancre with indurated borders at the site of entry on the genitals or mouth (Fig. 17-35, *A*). In men the most common location is on the shaft of the penis (see Fig. 17-35, *B*). This ulcer typically appears about 21 days after infection and usually heals within 3 to 6 weeks. Secondary syphilis occurs 6 to 12 weeks after the initial lesion. Individuals develop a rash characterized by

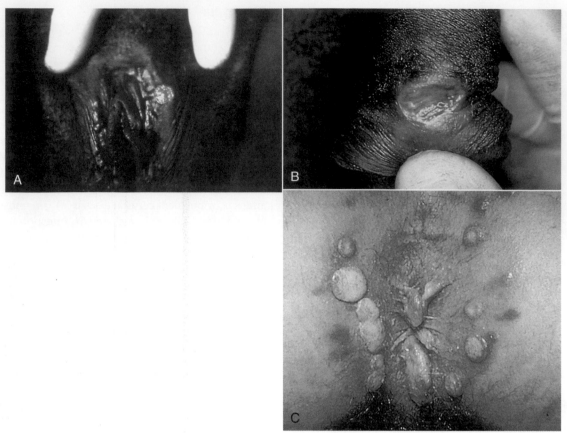

FIG. 17-35 **A,** Syphilis chancre on vulva. **B,** Syphilis chancre on the penis. **C,** Secondary syphilis lesions (condylomata lata) around the anus. (**A** Courtesy CDC Public Health Image Library; **B** and **C** from Goldstein and Goldstein, 1997.)

red macules and papules over the palms of the hands and soles of the feet. Round or oval flat, grayish lesions known as *condyloma latum* develop in the anogenital area (see Fig. 17-35, *C*).Latent syphilis follows the secondary stage and can last from 2 to 20 years; during this period the patients are asymptomatic. Tertiary infection has destructive effects on the neurologic, cardiovascular, ophthalmic, and musculo-skeletal systems. **Clinical Findings, Neonates:** Infected neonates are often premature with intrauterine growth retardation. Manifestations include retinal inflammation, glaucoma, destructive bone and skin lesions, and central nervous system involvement.

Trichomoniasis

Trichomoniasis is a highly contagious STD caused by the protozoan *Trichomonas vaginalis,* which inhabits the vagina and lower urinary tract, particularly the Skene's ducts. **Clinical Findings:** Although some women are asymptomatic, the primary symptom is a malodorous greenish-yellow vaginal discharge often accompanied by vulvar irritation.[3] The walls of the vagina and the cervix may have petechial "strawberry patches" (Fig. 17-36).

Herpes Genitalis

Herpes is a sexually transmitted viral infection caused by the herpes simplex virus. Herpes simplex virus type 1 (HSV1)

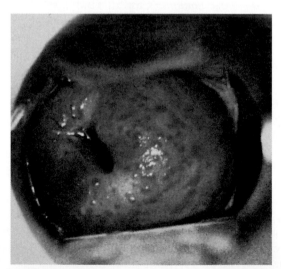

FIG. 17-36 Trichomoniasis. The vaginal mucosa and cervix are inflamed and speckled with petechial lesions. (From Seidel et al., 2011.)

and herpes simplex virus type 2 (HSV2) are two different antigen subtypes of the herpes simplex virus. HSV1 is more commonly associated with gingivostomatitis and oral ulcers (fever blisters), whereas HSV2 is usually associated with genital lesions. However, both types can be transmitted to both sites through genital-oral contact (Box 17-7).

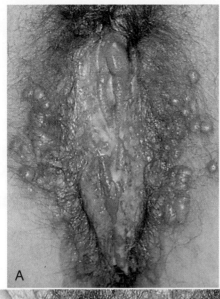

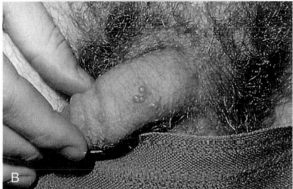

FIG. 17-37 Herpes lesions. **A,** Female. **B,** Male. (**A** from Swartz, 2010. **B** from Goldstein and Goldstein, 1997.)

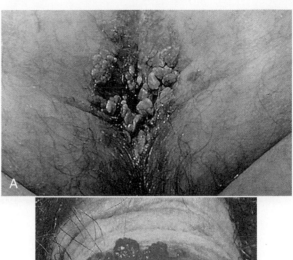

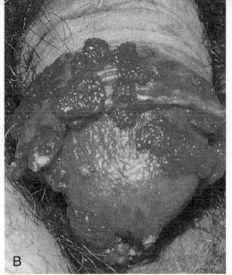

FIG. 17-38 Condyloma acuminatum. **A,** Female. **B,** Male. (Courtesy Lemmi and Lemmi, 2013.)

BOX 17-7 CLINICAL NOTE

Sexually transmitted disease (STD) can occur on the genitalia, on the anus, and in the oral cavity. Furthermore, STD can be present concurrently in more than one location. Therefore, if STD is suspected, examination of other areas is warranted.

Clinical Findings, Women: Herpes genitalis is far more common among women than in men, and women usually have a more severe clinical course. Typical early symptoms include burning or pain with urination, pain in the genital area, and fever. Examination findings reveal single or multiple vesicles that can be found on the genital area or the inner thigh. After vesicles rupture, small, painful ulcers are observed (Fig. 17-37, *A*). **Clinical Findings, Men:** The typical clinical manifestations for men include lesions that appear anywhere along the shaft of the penis or near the glans (see Fig. 17-37, *B*). The lesion is identified because of the red superficial vesicles, which are frequently quite painful. Many men with HSV2 are unaware that they have an infection because the symptoms may be mild.

Human Papillomavirus (Genital Warts, Condylomata Acuminatum)

One of the most common STDs is human papillomavirus (HPV) because it is highly contagious and because these infections are often asymptomatic or unrecognized.[3] HPV infection is associated with early onset of sexual activity, multiple sex partners, and infrequent use of barrier protection. Although it previously was considered benign, HPV has been linked to malignancies of the cervix and penis. **Clinical Findings:** HPV can cause wartlike growths that are termed *condylomata acuminata* (Fig. 17-38, *A* and *B*). The warts typically appear as soft, papillary, pink-to-brown, elongated lesions that may occur singularly or in clusters on the internal genitalia, the external genitalia, and the anal-rectal region. When in clusters, they take on a cauliflower-like appearance.

Pediculosis Pubis (Crabs, Pubic Lice)

Pediculosis pubis is a parasitic infection usually transmitted by sexual contact. **Clinical Findings:** The primary symptom of pubic lice infestation is severe pruritus in the perineal area. Patients may also notice the lice or nits (eggs) in the pubic hair. Examination findings include excoriation and an area of erythema; on close inspection the lice and nits can be seen.

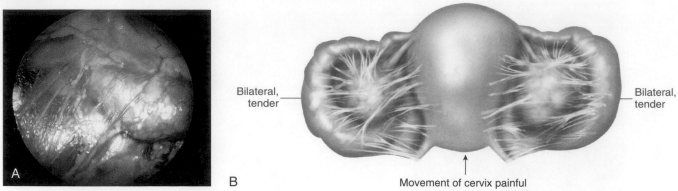

Bilateral, tender

Bilateral, tender

Movement of cervix painful

FIG. 17-39 Pelvic inflammatory disease. (**A** from Symonds and MacPherson, 1994. **B** from Seidel et al., 2011.)

Nits are tiny, yellow-white eggs that are attached to the hair shaft. The adult lice are larger, are tan-to–grayish-white in color, and have a crablike appearance when viewed under a magnifying glass. Lice feces appear as tiny dark spots (resembling pepper) and may be seen adjacent to the hair shafts.

Pelvic Inflammatory Disease (Women)

Pelvic inflammatory disease (PID) is a polymicrobial infection of the upper reproductive tract affecting any or all of the following structures: endometrium, fallopian tubes, ovaries, uterine wall, or broad ligaments. It usually is caused by untreated gonococcal and chlamydia infections. PID is a leading cause of infertility in the United States.[8] **Clinical Findings:** PID can occur as an acute or chronic disease; thus symptoms may vary. Acute PID is associated with very tender adnexal areas (ovaries and fallopian tubes). Typically the pain is so severe that the patient is unable to tolerate bimanual pelvic examination. Other symptoms include fever, chills, dyspareunia, and abnormal vaginal discharge. Chronic PID is associated with tender, irregular, and fixed adnexal areas (Fig. 17-39).

Epididymitis

An inflammation of the epididymis and vas deferens is referred to as *epididymitis*. It is usually caused by the spread of infection from the urethra or bladder. Among sexually active men under the age of 35, it is most often associated with STDs involving chlamydia and gonorrhea.[3] **Clinical Findings:** Classic symptoms include dull, unilateral scrotal pain that develops over a period of hours to days. The scrotum becomes erythematous and edematous (Fig. 17-40). Associated symptoms may include fever and dysuria. A hydrocele may be seen with transillumination.

BENIGN REPRODUCTIVE CONDITIONS AFFECTING WOMEN

Premenstrual Syndrome

Premenstrual syndrome (PMS) is a group or cluster of recurrent symptoms experienced by women associated with their menstrual cycle. It is thought to be associated with

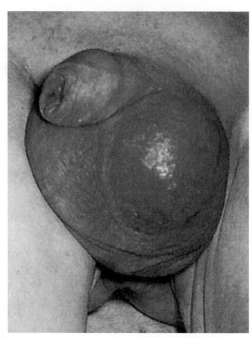

FIG. 17-40 Epididymitis. (From Lloyd-Davies et al., 1994.)

fluctuations in hormone levels and changes in altered sensitivity of the neurotransmitter serotonin.[13] A history of sexual abuse as an adolescent is also associated with PMS in adulthood.[14] **Clinical Findings:** A combination of emotional, cognitive, and physical symptoms begins during the last half of the menstrual cycle and diminishes after menstruation begins. Common emotional symptoms include mood swings, depression or sadness, irritability, tension, anxiety, restlessness, and anger. Common cognitive symptoms include difficulty concentrating, confusion, forgetfulness, and being accident prone. Physical symptoms may include excessive energy or fatigue, nausea or changes in appetite, insomnia, back pain, headaches, general muscular pain, breast tenderness, and fluid retention.

Endometriosis

Endometriosis is a benign, progressive disease process characterized by the presence and growth of uterine tissue outside

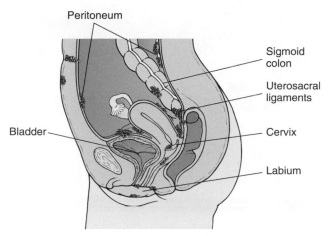

FIG. **17-41** Common sites of endometriosis. (From Lewis et al., 2011.)

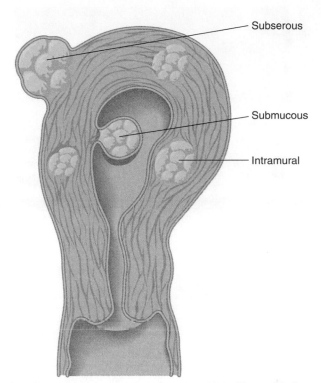

FIG. **17-42** Uterine leiomyomas (fibroids). (From McCance et al., 2010.)

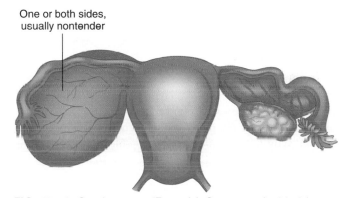

FIG. **17-43** Ovarian cyst. (From McCance et al., 2010.)

the uterus (Fig. 17-41). It is found primarily in women of reproductive age in all ethnic and social groups.[8] **Clinical Findings:** Common symptoms include pelvic pain, dysmenorrhea, and heavy or prolonged menstrual flow. In some women clinical examination findings include small, firm, nodular like masses palpable along the uterosacral ligaments. The uterus may be tender. However, in many women with endometriosis, a clinical examination does not detect any abnormality.

Uterine Leiomyomas

Leiomyomas (also called fibroids) are common benign uterine tumors that most commonly affect women over age 35. The tumors can occur singly or in multiples and can range in size from microscopic lesions to large tumors that fill the entire abdominal cavity. Leiomyomas are most prominent during reproductive years and tend to shrink after menopause. **Clinical Findings:** Most women with leiomyomas are asymptomatic. Those who have symptoms often report pelvic pressure and heaviness, urinary frequency, dysmenorrhea, pelvic or back pain, and abdominal enlargement. If large enough, the leiomyomas can be detected by palpation during a pelvic examination. The tumors typically feel firm, smooth, and irregular in shape (Fig. 17-42).

Ovarian Cysts

Ovarian cysts are benign cystic growths within the ovary. Cysts may be solitary or multiple; they can occur unilaterally or bilaterally. Ovarian cysts occur most commonly in young menstruating women.[8] **Clinical Findings:** Most ovarian cysts are asymptomatic. When symptoms occur, they often include tenderness and a dull sensation or feeling of heaviness in the pelvis. If a cyst ruptures, a sudden onset of abdominal pain occurs. Examination findings for an ovarian cyst include a nontender, fluctuant, mobile, and smooth mass on the ovary (Fig. 17-43).

MALIGNANT REPRODUCTIVE CONDITIONS AFFECTING WOMEN

Cervical Cancer

Cancer of the cervix is usually caused by HPV infection. **Clinical Findings:** The most common symptom is abnormal vaginal bleeding such as bleeding between normal menstrual periods, bleeding after intercourse, or menstrual bleeding that is heavier or lasts longer than normal. On examination a lesion may be visible; the lesion usually has a hard granular surface that bleeds easily and has irregular borders (Fig. 17-44).

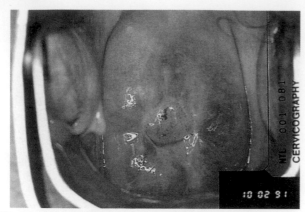

FIG. 17-44 Cervical cancer. The lesion is seen on the cervical os. (From Symonds and Macpherson, 1994.)

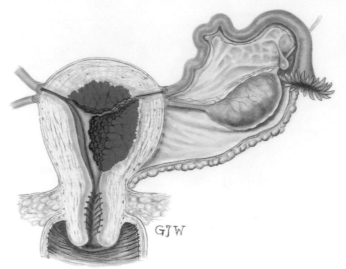

FIG. 17-45 Endometrial cancer. (From Belcher, 1992.)

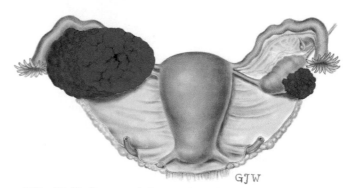

FIG. 17-46 Cancer of the ovaries. (From Belcher, 1992.)

 ETHNIC, CULTURAL, AND SPIRITUAL VARIATIONS

Cancer Screening

One of the four overarching goals of *Healthy People 2020* is to achieve health equity, eliminate disparities, and improve the health of all population groups. Eliminating racial and ethnic disparities in health requires enhanced efforts at preventing disease, promoting health, and delivering appropriate care. One of the focus areas in which racial and ethnic minorities experience disparity in health access and outcome is cancer screening and management. African American women are more than twice as likely to die of cervical cancer than are white women.

Data from Centers for Disease Control and Prevention, 2011, available at http://www.cdc.gov/cancer/cervical/statistics/race.htm.

Endometrial Cancer

The most common gynecologic malignancy is endometrial cancer. It occurs most often in postmenopausal women, especially women taking estrogen. **Clinical Findings:** The cardinal symptom is abnormal uterine bleeding or spotting, although a watery vaginal discharge is frequently noted several weeks to months before the bleeding (Fig. 17-45).

Ovarian Cancer

Ovarian cancer has the highest mortality rate of the gynecologic cancers because it is typically undetected; thus it is known as the "whispering disease." It most commonly occurs among white women over age 50 who live in Western industrialized nations. **Clinical Findings:** There are usually no symptoms until advanced stages of the disease. The most common symptom of ovarian cancer is abdominal distention or fullness. By the time ovarian malignancies are palpable, the disease is usually advanced (Fig. 17-46).

CONDITIONS OF THE SCROTUM/TESTICLES

Testicular Torsion

This condition is caused by the twisting of the testicle and spermatic cord, cutting off blood supply; it is considered a surgical emergency. It may occur at any age, but the prevalence is highest during adolescence. **Clinical Findings:** The hallmark finding of testicular torsion is a history of sudden onset of severe testicular pain and scrotal swelling. The testicle often becomes slightly discolored. It is not associated with physical activity or trauma.

Hydrocele

A hydrocele is an accumulation of fluid within the scrotum. In infants hydroceles often resolve on their own, but occasionally surgical intervention is required.[15] In adults the cause of hydrocele is often unknown but may result from infection or a malignancy. **Clinical Findings:** Gradual scrotal enlargement is the most common symptom. The scrotum appears enlarged; edema appears on the anterior surface of the testis but may also extend up into the spermatic cord area (Fig. 17-47, *A* and *B*). Transillumination of the scrotum is indicated when a hydrocele is suspected. A light red glow indicates the presence of fluid; failure to glow suggests a mass.

Spermatocele

A spermatocele is a cystic mass that occurs within the epididymis or spermatic cord. It is filled with sperm and seminal fluid. **Clinical Findings:** This condition is usually painless but is characterized by significant testicular edema in the involved

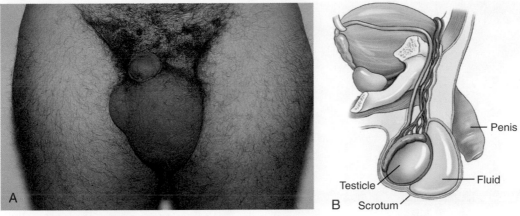

FIG. 17-47 A, Hydrocele. **B,** Cross-section of hydrocele. (**A** from Korting, 1980. **B** from LaFleur Brooks, 2009.)

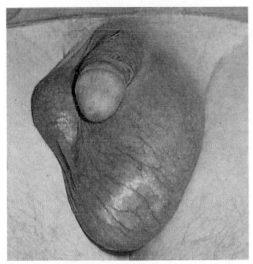

FIG. 17-48 Spermatocele. (From Lloyd-Davies et al., 1994.)

testicle. A separate mass is palpated within the testis adjacent to the epididymis or spermatic cord. Because the lesion is a cyst, it transilluminates (Fig. 17-48).

Varicocele

This condition is caused by an abnormal dilation and tortuosity of the veins along the spermatic cord (Fig. 17-49, *A* and *B*). The cause is often multifactorial; the dilation is thought to be caused by differences in venous drainage between the right and left sides. Varicocele is a condition primarily affecting boys and young men; most often it affects the left side. **Clinical Findings:** The patient may describe a pulling sensation or a dull ache or have scrotal pain. The veins above the testis tend to feel thickened; a palpable mass is usually detected in the scrotum. Ninety percent of varicoceles occur on the left side.[15]

Testicular Cancer

The most common malignancy in men ages 20 to 34 is testicular cancer. **Clinical Findings:** The classic manifestation is a painless testicular mass that is usually discovered by the patient or his sexual partner. When pain is an initial symptom, it is usually an indication that the mass has caused bleeding within the testicle or testicular torsion. On examination a hard and irregular mass is felt within the testis. If the mass is large enough, deformity of the scrotum may be observable (Fig. 17-50).

CONDITIONS OF THE PROSTATE

Benign Prostatic Hyperplasia

Benign prostatic hyperplasia (BPH) is an enlargement of the prostate gland that usually affects older men (Fig. 17-51). At least some degree of BPH will eventually develop in all men with advanced age, causing minor-to-moderate symptoms. **Clinical Findings:** The American Urological Association symptom index is a tool used to assess voiding symptoms associated with obstruction of the urethra by the prostate (see Table 17-1). The higher the score, the more likely BPH is present. In addition to symptoms, prostate examination may reveal hyperplasia. When palpated, the prostate feels smooth, firm, and rubbery; and the prostate projects more than 1 cm into the rectum.

Prostatitis

An inflammation of the prostate gland is termed *prostatitis* (Fig. 17-52). It is the most common urologic diagnosis in men under age 50 and the third most common in men over age 50.[16] There are four recognized categories of prostatitis: acute bacterial prostatitis (ABP); chronic bacterial prostatitis (CBP); chronic pelvic pain syndrome (CPPS); and asymptomatic inflammatory prostatitis. **Clinical Findings:** The clinical manifestation of prostatitis varies. The patient with ABP classically has fever, chills, pain in the back and rectal or perineal area, and obstructive symptoms; examination reveals an enlarged prostate that is usually tender with induration. CBP commonly causes recurrent urinary tract infection, pain, dysuria, and scrotal or penile pain; examination findings may be nonspecific or reveal an enlarged, tender, and boggy prostate. CPPS is characterized by urinary urgency,

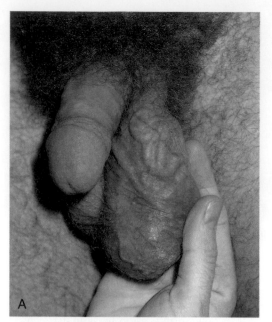
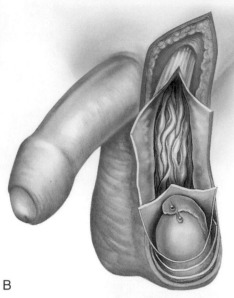

A

B

FIG. 17-49 Varicocele. (**A** from Swartz, 2010. **B** from Seidel et al., 2011.)

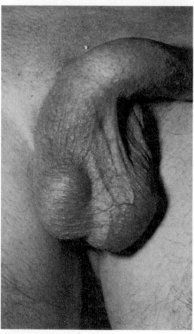

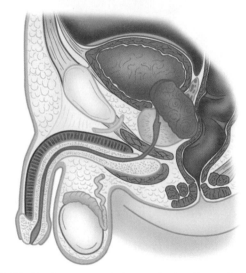

FIG. 17-51 Benign prostatic hyperplasia. (From Seidel et al., 2011.)

FIG. 17-50 Scrotal asymmetry caused by testicular cancer. (From 400 Self-assessment picture tests in clinical medicine, 1984.)

frequency, nocturia, dysuria, and pain or discomfort; examination findings may be normal or may include a soft and boggy prostate. Asymptomatic prostatitis has no symptoms and is often detected based on abnormal urinalysis (increased white cells) or a digital examination finding, such as a boggy prostate.

Prostate Cancer

Cancer of the prostate is the leading site of cancer in men. Approximately 80% of men who reach age 80 have evidence of prostate cancer at autopsy.[17] **Clinical Findings:** The patient

is usually asymptomatic until the cancer begins causing urinary obstruction, resulting in difficulty urinating. On palpation the prostate feels hard and irregular. The median sulcus is obliterated as the prostate tumor grows (Fig. 17-53).

CONDITIONS OF THE ANUS AND RECTUM

Pilonidal Sinus

A pilonidal sinus is a small sinus tract under the skin in the sacrococcygeal region. The sinus is lined with epithelium and hair. If the hair penetrates the skin and becomes infected, a pilonidal cyst or abscess results. Nearly 80% of those affected are males; the peak ages are between 15 and 24 years. **Clinical Findings:** A pilonidal cyst or sinus is usually seen as a dimpled area with a small sinus opening that may contain a tuft of

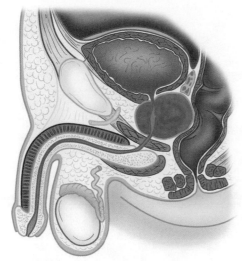

FIG. 17-52 Prostatitis. (From Seidel et al., 2011.)

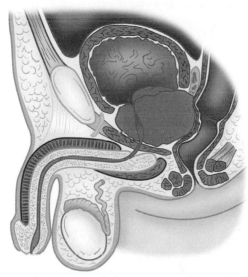

FIG. 17-53 Carcinoma of the prostate. (From Seidel et al., 2011.)

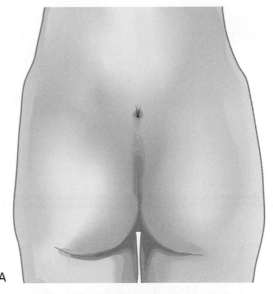

A

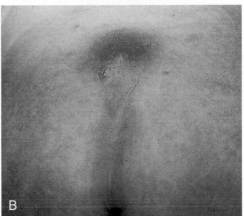

B

FIG. 17-54 A, Pilonidal sinus. **B,** Inflamed pilonidal cyst. (**B** from Zitelli, McIntire, and Nowalk, 2012.)

hair in the sacrococcygeal area. It is usually diagnosed in young adulthood, although occasionally it is recognized at birth by a depression in the sacral area. Generally the individual is asymptomatic unless the area becomes infected. Once infected, the area becomes red and tender, and a cyst may be palpable. The cyst often drains a mucoid or purulent discharge. The patient may complain of pain and swelling at the base of the spine (Fig. 17-54, *A* and *B*).

Hemorrhoids

Hemorrhoids are dilated veins of the hemorrhoidal plexus resulting from increased portal venous pressure. Both genders are thought to be affected equally. **Clinical Findings:** External hemorrhoids originate outside the external rectal sphincter and appear as flaps of tissue. If they become irritated or thrombosed, symptoms include localized itching and perhaps bleeding; and they may appear as blue or purple shiny masses at the anus. Internal hemorrhoids originate above the interior

sphincter. Although they may be present in the rectum, they may not be seen unless they become thrombosed, prolapsed, or infected (Fig. 17-55, *A* and *B*).

Anorectal Fissure

An anorectal fissure is a tear of the anal mucosa causing intense pain. It occurs in all age-groups but is seen most often in young healthy adults; the incidence is similar between genders. **Clinical Findings:** The fissure appears as a crack within the anus usually located midline in the posterior wall of the rectum (Fig. 17-56). The patient experiences severe rectal pain, itching, and rectal bleeding.

Anorectal Abscess and Fistula

A pus-filled cavity in the anal or rectal area is referred to as an *anorectal abscess*. A fistula is an inflamed tract that forms an abnormal passage from within the anus or the rectum to the outside skin surface, usually in the perianal area. Typically the fistula is caused by the drainage of an abscess. **Clinical Findings:** The principal symptom of an abscess is rectal pain; frequently the patient also has a fever. An area of

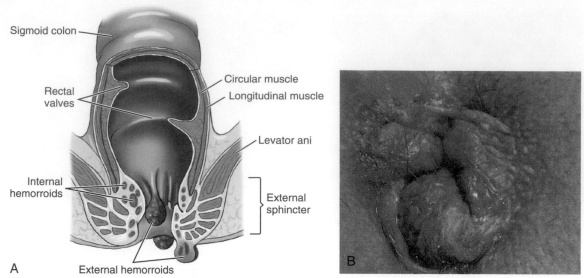

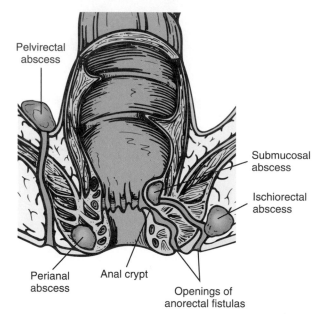

FIG. 17-55 A, Internal and external hemorrhoids. **B,** External hemorrhoid. (**A** from LaFleur Brooks, 2009. **B** from Seidel et al., 2011. Courtesy Gershon Efron, MD, Sinai Hospital of Baltimore.)

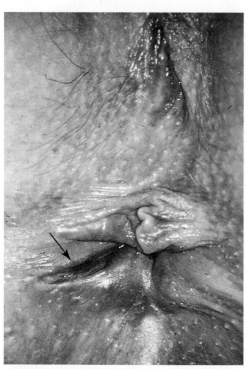

FIG. 17-56 Lateral anal fissure. (From Seidel et al., 2011. Courtesy Gershon Efron, MD, Sinai Hospital of Baltimore.)

FIG. 17-57 Common sites of anorectal fistula and abscess formation. (From Lewis et al., 2011.)

inflammation adjacent to or within the anus is observed with edema, erythema, and induration. Often the pain is so severe that the patient cannot tolerate palpation of the area. If a fistula is present, the opening on the skin usually appears as red, raised granulation tissue; the drainage is serosanguineous or purulent (Fig. 17-57).

Rectal Polyp

A rectal polyp is a protruding growth from the rectal mucosa. It may grow outward, as on a stalk (pedunculated), or

adhering to the mucosa (sessile) (Fig. 17-58, *A* and *B*). Most colorectal cancers arise from mutated adenomatous polyps. **Clinical Findings:** A common symptom is rectal bleeding, although often the patient is unaware that a polyp exists. Occasionally a polyp may protrude from the anus and appear as small, soft nodules. Polyps are often difficult to palpate and are most often identified during a colonoscopy examination.

Carcinoma of the Rectum and Anus

Rectal and anal cancer occurs when a malignant tumor grows within the rectal mucosa, anal canal, or anus. **Clinical Findings:** Patients may or may not have symptoms; however, the

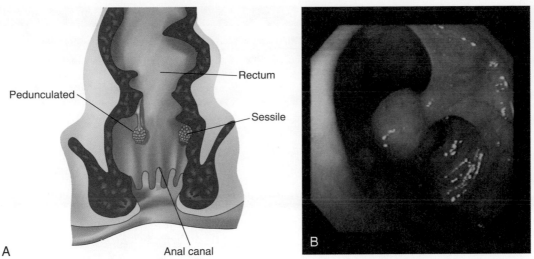

FIG. 17-58 **A,** Types of rectal polyps. **B,** Endoscopic image of a pedunculated polyp. (**B** from McCance and Huether, 2010. Courtesy David Bjorkman, MD, University of Utah School of Medicine, Department of Gastroenterology.)

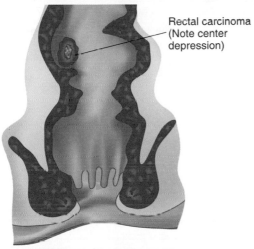

FIG. 17-59 Rectal carcinoma.

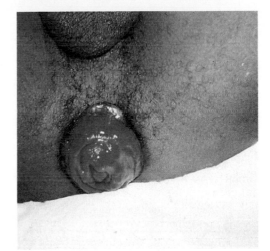

FIG. 17-60 Prolapse of the rectum. (From Seidel et al., 2006. Courtesy Gershon Efron, MD, Sinai Hospital of Baltimore.)

most common symptom is rectal bleeding. If palpable, a malignant rectal tumor manifests as an irregular mass on the rectal wall with nodular, raised edges (Fig. 17-59).

PROLAPSE OR HERNIATION

Hernia

A hernia is a protrusion of part of the peritoneal-lined sac through the abdominal wall. The three most common types of hernias seen when examining the inguinal area are indirect inguinal, direct inguinal, and femoral. **Clinical Findings:** Signs and symptoms of the various types of hernias are presented in Table 17-4.

Rectal Prolapse

Rectal prolapse is a full-thickness protrusion of the rectal wall though the anus (turning inside out). The incidence is hard to determine because many people have mild forms of this

condition and never seek treatment. It can occur at any age, but most cases involve women over age 60. **Clinical Findings:** Symptoms of rectal prolapse include rectal bleeding, a mass, and change in bowel habits (e.g., fecal incontinence or soiling with mucous discharge). The patient may report that an intestine or a hemorrhoid is hanging out of the anus. The prolapsed rectum appears as a pink mucosal bulge that is described as a "doughnut" or "rosette" (Fig. 17-60).

Uterine Prolapse

Uterine prolapse is associated with a retroverted uterus that descends into the vagina. In first-degree prolapse the cervix remains within the vagina (Fig. 17-61, *A*). In second-degree prolapse the cervix is in the introitus (see Fig. 17-61, *B*). In third-degree prolapse the cervix and vagina drop outside the introitus (see Fig. 17-61, *C*). **Clinical Findings:** The primary symptoms described by individuals with uterine prolapse include a feeling of heaviness, fullness, or the sensation of

TABLE 17-4　COMPARISONS OF HERNIAS

	DESCRIPTION	CLINICAL SIGNS
Indirect Hernia Internal ring / External ring / Indirect inguinal hernia Most frequent type of hernia; may occur in both sexes and in children (mostly males)	The sac herniates through the internal inguinal ring. It can remain in the inguinal canal, exit through the external canal, or actually pass into the scrotum.	The hernia feels like a soft swelling against the nurse's fingertips. The patient usually complains of pain with straining. The hernia may decrease when the patient lies down.
Direct Hernia Internal ring / External ring / Direct inguinal hernia Less common; occurs most frequently in males over age 40; uncommon in women	The sac herniates through the external inguinal ring. The hernia is located in the Hesselbach triangle region. It rarely enters the scrotum.	The patient has a bulge in the Hesselbach triangle area that is usually painless. The hernia pushes against the nurse's fingertips when the patient bears down. The hernia may decrease when the patient lies down.
Femoral Hernia Internal ring / External ring / Femoral hernia Least common type of hernia; occurs most frequently in women	The sac extends through the femoral ring, canal, and below the inguinal ligament.	There is pain in the inguinal area. The right side is more frequently affected than the left side. Pain may be severe.

Illustrations from Seidel et al., 2011.

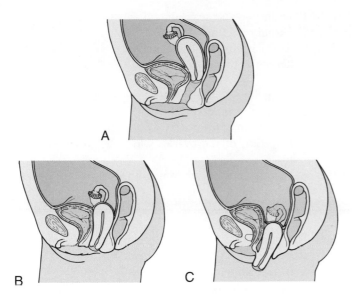

FIG. 17-61 Uterine prolapse. **A,** First-degree prolapse of the uterus. **B,** Second-degree prolapse of the uterus. **C,** Third-degree prolapse of the uterus. (From Lewis et al., 2011.)

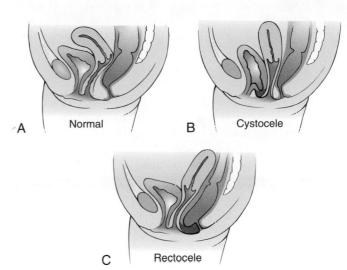

FIG. 17-62 A, Normal anatomical position. **B,** Cystocele (protrusion of the urinary bladder wall through the vagina). **C,** Rectocele (protrusion of the rectal wall through the vagina). (From Swartz, 2010.)

"falling out" in the perineal area. The cervix is visualized low within the vagina, at the vaginal opening, or protruding from the vaginal opening.

Cystocele

Cystocele is a protrusion of the urinary bladder against the anterior wall of the vagina. **Clinical Findings:** The woman may experience a sensation of fullness or pressure, stress incontinence, occasional urgency, and a feeling of incomplete emptying after voiding. A soft bulging mass of the anterior vaginal wall is usually seen and felt as the woman bears down (Fig. 17-62, *A* and *B*).

Rectocele

Rectocele is a hernia-type protrusion of the rectum against the posterior wall of the vagina. **Clinical Findings:** The woman often complains of a heavy feeling within the vagina. Other commonly reported symptoms include constipation, a feeling of incomplete emptying of the rectum after a bowel movement, and a feeling of something "falling out" in the vagina. Bulging of the posterior vagina is observed as the woman bears down (see Fig. 17-62, *C*).

CLINICAL APPLICATION AND CLINICAL REASONING

See Appendix D for answers to exercises in this section.

REVIEW QUESTIONS

1. Which finding does the nurse recognize as abnormal when examining a male patient?
   1. Testes that are palpable and firm within the scrotal sac bilaterally
   2. Discharge from the penis when the glans is compressed
   3. Foreskin that lies loosely over the penis
   4. Glans a lighter skin tone than the rest of the penis

2. A 22-year-old white male comes to the emergency department with a concern about a mass in his testicle. In addition to his age and race, which fact is a known risk factor for testicular cancer?
   1. He had an undescended testicle at birth.
   2. His mother had breast cancer.
   3. He was treated for gonorrhea 18 months ago.
   4. He had a hydrocele during infancy.

3. Which instructions should the nurse provide to the patient before a visit for a pelvic examination and Pap test?
   1. Avoid sexual intercourse for 2 days before the examination.
   2. If menstruating, avoid using tampons before the examination.
   3. Take a tub bath shortly before the examination.
   4. Avoid douching for 24 hours before the examination.

4. While taking the health history of a 23-year-old female patient, the nurse considers risk factors for STD. Which data from the patient suggest a need for patient education?
   1. The patient states that she has been in a monogamous sexual relationship for 2 years.
   2. The patient states that she has been sexually involved with one man for the last 2 weeks; she uses spermicidal gel to prevent pregnancy.
   3. The patient has a Pap test each year.
   4. The patient uses oral contraceptives to prevent pregnancy.

5. A patient has a herpes lesion on her vulva. While examining her, the nurse should take which measures?
   1. Wear examination gloves while in contact with the genitalia
   2. Place the patient in an isolation room
   3. Wash the genitalia with alcohol or povidone-iodine (Betadine) before the examination
   4. Inspect the genitalia only; reschedule the patient for a full examination after the lesion has healed

6. To inspect the glans penis of the uncircumcised male, the nurse retracts the foreskin. After inspection he or she is unable to replace the foreskin over the glans. The nurse recognizes that this situation could potentially lead to which complication?
   1. Decreased sperm production
   2. Urinary tract infection
   3. Tissue necrosis of the penis
   4. Testicular cancer

7. Examination of the ovaries is performed by which assessment technique?
   1. Inspection of the ovaries while a speculum is in place
   2. Palpation of the ovaries while the speculum is in place
   3. Percussion of the abdomen directly over the ovaries
   4. Palpation of the ovaries using a bimanual palpation technique

8. The nurse recognizes which symptom as commonly associated with prostate enlargement?
   1. Constipation
   2. Rectal bleeding
   3. A weak urinary stream
   4. Penile discharge

9. During an examination the nurse palpates the Skene's glands. Which technique best describes this process?
   1. Exerting pressure over the clitoris, slide the finger downward (posteriorly) toward the vaginal opening.
   2. Palpate the fourchette and slide the finger forward (anteriorly) toward the vaginal opening.
   3. Exert pressure on the anterior vaginal wall and slide the finger outward toward the vaginal opening.
   4. Grasp the labia majora between the index finger and thumb and milk the labia outward.

10. A patient tells the nurse that her stools have bright red blood in them. The nurse suspects which problem?
    1. Gallbladder disease
    2. Hemorrhoids
    3. Rectal polyps
    4. Upper intestinal bleeding

CASE STUDY

Mia Richards is a 33-year-old woman who comes to the urgent care center. The nurse collects the following data.

Interview Data

Ms. Richards tells the nurse, "I have a really bad pain in front of my butt. It hurts so much that I can't even wipe with a tissue after I go to the bathroom. There is no way I could have a bowel movement right now." Ms. Richards states that the pain started 2 days ago and is "much worse now." When asked about her sexual activity, she says, "I'm with a guy, but it's not exclusive or anything. We see other people and try not to be real serious."

Examination Data

- *External examination:* Typical hair distribution, urethral meatus intact, no redness or discharge. Perineum intact.

Extreme pain response to palpation of vaginal opening; edema, redness, and mass detected on right side. Spontaneous, foul-smelling, dark yellow discharge noted with palpation over Bartholin's glands.
- *Internal examination:* Deferred because of extreme pain associated with inflammation.

Clinical Reasoning

1. Which data deviate from normal findings, suggesting a need for further investigation?
2. For which additional information should the nurse ask or assess?
3. Based on the data, which risk factors for STD does Ms. Richards have?
4. With which additional health care professionals should you consider collaborating to meet her health care needs?

Developmental Assessment Throughout the Life Span

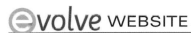 WEBSITE

http://evolve.elsevier.com/Wilson/assessment

Physical, behavioral, and cognitive development of patients is a vital part of assessment. Nurses compare and contrast a patient's actual characteristics with those described by standardized norms. For example, the growth of infants is assessed to determine if their bones and muscles are developing as expected for a specific age. Deviations from these expectations or the norm may indicate a health problem that nurses can address with the parents or caregivers. Nurses also collect data related to behavioral and cognitive development from patients and compare these data with the developmental tasks that have been identified for those age-groups. When deviations from the norm are found, nurses discuss the findings with patients, parents, or caregivers. Patients are asked about actions they take to prevent illness. The patient's responses are compared with recommendations such as those by the U.S. Preventive Services Task Force and the immunization schedule found in Table 18-6.

This chapter is organized by chronologic age divisions that correlate with developmental periods. Each division discusses physical, behavioral, and cognitive development and developmental tasks for that age-group. However, during the first 6 years, physical growth and development are so dramatic that additional data are used to describe motor development, social-adaptive behaviors, and language development.

- *Motor development* has two components: gross and fine motor behavior. Gross-motor behavior refers to postural reactions such as head balance, sitting, creeping, standing, and walking. Fine-motor behavior refers to the use of hands and fingers in the prehensile approach to grasping and manipulating an object.
- *Social-adaptive behavior* refers to the interactions of the infant or child with other people and the ability to

organize stimuli, perceive relationships between objects, dissect a whole into its component parts, reintegrate these parts in a meaningful fashion, and solve practical problems. Examples are smiling at other people and learning to feed self.
- *Language behavior* is used broadly to include visible and audible forms of communication, whether facial expression, gesture, postural movements, or vocalizations (words, phrases, or sentences). Language also includes the comprehension of communication by others.

THEORIES OF DEVELOPMENT

By using theories of development, nurses can describe and predict the growth and development of patients throughout the life span. Two widely used theories of behavioral and cognitive development are described briefly. These theories were developed by Erik Erikson and Jean Piaget.

Personality Development: Erikson's Theory

Erik Erikson (1902-1994) believed that the ego was the primary seat of personality functioning.[1] In addition to the ego, he believed that society and culture influenced behavior. Erikson believed that people developed through a predetermined unfolding of their personalities in eight stages. An analogy of a rosebud unfolding may be useful in thinking about development. Each petal opens at a certain time in a certain order, which is predetermined. If the natural order is disturbed by pulling off a petal prematurely or out of order, the development of the mature rose is affected.[2] Each stage involves certain developmental tasks that are psychosocial in

TABLE 18-1 ERIKSON'S EIGHT STAGES OF HUMAN DEVELOPMENT

STAGE (APPROXIMATE)	PSYCHOSOCIAL STAGE	LASTING OUTCOMES
Infancy	Basic trust versus basic mistrust	Drive and hope
Toddlerhood	Autonomy versus shame and doubt	Self-control and will power
Preschool	Initiative versus guilt	Direction and purpose
Middle childhood (school age)	Industry versus inferiority	Method and competence
Adolescence	Identity versus role confusion	Devotion and fidelity
Young adulthood	Intimacy versus isolation	Affiliation and love
Middle adulthood	Generativity versus stagnation	Production and care
Older adulthood	Ego integrity versus despair	Renunciation and wisdom

"Figure of Erickson's Stages of Personality Development" from Childhood and Society by Erik H. Erikson. Copyright 1950, © 1963 by W.W. Norton & Company, Inc., renewed © 1978, 1991 by Erikson. Used by permission of W.W. Norton & Company, Inc.

nature and described as polar opposites or conflicts (Table 18-1). For example, in the first stage, during infancy the conflict is trust versus mistrust. Infants learn that they can depend on their caregivers to meet their needs for food, protection, comfort, and affection. When the infant develops trusting relationships with others, usually the mother, the lasting outcome tends to be ambition, enthusiasm, and motivation. By contrast, when trust is not developed, the person tends to develop apathy and indifference. However, Erikson believed that a balance was needed at each stage. For example, infants need to learn to trust, but they also need to learn a little mistrust so they do not grow up to become gullible.[2] Accomplishing each successive task provides the foundation for a healthy self-identity. Each stage builds on the previous stages and must be accomplished for the person to successfully complete the next one. People with whom a person interacts and environmental factors influence the accomplishment of these tasks; however, the motivation to achieve a healthy identity arises from within each person. Although each conflict is described at a particular developmental stage, all of the conflicts exist in each person to some extent throughout life. Even though the conflict may be resolved at one time in a person's life, it may recur in similar circumstances.[1]

Cognitive Development: Piaget's Theory

Jean Piaget (1896-1980) described stages of cognitive development from birth to approximately 15 years of age. *Cognition* is defined as how a person perceives and processes information. He believed the child's main goal was to establish equilibrium between self and environment.

Piaget believed that the child's view of the world developed from simple reflex behavior to complex logical and abstract thought. To fully develop cognition, the child needs a functioning neurologic system and sufficient environmental stimuli. Piaget described four distinct, sequential levels of cognitive development (Table 18-2). Each stage represents a change in how children understand and organize their environment, and each stage is characterized by more sophisticated types of reasoning. All children move through the stages in sequential order but not necessarily at the same age.[3]

TABLE 18-2 PIAGET'S LEVELS OF COGNITIVE DEVELOPMENT

STAGE	AGE	CHARACTERISTICS
Sensorimotor	0-2 yr	Thought is dominated by physical manipulation of objects and events.
Preoperational	2-7 yr	Function is symbolical, using language as major tool.
Concrete operations	7-11 yr	Mental reasoning processes assume logical approaches to solving concrete problems.
Formal operations	11-15 yr	True logical thought and manipulation of abstract concepts emerge.

Modified from Schuster C, Ashburn S: *The process of human development: a holistic life-span approach,* Boston, 1992, Lippincott.

Adult Intelligence

Although Piaget's work represents the most complete work in cognitive development, it does not progress through adulthood. Theorists of adult intelligence suggest assessing the "practical" intelligence of adults. They believe that intelligence develops through an interaction of biologic and environmental factors. Intellectual abilities of adults can be sustained or improved until late adulthood. Two types of adult intelligence have been described: fluid and crystallized. Fluid intelligence represents the ability to perceive complex situations and engage in short-term memory, concept formation, reasoning, and abstraction. This type of intelligence develops through central nervous system function and declines with age and physiologic change. Crystallized intelligence is associated with skills and knowledge learned as a part of growing up in a given culture such as verbal comprehension, vocabulary, and ability to evaluate life experiences. This type of intelligence develops through life experiences and education and remains stable or increases with maturity.[4] Although fluid intelligence begins to decline at approximately ages 35 to 40, crystallized intelligence is maintained longer.[5] In addition to innate ability, adult intelligence is also affected by other factors such as social class, illness, personality, and motivation. For example, adults of average intelligence who have the opportunities for education and are sufficiently motivated reveal greater increases in intelligence throughout adulthood.

Several theorists believe that the academic type of testing used to assess intelligence in children is not appropriate for adults. Intelligence in adults is gained from "real world" experiences that are difficult to measure by standardized tests. Sternberg[6] is a theorist who proposed a three-pronged theory of intelligence. The first prong (componential subtheory) was described as the internal analytic mental mechanism. The second (experiential subtheory) focused on how a person's learning through life experiences, combined with insight and creativity, affects his or her thinking. The third (contextual subtheory) focused on the role of the external environment in determining what constitutes intelligence in a particular situation. Diminished vision and slower response time may contribute to an intellectual decline in older adults.

DEVELOPMENTAL TASKS

Developmental tasks evolve from physical growth and cultural influences. As individuals grow, they are able to perform more complex tasks. For example, as infants' bones, muscles, and nervous systems mature, they progress from sitting to standing to walking. This progression increases the tasks that they are able to accomplish. Likewise, as their nervous system matures, they are able to interact with family members to develop communication skills. Infants who live in an environment with many family members may have more opportunity to develop communication skills earlier because of the increased number of people with whom they interact. Families, peers, and associates expect individuals in their spheres of influence to conform in certain ways. These expectations are culturally appropriate and influence individuals' functioning in various roles and statuses for their age and gender.[7] For example, the developmental task of working toward a vocation may be expected of adolescent males in some cultures but in young male adults in other cultures.

Each culture has its own developmental tasks and expectations. These tasks also vary from region to region in the United States and even from one socioeconomic class to another within one geographic area, which may account for differences among people of various ethnic and cultural backgrounds. A developmental task is a drive from within the individual to develop in such a way as to attain a goal. The thrust to change usually comes from within the person, but it may be motivated by the demands and expectations of others.[7] A conflict may arise in families who move to the United States from foreign countries. Their children are expected to follow the culture of the parent's country of origin, but they also are influenced by the American culture. The developmental tasks presented in this chapter are intended to be used as a guide because there are many normal variations based on ethnic and cultural influences. The boxes in this chapter describe developmental tasks throughout the life span:

- Infants (birth to 1 year)
- Toddlers (1 to 3 years)
- Preschoolers (3 to 5 years)
- School-age children (6 to 12 years)
- Adolescents (13 to 18 years)
- Young adults (19 to 35 years)
- Middle adults (36 to 65 years)
- Older adults
  - Young-old (66 to 74 years)
  - Middle-old (75 to 84 years)
  - Old-old (over 85 years)

EXPECTED GROWTH AND DEVELOPMENT BY AGE-GROUP

Infants

Infancy refers to the first year of life. The rapid growth and development that occur during these first 12 months are evident from the data given in Table 18-3, which lists changes in the infant by month, whereas subsequent tables document changes by intervals of 6 months to 1 year. During this time extensive physical development occurs in addition to the acquisition of psychosocial skills.

Physical Growth

Height, weight, and head circumference are measured to assess infant growth. Growth proceeds from head to toe (cephalocaudal) as evidenced by the infant's development of head control before sitting and mastery of sitting before standing. Healthy newborns weigh between 5 lb 8 oz and 8 lbs 13 oz (2500 and 4000 g). The newborn period is the first 28 days of life. Commonly newborns lose 10% of their birth weight in the first week but regain it in 10 to 14 days. In general they double their birth weight by 4 to 5 months of age and triple it by 12 months of age. The infant grows 1 inch (2.5 cm) each month for the first 6 months, followed by 0.5 inch (1.3 cm) a month from ages 6 to 12 months. Expected head circumference for term newborns averages from 13 to 14 inches (33 to 36 cm) and increases 0.5 inch (1.3 cm) monthly for the first 6 months. By 6 months teeth begin to erupt, with a total of six to eight teeth by the end of the first year.

Behavioral and Cognitive Development

A summary of the expected developmental milestones of infants is found in Table 18-3. Erikson's developmental task of infancy, or the oral-sensory stage, is to develop trust without completely eliminating the capacity for mistrust.[2] Infants develop trust relationships with the mother or primary caregiver. Important criteria are the quality and consistency of the mother-infant relationship. Infants who receive consistent, loving care learn that they can depend on people around them to meet their needs. By contrast, care that is

TABLE 18-3 EXPECTED DEVELOPMENT OF INFANTS

AGE	FINE-MOTOR	GROSS-MOTOR	SOCIAL-ADAPTIVE	LANGUAGE
1 mo	Follows with eyes to midline Hands predominantly closed Strong grasp reflex	Turns head to side Keeps knees tucked under abdomen When pulled to sitting position, has gross head lag and rounded, swayed back	Regards face	Responds to bell Cries in response to displeasure Makes sounds during feeding
2 mo	Follows objects well; may not follow past midline Hands frequently open	Holds head in same plane as rest of body Can raise head and maintain position; looks downward	Smiles responsively	Vocalizes (not crying) Cries become differentiated Coos
3 mo	Follows past midline When in supine position puts hands together; holds hands in front of face Pulls at blanket and clothes	Raises head to 45-degree angle Maintains posture Looks around with head May turn from prone to side position When pulled into sitting position, shows only slight head lag	Shows interest in surroundings	Laughs Coos, babbles, chuckles
4 mo	Grasps rattle Plays with hands together Inspects hands Carries objects to mouth	Actively lifts head up and looks around (Fig. 18-1) Rolls from prone to supine position When pulled to sitting position, no longer has head lag When held in standing position, attempts to maintain some weight support	Becomes bored when left alone Begins to show memory	Squeals Vocalizations change with mood
5 mo	Can reach and pick up object May play with toes	Able to push up from prone position and maintain weight on forearms Rolls from prone to supine and back to prone Maintains straight back when in sitting position	Smiles spontaneously Playful, with rapid mood changes Distinguishes family	Uses vowel-like cooing sounds with consonantal sounds (e.g., *ah-goo*)
6 mo	Holds spoon or rattle Drops object and reaches for second offered object Holds bottle	Begins to raise abdomen off table Sits, but posture still shaky May sit with legs apart; holds arms straight as prop between legs Supports almost full weight when pulled to standing position	Recognizes parents Holds out arms to be picked up	Begins to imitate sounds Uses one-syllable sounds (e.g., *ma, mu, da, di*)
7 mo	Can transfer object from one hand to other Grasps objects in each hand Bangs cube on table	Sits alone; still uses hands for support When held in standing position, bounces Puts feet to mouth	Fearful of strangers Plays peekaboo Keeps lips closed when dislikes food	Says four distinct vowel sounds "Talks" when others are talking
8 mo	Beginning thumb-finger grasping Releases object at will Grasps for toys out of reach	Sits securely without support Bears weight on legs when supported May stand holding on	Responds to word *no* Dislikes diaper changes	Makes consonant sounds *t, d, w* Uses two syllables such as *da-da* but does not ascribe meaning to them
9 mo	Continued development of thumb-finger grasp May bang objects together Use of dominant hand evident	Steady sitting; can lean forward and still maintain position Begins creeping (abdomen off floor) Can stand holding onto established object when placed in that position	Seems interested in pleasing parent Shows fears of going to bed and being left alone	Responds to simple commands Comprehends *no-no*

TABLE 18-3 EXPECTED DEVELOPMENT OF INFANTS—cont'd

AGE	FINE-MOTOR	GROSS-MOTOR	SOCIAL-ADAPTIVE	LANGUAGE
10 mo	Practices picking up small objects Points with one finger Offers toys to people but unable to let go of objects	Can pull self into sitting position; unable to let self down again Stands while holding on to furniture	Inhibits behavior in response to command *no-no* Repeats actions that attract attention Plays interactive games such as pat-a-cake Cries when scolded	Says *da-da*, *ma-ma* with meaning Comprehends *bye-bye*
11 mo	Holds crayon to mark on paper Drops object deliberately for it to be picked up	Moves about room holding onto objects Prepares to walk independently; wide-base stance Stands securely, holding on with one hand	Experiences satisfaction when task is accomplished Reacts to restrictions with frustration Rolls a ball to another on request	Imitates speech sounds
12 mo (1 yr)	May hold cup and spoon and feed self fairly well with practice Can offer toys and release them Releases cube in cup	Able to twist and turn and maintain posture Able to sit from standing position May stand alone, at least momentarily	Shows emotions of jealousy, affection, anger, fear May develop habit of "security blanket" or favorite toy	*Da-da* or *ma-ma* specific Recognizes objects by name Imitates animal sounds Understands simple verbal commands (e.g., "Give it to me")

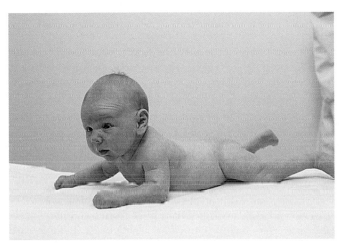

FIG. 18-1 At 4 months infant actively lifts head and looks about.

inconsistent, abusive, or undependable may result in mistrust of people.

Piaget identifies sensorimotor development as the primary task at this age. Infants use their sensorimotor abilities to master motor milestones and launch relationships with others.[3] Not only can infants advance from crawling to walking and eating some foods, but they also have the ability to win the hearts and attention of others with an intentional smile and showing preference for familiar caregivers. Bonding takes place with caregivers; at about 1 month different cries can be identified as being related to different needs, expressive language progresses to the first word, and receptive language is developed enough to understand and briefly respond to

BOX 18-1 DEVELOPMENTAL TASKS OF INFANTS

- Achieving physiologic equilibrium following birth
  - Learning to take food satisfactorily
- Learning to adjust to other persons
  - Reacting positively to both familiar and strange persons
- Learning to love and be loved
  - Responding affectionately to others through cuddling, smiling, and loving
  - Beginning to give self spontaneously and trustingly to others
- Developing system of communication
  - Learning patterns of recognition and responses
  - Establishing nonverbal, preverbal, and verbal communication
- Learning to express and control feelings
  - Developing a sense of trust and confidence with the world
- Laying a foundation for self-awareness
  - Seeing oneself as a separate entity
  - Finding personal fulfillment with and without others

From Duvall EM, Miller BC: *Marriage and family development,* ed 6, New York, 1985, Harper & Row.

simple commands. Learning at the sensorimotor level of cognitive development occurs through the five senses as infants interact with the environment. Infants learn object permanence, which means that objects and people still exist when they are out of sight. The developmental tasks of infancy are listed in Box 18-1.

Assessment tools for the infant focus on physical growth, psychosocial development, and determining the mother's and father's interactions with the infant. The most widely used developmental screening test for young children is the Denver II, used for children ages 1 month to 6 years. This test provides assessment for gross-motor movement, language, fine-motor movement, and personal-social skills.[8] Training is needed to use this tool. A tool that surveys parents about their child's development is the Ages and Stages Questionnaire (ASQ), which identifies developmental delays in children from 4 to 60 months. The ASQ has 19 age-specific questionnaires that gather data from parents about their child's communication, fine-motor movement, gross-motor movement, problem solving and personal-social skills. The ASQ is available from www.brookespublishing.com by typing "ASQ" in the Search box. Preventive services recommended for infants are in Table 18-6 in the column labeled "Birth to 6 years."

Toddlers

Toddlerhood is the period of growth and development from 12 to 36 months. During this period the child moves about more independently. Toddlers have a strong need to explore and master their environment. Parents who want to encourage their children's exploratory and inquiring spirit, along with the mastery of motor skills, often feel overwhelmed and exhausted at the end of the day. This exhaustion may occur when parents try to keep up with the toddlers to encourage exploration while keeping them safe.

Physical Growth

A slower but steady growth in height and weight occurs during toddlerhood. By 24 months chest circumference exceeds head circumference. Children are half their adult height by age 2. By 30 months the birth weight is quadrupled. The usual appearance of a toddler includes a potbelly, swayback, and short legs. The toddler may be ready for daytime control of bowel and bladder function by age 24 months. Teeth continue to erupt, with 20 teeth expected by 30 months.

Behavioral and Cognitive Development

The developmental task for toddlers is to achieve a degree of autonomy while minimizing shame and doubt. The terms *holding on* and *letting go* are used to describe this stage. Now that toddlers are walking and talking, they yearn for independence; however, they lack judgment to maintain their safety. They learn when it is safe to hold on to furniture and when to let go. The parents or caregivers try to balance their control between allowing independent exploration of the environment and keeping the toddlers safe from injury. Holding on and letting go also apply to bowel control established at this time. In their attempts to be independent, toddlers may fail to achieve their goals. Repeated failures may lead to feelings of shame and doubt in their abilities, particularly when parents try to help them do what the children should learn to do independently. When parents do not have enough patience to allow children to accomplish tasks such as tying

---

BOX 18-2 DEVELOPMENTAL TASKS OF TODDLERS

- Achieving physiologic equilibrium following birth
  - Learning the know-how and where-when of elimination
  - Learning to manage one's body effectively
- Learning to adjust to other people
  - Responding to others' expectations
  - Recognizing parental authority and controls
  - Learning the do's and don'ts of the immediate world
- Learning to love and be loved
  - Meeting emotional needs through widening spheres and variety of contacts
- Developing system of communication
  - Acquiring basic concepts such as yes/no
  - Mastering basic language fundamentals
- Learning to express and control feelings
  - Healthy management of feelings of fear and anxiety
  - Handling feelings of frustration, disappointment, and anger appropriately for age
  - Moderating demanding attitudes
- Laying a foundation for self-awareness
  - Exploring the rights and privileges of being an individual

From Duvall EM, Miller BC: *Marriage and family development*, ed 6, New York, 1985, Harper & Row.

---

shoes alone, the children may doubt their ability to accomplish tasks.[2]

Cognitive development of toddlers remains in the sensorimotor level. Piaget's preoperational stage begins at approximately 2 years of age, when toddlers learn by trial and error and exploration. Using their motor skills, they move around the environment and pick up objects; using their senses, they see, feel, smell, taste, and hear what they find.[3]

Developmental tasks of toddlers are listed in Box 18-2. A summary of the expected development milestones, including fine- and gross-motor, social-adaptive, and language behaviors, is found in Table 18-4 and Fig. 18-2. The Denver II and ASQ may be used with toddlers to assess development. Preventive services recommended for toddlers are in Table 18-6 in the column labeled "Birth to 6 years."

Preschoolers

The preschooler ranges in age from 3 to 5 years. As children's locomotion and language mature, they move away from the protective yet confining care of parental figures. They begin to understand concepts and meanings in a more "real" sense and begin increased forms of independent play and decision making.

Physical Growth

Typical preschoolers grow 2 to 2.75 inches (5 to 7 cm) a year. By age 4 birth length has doubled, and weight increases by 3 to 5 lb (1.4 to 2.3 kg) a year. Appearance changes as the long bones grow more than the trunk and preschoolers lose their baby fat and potbellies. By age 5 children begin to lose deciduous teeth, and the first permanent teeth erupt.

TABLE 18-4	EXPECTED DEVELOPMENT OF TODDLERS			
AGE	**FINE-MOTOR**	**GROSS-MOTOR**	**SOCIAL-ADAPTIVE**	**LANGUAGE**
15 mo	Can put raisins into bottle Takes off shoes and pulls toys Builds tower of two cubes Scribbles spontaneously Uses cup well but rotates spoon	Walks alone well Able to seat self in chair Creeps up stairs Cannot throw ball without falling	Tolerates some separation from parents Begins to imitate parents' activities (e.g., sweeping, mowing lawn)	Says 10 or more words "Asks" for objects by pointing Uses *no* even when agreeing with request
18 mo	Builds tower of three to four cubes Turns pages in book two or three at a time Manages spoon without rotating	May walk up and down stairs holding hand May show running ability	Imitates housework Temper tantrums may be more evident Has beginning awareness of ownership (e.g., *my toy*)	Says 10 or more words Points to two or three body parts
24 mo (2 yr)	Able to turn doorknob Able to take off shoes and socks Able to build seven- to eight-block tower (see Fig 18-2) Dumps raisins from bottle following demonstration Turns pages in book one at a time	May walk up stairs by self, two feet on each step Able to walk backward Able to kick ball	Demonstrates parallel play Pulls people to show them something Increased independence from mother	Has vocabulary of 300 words Uses two- or three-word phrases Uses pronouns *I, you* Uses first name Refers to self by name
30 mo (2½ yr)	Able to build eight-block tower Scribbling techniques continue Feeds self with increased neatness Dumps raisins from bottle spontaneously	Able to jump from object Walking becomes more stable; wide-base gait decreases Throws ball overhanded	Separates easily from mother In play helps put things away In toileting only needs help to wipe Begins to notice sex differences	Gives first and last name Uses plurals Refers to self by appropriate pronoun Names one color

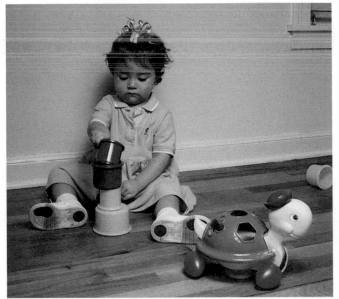

FIG. 18-2 The toddler takes great pleasure in building a tower of four blocks.

Behavioral and Cognitive Development

During the preschool years children have become more autonomous, can communicate easily, achieve bowel and bladder continence, have an active imagination, can demonstrate basic social skills, can delay gratification, use more acceptable outlets to express frustration, and can expand their environment beyond home. The task of this age-group is to learn initiative without an overabundance of guilt. Preschoolers continue to explore their environments with greater skills and a new enthusiasm and motivation. When children are praised for their activities, they learn that they are meeting others' expectations and become independent and self-sufficient. At this stage their conscience (i.e., that inner voice that provides a sense of right and wrong) develops.

Cognitive development continues at the preoperational level. Children begin the symbolic function, in which they develop concepts and classifications to associate one event, object, or person with a similar one. Children demonstrate this when they act out an event they have seen or experienced but emphasize only one aspect of the event. At this level children become egocentric, (i.e., they are self-centered and unable to understand others' viewpoints).[3]

BOX 18-3   DEVELOPMENTAL TASKS OF PRESCHOOLERS

- Settling into healthy daily routines
  - Enjoying a variety of active play
  - Being more flexible and capable of accepting change
  - Mastering good eating habits
  - Mastering the basics of toilet training
  - Developing physical skills
- Becoming a participating member of the family
  - Assuming responsibility within the family
  - Giving and receiving affection and gifts freely
  - Identifying with the parent of the same sex
  - Developing an ability to share parents with others
  - Recognizing the family's unique ways
- Beginning to master impulses and conform to expectations of others
  - Outgrowing impulsivity
  - Learning to share, take turns, enjoy companionship
  - Developing sympathy and cooperation
  - Adopting situationally appropriate behavior
- Developing healthy emotional expressions
  - Acting out feelings during play
  - Delaying gratification
  - Expressing hostility/making up
  - Discriminating between a variety of emotions and feelings
- Learning to communicate effectively with others
  - Developing a vocabulary and speech ability
  - Learning to listen, follow directions, increase attention span
  - Acquiring social skills that allow more comfortable interactions with others
- Developing ability to handle potentially dangerous situations
  - Respecting potential hazards
  - Effectively using caution and safety practices
  - Being able to accept assistance when needed
- Learning to be autonomous with initiative and a conscience of his or her own
  - Becoming increasingly responsible
  - Taking initiative to be involved in situations
  - Internalizing expectations, demands of family and culture
  - Being self-sufficient for stage of development
- Laying foundation for understanding the meaning of life
  - Developing gender awareness
  - Trying to understand the nature of the physical world
  - Accepting religious faith of parents, learning about spirituality

From Duvall EM, Miller BC: *Marriage and family development,* ed 6, New York, 1985, Harper & Row.

The developmental tasks of preschoolers are listed in Box 18-3. A summary of the expected development of preschoolers, including fine- and gross-motor, social-adaptive, and language behaviors, is found in Table 18-5. The Denver II and ASQ may be used with preschoolers to assess development. Preventive services recommended for preschoolers are in Table 18-6 in the column labeled "Birth to 6 years."

School-Age Children

The beginning of school is a developmental landmark for children. Entering school brings a new influential environment into their lives. Information about concepts, life, and interpersonal relationships expands beyond the confines of the home. Teacher and peer influences may be noticed in school-age children's reactions and behavior. The school-age period lasts from approximately 6 to 12 years of age.

Physical Growth

The growth continues at a slow pace, with about a 5-lb (2.3 kg) weight gain and 2-inch (5 cm) height increase per year. Growth rates for boys and girls are similar until the growth spurt starts between 10 and 12 years of age. By age 8 or 9 there is increased smoothness and speed in motor control, making the child more agile and graceful. Bone replaces cartilage and continues to harden. Bones of the face and jaw grow at a faster rate than they have in previous years. The school-age child is slimmer, with less body fat and a lower center of gravity. Eyes and hands are well coordinated, and muscles are stronger and more developed. These changes

in growth improve fine-motor activities such as drawing, needlework, and playing musical instruments and gross-motor activities such as jumping, biking, and swimming. By age 12 the rest of the teeth (except the wisdom teeth) erupt.

Behavioral and Cognitive Development

The task for this age-group is to develop a capacity for industry while avoiding an undue sense of inferiority. Interactions with children and teachers at school broaden children's social contacts. Industry influences a desire to achieve. Children learn how to compete and cooperate with others. School relationships provide social support outside the home environment, and peer approval becomes important. A sense of inferiority develops when the child is allowed little success because of interactions with rejecting teachers, peers, or parents. Feelings of racism, sexism, and other forms of discrimination contribute to feelings of inferiority. A maladaptation that may occur is inertia, in which the child feels so inferior that he or she stops making the effort to achieve goals or accomplish tasks.[2]

The cognitive development described by Piaget for this age is concrete operations, when children learn inductive reasoning and logical operations. In school they learn to use numbers, read, and classify.[3] By the time children enter school, their development of fine- and gross-motor, social-adaptive, and language skills changes more gradually (Fig. 18-4). Tasks for the school-age child are listed in Box 18-4. Assessment tools for school-age children focus on mental

TABLE 18-5	EXPECTED DEVELOPMENT OF PRESCHOOLERS			
AGE	**FINE-MOTOR**	**GROSS-MOTOR**	**SOCIAL-ADAPTIVE**	**LANGUAGE**
36 mo (3 yr)	Can unbutton front buttons Copies vertical lines within 30 degrees Copies zero Begins to use fork	Walks up stairs, alternating feet on steps Walks down stairs, two feet on each step Pedals tricycle Jumps in place Able to perform broad jump	Dresses self with help with back buttons Pulls on shoes Parallel play Able to share toys	Vocabulary of 900 words Uses complete sentences Constantly asks questions
48 mo (4 yr)	Able to copy plus sign (+) Picks longer line three out of three times Uses scissors Can lace shoes	Walks down stairs, alternating feet on steps Able to button large front buttons Able to balance on one foot for approximately 5 seconds Catches ball	Associative play Imaginary friend common Boasts and tattles Selfish, impatient, rebellious	Gives first and last name Has 1500-word vocabulary Uses words without knowing meaning Questioning is at a peak
60 mo (5 yr)	Able to dress self with minimal assistance (Fig. 18-3) Able to draw three-part human figure Draws square (■) following demonstration Colors within lines	Hops on one foot Catches ball bounced to him or her two out of three times Able to demonstrate heel-toe walking Jumps rope	Eager to follow rules Less rebellious Relies on outside authority to control the world	Has 2100-word vocabulary Recognizes three colors Asks meanings of words Uses sentences of six to eight words

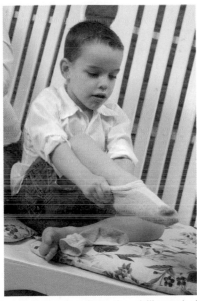

FIG. 18-3 Preschooler develops the ability to help dress self. (©Andy Dean Photography/Shutterstock.com.)

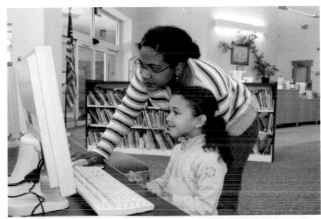

FIG. 18-4 School-age children learn the basic skills required for school. (©Rob Marmion/Shutterstock.com.)

abilities and social and emotional behaviors. Preventive services recommended for school-age children are in Table 18-6 in the columns labeled "Birth to 6 years" and "7 to 18 years."

Adolescents

The hallmark of adolescence is puberty, which marks the end of childhood and the onset of adulthood. Adolescence occurs from approximately 13 to 18 years of age.

Physical Growth

The growth spurt that occurs during puberty varies greatly and accounts for 20% to 25% of the final adult height. Growth frequently occurs during spring and summer months. The peak height velocity (PHV) occurs at approximately 12 years of age in girls, 6 to 12 months before menarche. The PHV is used as a predictor of menarche. On average girls gain 2 to 8 inches (5 to 20 cm) in height and 15.5 to 55 pounds (7 to 25 kg) in weight during adolescence. By contract, boys usually reach PHV at approximately 14 years of age, after growth of testicles and penis and appearance of axillary and mature pubic hair. On average boys gain 4 to 12 inches (10 to 30 cm) in height and 15 to 66 pounds (7 to 30 kg) in weight during adolescence.[9]

BOX 18-4　DEVELOPMENTAL TASKS OF SCHOOL-AGE CHILDREN

- Learning the basic skills required for school (see Fig. 18-4)
  - Mastering reading and writing
  - Developing reflective thinking
  - Mastering physical skills
- Mastering money management
  - Obtaining money through socially acceptable ways
  - Buying wisely
  - Saving
  - Delaying gratification
  - Understanding role of money and place in life
- Becoming an active and cooperative member of the family
  - Participating in family discussions
  - Joining in family decision making
  - Being responsible for household chores
  - Participating in reciprocal gift giving
- Extending abilities to relate to others
  - Asserting rights
  - Developing leadership skills
  - Following social mores and customs
  - Cooperating in group situations
  - Maintaining close friendships
- Managing feelings and impulses
  - Coping with frustrations
  - Managing anger appropriately
  - Expressing feelings in the right time, place, and manner and to the right person
- Identifying the sex and gender role
  - Differentiating expectations based on gender
  - Understanding reproduction and gender-specific physical development
  - Managing physical growth spurts
  - Conceptualizing life as a mature man or woman
- Identifying self as worthy individual
  - Gaining status and respect
  - Growing in self-esteem and self-confidence
  - Establishing unique identity
- Developing conscience and morality
  - Determining right from wrong
  - Developing moral-guided control over behavior
  - Learning to live according to identified values

From Duvall EM, Miller BC: *Marriage and family development*, ed 6, New York, 1985, Harper & Row.

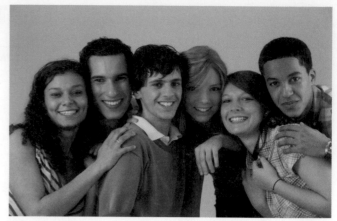

FIG. 18-5 The peer group is a major influence in adolescent development. (©auremar/Shutterstock.com.)

Behavioral and Cognitive Development

The task during adolescence is to achieve ego identity and avoid role confusion. The adolescent reviews the learning, experiences, and values that he or she accepted in earlier stages and modifies them into a unique and personalized identity. During this identity clarification process adolescents may decide that previously accepted ideas and beliefs need to be changed. They may behave in new and different ways, much to the chagrin of their parents, as they "try on" differing roles and values. Adolescents begin testing and evaluating previously accepted notions about life, living, spirituality, relating, and being. Some influences to change may come from peers (Fig. 18-5). The early values of the child often are the accepted values from the parental authority in the family. Role confusion develops for adolescents who are unsuccessful in developing their own identity. They may develop low self-esteem, have poor-to-no direction in their lives, and have difficulty making career choices.

Formal operations is the term Piaget gave to the adolescent years. Adolescents are able to perform abstract reasoning and form logical conclusions. They can form hypotheses and devise ways to test them. They use analytic skills in making judgments about their actions and future lives. Advanced intellectual skills allow them to reexamine accepted ideas, which can be a strain within the family but leads to a stronger sense of self and independence.[3] Developmental tasks for the teen years include those listed in Box 18-5.

Assessment tools for this age-group focus on social and emotional behaviors, in addition to identifying and reducing stress. Preventive services recommended for adolescents are in Table 18-6 in the column labeled "7 to 18 years."

Young Adults

Young adults (approximately 20 to 35 years of age) move away from the dependent role in the family of origin to establishing their own lifestyle. The task of young adults is to achieve some degree of intimacy as opposed to remaining isolated. These individuals begin to express their identity through work, recreation, and interpersonal relationships. Productivity, self-sufficiency, and intimacy in love relationships are driving tasks for young adults, even though they may shift back and forth in career choices, commitment, and goals as they continually redefine themselves. The young adult is ready to enter the adult world and assume a position as a responsible citizen. Achievements are the result of self-direction, with goals that may change as an outcome of reevaluation. Mature relationships with others are important in both the work and home environments. Many young adults choose to marry and start a family. Role confusion may develop when young adults have difficulty moving from adolescence and their dependence on parents or family to developing their own identity and adult role responsibilities.

BOX 18-5 DEVELOPMENTAL TASKS OF ADOLESCENTS

- Accepting physical changes
  - Coming to terms with physical maturation
  - Accepting one's own body
- Achieving a satisfying and socially accepted role
  - Learning masculine/feminine role
  - Realistically understanding gender role
  - Adopting acceptable practices
- Developing more mature peer relationships
  - Being accepted by peer group (see Fig. 18-5)
  - Making and keeping friends of both sexes
  - Dating
  - Loving and being loved
  - Adapting to variety of peer associations
  - Developing skills in managing and evaluating peer relationships
- Achieving emotional independence
  - Outgrowing childish parental dependence
  - Developing mature affection for parents
  - Being autonomous
  - Developing mature interdependence
- Getting an education
  - Acquiring basic knowledge and skills
  - Clarifying sex-role attitudes toward work and family roles
- Preparing for marriage and family life
  - Formulating sex role attitudes
  - Enjoying responsibilities
  - Developing responsible attitudes
  - Distinguishing between infatuation and mature love
  - Developing mutually satisfying personal relationships
- Developing knowledge and skills for civic competence
  - Communicating as a citizen
  - Becoming involved in causes outside oneself
  - Acquiring problem-solving skills
  - Developing social concepts
- Establishing one's identity as a socially responsible person
  - Developing philosophy of life
  - Implementing worthy ideals and standards
  - Assuming social obligations
  - Adopting mature sense of values and ethics
  - Dealing effectively with emotional responses

From Duvall EM, Miller BC: *Marriage and family development,* ed 6, New York, 1985, Harper & Row.

Developmental tasks listed in Box 18-6 are usually accomplished during this stage.

The focus of assessment for young adults is on career choice and mate selection.

Career Choice

Many assessment tool inventories have been developed for young adults contemplating career choices. In these inventories basic interest areas are compared with occupational themes. The inventory responses cluster similar interest areas and relate them to an occupation or vocational choice. Stability in interest areas is important to the predictive power of these inventories. If an individual has many, varied interests, the inventory scores may be less reliable and less valid.

BOX 18-6 DEVELOPMENTAL TASKS OF YOUNG ADULTS

- Establishing one's autonomy as an individual
- Planning a direction for one's life
- Getting an appropriate education
- Working toward a vocation
- Appraising love and sexual feelings
- Becoming involved in love relationships
- Selecting a mate
- Getting engaged
- Being married

From Duvall EM, Miller BC: *Marriage and family development,* ed 6, New York, 1985, Harper & Row.

Mate Selection

Along with career choice, mate selection is a primary interest area for many individuals in early adulthood. The field of premarital and couple counseling has rapidly expanded since the 1940s, along with the increasing divorce rate in America. Various tools and Internet services are used to match couples based on compatibilities. Preventive services recommended for young adults are in Table 18-6 in the column labeled "19 to 64 years."

Middle Adult

Entry into the middle years, between ages 36 and 65, may be met with the feeling that one's best years have passed, especially in light of today's emphasis on youth.

Physical Growth

There are obvious physical signs of aging such as wrinkling of the skin, graying or loss of hair, and changes in muscle tone and mass. Changes in vision and hearing may affect social relationships and learning unless corrective actions are taken.

Behavioral and Cognitive Development

During this time many decisions are made concerning career, partner, children, lifestyle, and living arrangements. The task is to reach a balance between generativity and stagnation. Generativity involves showing concern for the generations to follow. This may be accomplished by raising children and grandchildren or may be in the form of writing, teaching, inventing, or performing community service projects to contribute to the welfare of those who follow. Stagnation develops when the person is so self-absorbed that he or she ceases to be a productive member of society. For persons who have successfully met the developmental tasks of earlier stages, this can be a period of stability, self-understanding, and self-actualization. For others this is the time of the midlife crisis, when they feel that life is stagnant or incomplete. Frustration drives them to search for new directions and goals in life. During middle age one reaps the benefits of career success, support of family and friends, and experiences of earlier years. Developmental tasks for this stage are listed in Box 18-7. Preventive services recommended for middle adults are in Table 18-6 in the column labeled "19 to 64 years."

TABLE 18-6 PREVENTIVE SERVICES THROUGHOUT THE LIFE SPAN*

	BIRTH TO 6 YEARS	7 TO 18 YEARS	19 TO 64 YEARS	OVER 65 YEARS
Screening	Height and weight Hemoglobinopathy at birth Phenylalanine level at birth Vision screen between ages 3 and 5 Hearing loss in newborns	Height and weight Blood pressure Papanicolaou (Pap) test/*Chlamydia* screening Obesity Vision screening	Height and weight Blood pressure Cholesterol screening Pap test (women) Mammogram (women) Vision screening Fecal occult blood test, sigmoidoscopy, or colonoscopy (men and women over 50) Rubella serologic tests or vaccination history (women of childbearing age)	Height and weight Blood pressure Cholesterol screening Pap test (women) Fecal occult blood test, sigmoidoscopy, or colonoscopy Mammogram Vision screening Hearing screening
Counseling	**Injury prevention:** Infant/child safety seats for children <5 years Lap-shoulder belt for children >5 years Smoke detector in home Bicycle helmet; bicycle safety Hot water heater temperature <120°-130° F (49°-54° C) Window and stair guards; pool fences Safe storage of drugs, toxic substances, firearms, and matches Syrup of ipecac, poison control numbers Cardiopulmonary resuscitation (CPR) training for parents and caretakers **Substance abuse:** Effects of passive smoke Antitobacco message **Diet and exercise:** Breast-feeding, iron-enriched formula and foods (infants and toddlers) Limit fat and cholesterol, maintain caloric balance; emphasize grain, fruits, vegetables (ages 2-10); regular physical activity	**Injury prevention:** Lap-shoulder seat belts Helmet use Smoke detector in home Safe storage of firearms **Substance abuse:** Avoid tobacco use Avoid underage drinking Avoid alcohol and drug use while driving, swimming, boating, etc. **Sexual behavior:** Sexually transmitted infection prevention: abstinence, avoid high-risk behavior; use condoms or female barrier with spermicide Unintended pregnancy: contraception **Diet and exercise:** Limit fat and cholesterol, maintain caloric balance; emphasize grain, fruits, vegetables; regular calcium intake; regular physical activity	**Injury prevention:** Lap-shoulder seat belts Helmet use Smoke detector in home Safe storage of firearms **Substance abuse:** Tobacco cessation Avoid alcohol and drug use while driving, swimming, boating, etc. **Sexual behavior:** Sexually transmitted infection prevention: abstinence, avoid high-risk behavior; use condoms or female barrier with spermicide Contraception **Diet and exercise:** Limit fat and cholesterol, maintain caloric balance; emphasize grain, fruits, vegetables; regular calcium intake (women) Regular physical activity	**Injury prevention:** Lap-shoulder seat belts Helmet use Fall prevention Smoke detector in home Safe storage of firearms Hot water heater temperature <120°-130° F (49°-54° C) **Substance abuse:** Tobacco cessation Avoid alcohol and drug use while driving, swimming, boating, etc. **Sexual behavior:** Sexually transmitted infection prevention: abstinence, avoid high-risk behavior; use condoms **Diet and exercise:** Limit fat and cholesterol, maintain caloric balance; emphasize grain, fruits, vegetables; regular calcium intake (women) Regular physical activity
Dental health	Regular visits to dental care provider Floss daily; brush with fluoride toothpaste daily Advice about baby bottle tooth decay	Regular visits to dental care provider Floss daily; brush with fluoride toothpaste daily	Regular visits to dental care provider Floss daily; brush with fluoride toothpaste daily	Regular visits to dental care provider Floss daily; brush with fluoride toothpaste daily

TABLE 18-6	PREVENTIVE SERVICES THROUGHOUT THE LIFE SPAN—cont'd			
	BIRTH TO 6 YEARS	**7 TO 18 YEARS**	**19 TO 64 YEARS**	**OVER 65 YEARS**
Immunizations[†]	Hep B, Rota, DTaP, Hib, PCV, IPV, influenza yearly, MMR, varicella, Hep A See www.cdc.gov for schedule	Tdap, HPV, MCV4, influenza annually See www.cdc.gov for schedule	Tetanus, varicella, influenza HPV (19-26 yrs), MMR See www.cdc.gov for schedule	Tetanus, varicella, influenza, pneumococcal, zoster See www.cdc.gov for schedule
Chemoprophylaxis	Ocular antibiotic prophylaxis at birth Multivitamin	Multivitamin with folic acid (females planning or capable of pregnancy)	Multivitamin with folic acid (women planning or capable of pregnancy)	

*U.S. Preventive Services Task Force–recommended interventions (i.e., screening tests, counseling interventions, immunizations, and chemoprophylactic regimens) for the prevention of more than 80 target conditions. The patients who receive these services are asymptomatic individuals of all age-groups and risk categories. The recommendations are based on a standardized review of current scientific evidence.
[†]Vaccine abbreviations: *DTaP*, diphtheria and tetanus toxoids and acellular pertussis vaccine; *HBV*, hepatitis B virus vaccine; *Hib, Haemophilus influenzae* type b conjugate vaccine; *HPV*, human papilloma virus; *IPV*, inactivated poliovirus vaccine; *MCV4*, meningococcal vaccine; *MMR*, measles, mumps, and rubella virus vaccine live; *Td*, adult tetanus toxoid (full dose) and diphtheria toxoid (reduced dose) for children older than 7 years and adults, *PCV*, pneumococcal conjugate vaccine; *rota*, rotavirus vaccine.
From http://www.uspreventiveservicestaskforce.org, 2010, accessed October 29, 2011. www.cdc.gov/vaccines/recs/schedule, December, 2010, accessed October 29, 2011.

Older Adult

For most adults the later years, beginning with age 65, are productive years met with a sense of pleasure and enjoyment. Older adults represent the fastest-growing population in the United States and probably the least understood. They are a highly diverse group.

Physical Growth

Although many physical changes accompany aging, most older adults are active members of society and have independent lifestyles. Chronic health problems are common but usually can be managed.

Behavioral and Cognitive Development

The task of development is to achieve ego integrity with a minimal amount of despair. Ego integrity is achieved when older adults can look back at their lives and accept the course of events and the choices they made as being necessary.

Despair may develop with the death of one's spouse and friends or the adjustment related to retirement. Society is becoming more aware of the presence of ageism and stereotyping of a person because of age. Older adults are encouraging positive attitudes about aging and making society aware of the developmental tasks they experience and the barriers to leading a healthy, happy life in a society that values youth. Ego integrity develops as older adults give back to society and interact with grandchildren (Fig. 18-6).

Cognitive development in the old-old adult was reported in a longitudinal study of subjects ranging from 73 to 99 years of age. Researchers found that, although many subjects reported some decline in abilities, more than half displayed no decline. A study of 18 people ages 100 to 106 found that these centenarians reported rich late-life learning experiences, the majority of which occurred through social interaction.[7]

BOX 18-7	**DEVELOPMENTAL TASKS OF MIDDLE ADULTS**

- Providing a comfortable and healthful home
- Allocating resources to provide security in later years
- Dividing household responsibilities
- Encouraging both husband and wife roles within and beyond the family
- Maintaining emotional and sexual intimacy
- Incorporating all family members into family circle as family enlarges and caring for extended family
- Participating in activities outside the home
- Developing competencies that maintain family functioning during crises and encourage achievement

From Duvall EM, Miller BC: *Marriage and family development*, ed 6, New York, 1985, Harper & Row.

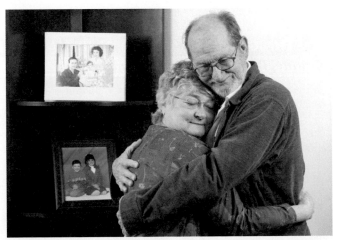

FIG. 18-6 Love and affection are important to older persons. (From Sorrentino and Gorek, 2007.)

Because of the variation between a 65-year old and an 85-year old, old age has been categorized into young-old from ages 65 to 74, middle-old from ages 75 to 84, and old-old as 85 years and older.[10] Developmental tasks with different age-groups are identified in Box 18-8. Preventive services recommended for older adults are in Table 18-6 in the column labeled "Over 65 years."

FAMILY DEVELOPMENT AND ASSESSMENT

Most individuals in America grow up within the social unit of a family. However, the definition and composition of

---

BOX 18-8 DEVELOPMENTAL TASKS OF YOUNG-OLD AND OLD-OLD ADULTS

Young-Old (Approximately 65 to 85 Years)
- Preparing for and adjusting to retirement
- Adjusting to lower and fixed income of retirement
- Establishing physical living arrangements
- Adjusting to new relationships with adult children and their offspring
- Managing leisure time
- Adjusting to slower physical and intellectual responses
- Dealing with death of parents, spouse, and friends

Old-Old (over 85 Years)
- Learning to combine new dependency needs with continued need for independence
- Adapting to living alone
- Accepting and adjusting to possible institutional living
- Establishing affiliation with age-group
- Adjusting to increased vulnerability to physical and emotional stress
- Adjusting to loss of physical strength, illness, and approach of one's own death
- Adjusting to losses of spouse, home, and friends

From Touhy TA: Gerontological nursing and an aging society. In Ebersole P et al: *Toward healthy aging: human needs & nursing response*, ed 7, St Louis, 2008, Mosby, pp 1-23.

---

family structures have changed over the years. Families are no longer only the traditional two married heterosexual parents with children who live under one roof. Blended families are composed of stepchildren and children from the current unit. Homosexual couples join as family units, some of which include children. There are single-parent families: some from divorce, some never married, and some formed because of adoption or artificial fertilization. There are also intergenerational families in which multiple generations live together under one roof or in which grandparents or even great-grandparents raise and care for their grandchildren. An Ethnic, Cultural, and Spiritual Variations box describes some cultures in which extended families may be maintained. For our purposes, a *family* is defined as two or more individuals who share bonds of commitment, loyalty, and affection. The family unit typically shares some degree of time, financial, and physical resources and responsibilities for the unit maintenance (Fig. 18-7). Developmental tasks of the family are summarized in Table 18-7.

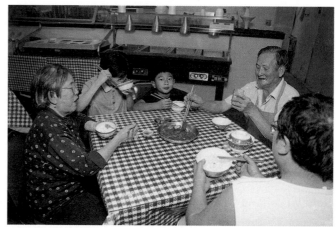

FIG. 18-7 The family unit typically shares some degree of time, financial, and physical resources and responsibilities for the unit maintenance.

⊕ ETHNIC, CULTURAL, AND SPIRITUAL VARIATIONS
Cultural Differences Within Families

In many cultures the extended family is important in the care of children. In African American families, when mothers are unable to provide emotional and physical support for their children, grandmothers, aunts, and extended family members readily provide assistance or take responsibility for the children. About 44% of all children living with grandparents today are African American. Of these, 66% have grandparents as the primary caregivers.

Chinese family members emphasize loyalty to the family and tradition. Personal independence is not valued. Often children live with grandparents or aunts and uncles so individual family members can obtain a better education or to reduce financial burden.

Mexican American families are patriarchal, with some evidence of a slow change to a more egalitarian pattern in recent years. Children are highly valued because they ensure the continuation of the family and cultural values.

Navajo families have separate dwellings but are grouped together by family relationships. The Navajo family unit consists of the nuclear family and relatives such as sisters, aunts, and their female descendants. The elderly play an important role in keeping rituals and instructing children and grandchildren.[9]

TABLE 18-7	DEVELOPMENTAL TASKS OF THE FAMILY
STAGES	**THEMES**
Married couple	Without children; establishing satisfying marriage; adjusting to pregnancy; fitting into kin network
Childbearing	Oldest child birth to 30 months; nurturing infants; establishing home
Family with preschoolers	Oldest child 2½ to 6; adapting to needs of children; decreased energy and privacy as parents
Family with school-age children	Oldest child 6 to 13; being part of community of school-age families; encouraging educational achievement of children
Family with teenagers	Oldest child 13 to 20; balancing freedom and responsibility; establishing postparental interests
Family launching young adults	First child gone until last child leaves home; maintaining supportive home base
Middle-age parents	Empty nest to retirement; refocusing on marriage; maintaining kin ties
Aging family members	Retirement to death of both spouses; coping with bereavement; adapting home for aging; adjusting to retirement; living alone

From Duvall EM, Miller BC: *Marriage and family development,* ed 6, New York, 1985, Harper & Row.

In stepfamilies a biologic parent lives elsewhere, and the children commonly move between the homes of two biologic families. Virtually all members of a stepfamily sustain primary relationship loss. The parent and stepparents must repeatedly deal with a part-time relationship with the stepchild if the stepchild is involved with the other biologic parent. The relationship between the adult parents outside of the stepfamily predates the new marriage and the relationship with the stepparent. This can create conflicts and loyalty divisions in parenting strategies and with the child. Children within a stepfamily struggle with being members of more than one household, whereas stepparents cope with parenting a child to whom they are not related.

Single-parent families are rising in number because of the increasing divorce rate in America and the decreasing social stigma related to unwed mothers. In single-parent families the child lives with one biologic parent. Both the child and the single parent sustain a loss from the absent biologic parent of the child. There is great variation in the involvement of the absent parent in the life of the child; some are actively involved, whereas others have minimal to no involvement. Other children may be added to the single-parent family from the same or different biologic parentage. Financial difficulties are a common stressor for single-parent families because only one adult is present to care for the children, maintain the home, and provide for the family.

CLINICAL APPLICATION AND CLINICAL REASONING

See Appendix D for answers to exercises in this section.

REVIEW QUESTIONS

1. Which immunizations does the nurse ask about when interviewing a 75-year-old patient?
   1. Measles, mumps, and rubella
   2. Tetanus and influenza
   3. Hepatitis B and varicella
   4. Inactivated polio vaccine

2. Which statement reflects an expected developmental task of a 40-year-old man?
   1. "I'll be completing my degree this year, and then I plan to marry my fiancé."
   2. "I'm staying active with plenty of volunteer activities every day of the week."
   3. "My wife and I have divided the chores with the children since we're both working."
   4. "My life is going to be different now that dad has died and the care of mom is my responsibility."

3. Which finding is expected when assessing an 11-year-old child?
   1. Five-pound (2.3 kg) weight gain and beginning of a growth spurt
   2. Loss of deciduous teeth and eruption of permanent teeth
   3. Development of mature relationships and beginning of dating
   4. Acting out feelings during play and sports

4. A nurse is assessing an infant who is able to pull up to a sitting position, turn from prone to side position, laugh and babble, and show interest in her surroundings. These behaviors are consistent with an infant of which age?
   1. 7 months old
   2. 5 months old
   3. 3 months old
   4. 1 month old

5. A 15-year-old boy approaches the school nurse and describes how uncomfortable he is around the girls because most of them are taller than he is. What is the nurse's best response to this adolescent?
   1. "Let's discuss your diet to determine if you are eating enough nutrients."
   2. "Genetics play an important part in height; if your parents are short, you may be short as well."
   3. "Sleep is necessary for growth. Are you getting adequate sleep?"
   4. "The growth spurt during adolescence occurs in girls 18 to 24 months before it occurs in boys."

CASE STUDY

Mrs. Caberra is a 78-year-old woman who is brought to the geriatric clinic by her son and daughter-in-law. Mrs. Caberra's son tells the nurse that his father died 5 months ago and ever since then his mother has "gone downhill." Mr. Caberra indicates that his mother is no longer keeping her house clean or cooking appropriate meals. Her personal hygiene habits have also dramatically changed. She has lost interest in getting her hair done, and she no longer likes to dress for the day. Mr. Caberra tells the nurse, "When I suggest a retirement home, she becomes very angry and tells me to mind my own business. I'm just worried about Mom, and I want to make sure that someone is taking care of her." During this conversation Mrs. Caberra sits quietly. She interjects only to say, "I've taken care of you, your brother, and your father. Now all of a sudden you think I'm helpless and want to lock me away." Mrs. Caberra appears clean, although her hair is matted and her

clothes are badly wrinkled and don't match. Her speech is clear, but her overall affect is very dull. She doesn't make eye contact with her son or the nurse. A physical examination demonstrates expected bodily functioning consistent with her age.

Clinical Reasoning
1. List the subjective data described in the case study.
2. List the objective data described in the case study.
3. Which of Erikson's developmental stages is Mrs. Caberra experiencing?
4. Based on what is known from the interview, with which developmental tasks of older adults may Mrs. Caberra be struggling?
5. Which additional assessment data are needed?

Assessment of the Infant, Child, and Adolescent

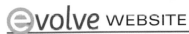

evolve WEBSITE

http://evolve.elsevier.com/Wilson/assessment

Pediatric nursing encompasses a wide range of ages, from birth through adolescence, making health assessment a challenge. To adequately assess children, the nurse considers differences in anatomy and physiology that occur with growth; developmental milestones specific to age; and the psychosocial issues unique to infants, toddlers, preschoolers, school-age children, and adolescents. Adding to this complexity is the fact that the children are assessed in the context of their family; thus nurses performing pediatric assessments must be skilled at interviewing and observing both families and children. In performing the physical examination, the nurse adjusts examination components and techniques to meet the unique needs of each age-group. Table 19-1 presents definitions for these age-groups.

ANATOMY AND PHYSIOLOGY

Children differ anatomically and physiologically from adults in many important ways; generally the younger the child, the greater these differences. Of particular importance are differences that exist at birth, including immaturities of the central nervous system, respiratory and cardiovascular function, and immune functions. These immaturities are evident in such things as heart and respiratory rate, reflexes, and pain response. Differences in anatomy and physiology also place young children at unique risk for certain illnesses such as otitis media because of their short, straight eustachian tube. Even the adolescent, who may be adultlike in size and appearance, is still undergoing maturation of body systems, including the reproductive and central nervous systems and cognitive function. Box 19-1 summarizes basic variations in anatomy and physiology in infants, children, and adolescents.

HEALTH HISTORY

Nurses interview patients to collect subjective data about their present health and any past medical experiences. The pediatric health history includes all age-groups (neonate through adolescence) and is adapted to the age and developmental status of the child. The basic format of the history is similar to that of the adult, with additional age-specific data in the areas of perinatal history, growth and development, and behavioral status. In addition, observing the interaction between parent and child throughout the history and examination is important. As in the adult, a complete history is obtained during well-child visits. A more limited, focused history is performed when the child presents with an illness.

Much of the pediatric history is obtained from the parent (or other adult) accompanying the child, but including the child as much as appropriate for his or her age is important (Fig. 19-1). After the parent's concerns are explored, additional health history questions can be asked directly to school-age children and adolescents using language and concepts appropriate to their age. Giving adolescents an opportunity to talk with the health care provider without the parent present is important. In many states adolescents have a legal right to confidential care for specific problems, including sexually transmitted infections, contraception and pregnancy, mental health issues, and substance abuse. For these reasons

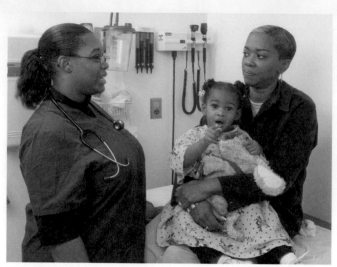

FIG. 19-1 Most data are obtained from the adult accompanying the child.

TABLE 19-1	PEDIATRIC AGE-GROUPS
NEWBORN (NEONATE)	**BIRTH-28 DAYS**
Infant	1-12 months
Toddler	1-3 years
Preschool	3-5 years
School Age	6-12 years
Adolescent	12-18 years

the adolescent should be given an opportunity to discuss these issues privately. The American Medical Association's *Guidelines for Adolescent Preventive Services* (GAPS)[1] includes health history questionnaires that can be completed by both the adolescents and their parents. These forms provide a valuable first step in data collection for these age-groups.

Quality Improvement Competencies for Nurses include providing patient-centered care to infants, children, or adolescents and their families or caregivers. Table 11-1 on p. 196 presents knowledge, skills, and attitudes to use when demonstrating this competency.

COMPONENTS OF THE PEDIATRIC HEALTH HISTORY

Biographic Data

In addition to the information included in the adult history (name, gender, age, date of birth, race, and culture), biographic data also include the name of the person giving the history (the informant) and that person's relationship to the child.

Reason for Seeking Health Care

Record the reason for the visit in the words of the parent or older child/adolescent. Many pediatric visits are for well-child care. If this is the case, record the reason for the visit (e.g., "6-month well-child care"). If the child is seen for acute or chronic illnesses, the reason for the visit is often a symptom (e.g., "cough and runny nose × 10 days"). The reason for seeking care should be brief (i.e., no more than a sentence or two).

History of Present Illness

The same information is recorded for the infant and child as for the adult. If illness is present, record a complete symptom analysis using the mnemonic OLD CARTS, which includes the *O*nset, *L*ocation, *D*uration, *C*haracteristics, *A*ggravating factors, *R*elated symptoms, *T*reatment, and *S*everity (see Box 2-3). In addition, it is important to include questions related to the sleeping and eating behaviors of the infant or child because these behaviors offer important clues regarding the severity of the illness. If the child is being seen for a well visit, an overall statement about his or her current health is included.

Present Health Status

As in the adult history, the nurse asks the parents or accompanying adult about the child's health conditions, including chronic illnesses such as asthma. In addition, the nurse asks about medications the child is taking and allergies the child has experienced.

Past Health History

For newborns, infants, and toddlers, the past health history includes the mother's health status during the course of the pregnancy and information about the birth and neonatal period. Collectively these data are referred to as the perinatal history and are presented in Box 19-2. The perinatal history may also be important for older children with congenital problems or other problems that may be related to pregnancy or birth complications (e.g., fetal alcohol syndrome or cerebral palsy). Also included in the past health history is a developmental history, which details the age of achievement for major developmental milestones. Specific questions asked depend on the age and developmental level of the child. Chapter 18 presents further information regarding developmental assessment and milestones.

Other components of the past health history are similar to the adult history and include a summary of childhood illnesses; chronic illnesses; hospitalizations and surgeries; accidents or injuries; medications; allergies; and the dates of the last medical, vision, and dental care. Particularly important in pediatrics is the immunization history, which should be reviewed at every well-child visit and at each visit for acute illness. The immunization schedule is presented in Table 18-6 on p. 450.

Family History

The family history includes the medical history of three generations, including the child and any siblings, the parents, and both sets of grandparents. The ages and health status of all family members are recorded, with particular attention to

BOX 19-1   SELECTED ANATOMIC AND PHYSIOLOGIC DIFFERENCES IN CHILDREN

Skin
- Newborns, especially preterms, have thinner, more permeable skin than older children and adults.
- Newborns and young infants have decreased subcutaneous fat and a large body surface area, which can lead to thermoregulation problems.
- Apocrine sweat glands and sebaceous gland activity increase in adolescents, resulting in more oily skin and acne.

Head
- The cranial bones are soft and not fused at birth. The posterior fontanelle closes by 2 months, and the anterior fontanelle closes by 18 months. This allows for continuing head growth.
- Infants' and small children's heads are larger in proportion to their body.
- The brain and CNS are immature at birth; major development occurs during the first year of life and continues throughout childhood. The immature brain is particularly vulnerable to injury.

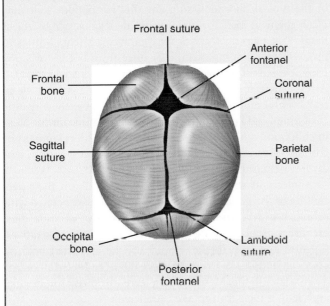

Frontal suture
Anterior fontanel
Frontal bone
Coronal suture
Sagittal suture
Parietal bone
Occipital bone
Lambdoid suture
Posterior fontanel

Ears, Nose, Throat, Mouth
- The eustachian tubes are shorter and straighter in infants and young children, increasing their susceptibility to ear infections.
- Newborns and young infants are obligate nose breathers.

- The airway is vulnerable to obstruction because the nasal passages are small, the trachea narrower and less rigid, and the tongue large.
- Twenty deciduous teeth appear between 6 and 24 months of age; permanent teeth begin to erupt at about age 6.

Lungs
- Young infants rely on the diaphragm and abdominal muscles for breathing; the chest wall is thinner and more flexible.
- The respiratory rate is faster in newborns, infants, and young children.

Heart
- Several anatomic shunts are present in the newborn heart, closing shortly after birth.
- The heart rate is faster in infants and young children; the rate frequently increases on inspiration (sinus arrhythmia).
- The heart lies more horizontally in the chest; the PMI is higher (fourth ICS) and more lateral in young infants and toddlers.
- Innocent murmurs are common throughout childhood.

Musculoskeletal
- Bones are softer in children, making them more vulnerable to fractures.
- Infants and young toddlers are usually bowlegged; preschoolers and young school-age children are often "knock-kneed."

Lymph System
- Lymph tissue increases during childhood, reaching a peak between 6 and 9 years. Children at this age often have large tonsils.

Neurologic
- Major growth of the nervous system occurs during the first year of life; motor control develops in a cephalocaudal direction, from head to trunk to extremities.
- Primitive reflexes are present at birth and disappear in a predictable pattern throughout early infancy.
- Infants, including preterm infants, perceive and react to pain. This pain response is manifested primarily by physiologic changes (heart rate, blood pressure, oxygen saturation).

Breasts
- Breasts remain undeveloped until the onset of puberty.

Reproductive System
- Genitalia of males and females do not undergo development until the onset of puberty.

CNS, Central nervous system; *ICS*, intercostal space; *PMI*, point of maximum impulse.
Image from Duderstadt K: *Pediatric physical examination: an illustrated handbook*, St Louis, 2006, Mosby.

congenital problems, infant and child deaths, and hereditary illnesses. As in the adult, a family history of chronic illness (including diabetes, cardiovascular disease, malignancy, or mental health disorders) is noted. Smoking among family members and problems with alcohol or substance abuse are particularly important to note.

Personal and Psychosocial History

The personal and psychosocial history includes an overview of the child's current level of function and data about social and family relationships, behaviors and health habits, and mental health. With young children these data are collected primarily from the parent. As children reach adolescence,

Diet and Nutrition

When taking a diet history, inquire about typical daily diet, intolerances or allergies, supplements (particularly vitamin D for breast-fed infants), family mealtime routines, snacks, and any concerns of the parent or child about diet or weight. For newborns and infants, determine the type (breast or formula) and amount/frequency of feeding, introduction of solid foods (cereal, fruits, vegetables, meats, eggs) and other liquids (e.g., water, juice, cow's milk). Note excess intake of milk or juice, which may impact appetite and decrease the intake of more nutritious foods.

The diet history of children should include a description of the typical diet, including any diet restrictions that may place them at risk for nutritional deficiencies. Ask about habits that increase the risk for dental caries (e.g., bottles in bed, constant sipping of milk or juice from bottles or sippy cups, consumption of soda and sweet and sticky foods). Assess where most meals are eaten (at home, school, or in restaurants) and identify children who frequently consume "fast food" and "junk food." Obesity is a significant problem in childhood and is associated with the later development of chronic diseases such as type 2 diabetes, hypertension, and cardiovascular disease.

Adolescents should be asked specifically about their perception of their current weight and behaviors associated with eating disorders, including food restrictions, extreme diet/exercise routines, binging or purging, and the use of laxatives. Calcium and iron intake should also be evaluated because poor calcium intake in adolescence has been linked to osteoporosis later in life. Menstruating teens are at risk for anemia, especially if their iron intake is deficient.

Sleep

The pediatric sleep history includes where and with whom the child sleeps; total amount of sleep, including naps; bedtime rituals; difficulty falling or staying asleep; and nightmares or night terrors. Parents should be asked about the sleep position of newborns and infants and the sleep environment (Box 19-3).

Sexuality

Ask about pubertal changes, which occur earlier in girls than in boys. Teenage girls should be asked about menstruation, including their last menstrual period and the frequency and duration of menses. Teens should be asked privately about sexual activity. Questions about sexuality should be approached with great sensitivity, and the nurse must not make assumptions about sexual orientation. The sexually

sensitive parts of the history should be obtained without the parent present. This provides the adolescent with the opportunity to give a confidential history and discuss issues privately.

Personal Status

Ask the parent to describe the child's personality and temperament. Engage older children in a conversation about how they think their life is going, things they like about themselves, and things they do well or not so well. Determine if the school-age child is in an age-appropriate grade and if there are any issues related to school performance. Ask about personal habits and behavior patterns such as nail biting, thumb sucking, rituals (e.g., "security blanket" or toy), and unusual behaviors (e.g., head banging, rocking, overt masturbation, walking on toes). Also ask for a description of the child's typical day.

active adolescent should be evaluated for risk of pregnancy and/or sexually transmitted infections. Determining that sexual activity is consensual and that no coercion or force is involved is important. See Chapter 17 for a complete discussion of the menstrual and sexual history.

Development

To assess the current developmental stage of infants and children, the nurse asks parents about new skills since the last well-child visit and the specific milestones that should be occurring. For example, ask the parent of a 5-year-old if the child is able to dress self, jump rope, identify colors, and follow rules when playing games, all of which are expected developmental achievements in a 5-year-old. Asking about school performance is another key component of developmental assessment. Include current grade level, any special educational needs, school problems, and truancy. Adolescents should be asked about future school and career plans.

Health Promotion Habits

To assess health habits, ask about diet; smoking; exercise; hobbies; and other activities, including amounts of television and computer time. Also evaluate the use of safety measures, including car seats, sunscreen, and bicycle helmets/sports equipment. Teenage males should be asked about testicular self-examination.

Social and Family Relationships

A comprehensive pediatric history includes assessment of social relationships, including family and friends, and a description of the home environment. Information to gather about this topic includes:

Family composition: Individuals who live in the home and their relationship to the child, the primary caregiver(s) in the family, recent changes in family composition, family members or other important persons who interact frequently with the child but live outside the home (noncustodial parents, grandparents, other extended family, nannies, or day care providers)

Family life: Family activities, impact of culture on family, parenting style and skills, discipline methods and their effectiveness, family rules, child care arrangements, parent and family support system, family conflict or chaos, family violence

Family Socioeconomic Status: Parents' occupation and employment; sources of income, including government assistance (Medicaid, food stamps, the Special Supplemental Nutrition Program for Women, Infants, and Children [WIC]); insurance coverage; history of homelessness or unstable living arrangements; ability of parents to meet child's basic physical needs (food, shelter, clothing, medical care, supervision)

Home Environment: Characteristics of the home, including facilities (heat, running water, cooking facilities, adequate space, sleeping arrangements) and home safety (child proofing; storage of firearms, medications, and chemicals; animals in the home; pool safety); characteristics of the community (available resources, crime, pollution, overcrowding, safety hazards)

Friends: Child's relationships with friends, classmates, and siblings; ages of friends; ability to make friends easily; activities shared with friends; history of bullying or being bullied; fighting; violence among peers. Adolescents should be asked specifically about peers, gang activity and violence in their school and peer group, alcohol and drug use, and dating and sexual activity.

Mental Health

Many factors that can impact mental health will have been previously noted in either the past medical history (maternal substance abuse in pregnancy, perinatal hypoxia, neurologic illness or injury) or the social history (e.g., developmental delays, family problems, body image disturbances, witnessed violence). The mental health history should explore the impact of these problems on the child, identify past psychiatric history, explore current stresses in the child's life, and identify signs and symptoms of mental health conditions. Questions should include frequent sense of boredom, suicidal thoughts or attempts, symptoms of depression or anxiety, and risk-taking behaviors (e.g., drug or alcohol use, fighting, risky sexual behaviors, school failure or truancy). Determine the child's usual ability to cope with stress and any recent changes in coping, mood, or behavior. Asking children to identify to whom they can talk about problems in their lives is also important. Children who have poor coping skills, many stressors, and no trusted adult in their lives and those who engage in multiple risk-taking behaviors are at particular risk. Note that the health care provider's duty to maintain confidentiality ends when a child or adolescent reveals that he or she is a danger to themselves or others.

The Pediatric Symptom Checklist (PSC)[3] can be used to identify parental concerns about behavioral and emotional issues in children ages 4 to 18. A second version of the form, the PSC Youth Report, is available for self-reporting of symptoms by older children and adolescents (Fig. 19-2). GAPS Questionnaires[1] (described previously) are also useful components of an adolescent mental health history.

Review of Systems

The review of systems for the infant, child, and adolescent is similar to that for an adult. The goal is to elicit symptoms and problems from the parent or caregiver that may not have been identified earlier in the history. Critical components of the review of systems in pediatrics include:

General Symptoms

- *Constitutional symptoms:* Fever, chills, night sweats, fatigue, tiring with feeding (infants), change in energy level or activity tolerance
- *Growth:* Recent weight gain or loss; concerns about height, weight, or head size
- *Pain:* Ask the parents of infants and toddlers if they think that their baby is in pain and which signs of pain they see;

Pediatric Symptom Checklist (PSC)

Emotional and physical health go together in children. Because parents are often the first to notice a problem with their child's behavior, emotions, or learning, you may help your child get the best care possible by answering these questions. Please indicate which statement best describes your child.

Please mark under the heading that best describes your child:

		NEVER	SOMETIMES	OFTEN
1. Complains of aches and pains	1			
2. Spends more time alone	2			
3. Tires easily, has little energy	3			
4. Fidgety, unable to sit still	4			
5. Has trouble with teacher	5			
6. Less interested in school	6			
7. Acts as if driven by a motor	7			
8. Daydreams too much	8			
9. Distracted easily	9			
10. Is afraid of new situations	10			
11. Feels sad, unhappy	11			
12. Is irritable, angry	12			
13. Feels hopeless	13			
14. Has trouble concentrating	14			
15. Less interested in friends	15			
16. Fights with other children	16			
17. Absent from school	17			
18. School grades dropping	18			
19. Is down on himself or herself	19			
20. Visits the doctor with doctor finding nothing wrong	20			
21. Has trouble sleeping	21			
22. Worries a lot	22			
23. Wants to be with you more than before	23			
24. Feels he or she is bad	24			
25. Takes unnecessary risks	25			
26. Gets hurt frequently	26			
27. Seems to be having less fun	27			
28. Acts younger than children his or her age	28			
29. Does not listen to rules	29			
30. Does not show feelings	30			
31. Does not understand other people's feelings	31			
32. Teases others	32			
33. Blames others for his or her troubles	33			
34. Takes things that do not belong to him or her	34			
35. Refuses to share	35			

Total score _____

Does your child have any emotional or behavioral problems for which she/he needs help? ( ) N ( ) Y
Are there any services that you would like your child to receive for these problems? ( ) N ( ) Y

If yes, what
services?_____

FIG. 19-2 Pediatric Symptom Checklist and Pediatric Symptom Checklist Youth Report. (Jellinek et al., 1994.)

Pediatric Symptom Checklist - Youth Report (Y-PSC)

Please mark under the heading that best fits you:

	Never	Sometimes	Often
1. Complain of aches or pains............................	—	—	—
2. Spend more time alone................................	—	—	—
3. Tire easily, little energy............................	—	—	—
4. Fidgety, unable to sit still.........................	—	—	—
5. Have trouble with teacher..................	—	—	—
6. Less interested in school...............	—	—	—
7. Act as if driven by motor............................	—	—	—
8. Daydream too much....................................	—	—	—
9. Distract easily......................................	—	—	—
10. Are afraid of new situations.........................	—	—	—
11. Feel sad, unhappy....................................	—	—	—
12. Are irritable, angry.................................	—	—	—
13. Feel hopeless..	—	—	—
14. Have trouble concentrating...........................	—	—	—
15. Less interested in friends...........................	—	—	—
16. Fight with other children............................	—	—	—
17. Absent from school...................................	—	—	—
18. School grades dropping.	—	—	—
19. Down on yourself.....................................	—	—	—
20. Visit doctor with doctor finding nothing wrong........	—	—	—
21. Have trouble sleeping................................	—	—	—
22. Worry a lot..	—	—	—
23. Want to be with parent more than before...............	—	—	—
24. Feel that you are bad................................	—	—	—
25. Take unnecessary risks...............................	—	—	—
26. Get hurt frequently..................................	—	—	—
27. Seem to be having less fun...........................	—	—	—
28. Act younger than children your age...................	—	—	—
29. Do not listen to rules...............................	—	—	—
30. Do not show feelings.................................	—	—	—
31. Do not understand other people's feelings.............	—	—	—
32. Tease others...	—	—	—
33. Blame others for your troubles.......................	—	—	—
34. Take things that do not belong to you................	—	—	—
35. Refuse to share......................................	—	—	—

FIG. 19-2, cont'd.

older children can be asked about pain using age-appropriate pain scales (Figs. 19-3 and 19-4, *A* to *C*).

Integumentary System

- *Skin:* Jaundice (newborn); rashes, birthmarks, or lesions; easy bruising; petechiae; itching; dry skin; acne (adolescents); piercings and tattoos (adolescents)
- *Hair:* Infestations (such as lice), hair loss, seborrhea (infants)
- *Nails:* Nail changes; nail biting; ingrown or painful nails

Head, Eyes, Ears, Neck, and Throat

- *Head:* Concerns about head size or shape (newborns, infants); headaches; recent trauma

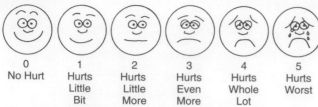

FIG. 19-3 Wong-Baker FACES Pain Rating Scale. Recommended for children 3 years of age and older. Ask the child to choose the face that best describes how he or she is feeling. (From Hockenberry MJ, Wilson D: *Wong's essentials of pediatric nursing,* ed 8, 2009, Mosby. Used with permission. Copyright © Mosby.)

BOX 19-4 TALKING WITH CHILDREN WHO REVEAL ABUSE

- Provide a private time and place to talk.
- Do not promise not to tell; tell the child that you are required to report the abuse.
- Do not express shock or criticize the family.
- Use the child's vocabulary to discuss the body part.
- Avoid using any leading statements that can distort the child's story.
- Reassure the child that he or she has done the right thing by telling.
- Tell the child that the touching or abuse is not his or her fault; he or she is not bad or to blame.
- Determine the child's immediate need for safety.
- Let the child know when you report the situation.

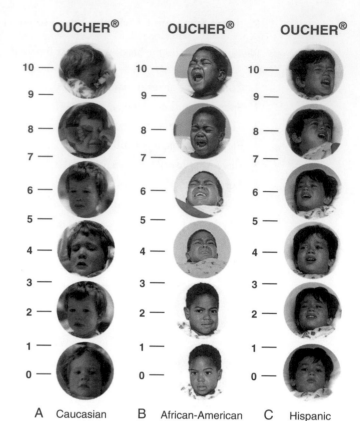

FIG. 19-4 Oucher Pain Scales. **A,** Caucasian, **B,** African American, **C,** Hispanic. (**A** developed and copyrighted by Judith E. Beyer, 1983. **B** and **C** Courtesy Denyes, Villaruel.)

- *Eyes:* Visual concerns, including not fixing on objects or following with eyes (newborns, infants), reading difficulty, sitting too close to television or computer screen, bumping into things; redness, drainage, or crusting; itching or pain; abnormal eye movement or alignment
- *Ears:* Hearing concerns, including not responding to sound (newborns, infants), unusual vocalizations (infants), loud speech or loud television, child's complaint of decreased hearing, ear pain, discharge
- *Nose:* Congestion, drainage, frequent nosebleeds (epistaxis), snoring
- *Mouth/throat:* Teeth (tooth pain, tooth loss, caries); mouth pain or lesions; unusual coatings of tongue or mouth; throat pain; difficulty swallowing; voice changes
- *Neck:* Lymph node enlargement, swelling or masses in neck, stiff neck, unusual head/neck position

Breasts

- Breast engorgement (newborns of both sexes); breast changes (school age and adolescents); pain

Respiratory System

- Cough; wheezing or noisy breathing; shortness of breath at rest or with activity; nighttime snoring; increased respiratory rate or effort; use of "inhalers"

Cardiovascular

- Cyanosis or pallor; edema; known murmur or cardiovascular disease; syncope

Gastrointestinal System

- Usual pattern of bowel movements; changes in bowel function, including constipation and diarrhea; abdominal pain; nausea; vomiting; change in appetite

Urinary System

- Number of wet diapers per day (newborns, infants); toilet training progress; bedwetting or daytime accidents in a previously toilet-trained child; signs of urinary tract infection (dysuria, urgency, frequency, foul odor); hematuria

Reproductive System

- Boys: Healing of circumcision, rash or irritation, penile discharge, pain, itching, development of secondary sexual characteristics, testicular masses, trauma
- Girls: Menstrual concerns (dysmenorrhea, irregular menses, heavy bleeding, amenorrhea); rash or irritation; discharge
- Questions need to be at an appropriate developmental level (Box 19-4)

Musculoskeletal System

- Symmetric movement and muscle tone (newborns/infants); pain in joints or muscles; deformity or asymmetry; range-of-motion limitations; muscle or joint trauma; curvature of the spine; concerns about legs or feet (e.g., bowlegged, intoeing, limp)

Neurologic System

- Unusual cry; irritability; speech problems (stuttering, articulation, language delay); fainting or dizziness; seizures; difficulty with coordination or gait

EXAMINATION

Because the process and findings associated with infant, child, and adolescent examinations vary, the presentation of the examination is organized by age-group (with the exception of vital signs and baseline measurements, which are presented across age-groups). For each age-group a separate discussion of examination issues and techniques is provided for each body system. Wash hands before beginning the examination.

VITAL SIGNS AND BASELINE MEASUREMENTS

Vital signs are measured with every visit.

Temperature

Procedure and Techniques. The recommended approaches for temperature measurement in newborns, infants, and children up to age 5 are axillary, tympanic membrane (TM), and temporal artery sites. Oral measurement using an electronic thermometer is permissible with older children, but the nurse must be sure that the probe is held correctly in the mouth (thermometer under the tongue with the mouth closed). To take a tympanic measurement in a child younger than 3 years of age, pull down on the earlobe to straighten the ear canal. For children older than 3, pull up on the ear to straighten the canal. Although research has shown that tympanic measurements in children may be unreliable,[4-5] it is possible that unreliable measurements are attained because the sensor beam is directed at the sides of the ear canal rather than at the TM.

Rectal temperatures should be taken as a last resort because children tend to fear intrusive procedures and because of the risk for rectal perforation. A convenient position for taking a rectal temperature is with the child in a side-lying position with knees flexed toward the abdomen. This position is maintained with one of the nurse's hands while the lubricated thermometer is held in the rectum a maximum of 2.5 cm (less in newborns and young infants).

Expected and Abnormal Findings. The temperature of the infant should be similar to that of the adult (98.6° F or 37° C). However, temperature variations may be found in newborns because they have less effective heat-control mechanisms. Elevated temperatures among infants, children, and adolescents are often related to viral or bacterial infections, dehydration, and environmental exposure to heat. Low body temperature is most commonly associated with environmental exposure.

Heart and Respiratory Rates

Procedure and Techniques. Heart and respiratory rates are assessed for the same qualities as in the adult. This assessment should take place when the infant is quiet. If the infant is quiet at the beginning of the assessment, the nurse listens to the apical pulse for a full minute and counts the respirations before proceeding to other parts of the assessment.

Respiratory rates are counted using the same procedure as for adults; however, infants usually breathe diaphragmatically, which requires observation of abdominal movement. Respirations are counted for a full minute because an infant's respiratory rate may be irregular as a normal variation.

Expected and Abnormal Findings. Expected heart, respiratory rate, and blood pressure for infants and children are listed in Table 4-1. Elevations in heart rate are most commonly seen with crying, fever, respiratory distress, and dehydration. Elevations in respiratory rate may be associated with crying, fever, or respiratory distress.

Blood Pressure

Blood pressure measurement should occur with every health visit for all children over the age of 3.[6] For an accurate blood pressure reading, the appropriate cuff size must be used (see Chapter 4). Measurements may be taken in the arm or leg of infants and younger children. Blood pressure standards for children ages 1 through 17 are based on gender, age, and height. Blood pressure tables that include both systolic and diastolic blood pressures according to blood pressure percentiles are available on the National Heart Lung and Blood Institute website (www.nhlbi.nih.gov/guidelines/hypertension/). Although not common, hypertension can develop in childhood and adolescence; thus the differentiation of two terms, prehypertension and hypertension, is worth noting. *Hypertension* in children is defined as average systolic blood pressure (SBP) and/or diastolic blood pressure (DBP) that is greater than or equal to the 95th percentile for gender, age, and height on three or more occasions. Any child whose SBP or DBP is 5 mm above the 99th percentile and is symptomatic (chest pain, shortness of breath, palpitations) needs immediate referral. *Prehypertension* in children is defined as average SBP or DBP levels that are greater than or equal to the 90th percentile but less than the 95th percentile on three or more occasions. As with adults, adolescents with blood pressure levels between 120/80 and 130/90 should be considered prehypertensive[6] (Box 19-5).

Height and Weight

Routine height and weight measurements are taken on all visits until the end of the growth spurt between ages of 18 and 20. The height or recumbent length for infants is recorded in inches or centimeters; the weight is measured in pounds and ounces, or kilograms. Height and weight are plotted on a growth chart and allow the nurse to track the child's growth in comparison with the population standard. Growth charts for infants through adolescence are available on the Centers for Disease Control and Prevention website (www.cdc.gov). A BMI should be calculated on all children beginning at age 2 and recorded as BMI percentile for age.

Height

Procedure and Techniques. Recumbent length of newborns and infants is measured from the top of the head to the heel with the infant in a supine position (Fig. 19-5). The length is recorded in inches or centimeters.

Devices such as measuring mats and boards can be used to measure recumbent length. An infant measuring mat consists of a soft rubber graduated mat attached to a plastic footboard. The infant lies on the mat with the head against the headboard. The infant's knees are held together and pressed gently against the mat with one hand while the footboard is moved against the heels. A measuring board has a

rigid headboard and a movable footboard. It is placed on a table, and the infant lies on the board so the head touches the headboard. The footboard is then moved until it touches the bottom of the infant's feet.

To measure the height of a child who can stand but is too short for the adult scale, the nurse uses a platform with a movable headboard. The child stands erect on the platform, and the headboard is lowered until it touches the child's head (Fig. 19-6, *A* and *B*). A tape measure also can be attached to a wall so the child's height can be measured by having the child stand against the wall.

Weight

Procedure and Techniques. The platform scale is used for weighing newborns, infants, and small children (Fig. 19-7).

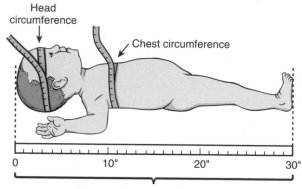

FIG. 19-5 Measurement of head and chest circumference and recumbent length. (Redrawn from Hockenberry et al., 2003.)

BOX 19-5 CLINICAL NOTE

The National Institute of Health recommends that blood pressure be measured in children from age 3 through adolescence as part of routine health care visits.[6]

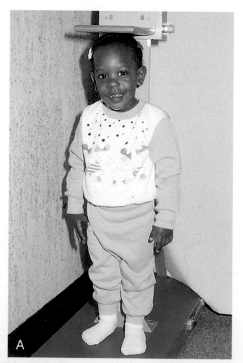

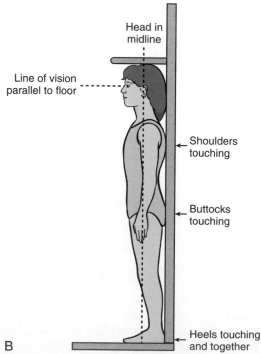

FIG. 19-6 A, Measure the height of a child using a platform with movable headboard. **B,** Side view showing correct posture for accurate measurement. (**A** from Seidel et al., 2011.)

The scale has curved sides to prevent the infant from rolling off. A paper is placed on the scale, and the unclothed newborn is laid on the paper. The newborn is weighed by balancing the scale. The weight is recorded to the nearest 0.5 oz.

Expected and Abnormal Findings. Healthy newborns typically weigh between 5 lb 8 oz and 8 lb 13 oz (2500 and 4000 g). Newborns may lose up to 10% of their birth weight in the first few days of life but regain it in 10 to 14 days. In general they double their birth weight by 4 to 6 months of age and triple it by 12 months of age.

EXAMINATION OF NEWBORNS AND INFANTS

The nurse should undress the infant completely for examination, keeping the diaper in place until the buttocks and genitalia are examined. Care must be taken to ensure that the infant remains warm during the examination period. Keep the room warm and cover areas not being examined to prevent excessive chilling. If the infant becomes chilled, the skin, hands, and feet may take on transient mottling (blotching or marbling) appearance.

Unlike the physical examination in adults, which for the most part proceeds in a head-to-toe sequence, the physical examination of an infant requires that the nurse conduct the least invasive portions of the examination before proceeding to the more invasive components. The nurse should observe the infant for any signs of distress and then proceed to auscultating heart and lungs, saving the ear and oral examination (more invasive procedures) for last. If the infant starts to cry, take time to comfort him or her because the examination of an infant who is crying can be very difficult.

In general the nurse should conduct the physical examination of young infants (<6 months) on an examination table. For the older infant (>6 months) and toddler, the nurse may find that having the caregiver hold the baby or toddler decreases fear and distress, thus making it easier for the nurse to conduct the examination.

Skin, Hair, and Nails

No special procedures or techniques are necessary when inspecting or palpating the skin, hair, and nails other than keeping the young infant warm during the examination.

Skin

Expected Findings. The skin color in the neonate depends partially on the amount of fat present. Preterm infants generally appear redder because they have less subcutaneous fat than full-term infants. In addition, the neonate may appear to have a red skin tone for a short period because of vasomotor instability. This color tends to fade within the first few days. In addition, immediately following birth the neonate's lips, nail beds, and feet may be dusky or appear cyanotic. Once the newborn is adequately warmed, the dusky color should fade, and a well-oxygenated pink tone should reappear. Dark-skinned newborns should also have a dark pink tone, which is most evident on the palms of the hands and the soles of the feet. Physiologic jaundice may be present in the newborn between the second and fifth day of life. The skin, mucous membranes, and sclerae may appear to have a yellow tone. This normal phenomenon occurs in almost half of all newborns and is secondary to the increased number of red blood cells that hemolyze following birth.[7]

Common primary skin lesions among newborns that are normal variations include the following:

- *Milia:* Small, whitish papules that may be found on the cheeks, nose, chin, and forehead of newborns (Fig. 19-8). These are benign and generally disappear by the third week of life.
- *Erythema toxicum:* A common rash among newborns (Fig. 19-9). It is a self-limited, benign rash of unknown etiology consisting of erythematous macules, papules, and pustules. The rash may appear anywhere on the body except the palms of the hands and the soles of the foot. Although it may be present at birth, it usually appears by the third or fourth day of life.

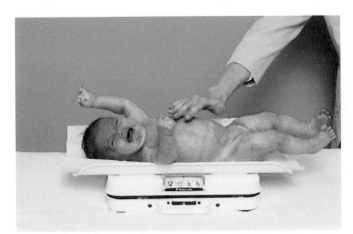

FIG. 19-7 Weighing an infant on an infant scale. (From Hockenberry and Wilson, 2011.)

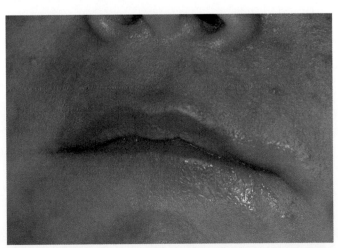

FIG. 19-8 Milia on the face of infant. (Courtesy Lemmi and Lemmi, 2013.)

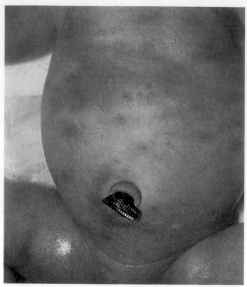

FIG. 19-9 Erythema toxicum on the trunk of an infant. (From Cohen, 1993.)

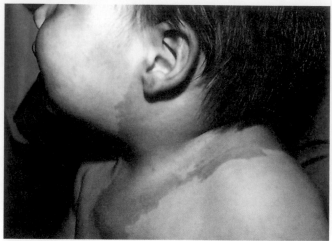

FIG. 19-11 Café-au-lait spot. (From Weston, Lane, and Morelli, 2002.)

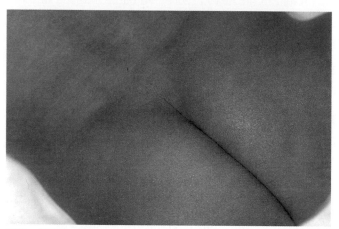

FIG. 19-10 Congenital dermal melanocytosis (mongolian spot). (From Lemmi, 2000.)

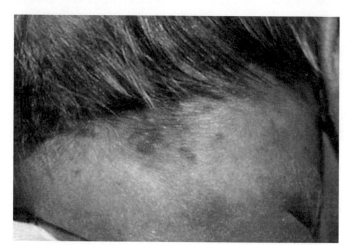

FIG. 19-12 Stork bite. (From Weston, Lane, and Morelli, 1996.)

Birthmarks in newborns may be pigmentation or vascular variations. Common birthmarks that are considered normal variations include:

- *Congenital dermal melanocytosis (mongolian spot):* An irregularly shaped, darkened flat area over the sacrum and buttocks (Fig. 19-10). They are most prevalent in African American, Hispanic, Native American, and Asian children and generally disappear by the time the child is 1 or 2 years of age.
- *Café-au-lait spot:* A large round or oval patch of light brown pigmentation that is generally present at birth (Fig. 19-11). Occasionally these spots may be associated with neurofibromatosis (a genetic disorder associated with tumor growth within the nervous system).
- *Stork bite (telangiectasis or flat capillary hemangioma):* This common vascular birthmark appears as a small red or pink spot that is often seen on the back of the neck or eyelids (Fig. 19-12). Stork bites usually disappear by 5 years of age.

Abnormal Findings. Some birthmarks considered abnormal include the following:

- *Port-wine stains (nevus flammeus):* Large, flat, bluish-purple capillary areas (Fig. 19-13, *A*). They are most frequently found on the face along distribution of the fifth cranial nerve. They do not disappear spontaneously.
- *Strawberry hemangioma:* Slightly raised, reddened areas with a sharp demarcation line (see Fig. 19-13, *B*). They may be 2 to 3 cm in diameter and usually disappear by 5 years of age.
- *Cavernous hemangioma:* Reddish-blue round mass of blood vessels (Fig. 19-14). They may continue to grow until the child reaches 10 to 15 months of age. They should be assessed frequently.

Hair and Nails

Expected Findings. Scalp hair on the newborn is generally fine and soft. Seborrheic dermatitis (cradle cap) is a scaly crust that may appear on the scalp of infants (Fig. 19-15). The newborn's skin may be covered with fine, soft, immature hair called *lanugo hair* (Fig. 19-16). It may be found anywhere on

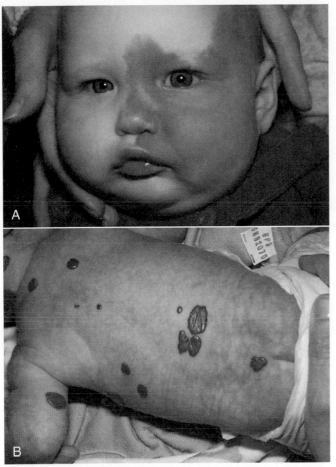

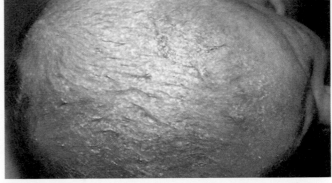

FIG. 19-15 Seborrheic dermatitis (cradle cap). (From Cohen, 1993.)

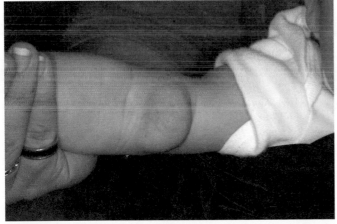

FIG. 19-13 **A**, Port-wine stain. **B**, Strawberry hemangioma. (From Zitelli, McIntire, and Nowalk, 2012.)

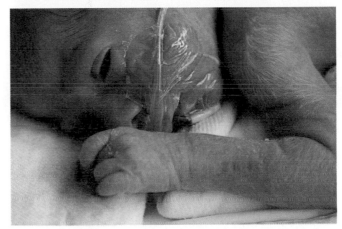

FIG. 19-16 Lanugo (silky body hair) in premature infant. (Courtesy Lemmi and Lemmi, 2013.)

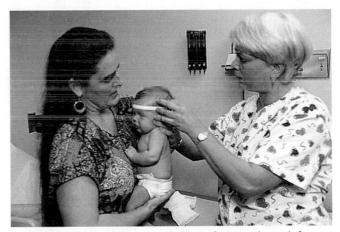

FIG. 19-14 Cavernous hemangioma. (From Rakel and Bope, 2004. Courtesy Richard P. Usatine.)

FIG. 19-17 Measuring head circumference in an infant.

the body but is most common on the scalp, ears, shoulders, and back. Postterm infants may have long fingernails at birth.

Head, Eyes, Ears, Nose, and Throat
Head

Procedure and Techniques. Inspect and palpate the infant's head. Palpate the anterior and posterior fontanelles

for fullness while the infant is in an upright position and calm. (If the infant is lying down or crying, a false fullness may be felt.) Head circumference should be measured at every well-baby visit through age 2. Head circumference is plotted on a growth chart as previously described for height and weight. To measure head circumference, a measuring tape is wrapped snugly around the infant's head at the largest circumference, usually just above the eyebrows, the pinna of the ears, and the occipital prominence at the back of the skull (Fig. 19-17). The tape measure is read to the nearest 0.5 cm. Head circumference is measured at least twice to check for accuracy; if the measurements differ, measure a third time.

Expected Findings. The neonate's head may be asymmetric as a result of *molding*, in which the cranial bones override each other. Molding may result when the head passes through the birth canal; this generally lasts less than a week. Another common finding in newborns is a cephalhematoma. This is a subperiosteal hematoma under the scalp that occurs secondary to birth trauma. The area, which appears as a soft, well-defined swelling over the cranial bone, generally is resorbed within the first month of life. The hematoma does not cross suture lines. The fontanelles should have a slight depression, should feel soft, and may have a slight pulsation. The anterior fontanelle in infants less than 6 months of age should not exceed 4 to 5 cm. It should get progressively smaller as the infant gets older and should be completely closed by 18 months of age. The infant's posterior fontanelle may or may not be palpable at birth. If it is palpable, it should measure no more than 1 cm, and it should close by 2 months of age. The infant should be able to turn his or her head from side to side by 2 weeks of age. Expected head circumference for term newborns averages from 33 to 36 cm and should be about 2 to 3 cm larger than chest circumference. By 4 months most infants demonstrate head control by holding the head erect and midline when in an upright position. By 2 years of age the child's head circumference is two thirds its adult size,

and the chest circumference should exceed the head circumference (Table 19-2 and Box 19-6).

Abnormal Findings. Marked asymmetry of the head is usually abnormal and may indicate craniosynostosis, a premature ossification of one or more of the cranial sutures. This condition occurs in 1 in 2500 live births; most cases involve male infants.[8] A deeply depressed fontanelle may indicate dehydration; a bulging fontanelle may indicate increased intracranial pressure. A head circumference that is increasing rapidly suggests increased intracranial pressure. A head circumference below the fifth percentile suggests microcephaly.

⊕ ETHNIC, CULTURAL, AND SPIRITUAL VARIATIONS

Infant Care

Native American and Alaskan Native infants may be secured to traditional cradle boards from birth, which may cause a cosmetic flattening of the posterior skull.

Eyes

Procedure and Techniques. Newborns may have edema of the eyelids, either from the trauma of birth or in response to prophylactic eyedrops or ointments. The edema may delay the examination for a few days. To begin the assessment, hold or rock the infant into an upright position to elicit eye opening. An alternative strategy is to hold the infant supine with the head gently lowered.

Observe if the eyes are small or of different sizes. Inspect the eyelids for edema, epicanthal folds, and position. Note the alignment and slant of the palpebral fissures. Draw an imaginary line through the corners of the eyes (from the medial to the outer canthi). Observe the space between the eyes for wide-spaced eyes. Inspect the sclera for color. Also test for pupillary reaction at this time. Using the ophthalmoscope, assess light reflex; also attempt to visualize the red reflex in each eye.

Expected Findings. Normal findings of the eye examination of an infant reveal eyes that are usually closed; often no eyebrows are present. The eyes are symmetric, and eyelashes may be long. Eyelids may have edema. The palpebral fissures lie horizontally (Fig. 19-18); in Asians an upward slant is normal. Infant sclerae may have a blue tinge caused by thinness; otherwise they are white. Tiny black dots (pigmentation) or a slight yellow cast may appear near the limbus of dark-skinned infants. Palpebral conjunctivae are pink and intact without discharge. There are no tears until about 2 to 3 months of age.

Infants should fix on and follow an object no later than 2 months age. The blink reflex also is present in normal newborns and infants. Pupils should constrict in response to bright light and are round, about 2 to 4 mm in diameter, and equal in size. A bilateral red reflex should be noted, which is a bright, round, red-orange glow seen through the pupil. It may be pale in dark-skinned newborns. Presence of the red

TABLE 19-2   AVERAGE CHEST AND HEAD CIRCUMFERENCE OF U.S. CHILDREN

AGE	CHEST CIRCUMFERENCE (CM)	HEAD CIRCUMFERENCE (CM)	
		MALES	FEMALES
Birth	35	35.3	34.7
3 mo	40	40.9	40.0
6 mo	44	43.9	42.8
12 mo	47	47.3	45.8
18 mo	48	48.7	47.1
2 yr	50	49.7	48.1
3 yr	52	50.4	49.3

Data from Lowrey GH: *Growth and development of children*, ed 8, Chicago, 1986, Mosby; and Waring WW, Jeansonne LO: *Practical manual of pediatrics*, ed 2, St Louis, 1982, Mosby.

BOX 19-6   HEAD CIRCUMFERENCE GROWTH RATES

- Full-term newborn to 3 months: 2 cm/month
- 3 to 6 months: 1 cm/month
- 6 months to 1 year: 0.5 cm/month

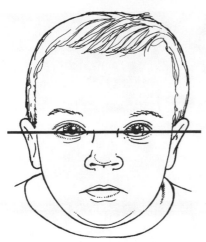

FIG. 19-18 Alignment of the outer canthus with the pinna of the ear is a normal finding. (From Seidel et al., 2011.)

reflex rules out most serious defects of the cornea, aqueous chamber, lens, and vitreous chamber.[7]

Specific age-related responses may be observed that indicate the infant's attention to visual stimuli.

- Birth to 2 weeks: Eyes do not reopen after exposure to bright light; there is increasing alertness to objects; the infant is capable of fixating on objects.
- Age 1 month: The infant can fixate on and follow a bright toy or light.
- Ages 3 to 4 months: The infant can fixate on, follow, and reach for a toy because binocular vision is normally achieved at this age.
- Ages 6 to 12 months: The infant is capable of fixating on and following a toy in all directions.

Corneal light reflex should be symmetric. Transient strabismus is common during the first few months of life because of lack of binocular vision. However, if it continues beyond 6 months of age, a referral to an ophthalmologist is needed because early recognition and treatment can restore binocular vision. Asian and Native American infants often have *pseudostrabismus*, the false appearance of strabismus caused by the flattened nasal bridge or epicanthal fold. Pseudostrabismus disappears at approximately 12 months of age.

Abnormal Findings. Abnormal findings may include a pronounced lateral upward slant of the eyes with an inner epicanthal fold, which may indicate Down syndrome; asymmetry of eyes; wide-set eyes (hypertelorism); or eyes that are close together (hypotelorism). Note any discoloration of the sclerae such as dark blue sclerae or any dilated blood vessels. Hyperbilirubinemia may cause jaundiced (yellow) sclerae in newborns. Asymmetric corneal light reflex may indicate abnormality of eye muscles.

Excessive tearing before the third month or no tearing by the second month is a deviation from normal. A purulent discharge from the eyes shortly after birth is abnormal. It may indicate ophthalmia neonatorum and should be reported. Redness, lesions, nodules, discharge, or crusting of the conjunctiva is abnormal. Birth trauma may cause conjunctival hemorrhage. If the pupillary response is not present after

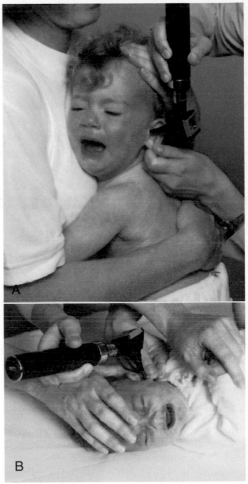

FIG. 19-19 Immobilization of young child or infant during otoscopic examination. Note that lower portion of pinna of ear is pulled down and slightly backward. **A,** Prone position. **B,** Supine position. (From Hockenberry and Wilson, 2011.)

3 weeks, the infant may be blind. A dilated, fixed, or constricted pupil may indicate anoxia or brain damage. Absence of the red reflex (white pupil) may indicate the presence of retinal hemorrhage; congenital cataracts; or retinoblastoma, a relatively rare congenital malignant tumor arising from the retina.[7]

Ears

Procedures and Techniques. Examine the infant's external ears as previously described for the adult. To examine the auditory canal and TM, the nurse must restrain the infant securely. Because the nurse must have both hands free to hold the ear and maneuver the otoscope, another individual must act as a "holder." The infant can be placed in either a prone or supine position. Instruct the holder to secure the infant's arms down at the sides with one hand and turn and hold the infant's head to one side with the other hand (Fig. 19-19). To optimize visualization of the ear canal and TM, the nurse must alter the method of holding the auricle of the ear. Grasp the lower portion of the pinna and apply gentle traction down and slightly backward (as opposed to pulling the pinna up and back for the adult). This maneuver straightens the ear canal.

Hearing screening is recommended for all newborns.[9] Two common hearing screening tools used in many newborn nurseries are the Auditory Brainstem Response (ABR) test and the Otoacoustic Emissions (OAE) test. The ABR and OAE tests do not actually test hearing but rather assess the structural integrity of the auditory pathway. For this reason hearing cannot be definitively considered normal until the child is old enough to perform an audiogram. In settings where special tools for screening are unavailable, a simple hearing screening can be performed and should also be included with an infant examination. This is easily done by eliciting a loud noise (e.g., clapping hands or ringing bell) and observing for a response from the infant such as sudden body movement, startle response, or crying.

Expected Findings. The ears should be symmetrically shaped and positioned. The top of the pinna of the ear should align directly with the outer canthus of the eye and be angled no more than 10 degrees from a vertical position.

The TM of the infant may be difficult to visualize because it is more horizontal than in older children and adults. It may appear slightly reddened secondary to crying. In addition, because the TM does not become conical for several months, the light reflex may appear diffuse. By age 6 months the infant's TM takes on an adult type of appearance and is easier to visualize and examine.

Hearing behaviors should be readily observed. By ages 4 to 6 months the infant should turn the head toward the source of a sound and respond to the parent's voice or other sounds. By 6 to 10 months the child should respond to his or her name and follow sounds.

Abnormal Findings. Low-set ears or ears with angulation greater than 10 degrees may indicate a congenital problem such as Down syndrome. An unusually small or absent auricle is referred to as *microtia*, a congenital anomaly of the external ear (Fig. 19-20, *A* and *B*). Microtia is classified from less severe (grade I) to the absence of an ear—termed *anotia* (grade IV).

Nose and Mouth

Procedures and Techniques. The examination of the nose and mouth is straightforward; the problem arises when the infant is uncooperative or unable to hold still. The infant must be restrained carefully and securely by a parent or other adult who acts as a "holder" to ensure the infant's safety and permit the full viewing of the examination area. The infant is usually restrained in a supine position, with the arms extended securely above his or her head (Fig. 19-21). The holder is then able to secure both the infant's arms and head. A second holder or the nurse may need to immobilize the infant's lower extremities.

The infant's nose is small and difficult to examine. Do not attempt to insert a speculum into the nares. Inspect the inside of the nose by tilting the infant's head back and shining a light into the nares. If an infant has nasal congestion, suction the nares with a bulb syringe or small-lumen catheter.

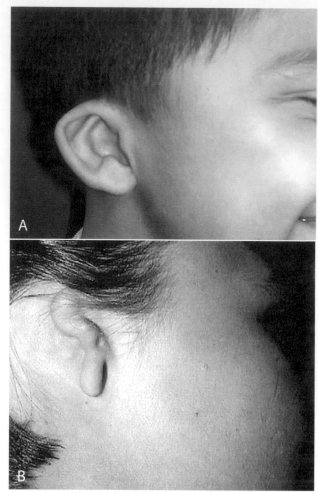

FIG. 19-20 Microtia. **A,** Grade I. **B,** Grade III. (From Bluestone et al., 2003.)

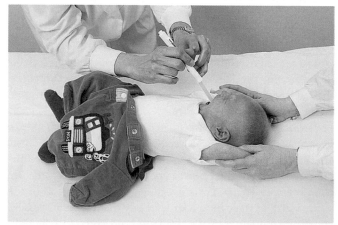

FIG. 19-21 Positioning of infant for examination of nose and mouth.

It is generally possible to examine the mouth while the infant is crying. Observe mucous membranes, posterior pharynx, tongue, gums, and any teeth. Palpate the buccal mucosa and gums using a gloved hand and light source. While a gloved finger is in the infant's mouth, check the strength of his or her suck and for an intact palate.

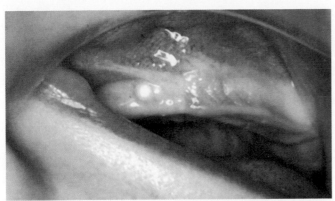

FIG. 19-22 Epstein's pearls (gingival cysts) in an infant. (From Scully and Welbury, 1994.)

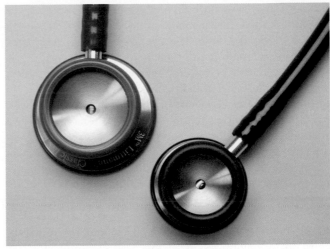

FIG. 19-23 The pediatric stethoscope has a smaller head compared to the adult stethoscope.

Expected Findings. Normally the base of the nose is appropriate to the size of the face. Milia may be present on the infant's nose. The infant's nares have only minimal movement with breathing. The buccal mucosa should appear pink, moist, and smooth. The infant's gums should appear smooth and full. Other normal findings may include the presence of small, white epithelial cells on the palate or gums. These are called *Bohn's nodules* or *Epstein's pearls* (Fig. 19-22). The infant's tongue should be appropriate to the size of the mouth and fit well into the floor of the mouth. The palate should be intact. The infant should have a strong suck with the tongue pushing upward against the nurse's finger.

Abnormal Findings. Abnormal findings include nasal flaring, which is a hallmark of respiratory distress.[7] Because infants are obligatory nose breathers, any obstruction of the nares secondary to a congenital abnormality such as choanal atresia (occlusion between pharynx and nose), foreign body, or nasal secretions causes the infant to be irritable or distressed. If whitish patches are seen along the oral mucosa, scrape the area with a tongue blade to differentiate between milk deposits and a lesion. Milk deposits can be scraped off easily; candidiasis lesions also scrape off but leave a red area that may bleed. Occasionally a natal loose tooth may be found. These teeth should be removed to prevent possible aspiration.

Neck

Procedures and Techniques. To examine the neck start with the infant in the supine position and pull his or her arms to lift the shoulders off the examining table. Permit the infant's head to lag back and inspect the neck for a midline trachea, abnormal skinfolds, and generalized neck enlargement. Return the infant to the supine position and palpate the neck for tone, presence of masses, and enlarged lymph nodes. The thyroid is not typically examined in the newborn.

Expected and Abnormal Findings. Normally the newborn's cervical and inguinal lymph nodes are not palpable. Significant head lag after 6 months of age is an abnormal finding requiring further evaluation.[7] If the infant's neck is proportionately short or has webbing (loose, fanlike skinfolds), he or she should be evaluated for congenital

abnormalities such as Down syndrome or Turner's syndrome. If an enlargement of the infant's anterior neck is palpated, the infant should be referred to a primary care provider for further evaluation.

Lungs and Respiratory System

Procedures and Techniques. Assessing the respiratory status of a newborn or infant usually follows the same sequence as for an adult. If possible, conduct the examination while the infant is calm because examination of a crying infant is difficult. Inspect the infant's chest to observe respiratory effort. Auscultation of the infant's breath sounds is performed in the same manner as for the older child and adult; however, the nurse should use a pediatric stethoscope with a small diaphragm (Fig. 19-23). An adult-size stethoscope diaphragm head covers at least half of the infant's chest and is inappropriate for an accurate assessment of the infant's respiratory status. Percussion and palpation are not routinely performed during infant assessment.

Chest circumference is not measured routinely unless an abnormal head or chest size is suspected. The chest circumference is measured at the nipples, pulling the tape measure firmly without causing an indentation in the skin. The measurement is noted between inspiration and expiration and recorded to the nearest $\frac{1}{8}$ inch (0.5 cm) (see Fig. 19-5). Chest circumference is plotted on a growth chart as previously described for height and weight.

Expected Findings. Inspection of the infant's thoracic cage should show a smooth, rounded, and symmetric appearance. Harrison's groove, a normal anatomic deviation, is a horizontal groove in the rib cage at the level of the diaphragm. It extends from the sternum to the midaxillary line. Unlike the adult, the infant has a round thorax with an equal anteroposterior and lateral diameter. The average chest circumference ranges from 30 to 36 cm. This measurement should be approximately 2 to 3 cm smaller than the child's head circumference. Infants are obligate nose breathers until about age 3 months. Should their nasal passages become occluded, they may have difficulty breathing. Sneezing is a common finding for an infant and is therapeutic because it helps to clear the nose. However, coughing is considered abnormal and indicates a problem.

The respiratory pattern in the newborn may be irregular, with brief pauses between breaths of no more than 10 to 15 seconds. The respiratory rate in the newborn ranges from 30 to 60 breaths/min (see Table 4-1). The infant has a thin chest wall, which makes breath sounds difficult to localize with auscultation. They are commonly transmitted from one auscultatory area to another. Because of this, the predominant breath sound heard in the peripheral lung fields is bronchovesicular. The thin chest wall also makes the newborn's xiphoid process more prominent than that of an older child or adult. At birth the infant's chest circumference may be equal to or slightly less than the head circumference (see Table 19-2).

Abnormal Findings. Several respiratory findings indicate that an infant is in respiratory distress. These include stridor, grunting, sternal or supraclavicular retractions, and nasal flaring. Any one of these findings warrants immediate medical attention because infants tire and become hypoxic quickly. Stridor is a high-pitched sound that is primarily heard in a distressed infant during inspiration. It occurs secondary to upper airway obstruction. The obstruction may cause the infant's inspiratory cycle to be three or four times longer than expiration. Respiratory grunting is a mechanism by which the infant tries to prolong expiration to maintain adequate alveolar inflation. Sternal and supraclavicular retractions and nasal flaring are indications of respiratory distress. Clinically this may be observed as "see-saw" type of breathing with alternating movements of the chest and abdomen. If any of these are observed, the infant is working very hard to try to maintain adequate breathing and should be referred to a primary care provider.

Heart and Peripheral Vascular System

Procedures and Techniques. Assessing the cardiovascular system of a newborn or infant usually follows the same sequence as for an adult. The apical pulse of the newborn normally is felt in the fourth or fifth intercostal space (ICS) just medial to the midclavicular line. Examine the heart within the first 24 hours of birth and again at 2 to 3 days to assess changes from fetal to systemic and pulmonic circulation. The heart must be auscultated when the infant is quiet. The stethoscope used must have a small diaphragm and bell to detect specific cardiac sounds of the newborn or infant. Palpate the femoral and brachial pulses and assess capillary refill.

Expected Findings. Normally the heart rate of infants is faster when they are awake and slower when they are asleep. Sinus dysrhythmia is an expected finding when the heart rate increases during inspiration and decreases during expiration. Murmurs are common in infants up to 48 hours after birth. Capillary refill in infants is very rapid (i.e., less than 1 second after the first day of life). Acrocyanosis (cyanosis of hands and feet) in the newborn without central cyanosis is

of little concern and usually disappears within hours to days of birth.

Abnormal Findings. Abnormal findings include changes in the skin and cardiovascular system. Central cyanosis may indicate congenital heart defects. Note if cyanosis increases with crying or sucking. Severe cyanosis that appears shortly after birth may indicate transposition of the great vessels, tetralogy of Fallot, a severe septal defect, or severe pulmonic stenosis. Cyanosis that appears after the first month of life suggests pulmonic stenosis, tetralogy of Fallot, or large septal defects. Murmurs that persist after 3 days or radiate must be referred for further evaluation. A pneumothorax shifts the apical impulse away from the area of the chest where the pneumothorax is located. The infant's heart may be shifted to the right by a diaphragmatic hernia commonly found on the left. Dextrocardia (location of the heart in the right hemithorax) causes the apical pulse to shift toward the right side. Weak or thin peripheral pulses may be associated with decreased cardiac output or peripheral vasoconstriction. Bounding pulses may indicate a patent ductus arteriosus creating a left-to-right shunt. Coarctation of the heart is suspected when the femoral pulses are absent or there is a difference in pulse amplitude between upper and lower extremities.

Abdomen and Gastrointestinal System

Procedures and Techniques. The abdominal examination is straightforward, with the infant lying supine on an examining table. Follow the same procedures for examining the abdomen as for adults.

Expected Findings. Inspecting the abdomen of a healthy infant finds a symmetric, soft, and round abdomen with no masses present. There is synchronous abdominal and chest movement with breathing. Diastasis rectus (a gap between the rectus muscles) may be noted during crying. Visible pulsations in the epigastric areas are common. Note any distention, masses, and concave, sunken, or flat appearance. A scaphoid, shaped abdomen suggests diaphragmatic hernia.

Inspect the umbilicus in the newborn. Immediately after the umbilical cord is cut, two arteries and one vein should be noted. After the cord is clamped, it changes from white to black as it dries; it should dry in 5 days and fall off spontaneously in 7 to 14 days. The abdomen of a newborn should be soft and nondistended on palpation. The edge of the infant's liver may be up to 1 to 2 cm below the right rib cage (costal margin). The spleen is generally not palpable, although the tip may be felt in the left upper quadrant (far left costal margin). Both kidneys may be noted with deep palpation, especially in newborns.

Abnormal Findings. Abnormal findings include discharge, odor, or redness around the umbilicus; a protrusion or nodular appearance of the umbilicus; thick Wharton's jelly; and a thin or green cord. Absence of bowel sounds may indicate a bowel obstruction. An enlarged liver 3 cm or more below the margin, palpable spleen, masses near the kidneys, and enlarged kidneys are considered abnormal findings.

Musculoskeletal System

Procedures and Techniques. Examine the infant undressed and lying supine. Palpate clavicles for evidence of fractures. Extend both arms and legs to compare muscle tone and length. Inspect the back and spine for alignment, tufts of hair, or bulges. Assess hip stability by performing the Barlow and Ortolani maneuvers. These maneuvers can be performed up until 3 months of age. With the infant supine, the nurse flexes the infant's knees, holding his or her thumbs on the inner midthighs and fingers outside on the hips touching the greater trochanters. Adduct the legs, exerting downward pressure (Barlow's maneuver) (Fig. 19-24, *A*). Then abduct, moving the knees apart and down toward the table and applying upward pressure with the fingers on the greater trochanter (Ortolani maneuver) (see Fig. 19-24, *B*). Allis' sign is another assessment of hip location. With the infant supine, flex the knees with the feet flat on the table and align the femurs. Observe the height of the knees. Assess the feet for shape and position. Observe the lateral and medial borders of the foot. If the borders are not straight, assess flexibility of the forefoot by gently moving it to a neutral position.

Expected Findings. Expected findings include stable and smooth clavicles without crepitus. Arms and legs should have spontaneous, equal movement and be of equal length. The feet should be flexible and not fixed. Note the relationship of the forefoot to the hindfoot. The hindfoot aligns with the lower leg, and the forefoot may turn inward slightly. The Barlow and Ortolani maneuvers should feel smooth and produce no clicks. When both knees are the same height, an Allis' test is negative. The spine should be flexible and straight without abnormal curvatures.

Abnormal Findings. Abnormal findings include limited shoulder range of motion and deformity if the clavicle is fractured. Erb's palsy (paralysis of shoulder and upper arm muscles) may be noted. Asymmetry of extremities, limited movement, syndactyly (fused digits), and polydactyly (extra digits) are also abnormal findings. Metatarsus adductus (an inward curve of the forefoot) or talipes equinovarus (clubfoot) may be noted. Hip dislocation may be identified by three procedures. A positive Barlow or Ortolani sign is reported when any click occurs with these maneuvers. When one knee is lower than the other, the Allis' sign is positive (Fig. 19-25). Uneven skinfolds are another sign that suggests hip dislocation (Fig. 19-26). Any asymmetric spinal curve, masses (hair tufts, dimples), and abnormal posture may indicate underlying spinal or vertebral malformations.

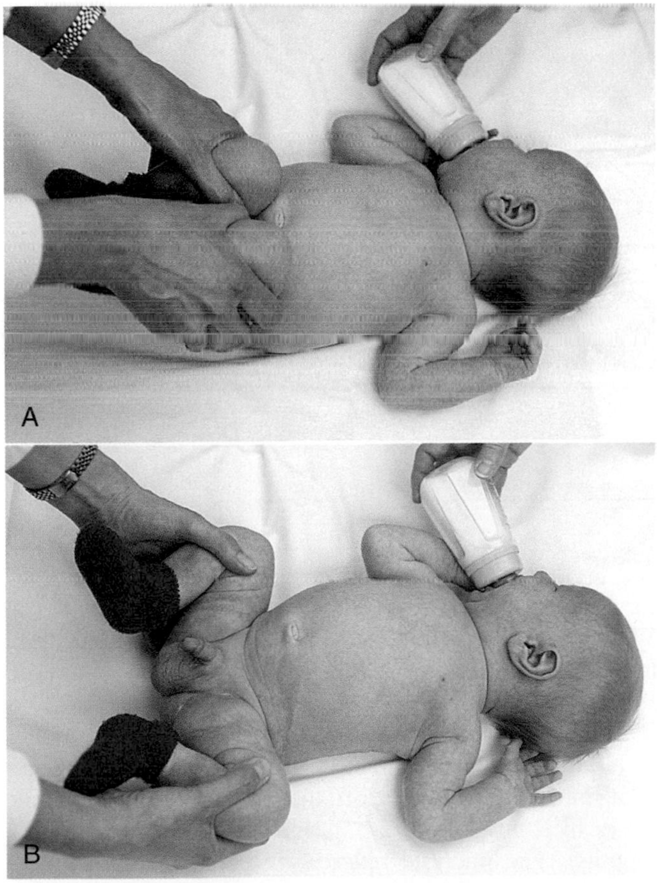

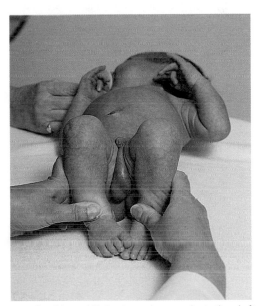

FIG. 19-25 Positive Allis' sign shows that the left leg is shorter than the right leg, indicating left hip dysplasia. (From Seidel et al., 2011.)

FIG. 19-24 Barlow and Ortolani maneuvers to detect hip dislocation. **A,** Phase I, adduction. **B,** Phase II, abduction. This is a negative finding because no dislocation is found.

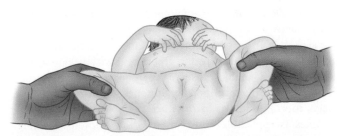

FIG. 19-26 Sign of hip dislocation: the three skinfolds on the left upper leg and limited abduction indicate left hip dysplasia. (Seidel et al., 2011.)

TABLE 19-3 INFANTILE REFLEXES

REFLEX	TECHNIQUE FOR EVALUATION	APPEARANCE AGE	DISAPPEARANCE AGE	NORMAL RESPONSE
Reflexes to Evaluate Position and Movement				
Moro's	Startle infant by making loud noise, jarring examination surface, or slightly raising infant off examination surface and letting him or her fall quickly back onto examining table	Birth	1 to 4 months	Infant abducts and extends arms and legs; index finger and thumb assume C position; then infant pulls both arms and legs up against trunk as if trying to protect self
Palmar grasp	Touch object against ulnar side of infant's hand; then place finger in palm of hand	Birth	3 to 4 months	Infant grasps finger; grasp should be tight, and nurse may be able to pull infant into sitting position by infant's grasp
Tonic neck	Infant supine; rotate head to side so chin is over shoulder	Birth to 6 weeks	4 to 6 months	Arm and leg extend on side to which head turns; opposite arm and leg flex; infant assumes fencing position (some normal infants may never show this reflex)
Plantar grasp	Touch object to sole of infant's foot	Birth	8 to 10 months	Toes flex tightly downward in attempt to grasp

Neurologic System

Procedures and Techniques. Observe spontaneous motor activity for symmetry. Palpate the infant's fontanelles for size and contour. Measure the infant's head circumference using a soft tape measure and compare it with previous measurements if available. Observe the infant's response to touch and pressure. Determine the presence of the Moro, tonic neck, rooting, sucking, palmar grasp, Babinski's, and plantar reflexes as applicable. Initial reflexes that should be evident in the newborn are shown in Table 19-3. Cranial nerves (CNs) are assessed by observing eye movements and blinking (CNs III, IV, and VI), sucking (CN V), wrinkling of the forehead (CN VII), turning the head toward a sound (CN VIII), and swallowing (CN IX). With the infant supine, pull to a sitting position holding the wrists; observe head control. Evaluate resting posture for muscle tone.

Expected Findings. Expected development of the infant by month is outlined in Table 18-3. Expected findings begin with fontanelles that are soft and flat (posterior fontanelle closes by 2 months and anterior fontanelle closes by 18 months). The infantile reflexes are present but disappear during the first year as the infant's nervous system matures. Babinski's reflex is an exception; it disappears by 18 months. Some head lag normally is present up to 4 months of age.

TABLE 19-3 INFANTILE REFLEXES—cont'd

REFLEX	TECHNIQUE FOR EVALUATION	APPEARANCE AGE	DISAPPEARANCE AGE	NORMAL RESPONSE
Babinski's	Stroke lateral surface of infant's sole, using inverted J curve from sole to great toe (see Fig. 15-9, *F*).	Birth	18 months	Infant response: positive response showing fanning of toes
Step in place	Infant in upright position, feet flat on surface	Birth	3 months	Paces forward using alternating steps
Clonus	Dorsiflex foot; pinch sole of foot just under toes	Birth	4 months	May get clonus movement of foot (not always present)
Feeding Reflexes				
Rooting response (awake)	Brush infant's cheek near corner of mouth	Birth	3 to 4 months	Infant turns head in direction of stimulus and opens mouth slightly
Suckling	Touch infant's lips	Birth	10 to 12 months	Sucking motion follows with lips and tongue

Three-month-old infants raise the head and arch the back; this reflex persists until 18 months of age. Spontaneous movement should be smooth and symmetric. The infant's knees should unfold gradually after being flexed to the chest.

Abnormal Findings. Abnormal findings may include fontanelles that feel full and distended. This finding, together with head circumference greater than expected and lethargy, irritability, shrill cry, weakness, and "sunset eyes," may indicate hydrocephalus (see Fig. 19-56). Motor activity abnormalities indicating brain damage include hypotonia, as evidenced by poor head control and limp extremities; hypertonia; stiff legs; jittery arm movements; and hands tightly flexed. An arched back (opisthotonos) with a stiff neck and extension of extremities may indicate meningitis. Any asymmetric posture is also abnormal. Note any spasticity, which may be an early sign of cerebral palsy. If present, the legs quickly extend and adduct, possibly even in a scissoring pattern.

Breasts

Procedures and Techniques. The examination of the newborn's and infant's breasts generally requires inspection only. The infant's chest should be exposed.

Normal and Abnormal Findings. Neonates of both genders may have full, slightly enlarged breasts secondary to the mother's estrogen level before the infant was born (Fig.

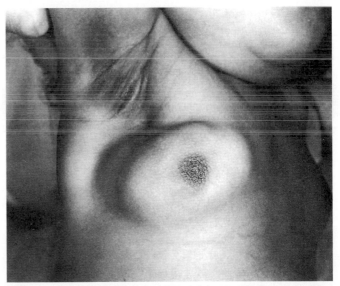

FIG. 19-27 Marked enlargement of breast bud in neonate. This is an exaggerated response to maternal hormones. (From Gallager et al., 1978.)

19-27). Maternal hormones are also responsible for the production of a small amount of watery or milky nipple discharge (referred to as *witch's milk*) during the first month of life in approximately 5% of neonates.[10] The nipples normally are located slightly lateral to the midclavicular line between

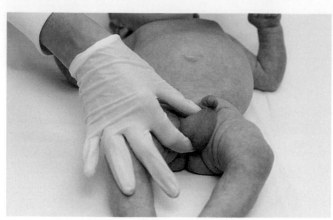

FIG. 19-28 Palpation of the scrotum in an infant.

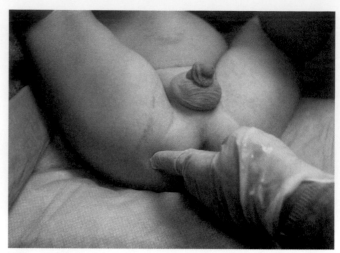

FIG. 19-29 Position for rectal examination of the infant. (From Seidel et al., 2011.)

the fourth and fifth ribs; the nipple should be flat and surrounded by a slightly darker pigmented areola.

Reproductive System and Perineum

Procedures and Techniques: Female Examination. During infancy the examination is limited to an evaluation of the external genitalia to determine if the structures are intact. The infant is placed on the examination table in frog-leg position (hips flexed with the soles of the feet together and up to the buttocks). Using gloved hands, place both thumbs on either side of the labia majora and gently push the tissue laterally while pushing the perineum down. This should permit visualization of the perineal area, the urethra, the clitoris, the hymen, and possibly the vaginal opening.

Expected Findings: Female Examination. Secondary to maternal hormones, the newborn's genitalia may appear somewhat engorged, with edematous labia majora and prominent and protruding labia minora. The clitoris also looks relatively enlarged, and the hymen may appear thick; the vaginal opening may be difficult to see. A mucoid, white vaginal discharge may be observed during the early period following birth but should disappear by 1 month. Vaginal discharges noted after the infant is 1 month old may occur secondary to diaper or powder irritation.

Procedures and Techniques: Male Examination. Inspect the penis and foreskin. If the infant is circumcised, the urinary meatus should be centered at the tip of the meatus. In uncircumcised males it may not be possible to visualize the meatus because of the tight foreskin. Do not attempt to retract the foreskin. Force may tear the prepuce from the glans, which in turn could cause binding adhesions to form between the prepuce and the glans.

Palpate the scrotum to determine presence of the testes (Fig. 19-28). If a mass other than a testicle or spermatic cord is palpated in the scrotum, transillumination is indicated to determine the presence of fluid (hydrocele) or mass (possible hernia) in the testicle.

Expected Findings: Male Examination. If the infant is uncircumcised, the foreskin (prepuce) should cover the glans.

The foreskin has little mobility. As the infant becomes older, the foreskin has more mobility. The foreskin should retract enough to permit unobstructed urinary stream; no general cleaning is necessary. The urinary meatus should be at the tip of the penis. If possible, observe the infant's urine stream. It should be full and strong. A weak stream with dribbling is an abnormal finding and may indicate stenosis of the urethral meatus. The full-term infant has a pendulous scrotum with deep rugae; the size of the scrotum usually appears large when compared with the penis. The scrotum appears pink in Caucasian infants and dark brown in dark-skinned infants. A testis should be palpable in each scrotum. If one or both testicles are not palpable, gently place a finger over the upper inguinal ring and gently push downward toward the scrotum. If the testicle can be pushed into the scrotum, it is considered descended even though it retracts into the inguinal canal. A hydrocele is a common finding in infants. A hydrocele transilluminates and usually becomes bigger as the child cries or becomes stressed. A mass such as a hernia will not transilluminate.

Perianal Examination

Procedures and Techniques. The external perianal examination is performed routinely with comprehensive assessment; however, an internal anal examination is not performed routinely. Generally the infant is placed on his or her back with the feet held in the nurse's hand and the infant's knees flexed upward toward the abdomen (Fig. 19-29). In the newborn inspect the perineum and anal region for presence of anus, lesions, and inflammation. Confirm anal contraction by lightly stroking the anal opening with a cotton-tipped applicator. Observe the lower back and buttocks for appearance and surface characteristics. If stool is present when the diaper is removed, note the characteristics, color, odor, and consistency.

Expected and Abnormal Findings. The perineal and perianal skin should be free of lesions or inflammation, although diaper rash is a common finding with infants. A patent

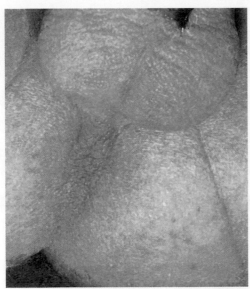

FIG. 19-30 Imperforate anus. (From Diagnostic picture tests in clinical medicine, 1984. By permission of Mosby International.)

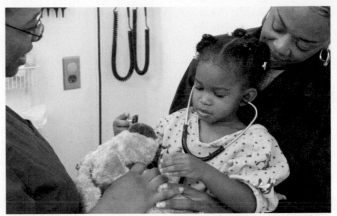

FIG. 19-31 Allow the child to touch examination equipment to reduce fear.

anus is the expected finding. Stroking the anus with the cotton-tipped applicator should produce an "anal wink" or contraction. The lower back and buttocks should be free of lesions. Normal variations include mongolian spots and birthmarks. Buttocks should be firm and rounded.

An imperforate anus is an abnormal finding that is assessed at birth (Fig. 19-30). Lack of anal contraction may indicate a lower spinal cord deformity. A tuft of hair or dimpling in the pilonidal (sacrococcygeal) area may indicate a lower spinal deformity or sinus tract.

EXAMINATION OF TODDLERS AND CHILDREN

If the young child is cooperative and does not appear to be fearful, the nurse can proceed with the physical examination in the same sequence as the adult examination, although examination of the ears and mouth are best left to the end of the examination in this age-group. Showing the equipment to the child, explaining the procedure, and allowing the child to use the equipment (e.g., a stethoscope) on a doll or teddy bear helps to enlist his or her cooperation (Fig. 19-31). Having the child blow bubbles or "blow out" the light of the otoscope or penlight before and during the examination may also help elicit his or her cooperation. This is particularly helpful when trying to auscultate lung sounds.

Skin, Hair, and Nails

No special procedures or techniques are necessary when examining the skin, hair, and nails other than keeping the young child warm during the examination.

Skin

Expected Findings. The skin should be smooth with consistent color and no lesions. As the child becomes mobile, bruising is common on the lower legs and perhaps even the face. When assessing skin turgor, the skin should move easily when lifted and return to place immediately when released.

Abnormal Findings. The most common abnormal lesions found in the young child are associated with communicable diseases and bacterial infections such as roseola, fifth's disease, tinea corporis (ringworm), impetigo, pediculosis corporis (body lice), and scabies. Less commonly, infants and children who are not fully immunized may present with varicella (chickenpox), rubella, and rubeola. Evidence of bruising that may be inconsistent with the child's developmental level or in an unusual area is cause for concern. Bruising in unusual areas (e.g., upper arms, back, buttocks, and abdomen) or multiple bruises found at different stages of healing should be investigated further to rule out abuse.[11] A child who is seriously dehydrated (more than 3% to 5% of body weight) has skin that appears "tented" after the abdominal skin is pinched.

Hair and Nails

Expected and Abnormal Findings. The young child should have very little body or facial hair. Nails should be intact and smooth. Common problems associated with the scalp and hair of the young child include alopecia, which may be secondary to hair pulling, twisting, or head rubbing; and lice, nits, and scabies. Nail biting is an abnormal behavior and finding. Evidence of cyanosis of the nail bed or nail clubbing requires careful evaluation. These may indicate a cardiac or respiratory disease or systemic disease such as cystic fibrosis.

Head, Eyes, Ears, Nose, and Throat
Head
Examination and findings of the head are similar to those of the adult. The anterior fontanelle should be closed by 18 months of age.

Eyes
Procedures and Techniques. Most of the examination of children's eyes is the same as that for adults. Vision can be assessed when performing developmental tests such as the Denver II (e.g., noting the child's ability to stack blocks or

identify animals). The assessment of vision and eyes should be appropriate for the developmental stage and age of the child.

Use the Allen Picture Cards to screen for visual acuity in children 2½ to 3 years of age. Show the large cards with pictures to the child up close to be sure that the child can identify them. Then present each picture at the appropriate distance (as directed per card instructions) from the child. Use Snellen's "E" chart for children 3 to 6 years of age (see Chapter 10). Have children point their fingers in the direction of the "arms" of the E. By 7 to 8 years of age, begin to use the standard Snellen's chart, as described for adults. Test each eye separately with and without glasses as appropriate. Be sure to screen children two separate times before referring them. Test for color vision once between ages 4 and 8. The red and green lines on Snellen's chart can be used as a gross screening tool for color blindness, to be followed with Ishihara's test as needed. Ask the child to identify each pattern seen in the cards.

Perform the corneal light reflex or Hirschberg at a distance of about 12 inches from the child's eyes. If the cover/uncover test is indicated, it should also be performed by having the toddler or child seated on the parent's lap. Have the child fixate on the light of the otoscope. If the child is uncooperative, it is often helpful to have him or her fixate on a toy. Use one hand to cover the eye and observe the uncovered eye for fixation on the object. Screen for nystagmus by inspecting the movement of the eyes to the six cardinal fields of gaze. The nurse may need to stabilize the child's chin with his or her hand to prevent the entire head from moving.

Prepare children for the ophthalmoscope examination by showing them the light, explaining how it shines in the eye, and explaining why the room must be darkened. As with the infant, it is important to elicit a bilateral red reflex using the ophthalmoscope.

Expected and Abnormal Findings. Visual acuity of 20/20 (line 7 on the chart) is achieved during toddler years, although 20/40 (line 5) is considered acceptable through age 8.[7] Normally the child is able to name three of the seven cards within three to five trials during the Allen Picture Cards test. A child with normal color vision sees the number or pattern embedded in Ishihara's test, whereas a color-blind child is unable to see the pattern. A symmetric corneal light reflex is an expected finding (Fig. 19-32). Early recognition and treatment of strabismus can restore binocular vision, whereas diagnosis of strabismus after age 6 has a poor prognosis. Children who are found to have strabismus need to be referred to an ophthalmologist.

Ears

Procedures and Techniques. The biggest challenge to examining the auditory canal and TM of the young child is his or her lack of cooperation. Restrain the child in either the supine or prone position as discussed previously with the infant (see Fig. 19-19). Inadequate restraint can result in pain to the child and also may cause injury to the ear canal. If the child is fearful, screaming, or uncooperative, the nurse should

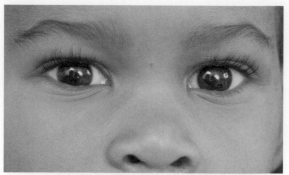

FIG. 19-32 Corneal light reflex.

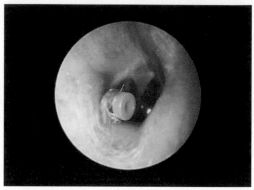

FIG. 19-33 Tympanotomy tube protruding from the right tympanic membrane. (From Bingham, Hawke, and Kwok, 1992.)

place his or her hand against the child's head to protect the ear canal from sudden movement or jolt. Because the young child may perceive the otoscope examination as traumatic, it may be deferred until the last procedure of the examination. If the child becomes upset during the examination, be sure to quickly return him or her to the parent for comforting.

As the child becomes older, the nurse should take the time to elicit his or her cooperation during the examination. If the nurse has any question regarding the child's ability to hold perfectly still during the otoscope examination, the parent or adult who is with the child should assist in restraining the child to ensure his or her safety.

The procedure for examination proceeds as previously discussed for the infant. If the child is younger than 1 year of age, the pinna should be pulled down during the examination as described for the infant. If the child is older, the pinna should be pulled up and backward as for the adult. Hearing screening may be indicated for children, particularly if risk factors were identified during infancy.

Expected and Abnormal Findings. The findings of the examination of the ears do not differ significantly for older children than those of the adult. The nurse should be aware that it is common to find foreign bodies in the ears of children.

Small polyethylene tubes (PE tubes) in the TM of a child who has recently had a myringotomy (Fig. 19-33) may be observed. These are surgically placed through the TM to relieve middle ear pressure and permit drainage of fluid or material collected behind the TM. They are most commonly put in the ears of young children because of recurrent ear infections. Usually the tubes spontaneously work their way out of the TM within 6 to 12 months after insertion.

Hearing evaluation of the young child is necessary if the parent or nurse perceives a lag in his or her development. Behavioral manifestations that may indicate hearing impairment include delay in verbal skills; speech that is monotone, garbled, or difficult to understand; inattentiveness during conversation; facial expressions that appear strained or puzzled; withdrawal and lack of interaction with others; asking "What?" a lot or asking for statements to be repeated; or having frequent earaches.

Nose and Mouth

Procedures and Techniques. A toddler or young child will probably tolerate the mouth and nose examination better while sitting on the parent's lap. Have the child sit on the adult's lap with his or her back to the parent. The parent may then restrain the child's legs by placing them between the adult's legs. The parent then has both hands free. One hand should be used to reach around the child's body to restrain his or her arms and chest. The other hand may be used to assist the nurse by restraining the child's head (Fig. 19-34). Once the child becomes too large for the parent's lap, the examination is best performed with the child in a supine position on the examination table.

The young child's nose should be assessed in the same manner as that of the infant. Use a thumb on the tip of the nose to improve visualization inside the nares. Palpation of the sinuses can be done after ages 7 or 8. When examining the teeth, note the eruption sequence; the timing, condition, positioning, and hygiene of the teeth; and the presence of debris around the teeth or gum line.

Expected Findings. The presence of a transverse crease at the bridge of the nose is called an *allergic salute,* which occurs when a child has a frequent runny nose or allergies and wipes

the nose with an upward sweep of the palm of the hand. The child's tonsils are larger than an adult's but should not interfere with swallowing or breathing. The child's tonsils should be dark pink and without vertical reddened lines, general erythema, edema, or exudate. Tooth eruption depends on the age of the child.

Abnormal Findings. Abnormal findings may include a foul odor and unilateral discharge from a nostril caused by a foreign body. Dryness, flaking, or cracking corners of the mouth may indicate excess licking of the lips, vitamin deficiency, or infection such as impetigo. The buccal mucosa should be pink, moist, and without lesions. Lesions such as Koplik's spots (as seen in measles) or candidiasis (thrush) may be observed (Fig. 19-35). An excessively dry mouth may indicate dehydration or fever. Excessive salivation may indicate gingivostomatitis or multiple dental caries. Excessive drooling after 12 months of age may indicate a neurologic disorder. Flattened edges on the teeth may indicate teeth grinding (bruxism). Darkened, brown, or black teeth may indicate decay or oral iron therapy. Mottled or pitted teeth may result from tetracycline therapy during tooth development. A strawberry-colored tongue may indicate scarlet fever. If the mouth has a fetid or musty smell, hygiene practices, local or systemic infections, or sinusitis should be investigated further.

Neck

Procedures and Techniques. The techniques for examining the neck of the child are the same as those for the adult. The thyroid of the child may be assessed using the same techniques as for the adult, but the challenge is to encourage the child to sit still and swallow as described so an adequate evaluation may be done. If the child is not able to cooperate, the thyroid examination may be deferred.

Expected and Abnormal Findings. Normally lymph nodes up to 3 mm may be palpable in children and may reach 1 cm in the cervical areas; but they are discrete, mobile, and nontender. The term *shotty* may be used to describe small, firm,

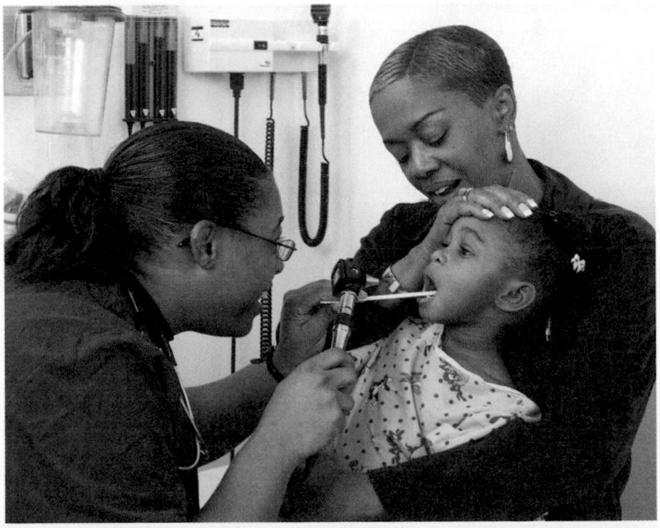

FIG. 19-34 Technique for immobilizing a young child's head for examination.

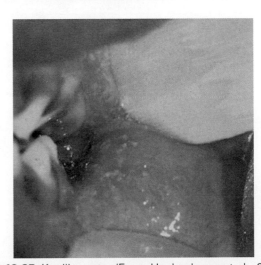

FIG. 19-35 Koplik spots. (From Hockenberry et al., 2003.)

and mobile nodes occurring as a normal variation in children. Enlarged postauricular and occipital nodes in children younger than 2 years of age are a normal variation. Likewise cervical and submandibular nodal enlargements are more frequent in older children. Thus the age of the patient should be considered in the decision to further evaluate lymph node enlargement. Abnormal findings are tender, fixed nodes greater than 1 cm. Enlarged, tender nodes may occur after immunizations or upper respiratory infection.[7]

Lungs and Respiratory System

Procedures and Techniques. The techniques for examining the lungs and respiratory system of the child are the same as those for the adult. By age 2 or 3 years, the child may be cooperative during the respiratory examination (Fig. 19-36). Even before that age, if the nurse takes the time to develop a relationship with the child, cooperation can usually be obtained.

If performing chest palpation, the nurse should adjust the number of fingers used to palpate the chest wall to be appropriate for the size of the chest. For example, if the child is small, the nurse may use only two or three fingers. On the other hand, if the child is large, three or four fingers may be used. Percussion is performed infrequently until the child is at least 10 years of age.

Expected Findings. By age 5 or 6 the rounded thorax of the child approximates the 1:2 ratio of anteroposterior-to-lateral diameter of the adult. By ages 6 or 7 the child's breathing pattern should change from primarily nasal and abdominal to thoracic in girls and abdominal in boys. The child's respiratory rate should gradually slow as he or she becomes older (see Table 4-1). Auscultation findings for the child range between the findings of the infant and those of the adult.

Depending on the size of the child and the musculature of the chest, slight variations may be found. Findings for a small or young child with undeveloped chest musculature may include more bronchovesicular breath sounds in the peripheral lung areas; whereas, if the child is larger and has started to develop more, the breath sounds are equivalent to those of the adult (vesicular in the peripheral lung fields). Palpation findings for the child are the same as those for the adult. If percussion is performed, the nurse should note that young children normally have a hyperresonance tone.

Abnormal Findings. Abnormal findings include increased respiratory rate, retractions, and adventitious sounds such as crackles, rhonchi, or wheezing. If the child's chest proportion remains rounded, it may be an outward indication of a significant problem such as asthma or cystic fibrosis.

Heart and Peripheral Vascular System

Procedures and Techniques. The child's heart is auscultated in the same areas as that of the adult (Fig. 19-37). Because it may take a considerably longer time to be sure of the sounds, explanations should be given in advance to the caregiver to avoid unneeded concern. All of the techniques used require that the child wear only underwear and sit on the table or the caregiver's lap. Cooperative children may recline at a 45-degree angle. If this is not possible, the child may lie supine to allow the nurse to hear more cardiovascular sounds.

If an irregular rhythm is noted, have the child hold his or her breath so only heart sounds are heard. Auscultate with the bell of the stethoscope over the right supraclavicular space at the medial end of the clavicle along the anterior border of the sternocleidomastoid muscle for a venous hum (Fig. 19-38). A venous hum is a vibration heard over the jugular

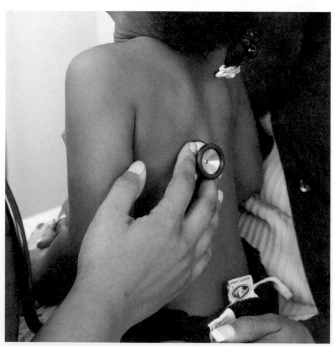

FIG. 19-36 Auscultation of lungs on a young child.

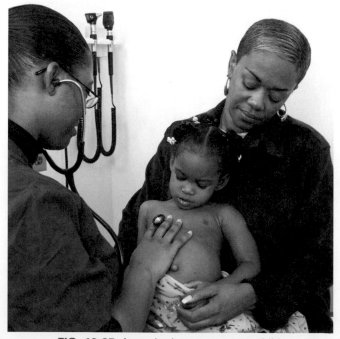

FIG. 19-37 Auscultation on a young child.

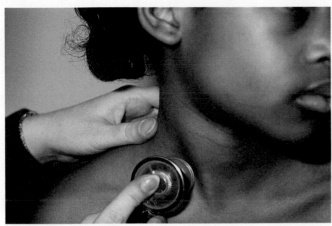

FIG. 19-38 Auscultation for venous hum. (From Seidel et al., 2003.)

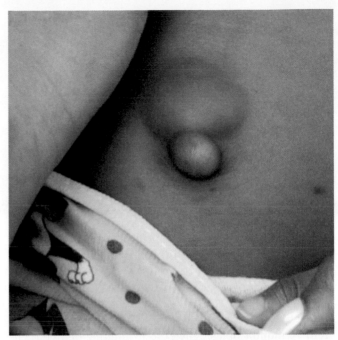

FIG. 19-39 Umbilical hernia on a toddler.

vein caused by turbulent blood flow; it has a continuous, low-pitched sound that is louder during diastole. It may be stopped by gentle pressure between the trachea and the sternocleidomastoid muscle at the level of the thyroid cartilage. Note differences (such as rate and amplitude) between pulses, particularly the radial and femoral.

Expected and Abnormal Findings. A child's rate and rhythm are consistent. A child's pulse may normally increase on inspiration and decrease on expiration. Changes in heart rates in children are listed in Table 4-1. A venous hum in the jugular vein is considered a normal variation.

Recording the abnormal findings observed during the child's activities is important. Squatting may be a compensatory position for a child with a heart defect. Cyanosis or pallor may indicate poor perfusion resulting from congenital heart defects. Note if there is more cyanosis with crying and if there is facial or ankle edema. Note signs of poor feeding (e.g., low weight) and reports of caregiver that the child stops eating to get his or her breath, which may indicate a heart problem. Labored respirations could indicate a cardiovascular problem. Weak or absent femoral pulses may indicate coarctation of the aorta.

Abdomen and Gastrointestinal System

Procedures and Techniques. Children may resist abdominal palpation because they are ticklish. Assessment of children is generally the same as that of adults, with the exception of the areas noted in the normal and abnormal findings.

Expected and Abnormal Findings. Toddlers normally exhibit a rounded (potbelly) abdomen while both standing and lying down. School-age children may show this rounded appearance until about 13 years of age when standing; when lying, the abdomen should be flat; generalized distention is an abnormal finding. An umbilical hernia is common in African American children until 7 years of age and in Caucasian children under 2 years of age[7] (Fig. 19-39). Note any hernia still present after these ages or any hernia that is not easily reducible.

Note movement of the abdomen during respiration. Until about age 7 children are abdominal breathers. Check the tenseness of the abdominal muscles. Diastasis recti abdominis (two rectus muscles fail to approximate one another) is common in African American children but should disappear during the preschool years.[7] The lower edge of the liver may be palpable in young children 1 to 2 cm below the right costal margin. Normally the liver descends during inspiration. It may not be palpable in older children. Abdominal pain is always considered an abnormal finding.

Musculoskeletal System

Procedures and Techniques. When evaluating children, compare data with tables of normal age and sequence of motor development. (Chapter 18 discusses expected motor development for children.) Measure the height of the child and compare values to tables of percentiles for growth to assess bone growth. Observe the gait for steadiness; inspect the spine for alignment. All joints and muscle groups are examined for range of motion, tone, and strength. Assess for Trendelenburg sign by inspecting the child standing on one leg, observing from behind. Observe for pelvic tilt.

⊕ ETHNIC, CULTURAL, AND SPIRITUAL VARIATIONS

Hip Dislocation

Navajo Indians and Canadian Eskimos are among the cultures with the highest incidence of hip dislocation. In these cultures newborns are tightly wrapped in blankets or strapped to cradle boards. Hip dislocation is virtually unknown in cultures in which infants are carried on their mother's backs or hips in the widely abducted straddle position such as in the Far East and Africa.[7]

Expected Findings. Toddlers have a wide stance and a wide-waddle gait pattern, which tends to disappear by age 24 to 36 months. The gait should become progressively stronger, steadier, and smoother as the child matures. The spine should be straight. By 12 to 18 months the lumbar curve develops as the child learns to walk; lumbar lordosis is common in toddlers; after 18 months the cervical spine is concave, the thoracic spine is convex (although less than that of adults), and the lumbar spine is concave (similar to that of adults). There should be no bulges or dimpling along the spine. Lordosis is seen more frequently in African American children but should not be seen in children over 6 years of age. The knees should be in a direct straight line between the hip, the ankle, and the great toe. Valgus (outward) rotation of the lower extremities (medial malleoli greater than 2.5 cm apart with knees touching) is normal in children 2 to 3.5 years of age and may be present up to 12 years of age. Varus (inward) rotation of the lower extremities (medial malleoli touching, with knees greater than 2.5 cm apart) requires further evaluation for tibial torsion; it may be normal until 18 to 24 months of age. The expected finding of Trendelenburg's sign is that the opposite thigh and hip elevate because the pelvic muscles to the greater trochanter are sufficient to elevate the hip not bearing weight. For example, when the patient stands on the left leg, the right thigh and hip should tilt upward.

Abnormal Findings. Any deviation from the pattern or a history of increasing falls or balance problems should be considered abnormal. A positive Trendelenburg's sign indicates hip dysplasia. When standing on the affected leg, no pelvic tilt is noted in the opposite thigh and hip. The patient with a Trendelenburg's sign shortens the step on the unaffected leg and has a lateral deviation of the entire trunk and affected side. This is one of the more common gait deviations.

Neurologic System

Procedures and Techniques. Follow the same sequence of evaluation as for adults when dealing with children. Observe the child carefully during spontaneous activity because he or she may not be able to cooperate with requests as an adult would. Making the examination a game helps in data collection. Observe the child for achievement of expected developmental milestones for fine- and gross-motor, social-adaptive, and language skills described in Table 18-4. Evaluate the child's general behavior while he or she is at play, interacting with parents, and cooperating with parents and with the nurse.

In testing cranial nerves, sense of smell usually is not tested; if it is, use a scent familiar to the child such as an orange or peanut butter. In testing visual fields and gaze (CNs II, III, IV, and VI), gently immobilize the head so the child cannot follow objects with the whole head but only with the eyes. When testing CN VII, approach it like a game, asking the child to make "funny faces" as the nurse models them (Fig. 19-40).

Using an appropriate developmental tool, assess fine-motor coordination in children under 6 years of age. For

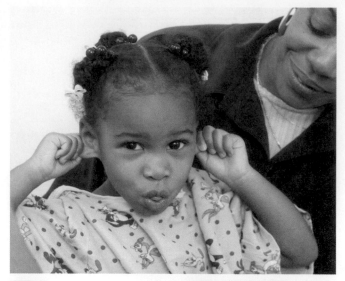

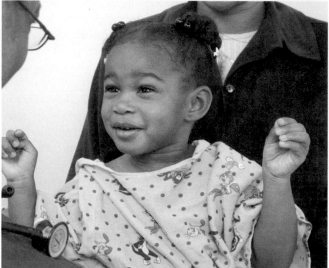

FIG. 19-40 Ask the child to make a "funny face" to assess cranial nerve VII.

children older than 6 years, use the finger-to-nose test, with the nurse's finger held 2.5 to 5 cm away from the child's nose.

Sensory function is not normally tested before age 5. Carefully explain what is being done when children are tested and use descriptions that the child can understand such as "this will feel like a tickle or a mosquito bite." Use simple numbers (such as 0, 7, 5, 3, or 1) for graphesthesia testing and X and O for younger children.

The screening for neurologic "soft" signs in school-age children is used to describe vague and minimal dysfunction signs such as clumsiness, language disturbances, motor overload, mirroring movement of extremities, or perceptual development difficulties (Table 19-4).

Typically deep tendon reflexes (DTRs) are not tested in young children unless they present with neurologic symptoms (i.e., muscle weakness, dizziness). However, if it is warranted, perform the DTR test in the same manner as in the adult examination.

TABLE 19-4 SCREENING ASSESSMENT OF NEUROLOGIC "SOFT" SIGNS

INSTRUCTIONAL TECHNIQUE	IMPORTANT OBSERVATIONS	VARIABLES AND CONSIDERATIONS
Evaluation of Fine-Motor Coordination Observe child during:		
a. Undressing, unbuttoning	Note child's general coordination.	
b. Tying shoe		
c. Rapidly touching alternate fingers with thumb	Note if similar movement on other side.	For items c to e and h and i, movement of other side noted as associated motor movements, adventitious overflow movements, or synkinesis
d. Rattling imaginary doorknob	Note if similar movement on other side.	
e. Unscrewing imaginary light bulb	Note if similar movement on other side.	
f. Grasping pencil and writing	Note excessive pressure on pen point; fingers placed directly over point, or placed greater than 2.5 cm up shaft.	May indicate difficulty with fine-motor coordination
g. Moving tongue rapidly		
h. Demonstrating hand grip	Note if similar movement on opposite side.	
i. Inverting feet	Note if similar movement on opposite side.	
j. Repeating several times "pa, ta, ka" or "kitty, kitty, kitty"	Accurate reproduction of these sounds indicates auditory coordination.	
Evaluation of Special Sensory Skills		
a. Dual simultaneous sensory tests (face-hand testing): First demonstrate technique, then instruct child to close eyes; nurse performs simultaneously: (1) Touch both cheeks (2) Touch both hands (3) Touch right cheek and right hand (4) Touch left cheek and right hand (5) Touch left cheek and left hand (6) Touch right cheek and left hand	Failure to perceive hand stimulus when face is simultaneously touched is referred to as *rostral dominance*.	Approximately 80% of normal children able to perform this test by age 8 years without rostral dominance
b. Finger localization test (finger agnosia test): Touch two spots on one finger or two fingers simultaneously; child has eyes closed; ask, "How many fingers am I touching, one or two?"	Evaluate number of correct responses with four trials for each hand. Six out of eight possible correct responses passes.	Approximately 50% of all children able to pass test by age 6 years Approximately 90% of all children able to pass test by age 9 Reflects child's orientation in space, concept of body image, sensation of touch, and position sense
Evaluation of Child's Laterality and Orientation in Space		
a. Imitation of gestures: Instruct child to use same hand as nurse and imitate the following movements ("Do as I do"): (1) Extend little finger. (2) Extend little and index fingers. (3) Extend index and middle fingers. (4) Touch two thumbs and two index fingers together simultaneously. (5) Form two interlocking rings—thumb and index finger of one hand, with thumb and index finger of other hand. (6) Point index finger of one hand down toward cupped finger of opposite hand held below.	Note difficulty with fine finger movements, manipulation, or reproduction of correct gesture. Note any marked right-left confusion regarding nurse's right and left hands.	Helps to evaluate child's finger discrimination; awareness of body image; and right, left, front, back, and up and down orientation Especially important after age 8 years if there continues to be marked right-left confusion

Continued

TABLE 19-4	SCREENING ASSESSMENT OF NEUROLOGIC "SOFT" SIGNS—cont'd	
INSTRUCTIONAL TECHNIQUE	**IMPORTANT OBSERVATIONS**	**VARIABLES AND CONSIDERATIONS**
b. Following directions: ask child to: (1) Show me your left hand. (2) Show me your right eye. (3) Show me your left elbow. (4) Touch your left knee with your left hand. (5) Touch your right ear with your left hand. (6) Touch your left elbow with your right hand. (7) Touch your right cheek with your right hand. (8) Note any difficulty with following sequence of directions. (9) Point to my left ear. (10) Point to my right eye. (11) Point to my right hand. (12) Point to my left knee.	Note any incorrect response. Note any difficulty with following sequence of directions.	Items 1 through 7 mastered by approximately age 6 years Items 8 through 11 mastered by age 8 years

Expected and Abnormal Findings. Normal findings should generally be the same as those for adults. Soft neurologic signs may be considered normal in the young child; but, as the child matures, the signs should disappear. Abnormal findings are the same as those for the adult. Spasticity; paralysis; or impaired vision, speech, or hearing may indicate neurologic abnormalities. The identification of soft signs as the child matures indicates failure of the child to perform age-specific activities (see Table 19-4), and the child should be referred to a health care professional for further evaluation. Inattention, motor restlessness, and easy distractibility may indicate attention deficit hyperactivity disorder.

Breasts

Procedures and Techniques. The examination of the child generally requires only inspection. The child's chest should be exposed.

Expected Findings. The nipples normally are located slightly lateral to the midclavicular line between the fourth and fifth ribs. For the prepubescent child the nipple should be flat and surrounded by a slightly darker pigmented areola. As the girl reaches prepubertal age, sometimes as young as age 8, her breasts show prepubertal budding. Precocious development of breasts in girls before age 8 should be investigated further.

Reproductive System and Perineum
Female Examination

Procedures and Techniques. The extent of the genitalia examination in children depends on their age and the report of problems during the history, but typically the examination is limited to inspection of the external genitalia to determine if the structures are intact and without obvious abnormalities. An inspection of a young girl's external genitalia should be included with each routine examination. If this examination is performed consistently, the child experiences less anxiety and embarrassment in later years when internal examination becomes necessary. Internal examination is not routinely performed because the internal female genitalia are underdeveloped in the prepubertal girl.

The nurse must take the time to gain the cooperation and understanding of the child; how this is done depends largely on the age of the child and previous experiences. By the time a child is 4 to 6 years of age, time is spent reassuring her that the procedure involves looking at her genitalia and touching her on the outside only. Approach the child in a matter-of-fact manner, informing her about the procedure and what to expect. It may be difficult to get her to understand the difference between a permissible genitalia examination by a nurse and inappropriate touching by others; it is important to include the parent in this discussion.

When nurses examine younger children, parents often are present and can participate by helping to position the child. In all cases ensure privacy for the child. She should participate in the decision about whether or not the parent should be present in the room during the examination. Some girls may want a parent present, whereas the preteen child may not. Confer with the child before the examination and, if appropriate, ask the parent to wait outside.

Position the child on her back and place her legs in a frog-leg position (hips flexed with the soles of the feet together and up to her buttocks), with the head slightly elevated so she can observe the nurse. The older girl may have difficulty obtaining adequate relaxation of the knees with the feet together; thus it may be necessary for her to assume the lithotomy position with feet in stirrups. The techniques of the external genitalia examination are the same as for the infant. Using gloved hands, gently spread the labia so the genitalia may be inspected.

Occasionally, situations warrant a more complete examination. The decision to do this is usually based on external examination findings or the history. For example, if the child has a history of urinary tract infections; vaginal discharge or irritation; or complaints of itching, rash, or pain, a more complete examination is necessary. A complete examination is also necessary if there is any indication of sexual abuse or mishandling of the child. (In this case such an examination is performed by a sexual assault nurse examiner.) If internal inspection of the vagina and cervix is necessary, a pediatric Pederson speculum may be used for an older girl. For young girls a nasal speculum with an attached light source is a useful instrument if the speculum is too large. A rectal examination is necessary if there is any suspected history of abuse, possibility of a foreign body in the rectum, or specific rectal symptoms. Internal inspection is considered an advanced skill and should only be attempted by nurses who have received adequate training for this type of examination.

Expected Findings. Until approximately age 7, the labia majora are flat, the labia minora are thin, and the clitoris is relatively small. Usually the hymen membrane has a visible opening, although there are a number of normal variations in the appearance of the hymen. In older girls the labia majora and minora appear thicker, and evidence of pubic hair may be seen by the time the child reaches pubescence—usually between ages 8 and 11. There should be no vaginal discharge, vaginal odor, or evidence of bruising.

Male Examination

Procedures and Techniques. The techniques for examining the male child's genitalia are the same as those for the infant. The major difference in the examination is the approach. In many cultures children are taught at a very early age that the genitalia should not be exposed or touched. In the presence of the child's parent, reassure him that his genitalia must be examined just as all of his other body areas. It is important to ask the parent to reassure the child that he needs to be examined to make sure that he is healthy. Whenever possible, reassure the child that he is growing up normally.

The examination can be performed with the child sitting or standing. If the child is sitting, he should be in a slightly reclining position with his knees flexed and heels near the buttocks (Fig. 19-41) or sitting with his knees spread and ankles crossed. If the child has not been circumcised, do not force the foreskin to be retracted. Retract the foreskin only to the point of tightness. Then evaluate whether it is retracted far enough to permit adequate urination and cleaning. Determine if the child has any discharge, crusting, or lesions around or under the foreskin. In addition, examine the scrotum for shape, size, and color and to determine the presence of testicles in the scrotum. Evidence of pubic hair may be seen by the time the child reaches pubescence.

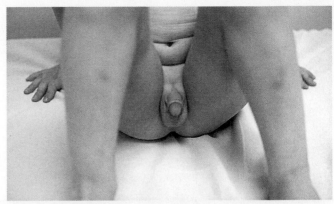

FIG. 19-41 Position of young child for examination of genitalia. (From Seidel et al., 2011.)

Expected and Abnormal Findings. The findings for children are the same as those for the infant. By ages 3 to 4 the foreskin can be retracted easily. If the scrotum has well-formed rugae, it indicates that the testes have descended into the scrotum. If the scrotum remains small, flat, and underdeveloped, it is considered an abnormal finding and may indicate cryptorchidism (undescended testes).

Perianal Examination

Procedures and Techniques. External perianal examination is routinely performed during a comprehensive assessment. For the external examination be sure to respect the child's modesty and apprehension; take the time to explain what is going to happen and what the child can expect. Children should be positioned so the perianal area is adequately exposed and the child is comfortable. The child should be positioned either in a knee-chest position or on the left side with the hips and knees flexed toward the abdomen (the same positioning as for the adult).

Internal rectal examination is not performed in children unless there are specific symptoms such as severe abdominal pain, constipation, or injury. If an internal rectal examination is warranted, the nurse should use the little finger to perform the examination. Even when this is done, there may occasionally be slight rectal bleeding. The parent should be told about this possibility before the examination. The procedure for the internal examination is the same as that for the adult.

Expected and Abnormal Findings. The findings for external examination are the same for the child as for the adult. The findings for the internal examination are the same as for the adult, with the exception that the prostate in the small child is not palpable. Variations are based on developmental maturity. Redness or irritation may be an indication of a bacterial or fungal infection or pinworms. Assess for signs of physical or sexual abuse such as bruising, anal tearing, rapid anal wink, anal dilation, or extreme or inappropriate apprehension from the child. If there is suspicion of child abuse or assault, report the findings to the appropriate local health authorities.

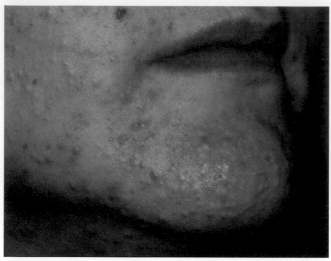

FIG. 19-42 Comedonal acne. (Courtesy Lemmi and Lemmi, 2013.)

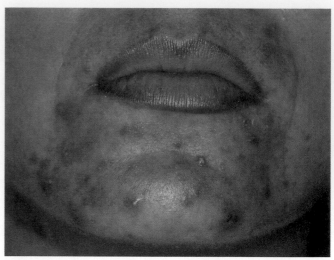

FIG. 19-43 Acne vulgaris. (Courtesy Lemmi and Lemmi, 2013.)

EXAMINATION OF ADOLESCENTS

Although the sequence of examination for the adolescent is the same as for the adult, the nurse needs to be aware that, as children enter their teen years, they should be given a choice about whether a parent is present during the physical examination. This ensures privacy and encourages teens to begin assuming responsibility for their health care.

Skin, Hair, and Nails

Although the examination of the skin, hair, and nails is thought to be straightforward, maturational changes and body hair development often make the adolescent more sensitive than children or adults. Provide adequate privacy and be sensitive to the patient's concerns during the examination.

Skin

Expected and Abnormal Findings. As the child becomes an adolescent, the skin undergoes significant maturational development. The skin texture takes on more adult characteristics. In addition, it has increased perspiration, oiliness, and acne secondary to an increase in sebaceous gland activity.

The most common abnormal finding and concern for the adolescent is acne. Acne may appear in children as young as 7 to 8 years of age but peaks in adolescence at approximately 16 years of age. Although most acne appears on the face, it may also be prevalent on the chest, back, and shoulders. Acne may appear as blackheads (open comedones) or whiteheads (closed comedones)[12] (Fig 19-42). Inflamed lesions of acne can be mild or severe. These lesions are painful and are of concern to the patient because of the appearance (Fig. 19-43).

Hair and Nails

Expected and Abnormal Findings. The presence and characteristics of facial hair in boys and body hair in both boys and girls change significantly; by the end of adolescence there is an adult hair distribution pattern (see Chapter 17). The examination findings are the same as those for the adult. Persistent nail biting may be a habit, indicating an abnormal or coping mechanism for dealing with stress. The nurse should take the time to evaluate why nail biting persists.

Head, Eyes, Ears, Nose, and Throat

The procedures, techniques, and examination findings for the adolescent are the same as for the adult.

Lung and Respiratory System

The procedures, techniques, and examination findings for the adolescent are the same as for the adult. The nurse should be sensitive to the possible modesty of the female adolescent and provide a drape for the breasts when the anterior chest is not being assessed.

Heart and Peripheral Vascular System

The procedures, techniques, and examination findings for the cardiovascular assessment are the same as for the adult.

Abdomen and Gastrointestinal System

The procedures, techniques, and examination findings for the gastrointestinal assessment are the same as for the adult.

Musculoskeletal System

Procedures and Techniques. Examination of the adolescent is the same as that of the adult. Observe the adolescent's posture. Adolescents are screened for scoliosis, kyphosis, and lordosis.

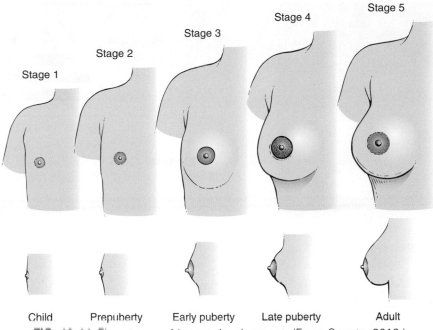

FIG. 19-44 Five stages of breast development. (From Swartz, 2010.)

Expected and Abnormal Findings. The normal findings for the adolescent are the same as those for the adult. A young person with low self-esteem or feelings of rejection may assume a slumped, careless, and apathetic posture. Poor posture, regardless of the cause (e.g., low self-esteem or heavy backpack), contributes to kyphosis. A curvature less than 10 degrees is considered a normal variation, and a curvature between 10 and 20 degrees is considered mild.[7] Curvature of the spine greater than 10 degrees needs further evaluation for early treatment. Postural kyphosis is almost always accompanied by a compensatory lordosis (i.e., an abnormally concave lumbar curvature).

Neurologic System

The procedures, techniques, and examination findings for the adolescent are the same as for the adult.

Breasts

Procedures and Techniques. Adolescent females may be sensitive about having their breasts exposed. The nurse should take time to reassure the patient that, although her privacy is important, exposing the chest for a complete breast examination is necessary. The breast examination should proceed in the same manner as for the adult female. Note the developmental stage of the patient.

Expected and Abnormal Findings. Breast development occurs in five stages over an average of 4 years[13] (Fig. 19-44). Menarche (the onset of menses) begins when the breasts reach stage 3 or 4, usually just after the peak of the adolescent growth spurt, which is approximately age 12 in most girls (Fig. 19-45). However, because there is variability in age of breast development across racial/ethnic groups, the nurse should consider the development stages as a general

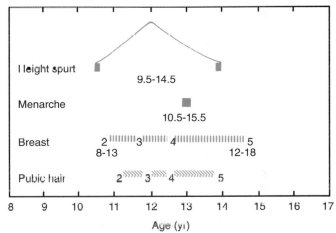

FIG. 19-45 Summary of maturational development of girls. The numbers 2 to 5 refer to the stage of development. (From Marshall and Tanner, 1969.)

guideline. For example, Harlan found that African American girls developed secondary sex characteristics earlier than Caucasian girls of the same age.[14] The right and left breasts may develop at different rates. It is important to reassure the patient that this is common and in time the development may equalize. The breast tissue in the adolescent female should feel firm and elastic throughout both breasts. By age 14 most females have developed breasts that resemble those of the adult female.

Male adolescents, especially obese males, may have transient unilateral or bilateral subareolar masses (Fig. 19-46). These firm and sometimes tender masses may be of great concern. Reassure the young adolescent that they are generally transient and should disappear within a year or

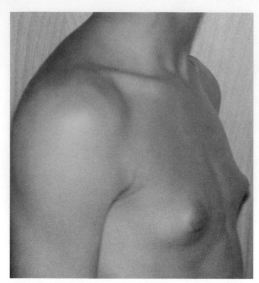

FIG. 19-46 Prepubertal gynecomastia. (Courtesy Wellington Hung, MD, Children's National Medical Center, Washington, DC. From Seidel et al., 2006.)

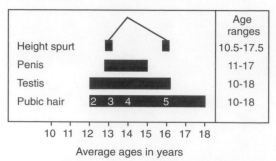

FIG. 19-47 Development of male genitalia and pubic hair associated with height spurt and age. (From Tanner, 1962.)

so. Gynecomastia, on the other hand, is an unexpected enlargement of one or both breasts in the male. It may be caused by hormonal or systemic disorders; however, it is most commonly a result of adipose tissue associated with obesity or the body change transition that occurs during early puberty.[7] Most adolescent males with gynecomastia are very self-conscious of this finding.

Reproductive System

Female Examination

Procedures and Techniques. If a parent is present, the adolescent should be given a choice to be examined alone, and she should be assured of privacy and confidentiality. Assess her menstrual history and sexual maturity. Sexual maturity is assessed through a gradual emergence of pubic hair (from straight, downy hair to dark, coarse, and thick hair) that gradually covers the pubic area to the inner thighs. Reassure the patient that the changes that her body is undergoing are normal. Because many preadolescents and adolescents are becoming interested in their own bodies and the changes that are taking place, they may want to take an active part in the examination. This may be a perfect opportunity to teach the patient about her own anatomy and the changes that she will experience. A mirror may be used during the examination for instruction.

The positioning and techniques for examination of the external genitalia are the same as for the adult. A pelvic examination should be performed beginning at age 21 or at any time the patient has signs of genital or vaginal irritation or infection. Routine pelvic examinations or Papanicolaou (Pap) tests are no longer recommended under the age of 21, even in sexually active females. A pelvic examination is not necessary before prescribing contraception to adolescents. The procedures to be followed are the same as for an adult woman, but additional time must be taken to explain the procedure, show the equipment, and tell the patient exactly

what she may expect. The size and type of vaginal speculum used is based on the size of the patient and the sexual history. The speculum most commonly used to reduce discomfort is a pediatric speculum with blades that are 1 to 1.5 cm wide.

Findings. All findings for the genitalia examination of the adolescent are the same as the findings previously described for the adult.

Male Examination

Procedures and Techniques. Genitalia assessment of the adolescent male is important to ensure that the maturational development is progressing and because testicular cancer occurs in this age-group. This is also the time when teen modesty is at its peak. The nurse must take time to develop a relationship with the patient and reassure him in a matter-of-fact manner that the examination of the genitalia is an essential part of a complete examination. Ensuring privacy and adequate draping when the genitalia are not being examined is important. Deferring the genitalia assessment to the last procedure of the examination is usually best. The process of examination is essentially the same as previously discussed for the adult.

Findings. Expected findings for the young adolescent male depend on the maturational stage of the patient. Maturational changes include a height spurt, gradual development of pubic hair, and gradual growth of the penis and scrotum (Fig. 19-47). In the preadolescent male there is an absence of pubic hair, and the penis and scrotum are proportionally similar as during childhood. The first sign of maturation includes the emergence of long and straight pubic hair, slight enlargement of the penis, and enlargement of the testes and scrotum with a darkening of the skin. As maturation continues, hair growth increases and becomes thick and coarse, the penis enlarges in both length and diameter, and the scrotum enlarges, with a darkening skin tone. Findings for the older adolescent are essentially the same as previously discussed for the adult.

Perianal Examination

Rectal examinations are not performed routinely unless warranted by symptoms (i.e., rectal bleeding). The prostate examination is not performed routinely in adolescent males. If performed, the procedures, techniques, and findings for the adolescent are the same as for the adult.

COMMON PROBLEMS AND CONDITIONS

SKIN CONDITIONS

Atopic Dermatitis

Atopic dermatitis is a chronic superficial inflammation of the skin with an unknown cause. It may be associated with allergies and asthma, and it is thought to be familial. It is most commonly seen in infancy and childhood. **Clinical Findings:** During infancy and early childhood, red, weeping, crusted lesions appear on the face, scalp, extremities, and diaper area. In older children lesion characteristics include erythema, scaling, and lichenification. The lesions are usually localized to the hands, feet, arms, and legs (particularly at the antecubital fossa and popliteal space) and are associated with intense pruritus (Fig. 19-48).

Diaper Dermatitis

One of the most common causes of irritant contact dermatitis, diaper dermatitis, is an inflammatory reaction to urine, feces, moisture, or friction. It is most common among infants between 4 to 12 months of age. **Clinical Findings:** This dermatitis is characterized by a primary irritant rash involving skin areas in contact with soiled diaper surfaces. The rash is composed of red macules and papules that may be raised and confluent in severe cases (Fig. 19-49).

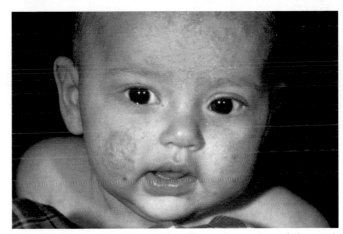

FIG. 19-48 Atopic dermatitis. (From Lemmi and Lemmi, 2013.)

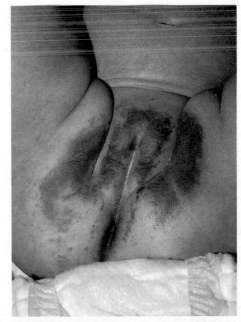

FIG. 19-49 Severe diaper rash. (From White, 2004.)

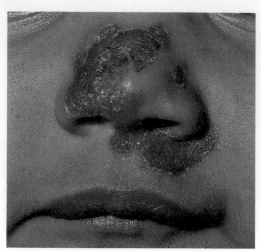

FIG. 19-50 Impetigo. (From Weston, Lane, and Morelli, 1996.)

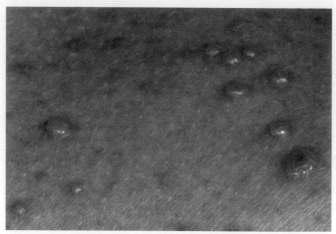

FIG. 19-51 Chickenpox (varicella). (Courtesy Lemmi and Lemmi, 2013.)

Impetigo

This is a common and highly contagious bacterial infection caused by staphylococcal or streptococcal pathogens. It is most prevalent in children, especially among individuals living in crowded conditions with poor sanitation. It occurs most commonly in mid-to-late summer, with the highest incidence in hot, humid climates. **Clinical Findings:** This infection appears as an erythematous macule that becomes a vesicle or bulla and finally a honey-colored crust after the vesicles or bullae rupture (Fig. 19-50).

Herpes Varicella (Chickenpox)

This is a highly communicable viral infection spread by droplets that most commonly occurs during childhood. **Clinical Findings:** The lesions first appear on the trunk and then spread to the extremities and the face. Initially the lesions are macules; they progress to papules and then vesicles, and finally the old vesicles become crusts. The lesions erupt in crops over a period of several days. For this reason lesions in various stages are seen concurrently (Fig. 19-51).

EAR CONDITIONS

Acute Otitis Media

Acute otitis media (AOM) is an infection of the middle ear with the presence of middle ear effusion that can be viral or bacterial in origin. It is one of the most common of all child-hood infections.[15] **Clinical Findings:** The major symptom associated with AOM is ear pain (otalgia). Infants, unable to verbally communicate pain, demonstrate irritability, fussiness, crying, lethargy, and pulling at the affected ear. Associated manifestations include fever, vomiting, and decreased hearing. On inspection in the early stages, the TM appears inflamed—it is red and may be bulging and immobile (Fig. 19-52). Later stages may reveal discoloration (white or yellow drainage) and opacification to the TM. Purulent drainage

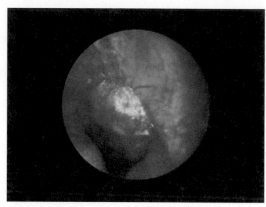

FIG. 19-52 Acute otitis media of the left ear with redness and edema of the pars flaccid. (From Bingham, Hawke, and Kwok, 1992.)

from the ear canal with a sudden relief of pain suggests perforation.

EYE CONDITIONS

Conjunctivitis

An inflammation of the palpebral or bulbar conjunctiva is termed *conjunctivitis*. It is caused by local infection of bacteria or virus and by an allergic reaction, systemic infection, or chemical irritation. **Clinical Findings:** The conjunctiva and sclera appear red, and there may be thick, sticky discharge on the eyelids.

MOUTH CONDITIONS

Tonsillitis

Tonsillitis is one of the most common oropharyngeal infections among children. It can be viral or bacterial in origin; common bacterial pathogens include beta-hemolytic

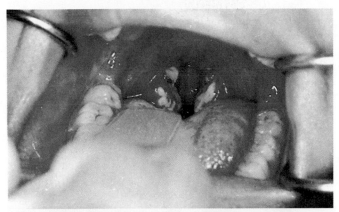

FIG. 19-53 Tonsillitis and pharyngitis. (Courtesy Dr. Edward L Applebaum, Head, Department of Otolaryngology. University of Illinois Medical Center.)

streptococci. **Clinical Findings:** The classic presentation of tonsillitis includes sore throat, pain with swallowing (odynophagia), fever, chills, and tender cervical lymph nodes. Some children may also complain of ear pain. On inspection the tonsils appear enlarged and red and may be covered with white or yellow exudates (Fig. 19-53).

Cleft Lip and Cleft Palate

Cleft lip and cleft palate are incomplete fusion of the maxillary process or the secondary palate during fetal development. These conditions are the most common congenital craniofacial defects and the fourth most common congenital defects seen in the United States. **Clinical Findings:** Usually diagnosed before or at birth, the defects are characterized by a defect in the upper lip or a complete separation extending to the floor of the nostril. This can be unilateral or bilateral (Fig. 19-54).

RESPIRATORY CONDITIONS

Cystic Fibrosis

This is an autosomal-recessive genetic disorder of the exocrine glands. It is a multisystem disease affecting most body systems but especially the lungs, pancreas, and sweat glands. It causes respiratory system dysfunction because of abnormally thick mucus production, which leads to a chronic, diffuse obstructive pulmonary disease (Fig. 19-55). Symptoms most commonly appear before the age of 4, although a milder form of disease may delay diagnosis until late childhood or early adolescence. **Clinical Findings:** The classic symptom of cystic fibrosis is the production of thick, sticky mucus. Stools of children with cystic fibrosis are often frothy, foul smelling, and greasy (steatorrhea). Respiratory signs and symptoms include a chronic moist productive cough with frequent respiratory infections. As the disease progresses, children develop a barrel chest and finger clubbing.

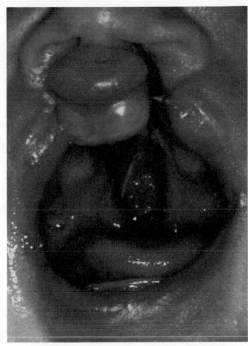

FIG. 19-54 Bilateral cleft lip and complete cleft palate. (From Zitelli, McIntire, and Nowalk, 2012.)

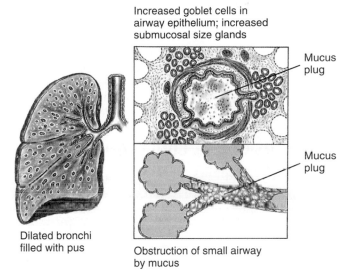

Increased goblet cells in airway epithelium; increased submucosal size glands

Mucus plug

Mucus plug

Dilated bronchi filled with pus

Obstruction of small airway by mucus

FIG. 19-55 Cystic fibrosis.

Childhood Asthma

This chronic respiratory disorder is characterized by airway obstruction and inflammation caused by multiple factors, including environmental exposures, viral illnesses, allergens, and genetic predisposition. Although it can occur anytime during childhood, most children develop symptoms in early childhood. **Clinical Findings:** The most common finding is a persistent cough that is worse at night. Exacerbations may present with increased respiratory rate with prolonged expiration, audible wheeze, shortness of breath, tachycardia, anxious appearance, possible use of accessory muscles, and cough.

Croup Syndromes

The term *croup* is used to describe a wide range of upper-airway illnesses that result from edema of the epiglottis and larynx that often extends into the trachea and bronchi. The three most common conditions—laryngotracheobronchitis, epiglottitis, and bacterial tracheitis—affect the greatest number of children across all age-groups (although it is most common in young children). **Clinical Findings:** The classic findings include inspiratory stridor, a barking-like cough, and hoarseness. In severe cases the child may display respiratory distress, including rapid, labored breathing with retractions and lethargy. Associated findings may include fever and runny nose.

CARDIOVASCULAR CONDITIONS

Congenital Heart Defects

There are a number of congenital heart defects; the most common involve an abnormal connection between the left and right side of the heart (septal defects) or between the great arteries (patent ductus arteriosus). Large defects are typically diagnosed before or shortly after birth, whereas smaller defects may be undiagnosed until the preschool years. **Clinical Findings:** Among infants and children, poor feeding and poor weight gain are often seen; elevations in heart and respiratory rates may be observed with feeding. A murmur is often auscultated, and splitting heart sounds may be noted. Children fatigue easily and often assume a squatting position to relieve cyanotic spells. Signs associated with congestive heart failure may be observed with larger defects.

MUSCULOSKELETAL CONDITIONS

Muscular Dystrophies

This is a group of inherited diseases characterized by progressive muscle wasting caused by degeneration of muscle fibers. The most common form in childhood is Duchenne's muscular dystrophy. **Clinical Findings:** In infancy, sucking and swallowing difficulties may be observed. In early childhood, weakness involving the lower extremities becomes evident with frequent tripping or toe walking. The muscle weakness progresses to muscle wasting; eventually the child loses the ability to walk.

Spina Bifida

Spina bifida is a type of neural tube birth defect characterized by a posterior vertebral defect. Types of spina bifida range from a defect in posterior vertebra only to protrusion of the spinal cord through the vertebral defect. These defects occur within the first month of gestation. **Clinical Findings:** At birth, a saclike protrusion may be noted on the infant's back along the spine, or there may be no obvious signs. These defects can occur anywhere from the upper thoracic to the sacral spine. A wide range of impairments (e.g., motor

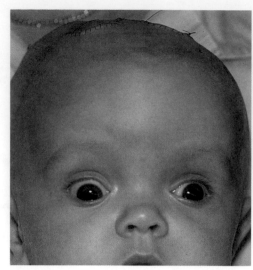

FIG. 19-56 Infantile hydrocephalus. (From Zitelli, McIntire, and Nowalk, 2012.)

impairment, sensory impairment of the lower extremities, and possibly sensory loss involving the anus and genitalia) are also noted.

NEUROLOGIC CONDITIONS

Hydrocephalus

Hydrocephalus is abnormal accumulation of cerebrospinal fluid (CSF). In infants, it is usually a result of an obstruction of the drainage of CSF in the ventricles. **Clinical Findings:** In infants, a gradual increase in intracranial pressure occurs, leading to an actual enlargement of the head (Fig. 19-56). As the head enlarges, the facial features appear small in proportion to the cranium, the fontanelles may bulge, and the scalp veins dilate.

Cerebral Palsy

This is a group of motor function disorders caused by permanent, nonprogressive brain injuries that occur during fetal development or near the time of birth. Classifications of cerebral palsy are spastic, accounting for 50% of cases; dyskinetic (athetoid), accounting for 20% of cases; ataxic, accounting for 10% of cases; and mixed, accounting for 20% of cases. **Clinical Findings:** Deficits may include spasticity; seizures; muscle contractions; delayed motor development; and impaired vision, speech, and hearing. Being mentally challenged may be an associated finding.

Attention Deficit Hyperactivity Disorder

Attention deficit hyperactivity disorder (ADHD) is a condition that begins in childhood characterized by inattentiveness, impulsivity, and hyperactivity that are developmentally inappropriate. ADHD is diagnosed three times more often in boys than girls. **Clinical Findings:** The manifestations may be numerous or few, mild or severe, and vary with the developmental level of the child. An important clinical manifestation is distractibility. The child seems to have selective attention and often does not seem to listen or follow through.

CLINICAL APPLICATION AND CLINICAL REASONING

See Appendix D for answers to exercises in this section.

REVIEW QUESTIONS

1. Which finding on a 2-month-old baby is considered abnormal and requires further follow-up?
   1. The anterior fontanelle is not palpable.
   2. The thyroid gland cannot be palpated.
   3. The head circumference is slightly greater than the chest circumference.
   4. Head lag is observed when the shoulders are lifted off the examination table.

2. A nurse is palpating the lymph nodes of an 18-month-old toddler and finds enlarged postauricular and occipital nodes. What is the significance of this finding?
   1. This is a normal finding at this age.
   2. The toddler may have an ear infection.
   3. The toddler may have an inflammation of the scalp.
   4. The toddler needs to be referred to a pediatrician.

3. While examining the ear of an infant with an otoscope, the nurse pulls down on the ear for which reason?
   1. Increases the depth that the otoscope can be inserted
   2. Stabilizes the ear to avoid injury if the infant moves the head suddenly
   3. Enhances visualization of the tympanic membrane by straightening the ear canal
   4. Facilitates drainage of cerumen from the ear canal, allowing better visualization of inner ear structures

4. What is an expected finding of the newborn's vision that the nurse teaches the parents?
   1. Small tears will be noted when their newborn cries.
   2. Peripheral sight does not develop until age 3 or 4 months.
   3. The newborn can only distinguish the colors of blue and green.
   4. The newborn is nearsighted and cannot see items unless they are close.

5. An adolescent tells a nurse that, while he was riding in a friend's car, the friend was stopped by the police for driving while intoxicated. Which assessment tool would be most appropriate to use with this adolescent?
   1. Denver II
   2. Pediatric Symptom Checklist (PSC)
   3. Guidelines for Adolescent Prevention (GAP)
   4. Oucher Scales

6. Which are expected findings of a newborn's respiratory assessment?
   1. Thoracic breathing
   2. A 1:2 ratio of anteroposterior-to-lateral diameter
   3. Flaring of the nares noted on inspiration
   4. Bronchovesicular breath sounds in the peripheral lung fields

7. Which finding of a preschooler during a cardiovascular system examination is abnormal?
   1. Heart rate of 106 beats/min
   2. Failure to gain weight because of fatigue while eating
   3. Continuous low-pitched vibration heard over the jugular vein
   4. Pulse increasing on inspiration and decreasing on expiration

8. What would be an abnormal finding for a 7-year-old African American boy?
   1. Potbelly
   2. Umbilical hernia
   3. Abdominal breathing
   4. Tenseness of abdominal muscles

9. When examining the genitalia of a 3-year-old boy, which position is ideal?
   1. Prone position
   2. Supine position
   3. Lithotomy position
   4. Sitting position with knees spread and ankles crossed

10. On assessment of the neurologic status of a 4-month-old infant, the nurse notes which finding as abnormal?
    1. The infant abducts and extends arms and legs when startled.
    2. When the infant's sole is touched, the toes flex tightly in an attempt to grasp.
    3. The infant steps in place when held upright with feet on a flat surface.
    4. When stroking the infant's foot from sole to great toes, there is fanning of the toes.

CASE STUDY

Megan Grady is an 8-year-old girl with cerebral palsy who is being treated for seizures.

Interview Data

Megan's mother states that Megan was at home watching television when she started "shaking and jerking all over." The seizure occurred several hours ago but lasted longer than 20 minutes. The mother is concerned because her daughter has never had a seizure that lasted this long. Megan denies recent headaches or problems with balance; she takes primidone 125 mg twice a day.

Examination Data

- *Vital Signs:* Blood pressure, 110/68 mm Hg; pulse, 84 beats/min; respiratory rate, 18 breaths/min; temperature, 98.6° F (37° C).
- *Cognition:* She is a cooperative, alert child with flat affect. She communicates slowly but appropriately.

- *Neurologic:* She has voluntary, symmetric, coordinated movement of all extremities with full range of motion; muscle strength is 5 bilaterally. Deep tendon reflexes are 2+ bilaterally. Sensation is present in arms and legs to vibration, cotton, and pinprick bilaterally.

Clinical Reasoning

1. Which data deviate from normal findings, suggesting a need for further investigation?
2. For which additional information should the nurse ask or assess?
3. Based on the data, which risk factors for injury does Megan have?
4. With which health care team members would you collaborate to meet this patient's needs?

Assessment of the Pregnant Patient

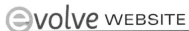 **WEBSITE**

http://evolve.elsevier.com/Wilson/assessment

Assessment of the pregnant patient warrants special attention because of the multiple hormonal, structural, and physiologic changes associated with pregnancy. This chapter builds on previous chapters regarding taking a health history and conducting an examination.

Ideally the pregnant woman is seen on a regular basis throughout pregnancy. Prenatal visits are recommended every 4 weeks up to 28 weeks; every 2 weeks from 28 to 36 weeks; and weekly after 36 weeks. The initial prenatal visit includes a comprehensive history and examination; follow-up visits are more limited in scope, monitoring the progress of the pregnancy and assessing for complications.

ANATOMY AND PHYSIOLOGY

Maternal physiologic adaptations during pregnancy result from hormonal changes and mechanical pressures caused by the enlarging uterus and changes in other tissues. These changes protect the woman's physiologic functioning, allow adaptation to the metabolic demands associated with pregnancy, and provide a protective environment for the growing fetus. Box 20-1 presents selected changes associated with pregnancy.

SIGNS OF PREGNANCY

A combination of laboratory tests and the clinical findings is used to determine the presence of a pregnancy. Laboratory tests used to determine pregnancy detect an antigen-antibody reaction between human chorionic gonadotropin (hCG) hormone and an antiserum within the urine or blood. Many physiologic changes are recognized as signs and symptoms of pregnancy. Some of these findings are categorized as: (1) presumptive symptoms (i.e., symptoms experienced by the woman); (2) probable signs (i.e., changes observed by the nurse); and (3) positive signs (i.e., findings that prove the presence of a fetus). Table 20-1 lists the signs of pregnancy by category and when they may become evident.

HEALTH HISTORY

COMPONENTS OF PRENATAL HEALTH HISTORY

A comprehensive history should be obtained at the first prenatal visit to establish baseline data; it can then be updated as needed during subsequent visits. The history is similar to that of the adult (see Chapter 2) but with a special emphasis on collecting data that could affect pregnancy outcomes. The physical and psychologic health of the mother and the presence of chronic diseases could affect her health and that of the fetus. Quality Improvement Competencies for Nurses include providing patient-centered care and interdisciplinary teamwork in the assessment of pregnant women. Table 11-1 on p. 196 presents knowledge, skills, and attitudes to use when demonstrating these competencies.

BOX 20-1 SELECTED ANATOMIC AND PHYSIOLOGIC CHANGES ASSOCIATED WITH PREGNANCY

Integumentary System

- Increased estrogen increases vascularity to the skin, causing itching and hands and feet to take on reddened appearance.
- Increased secretion of melanotropin causes pigmentation changes to the skin, including chloasma (mask of pregnancy); linea nigra (dark-pigmented line on abdomen); and increased pigmentation to nipples, areolae, axillae, and vulva.
- Increasing size of breasts and abdomen contribute to striae gravidarum (stretch marks) over abdomen and breasts.
- Increased hair or nail growth is reported by some individuals.

Respiratory System

- Uterine enlargement pushes up on diaphragm, causing periodic shortness of breath.
- Respiratory rate may increase slightly; tidal volume increases; breathing becomes more thoracic than abdominal; thoracic cage widens.

Cardiovascular System

- Blood volume increases by 1500 mL to meet the need of an enlarged uterus and fetal tissue, causing increased cardiac workload (increased heart rate).
- Uterine enlargement pushes up on the heart, causing it to shift upward and forward.
- Enlarged uterus increases pelvic pressure, causing decreased venous return, which results in varicosities and edema in lower extremities.

Gastrointestinal System

- Rise in human chorionic gonadotropin early in pregnancy causes nausea and vomiting (morning sickness).
- Uterine enlargement results in displacement of intestines and decreased peristalsis, causing heartburn and constipation, respectively.

- Increased pelvic pressure and vascularity cause hemorrhoids.
- Increased estrogen increases vascularity and tissue proliferation of gums, resulting in swollen and bleeding gums.

Urinary System

- Increased pressure of growing uterus on bladder in early pregnancy and fetal head exerting pressure on bladder in late pregnancy result in nocturia and urinary frequency.

Musculoskeletal System

- Increased size of uterus and growing fetus results in the center of gravity moving forward, causing lordosis (increased spinal curvature) and back discomfort; waddling gait and balance problems may occur.
- Abdominal wall muscles stretch and lose tone, which may lead to separation of abdominal muscles (diastasis recti) in the third trimester.

Reproductive System

- Uterus enlarges, and fundus becomes palpable because of growing fetus.
- Vagina, vulva, and cervix take on bluish color caused by increased vascularity.

Breasts

- Breasts become full and tender early in pregnancy.
- Breasts enlarge as pregnancy progresses.
- Nipples and areolae are more prominent and deeply pigmented.
- Increased mammary vascularization causes veins to become engorged; visible under skin surface.

TABLE 20-1 SIGNS OF PREGNANCY

CATEGORY	SIGN	TIME OF OCCURRENCE (WEEKS OF GESTATION)
Presumptive signs	Breast fullness/tenderness	3-4
	Amenorrhea	4
	Nausea, vomiting	4-12
	Urinary frequency	6-12
	Quickening (fetal movement)	16-20
Probable signs	Chadwick's sign (violet-blue color to cervix)	6-8
	Goodell's sign (softening of cervix)	5
	Hegar's sign (softening of lower uterine segment)	6-12
	Positive pregnancy test (hCG):	
	Serum	4-12
	Urine	6-12
	Ballottement	16-28
Positive signs	Visualization of fetus by ultrasound	5-6
	Auscultation of fetal heart tones:	
	Doppler	8-17
	Fetoscope	17-19
	Palpation of fetal movements	19-22
	Observable fetal movements	Late pregnancy

hCG, Human chorionic gonadotropin.

Reason for Seeking Care

The pregnant woman may be seeing her health care provider for routine prenatal care or for a specific problem that may or may not directly relate to the pregnancy. Prenatal visits are needed to monitor the health of the mother and the growth of the fetus and to educate the mother and family about the care of mother and neonate during the delivery process and neonatal period.

Present Health Status

Data collected are the same as those discussed in Chapter 2. Data specific to the pregnant woman include her present general physical and psychologic well-being and motherhood-coping abilities. In addition, it is essential to determine which medications the patient uses. Many pregnant women assume that the use of over-the-counter medications is safe and are not aware of the potentially harmful effects on the fetus.[1]

Past Health History

Data collected in this section are the same as those discussed in Chapter 2. It is important to document any chronic illness (such as diabetes mellitus, thyroid or cardiovascular conditions, renal disease, and depression) and other current risks that the pregnant patient may have.

Gynecologic and Obstetric History

General information regarding the reproductive system (e.g., problems with menstruation, infections, painful intercourse, and sexual patterns) should be included (see Chapter 17).

The history includes information regarding the current and past pregnancies. Determine the exact date of the last menstrual period (LMP) to estimate expected delivery date (Box 20-2).

An obstetric history includes gravidity (G) (number of pregnancies, including current pregnancy); the number of full-term births (T); the number of preterm births (P); the number of abortions (A) (both spontaneous "miscarriages" and "therapeutic" pregnancy interruptions); and the number of living children (L). The acronym GTPAL may be of help in remembering this system of documentation (Table 20-2).

The obstetric history also includes specific data regarding each pregnancy. Document the following information:

- The course of each pregnancy (including the duration of gestation, date of delivery, and significant problems or complications)
- The process of labor (including manner in which labor was started [i.e., spontaneous or induced], length of labor, and complications associated with labor)
- The delivery (presentation of the infant, method of delivery [i.e., vaginal or cesarean section], and pain management strategies used for delivery, if any)
- Condition of the infant at birth (including weight)
- Postpartum course (including any maternal or infant problems)

BOX 20-2 ESTIMATED DATE OF BIRTH

Nägele's Rule
Determine the first day of the last menstrual period (LMP), subtract 3 months, and then add 7 days.

Example:
First day of LMP	= November 1
− 3 months	= August 1
+ 7 days	= August 8 EDB*

EDB, Estimated date of birth.

*NOTE: Most women give birth during the period extending from 7 days before to 7 days after the EDB.

TABLE 20-2 DETERMINING GRAVIDITY AND PARITY USING A FIVE-DIGIT (GTPAL) SYSTEM

CONDITION	G GRAVIDA	T TERM BIRTH	P PRETERM BIRTH	A ABORTIONS	L LIVING CHILDREN
Woman who is pregnant for the first time	1	0	0	0	0
Woman who has carried her first pregnancy to term and the infant survived	1	1	0	0	1
Woman who is currently pregnant for the second time; has one child from the first pregnancy born full term	2	1	0	0	1
Woman who has been pregnant twice; has one child who was born preterm and had one miscarriage	2	0	1	1	1
Woman who has been pregnant once and delivered full-term twins	1	1	0	0	2

Modified from Lowdermilk DL, et al: *Maternity and women's health care,* ed 10, St Louis, 2012, Mosby.

Family History

In addition to the family history described in Chapter 2, a pregnant woman's family history should specifically address the childbearing history of her mother and sister(s), including multiple births, chromosome abnormalities, genetic disorders, congenital disorders, and chronic illnesses such as diabetes mellitus or renal disease and cancer.

Personal and Psychosocial History
Attitude Toward the Pregnancy

Inquire how the woman and her partner feel about the pregnancy. Was it planned? What kind of expectations does she have regarding being pregnant, the process of labor, childbirth, and parenthood? Explore if the patient has any fear (such as fear of pain) regarding the pregnancy and delivery process (Box 20-3). Adjustments to parenthood such as role changes within the family should also be explored. Emotional stability data are collected, which includes the incidence of excessive crying, social withdrawal, or decisions related to infant care.

Nutritional History

A woman's nutritional status during pregnancy affects maternal and fetal health. An understanding of the woman's usual dietary practices is essential for nutritional assessment. Cultural diversity should be taken into account when evaluating dietary practices. Patients should be interviewed regarding food allergies or intolerance. Development of an individualized meal pattern may be necessary to ensure that nutrient needs are met if the patient must avoid particular foods or food groups. Lactose intolerance is a commonly reported problem. Inadequate intake of iron in pregnancy commonly results in anemia of pregnancy because of the high fetal demands for iron.[2]

BOX 20-3 CLINICAL NOTE

Most women have some concerns about pain during the childbirth process. The discomfort and pain associated with childbirth are unique not only to each woman but also as a pain experience in itself. Compared with other known painful events or experiences, the potential for achieving satisfactory pain relief is high because of the uniqueness of this pain experience. Unique points include the following:

- The woman knows that the pain will happen.
- The woman knows approximately when (within a week or so) the pain will happen.
- The woman knows that there will be a predictable pattern to the pain.
- The woman knows that there is a time limit to the pain experience (hours as opposed to days or weeks) and that it will end.
- The woman knows that there is a tangible end product associated with the birth (i.e., the birth of her child).

Dietary assessment should also include questions regarding ingestion of nonnutritive substances known as pica. Clay, starch, baking soda, and dirt are some of the reported cravings during pregnancy.[3] To assess potentially harmful effects of eating nonnutritive substances, determine what is being ingested, the quantity, and the frequency.

⊕ ETHNIC, CULTURAL, AND SPIRITUAL VARIATIONS
Dietary Beliefs During Pregnancy

Cultural diversity should be taken into account with dietary assessment. An understanding of how different foods are viewed is important. Specific foods may be considered healthful or harmful during pregnancy and lactation by some cultures. For example, in some cultures eating hot foods is believed to provide warmth for the fetus and enable the baby to be born into a warm, loving environment. In addition, many cultural groups believe that certain cravings for foods should be met while pregnant to avoid harm to the baby.

Tobacco, Alcohol, and Illicit Drug Use

Some behaviors may contribute to a high-risk pregnancy. The nurse identifies high-risk behaviors and targets these areas for teaching. Some of the specific habits to discuss are tobacco, alcohol, and drug use.

Tobacco use should be assessed. Smoking during pregnancy is associated with premature and low–birth-weight (LBW) infants. However, women who stop smoking by the sixteenth week of pregnancy minimize the increased risk of having an LBW infant.[4] Furthermore, smoking increases the need for vitamin C, a nutrient that has increased intake requirements during pregnancy. For these reasons smoking is an important modifiable risk factor targeted by nursing interventions. Researchers reported that smoking cessation efforts among pregnant women are less successful among older women, those reporting Medicaid coverage, and those who have a partner/husband who also smoked.[5]

All pregnant women should be questioned about alcohol intake. Alcohol is a teratogen. No safe level of alcohol ingestion has been identified for the pregnant woman.[6] Advise the woman to avoid drinking alcoholic beverages entirely while pregnant. Fetal alcohol syndrome (birth defects in an infant born to a mother who consumed excessive amounts of alcohol during pregnancy) is a major public health problem.

The use of street drugs should also be explored with pregnant women. Many drugs (e.g., cocaine) are known teratogens; others have significant long-term effects on the infant after birth. Stimulants may affect the patient's appetite and therefore lead to decreased nutrient intake. Barbiturates and opiates may impair the patient's desire and ability to obtain food; in fact, in some cases the patient's resources may be used to obtain drugs instead of food. Patients who admit to drug use should be counseled and possibly referred to a drug treatment program. One study found that women who continue to use alcohol or other drugs are more frequent users, are more likely to smoke cigarettes, and have more psychosocial stressors than women who quit drug use with pregnancy.[7]

Environment

Pregnant women should be questioned about safety issues, including activities at work and in the home, routine safety practices such as use of seat belts while in a car, and the presence of physical abuse and violence in the home.

Problem-Based History

The health history includes questions related to the function of body systems. Following is an outline of common problems organized by body systems. Conduct a symptom analysis using the mnemonic OLD CARTS which includes Onset, Location, Duration, Characteristics, Aggravating factors, Related symptoms, Treatment measures, and Severity (see Box 2-3).

Fetal Assessments

- Report of fetal movements; frequency, time of day

Integumentary System

- Skin marks, lines, varicosities
- Pruritus

Nose and Mouth

- Nose bleeding or stuffiness
- Gum bleeding or swelling

Ears

- Changes in hearing
- Sense of fullness in ears

Eyes

- Excessive dryness
- Visual changes

Respiratory System

- Shortness of breath

Cardiovascular System

- Palpitations
- Edema of extremities
- Orthostatic hypotension (dizziness when standing up)

Breasts

- Enlargement, engorgement, tenderness
- Nipple discharge

Gastrointestinal System

- Nausea, vomiting (morning sickness), loss of appetite, food aversions
- Heartburn (gastric reflex), epigastric pain (second and third trimesters)
- Constipation (second and third trimesters)
- Hemorrhoids (second and third trimesters)

Genitourinary System

- Urinary pain, frequency, and urgency
- Vaginal discharge or bleeding

Musculoskeletal System

- Backache
- Leg cramps

Neurologic System

- Headaches

HEALTH PROMOTION FOR EVIDENCE-BASED PRACTICE

Maternal-Infant Health

Prenatal care can contribute to reductions in maternal and perinatal illness, disability, and death by identifying and minimizing potential risks and helping women address behavioral factors such as smoking and alcohol use that contribute to poor outcomes. Major maternal complications of pregnancy include hemorrhage, ectopic pregnancy, pregnancy-induced hypertension, embolism, and infection. The maternal mortality rate among African American women consistently has been three to four times that of Caucasian women. Prematurity and low birth weight (LBW) are among the leading causes of neonatal death. LBW is also associated with long-term disabilities.

Goals and Objectives—*Healthy People 2020*

The *Healthy* People *2020* goal related to maternal-fetal health is to improve the health and well-being of women, infants, children, and families. Objectives related to maternal-infant health generally fall into three categories: reduction of maternal

complications (maternal anemia, maternal illness, cesarean birth, maternal death), reduction of fetal or infant complications (LBW infants, preterm births, fetal/infant deaths), and enhanced health behaviors (increased number of women who receive prenatal care; increased number of women taking folic acid during pregnancy; and increased abstinence from alcohol, cigarettes, drug use).

Recommendations to Reduce Risk (Primary Prevention)
American College of Obstetricians and Gynecologists

- Counsel pregnant women about eating a healthy diet; encourage all women planning or capable of pregnancy to take daily multivitamins with folic acid to reduce risk of neural tube defects.
- Encourage healthy body weight during pregnancy.
- Encourage regular exercise while pregnant.
- Counsel patients regarding need to abstain from smoking, drug use, and alcohol use while pregnant. Remind patients

Continued

HEALTH PROMOTION FOR EVIDENCE-BASED PRACTICE

Maternal-Infant Health—cont'd

that over-the-counter medications are potentially harmful and to consult with health care provider.

- Counsel patients to avoid exposure to chemicals while pregnant.

Screening Recommendations (Secondary Prevention)
U.S. Preventive Services Task Force

- *Ultrasound:* It is unknown if routine ultrasound examination of the fetus in the second trimester is beneficial in low-risk pregnant women. Routine third-trimester ultrasound examination is not recommended.
- *Preeclampsia:* Screening for preeclampsia with blood pressure measurement in all pregnant women at first prenatal visit and throughout pregnancy is recommended.
- *Rh incompatibility:* Rh typing and antibody screening for all pregnant women at first prenatal visit are recommended.

Repeat screening is recommended at 24 to 28 weeks of gestation for unsensitized Rh-negative women.

- *Down syndrome:* Offering amniocentesis or chorionic villus sampling for chromosome studies for pregnant women age 35 or older and those at high risk for having a Down syndrome infant is recommended.
- *Neural tube defects:* Offering screening for neural tube defects by maternal serum alpha fetoprotein measurement at 16 to 18 weeks of gestation is recommended.
- *Anemia:* Screening for anemia among all pregnant women is recommended.
- *Sexually transmitted infection:* Screening for hepatitis B, human immunodeficiency virus, and syphilis among all pregnant women and for gonorrhea and chlamydial infections for pregnant women who are at high risk is recommended.

Data from American College of Obstetricians and Gynecologists website, available at *www.acog.org*; US Department of Health and Human Services: *Healthy People 2020,* available at *www.healthypeople.gov*); *US Preventive Services Task Force Recommendations*, available at http://www.uspreventiveservicestaskforce.org/recommendations.htm.

EXAMINATION

Positioning the pregnant patient for an examination is the same as discussed in previous chapters, with one exception: Be sure not to position the pregnant woman flat on her back for an extended length of time. The examination follows the same general process as a head-to-toe approach, although many nurses examine the abdomen just before the genitalia. Wash hands before beginning the examination.

PROCEDURES AND TECHNIQUES WITH EXPECTED FINDINGS	ABNORMAL FINDINGS

CLEAN hands.

VITAL SIGNS AND BASELINE MEASUREMENTS

MEASURE temperature, blood pressure, pulse, and respiration.

Vital signs are measured with every visit.
Pulse: The heart rate increases as much as 10 to 15 beats/min.

Respiration: Respiratory rate may increase slightly, especially during the third trimester; the patient may also experience shortness of breath.

Excessive shortness of breath and dyspnea are of concern and may indicate pulmonary complications such as embolus.

Blood pressure: Document blood pressure trends throughout pregnancy. Blood pressure should remain fairly consistent during pregnancy. It may decrease slightly in the second trimester and then return to the usual level during the third trimester. The approach to BP measurement should be consistent throughout pregnancy for accurate comparisons over time. Specifically, use the same arm, with an appropriate size cuff, with the patient in a sitting position.

Preexisting hypertension in pregnancy significantly increases risk of preterm delivery and infant mortality. Pregnancy-induced hypertension (PIH), also known as gestational hypertension, is a serious disorder that requires prompt and close medical management. It is characterized by systolic blood pressure of at least 140 mm Hg, a rise of 30 mm Hg or more above the usual level in two readings 6 hours apart, diastolic blood pressure of 90 mm Hg or more, or a rise of 15 mm Hg above baseline in two readings done 6 hours apart.

| **PROCEDURES AND TECHNIQUES WITH EXPECTED FINDINGS** | **ABNORMAL FINDINGS** |

MEASURE height and weight.

Height should be measured on the first visit. Weight should be measured with every visit. Prepregnancy weight may give the nurse insight into the woman's nutritional status. On the initial visit complete a weight-for-height assessment or body mass index (BMI) to determine an appropriate weight gain goal for pregnancy. Women with a normal prepregnancy BMI and those who meet appropriate weight gain goals are healthier and have healthier children.[8]

Evaluate the rate of weight change at each prenatal visit in addition to assessment of overall weight change. Expected patterns of weight gain are presented in Box 20-4. Generally, a total weight gain of 25 to 35 lbs (11.4 to 16 kg) is associated with positive pregnancy outcome for women with normal prepregnancy weight. Underweight women should gain more weight, whereas overweight women should gain somewhat less weight.

BOX 20-4	**EXPECTED WEIGHT GAIN DURING PREGNANCY**
First trimester	3-5 lbs (1.6-2.3 kg)
Second trimester	12-15 lbs (5.5-6.8 kg) ⎤
Third trimester	12-15 lbs (5.5-6.8 kg) ⎦ —Additional pounds

A prepregnancy BMI over 29 increases the risk of both inadequate and excessive weight gain during pregnancy.[9] A rapid increase in weight could indicate multiple gestation, preeclampsia, or diabetes associated with pregnancy (see Common Problems and Conditions on p. 512). If a woman gains more than 2 lbs (0.9 kg) in any 1 week or more than 6 lbs (2.7 kg) in 1 month, preeclampsia should be suspected.[10]

During the first trimester a weight loss of up to 5 lbs (2.3 kg) may be caused by nausea and vomiting. Poor weight gain or weight loss may be associated with a small-for–gestational age (SGA) infant or more serious complications such as placental dysfunction or fetal death in utero. LBW infants have more health problems than normal-weight infants; in one study low-birth-weight infants were 37 times more likely to die than normal-birth-weight infants.[11]

EXAMINATION OF THE EXTREMITIES

INSPECT the hands and nails for color, surface characteristics, edema, movement, and sensation.

Pinkish-red blotches or diffuse mottling of the hands caused by an increase in estrogen is termed *palmar erythema* and is considered an expected finding. The patient's nails may become thin and brittle. Women who take prenatal vitamins may report fast-growing, strong nails. Movement and sensation of fingers and hands should remain the same as previously discussed for the adult.

Although some edema is considered normal, excessive edema (particularly if noted on the hands, face, and lower extremities) is considered pathologic and may be an indication of PIH. Some pregnant patients may periodically report numbness of the fingers caused by a brachial plexus traction syndrome (caused by drooping shoulders associated with increased breast size and weight). A carpal tunnel syndrome caused by compression of the median nerve in the wrist and the hand may lead to symptoms of numbness, tingling, burning, and impaired finger movement. This typically affects the thumb and the second and third fingers (see Figs. 14-39 and 14-40).

INSPECT and PALPATE the lower extremities for edema, surface characteristics, redness, and tenderness.

Edema in the lower extremities is seen almost universally during the later stages of pregnancy. Typically women notice it late in the day or after long periods of standing. Palpating the legs helps to determine the extent of the edema (see Fig. 12-18). Vascular spiders or varicosities may appear on the lower legs and thighs and are considered normal findings. The legs should be free from redness and tenderness.

Edema not associated with preeclampsia or normal lower-extremity swelling should be evaluated for adequate protein intake. Redness in the legs, particularly if accompanied by tenderness, may be an indication of thrombophlebitis.

PROCEDURES AND TECHNIQUES WITH EXPECTED FINDINGS	ABNORMAL FINDINGS

EXAMINATION OF THE HEAD

INSPECT the head and face for skin characteristics, pigmentation, and edema.

Blotchy, brownish pigmentation of the face (i.e., chloasma, or the mask of pregnancy) is an expected finding (Fig. 20-1). There should be no facial edema. Fine, lanugo-type hair may be observed on the face and is an expected finding.

Facial edema is considered an abnormal finding and should be reported.

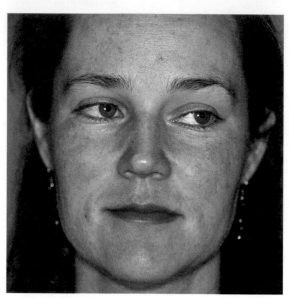

FIG. 20-1   Mask of pregnancy. (Courtesy Lemmi and Lemmi, 2013.)

INSPECT the eyes and TEST vision for acuity.

The eye examination should proceed as discussed in Chapter 10. Findings generally remain the same as previously discussed for the adult; however, the eyelids of some women may darken from melanin pigment. Visual acuity should be tested with the first visit to establish a baseline. Visual checks should be repeated if the patient verbalizes a change in vision during the pregnancy. Contact lenses may be uncomfortable to wear because of increased dryness. Both eyesight and the corrective prescription may change.

Pale conjunctivae may indicate anemia.

PIH may cause blurred vision. Chromatopsia may be noted, characterized by unusual color perception, seeing spots, or blindness in the lateral visual field. This requires immediate follow-up. Retinal arteriole constriction, disc edema, and retinal detachment (which is an emergency) are concerns; these may be caused by PIH.

INSPECT the ears, nose, and mouth.

The examination of the ears, nose, and mouth should proceed as discussed in Chapter 10. Findings generally are the same as previously discussed for the adult. However, the nurse may note an increase in vascularization of the external ear, the auditory canal, and the tympanic membrane. The nose and mouth of the pregnant woman also are associated with an increase in vascularization, causing redness in the nose, pharynx, and gums; the gums become edematous and spongy and may bleed easily. A normal variation seen in many women toward the end of the third trimester is an epulis. An epulis is hypertrophied gum tissue that presents as a small painless raised nodule.

Some women develop a pregnancy-induced tumor in the mouth. With the exception of hypertrophied gum tissue, any growth in the mouth is an abnormal finding.

PROCEDURES AND TECHNIQUES WITH EXPECTED FINDINGS	ABNORMAL FINDINGS

INSPECT and PALPATE the neck.

The examination of the neck and thyroid should proceed as discussed in Chapter 10. Findings generally are the same as previously discussed. There may be transient thyroid enlargement that makes the thyroid more easily palpable, but this disappears following delivery.

Excessive or asymmetric enlargement of the thyroid gland or nodules on the thyroid gland is an abnormal finding.

EXAMINATION OF THE ANTERIOR AND POSTERIOR CHEST

INSPECT, PERCUSS, PALPATE, and AUSCULTATE the anterior and posterior chest.

The examination of the anterior and posterior chest proceeds as discussed in Chapters 11 and 12. The findings are the same as in the adult female except as indicated below. If the patient is near term or has difficulty breathing when lying down, perform chest examination when she is in a sitting position.

The breathing pattern changes from abdominal to costal or lateral; likewise, it may be shallow with an increased respiratory rate. A wide thoracic cage and increased costal angle may be noted. Diaphragmatic excursion may decrease secondary to the growing fetus.

The heart shifts laterally in response to the positions of the uterus and diaphragm (Fig. 20-2). The point of maximum impulse also shifts upward and rotates slightly to the left. Murmurs, splitting of S_1 and S_2, and the presence of S_3 may be heard after the twentieth week of gestation.

Abnormal findings as discussed in Chapters 11 and 12 also apply to the pregnant patient. Dyspnea, orthopnea, fatigue, and palpitations may be attributed to the pregnancy but should be evaluated for other causes. Preexisting cardiac conditions may have pronounced symptoms because of the increased blood volume. Note any signs of heart failure. Note low blood pressure or tachycardia that occurs during this period.

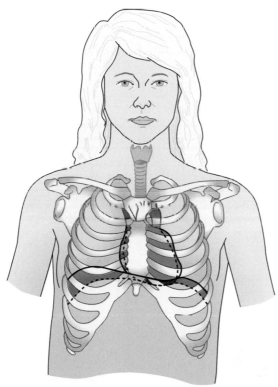

FIG. 20-2 Changes in position of heart, lungs, and thoracic cage during pregnancy. *Broken line,* nonpregnant; *solid line,* changes during pregnancy. (From Lowdermilk, Perry, and Cashion, 2010.)

PROCEDURES AND TECHNIQUES WITH EXPECTED FINDINGS	ABNORMAL FINDINGS

EXAMINATION OF THE BREAST

INSPECT and PALPATE the breast for surface and tissue characteristics.

Examine the breasts as described in Chapter 16. During the first trimester the breasts become fuller and have transient tenderness. As the pregnancy advances the breasts increase in size, and striae may develop. A subcutaneous venous pattern may be seen as a network of blue tracings across the breasts (Fig. 20-3). Palpation of the breasts reveals fullness and coarse nodularity. Following delivery breast engorgement peaks at about the third to fifth day. Engorged breasts may be very uncomfortable and painful. This is more pronounced in women who are not breastfeeding.

Note any asymmetry or appearance of attachment (fixation), bulging, or retraction of either breast. Abnormal findings during the breast palpation include masses or isolated areas of tenderness or pain.

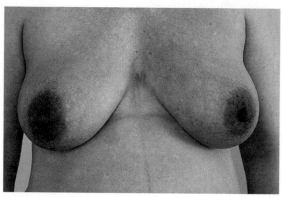

FIG. 20-3 Enlarged breasts in pregnancy with venous network and darkened areolae and nipples. (From Seidel et al., 2011.)

INSPECT and PALPATE the nipples for surface characteristics and nipple shape.

During the first trimester the nipples may become somewhat flattened or inverted. As pregnancy progresses the areolae become darker, and Montgomery's tubercles may appear. The nipples often protrude (Fig. 20-4). Press on the nipple just behind the areola to express any discharge and note whether the nipple protracts or inverts. Following the first trimester, colostrum may be expressed from the breast (a yellowish discharge).

Thickening of the nipple tissue, a mass, and loss of elasticity are signs consistent with malignancy. Nipple discharge is considered an abnormal finding (except for expression of colostrum as described).

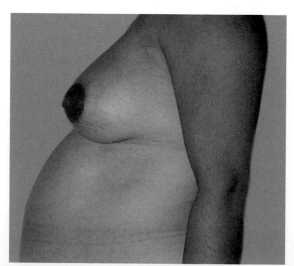

FIG. 20-4 Full-term pregnancy. Note enlargement of breasts, darkening of nipples, and lordotic curve. (Courtesy Lemmi and Lemmi, 2013.)

| PROCEDURES AND TECHNIQUES WITH EXPECTED FINDINGS | ABNORMAL FINDINGS |

EXAMINATION OF THE MUSCULOSKELETAL SYSTEM

INSPECT and PALPATE the spine, extremities, and joints.

Examination of the musculoskeletal system proceeds as described in Chapter 14. Changes that are expected during pregnancy include progressive lordosis, anterior cervical flexion, kyphosis, and slumped shoulders (Fig. 20-5). A characteristic "waddling" gait develops at the end of pregnancy.

Exaggerated posture or excessive activity can cause muscle strain. Pre-existing musculoskeletal conditions (e.g., chronic back pain) may become worse both during the pregnancy and after delivery. Muscle cramps, numbness, and weakness of the extremities are considered abnormal findings.

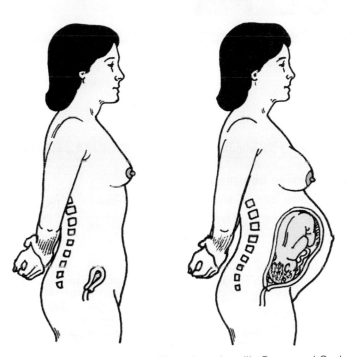

FIG. 20-5 Lordosis during pregnancy (From Lowdermilk, Perry, and Cashion, 2010.)

EXAMINATION OF THE NEUROLOGIC SYSTEM

EXAMINE the patient for neurologic changes.

Examine the patient as described in Chapter 15. Although the examination proceeds as for other adults, pregnancy alters balance. Assessment of deep tendon reflexes may also provide valuable data if the nurse suspects eclampsia.

Seizures or increased frequency of seizures associated with pregnancy is abnormal. Other abnormal findings are signs of myasthenia gravis, carpal tunnel syndrome (burning, pain, tingling in hand, wrist, or elbow), or hand numbness as a result of brachial plexus traction. These conditions return to prepregnant state after delivery. Hyperreflexia is an abnormal finding that may indicate eclampsia.

EXAMINATION OF THE ABDOMEN

INSPECT the abdomen for surface characteristics and fetal movement.

Common changes to the skin on the abdomen are linea nigra (Fig. 20-6), striae gravidarum, and venous patterns. After the twenty-eighth week, fetal movements may be observed.

Absence of fetal movement could indicate fetal demise.

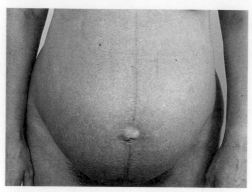

FIG. 20-6 Linea nigra on abdomen. (From Seidel et al., 2011.)

PROCEDURES AND TECHNIQUES WITH EXPECTED FINDINGS	ABNORMAL FINDINGS

PALPATE the abdomen for fetal movement and uterine contraction.

The mother should report fetal movements (also known as quickening) by approximately 20 weeks of gestation. Fetal movement and uterine contraction can be evaluated by placing the hands directly on the abdomen.

The absence of palpable fetal movement after 22 weeks is an abnormal finding.

MEASURE the fundus for height.

Enlargement of the uterus results in significant abdominal protrusion (see Fig. 20-4). Measure fundal height from the top of the symphysis pubis to the top of the fundus (Fig. 20-7). From the twentieth to thirty-sixth week of gestation, the expected pattern of uterine growth is an increase in fundal height of about 1 cm per week (Fig. 20-8). Uterine size should correlate roughly with gestational age. Measurement of fundal height is an estimate and may vary among nurses by 1 to 2 cm.

Any discrepancy greater than 2 cm between fundal height and the estimate of gestational age (based on last menstrual period) should be evaluated further. A uterus that is larger than expected may be caused by inaccurate dating of the pregnancy, more than one fetus, gestational diabetes, or polyhydramnios (excessive fluid in the uterus). A uterus that is smaller than expected for gestational age may be caused by inaccurate dating of the pregnancy or growth retardation of the fetus.

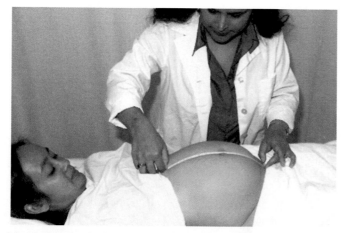

FIG. 20-7 Measuring fundal height. (Courtesy Chris Rozales, San Francisco, Calif. In Perry et al., 2010.)

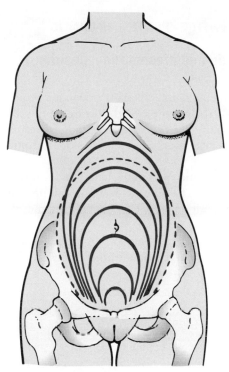

FIG. 20-8 Changes in fundal height during pregnancy. Weeks 1 through 12, the uterus is within the pelvis. Weeks 36 through 40, fundal height drops as the fetus begins to engage in the pelvis (lightening). (From Seidel et al., 2011.)

PROCEDURES AND TECHNIQUES WITH EXPECTED FINDINGS	**ABNORMAL FINDINGS**

AUSCULTATE the abdomen for fetal heart sounds.

Auscultation of fetal heart tones is performed by use of a Doppler ultrasonic stethoscope after 10 to 12 weeks of gestation or with a fetoscope after 17 to 19 weeks (Fig. 20-9). The fetal heart rate is usually heard over the lower abdomen for fetuses that are in a head-down position. The expected fetal heart rate ranges between 120 and 160 beats/min. (The Doppler and fetoscope are discussed in Chapter 3.)

Increases and decreases in fetal heart rate can be caused by multiple factors stressing the fetus. A fetal heart rate over 100 beats/min or below 120 beats/min requires further investigation. Absence of fetal heart tones is always abnormal and usually indicates fetal demise.

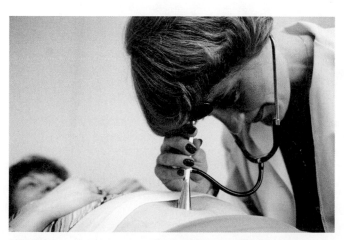

FIG. 20-9 Auscultating fetal heart tones with a fetoscope.

PROCEDURES AND TECHNIQUES WITH EXPECTED FINDINGS	ABNORMAL FINDINGS

★ PALPATE fetal position for fetal lie and presentation, position, and attitude.

The outline of the fetus can be determined after 26 to 28 weeks through a technique known as Leopold's maneuvers (Fig. 20-10). The patient should be lying supine, with head slightly elevated and knees flexed slightly. The fetal lie, presentation, position, and attitude can be determined through these maneuvers. See Table 20-3 for description of these terms.

Fundal palpation: This is done to determine which part of the fetus is at the fundus. Typically the feet or buttocks are at the fundus. The buttocks feel firm but not hard and slightly irregular. If the head is at the fundus, you will palpate a firm, movable part (see Fig. 20-10, *A*).

Lateral palpation: Palpate the sides of the uterus to identify the spine of the fetus. It is smooth and convex compared with the irregular feel on the other side of the fetus (i.e., the hands, elbows, knees, and feet) (see Fig. 20-10, *B*).

Inability to palpate the fetal position could be associated with polyhydramnios. A fetus with breech presentation or a transverse lie before delivery is of concern because of higher risks during the labor and delivery process.

★ Advanced practice.

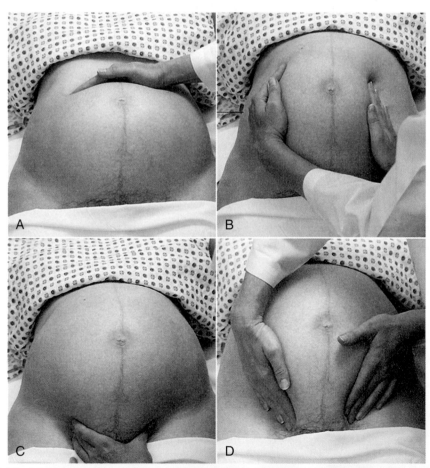

FIG. 20-10 Leopold's maneuvers. **A,** First maneuver. Place hand(s) over fundus and identify the fetal part. **B,** Second maneuver. Use palmar surface of one hand to locate the back of the fetus. Use other hand to feel the irregularities such as hands and feet. **C,** Third maneuver. Use thumb and third finger to grasp presenting part over the symphysis pubis. **D,** Fourth maneuver. Use both hands to outline the fetal head. With a head presenting deep in the pelvis, only a small portion may be felt. (Modified from Seidel et al., 2011.)

| **PROCEDURES AND TECHNIQUES WITH EXPECTED FINDINGS** | **ABNORMAL FINDINGS** |

Symphysis pubis palpation: This is done to assess which part of the fetus is in or just above the pelvic inlet and helps to determine if the presenting part is engaged. Gently grasp the presenting anatomic part over the symphysis pubis using your dominant hand. If the head is the presenting part, it feels very smooth, round, and firm. If it is movable from side to side and you are able to palpate all the way around it, the head is not engaged in the pelvis. If engaged, the head is not movable and is below the level of the symphysis, preventing palpation all the way around the head. The presenting part could also be the buttocks. The buttocks feel softer and irregular (see Fig. 20-10, *C*).

Deep pelvic palpation: If the head is the presenting part, palpation allows you to determine the position and attitude (see Fig. 20-10, *D*). Use both hands to identify the outline of the fetal head. Depending on the fetal position, the cephalic prominence can be either the forehead or the occiput.

EXAMINATION OF THE GENITALIA

INSPECT the external and internal genitalia for general appearance and discharge.

Follow the guidelines described in Chapter 17; the patient is placed in the lithotomy position for examination.

By the second month of pregnancy the cervix, vagina, and vulva take on a bluish color (Chadwick's sign); and there are increased vaginal secretions.

Note presence of infection of genitalia, including lesions or vaginal discharge with a foul odor. Leakage of watery fluid may be associated with preterm labor. During early pregnancy slight bleeding may occur for unknown reasons and be of no consequence, or it could indicate an impending abortion. During late pregnancy bleeding could be caused by abruptio placentae or placenta previa (discussed later in this chapter). Bleeding should never be considered a normal finding in pregnancy and should always be investigated thoroughly.

TABLE 20-3 FETAL ASSESSMENT TERMS

TERM	ILLUSTRATION
Fetal Lie The lie is the relationship of the long axis of the fetus to the long axis of the uterus. **A,** Longitudinal lie. **B,** Oblique lie. **C,** Transverse lie.	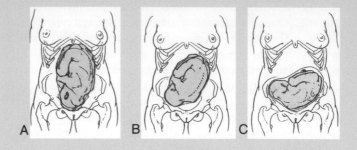
Presentation The presentation is determined by the fetal lie and by the body part of the fetus that enters the pelvic passage first. The presentation may be vertex, brow, face, shoulder, or breech. **A,** Vertex. **B,** Brow. **C,** Face. **D,** Shoulder. **E,** Breech.	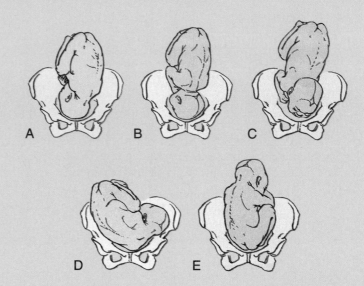
Position Position refers to the relationship of the landmark on the presenting fetal part to the front, sides, or back of the maternal pelvis. The landmark on the fetal presenting part is related to four imaginary quadrants of the pelvis: left anterior, right anterior, left posterior, and right posterior. These quadrants indicate whether the presenting part is directed toward the front, back, left, or right of the pelvic passage. **A,** Left occiput anterior. **B,** Left occiput transverse. **C,** Left occiput posterior.	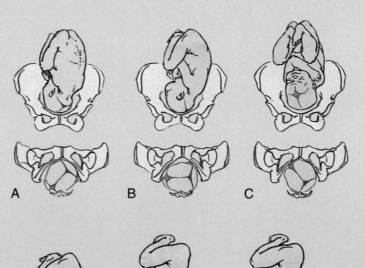
Attitude The attitude is the relationship of the fetal head and limbs to the body. **A,** Fully flexed. **B,** Poorly flexed. **C,** Extended.	

Illustrations from Barkauskas VH et al: *Health and physical assessment,* ed 3, St Louis, 2002, Mosby.

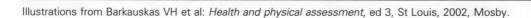

| **PROCEDURES AND TECHNIQUES WITH EXPECTED FINDINGS** | **ABNORMAL FINDINGS** |

★ PALPATE the cervix to determine length (effacement) and dilation.

During the last 4 weeks the cervix shortens (known as effacement) as the fetal head descends. Palpating for effacement and dilation is done near the expected date of delivery and once labor begins. The cervix should not efface until about the thirty-sixth week. The cervical os should remain closed until near delivery. The cervical os softens and is pulled upward, becoming incorporated into the isthmus of the uterus. As the cervix shortens, it also begins to dilate. Cervical dilation is measured in centimeters from 0 cm when completely closed to 10 cm when completely open. The effacement and dilation of the cervix are estimated by palpation (Fig. 20-11).

Effacement and dilation of the cervix before the thirty-sixth week may result in premature delivery. Failure of the cervical os to efface and dilate impedes the progression of labor. If the cervix has inadequate effacement and dilation at the onset of delivery, trauma to the cervix often results.

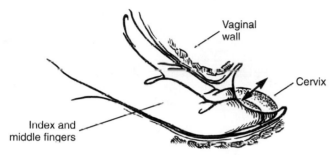

FIG. 20-11 Measurement of cervical length (effacement) and dilation. (From Barkauskus et al., 2002.)

EXAMINATION OF THE RECTUM AND ANUS

INSPECT and PALPATE the anus and rectum.

The perianal and rectal examination should be carried out in the pregnant woman as described in Chapter 17. The rectum and anus are commonly examined while the patient is in the lithotomy position with her legs up in stirrups. Early during pregnancy the patient should have minimal difficulty attaining and maintaining the position for the examination. However, later in pregnancy positioning for the rectal examination could be uncomfortable.

The presence of hemorrhoids, a common variation, is usually considered normal with pregnancy. The patient may not have hemorrhoids during the early phase of pregnancy, but toward the last trimester the hemorrhoids may appear secondary to pressure on the pelvic floor or possible constipation with straining when having a bowel movement. The hemorrhoids may be either internal in the lower segment of the rectum or prolapsed as external hemorrhoids.

Presence of lesions or rectal bleeding is considered an abnormal finding.

★ Advanced practice.

COMMON PROBLEMS AND CONDITIONS

RISK FACTORS
High-Risk Pregnancy

Maternal Characteristics
- Under 16 or over 35 years of age
- Marital status: Single (or lack of supporting relationship) (M)
- Short stature (less than 5 feet [150 cm] tall)
- Weight less than 100 lbs (45 kg) or over 200 lbs (91 kg) (M)
- Socioeconomic: Poverty, low education level (M)
- Lives at a high altitude (M)

Maternal Habits
- Alcohol consumption (M)
- Illicit drug use (M)
- Failure to obtain early prenatal care (M)
- Smoking (M)
- High-risk sexual behaviors (M)
- Poor diet (M)

Obstetric History
- Previous birth to infant weighing less than 2500 g
- Previous birth to infant weighing more than 4000 g
- Previous pregnancy ending in perinatal death
- More than two previous spontaneous abortions

- Birth to infant with congenital or perinatal disease
- Birth to infant with isoimmunization or ABO incompatibility

Current Medical Problems
- Chronic illnesses, including diabetes mellitus, thyroid disorder, heart disease, hypertension, pulmonary disease, renal failure, anemia, sickle cell disease
- Sexually transmitted disease
- Infectious disease (e.g., rubella or cytomegalovirus)

Problems with Current Pregnancy
- Bleeding
- Pregnancy-induced hypertension
- Eclampsia or preeclampsia
- Fetal position breech or transverse at term
- Polyhydramnios
- Multiple fetus (e.g., twins, triplets)
- Postmaturity (gestation >40 weeks)
- Premature rupture of membranes
- Weight gain that is inadequate or excessive

M, Modifiable risk factor.

ABRUPTIO PLACENTAE

The premature separation of the implanted placenta before the birth of the fetus is referred to as abruptio placentae (Fig. 20-12). This usually occurs during the third trimester, but it could occur as early as 20 weeks. The most important risk factor for abruptio placentae is maternal hypertension.[12] Because it is the most common cause of intrapartum fetal death, abruptio placentae is considered an obstetric emergency. **Clinical Findings:** Bleeding, abdominal pain, and uterine contractions are the three classic features of this complication. The blood is usually described as dark red, and the pain can range from mild to excruciating.

PLACENTA PREVIA

A placenta attachment in the lower uterine segment near or over the cervical os (as opposed to a more typical attachment higher in the uterus) is referred to as placenta previa (Fig. 20-13, *A* and *B*). This condition is often associated with premature rupture of membranes, preterm birth, anemia, infections, and postpartum hemorrhage.[10] **Clinical Findings:** The classic finding is painless vaginal bleeding most commonly during the third trimester, but bleeding can occur any time after 24 weeks. In a small percentage of women the bleeding is accompanied by mild uterine contractions. On palpation the uterus is typically soft and nontender.

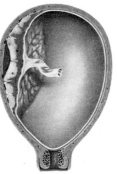
Partial separation
(concealed hemorrhage)

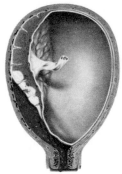
Partial separation
(apparent hemorrhage)

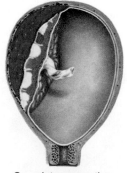
Complete separation
(concealed hemorrhage)

FIG. 20-12 Abruptio placentae. Premature separation of normally implanted placenta. (From Lowdermilk, Perry, and Cashion, 2010.)

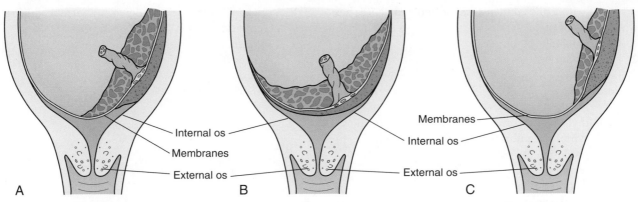

FIG. 20-13 Types of placenta previa after onset of labor. **A,** Low-lying placenta in second trimester. **B,** Placenta previa. **C,** Marginal placenta previa. (From Perry et al., 2010.)

HYDRAMNIOS (POLYHYDRAMNIOS)

An excessive quantity of amniotic fluid is referred to as *hydramnios*. It occurs in 1% to 2% of pregnancies; approximately half of the cases are idiopathic.[13] This is common in pregnancies with more than one fetus. In single-fetus pregnancies, it is associated with fetal malformation of the central nervous system and gastrointestinal tract. Hydramnios may result in perinatal death from premature labor and fetal abnormalities. **Clinical Findings:** Excessive uterine size, tense uterine wall, difficulty palpating fetal parts, and difficulty hearing fetal heart tones are common findings associated with this condition. The woman may also experience dyspnea, edema, and discomfort caused by pressure on the surrounding organs.

PREGNANCY-INDUCED HYPERTENSION

Pregnancy-induced hypertension (PIH) involves a group of hypertensive conditions during pregnancy in a previously normotensive patient. *Preeclampsia* refers to a condition of PIH with proteinuria and edema. *Eclampsia* is the occurrence of seizures precipitated by PIH in a preeclamptic patient. **Clinical Findings:** Hypertension in pregnancy is defined as follows: Systolic blood pressure is 140 mm Hg or higher; *or* there is an increase of more than 30 mm Hg of systolic blood pressure from baseline in the first half of pregnancy; *or* diastolic blood pressure is more than 90 mm Hg; *or* there is an increase of more than 15 mm Hg of diastolic blood pressure from baseline.[14]

PREMATURE RUPTURE OF MEMBRANES

A spontaneous rupture of uterine membranes before the onset of labor is referred to as *premature rupture of membranes (PROM)*. It can occur at any time during the pregnancy, but it is usually seen with term pregnancy. This situation is associated with a high risk of perinatal and maternal morbidity and mortality.[15] The cause of PROM is not known, although infection and hydramnios are thought to be associated factors. **Clinical Findings:** PROM manifests as passage of amniotic fluid from the vagina before labor

CLINICAL APPLICATION AND CLINICAL REASONING

See Appendix D for answers to exercises in this section.

REVIEW QUESTIONS

1. The nurse specifically assesses for which finding on every prenatal visit?
   1. Blood pressure
   2. Diastasis recti
   3. Personal habits (smoking, alcohol consumption)
   4. Visual acuity

2. During an initial prenatal visit the nurse identifies which factor as consistent with a high-risk pregnancy?
   1. Patient is 18 years old
   2. Patient height is 5 feet 4 inches
   3. Birth weight of infant with last pregnancy was 2800 g
   4. Patient smokes one-half pack of cigarettes a day

3. A patient with a missed menstrual period and nausea has which signs of pregnancy?
   1. Questionable
   2. Presumptive
   3. Probable
   4. Positive

4. What is the nurse assessing when measuring from the patient's symphysis pubis to the top of the fundus?
   1. Fetal development
   2. Fetal lie and position
   3. Attitude of the fetus
   4. Gestational age

5. Which finding is considered abnormal during late pregnancy?
   1. Watery vaginal discharge
   2. Hemorrhoids
   3. Lordosis
   4. Abdominal striae

CASE STUDY

Kristin Walters is a 17-year-old pregnant patient (G^1, T^0, P^0, A^0, L^0) who is in her thirtieth week of pregnancy. She comes to the clinic for a routine prenatal visit. The following data are collected by the nurse.

Interview Data

Ms. Walters tells the nurse, "I've been feeling pretty good the last few weeks; but I've noticed that my feet, hands, and face are getting so puffy. I feel like I'm full of water." When asked about other symptoms or problems, Kristin responds, "I have a backache sometimes." Ms. Walters indicates that she feels the baby move "all the time now." She conveys to the nurse that she is excited about the baby but is very worried about how bad the labor pain will be. "My friend Shawna told me that the pain is so bad that I'll want to be knocked out when it's time to have the baby."

Examination Data

*   *Vital signs:* BP, 154/96 mm Hg (prepregnancy BP reading, 114/70 mm Hg—within normal limits up until this visit);

pulse, 92 beats/min; respiration rate, 18 breaths/min; temperature, 98.3° F (36.8° C).
*   *Weight:* 152 lbs (69 kg) (prepregnancy weight, 116 lbs [52.7 kg]). She has had an increase of 10 lbs (4.5 kg) in last month.
*   *Fundal height:* 31 cm.
*   *Urine dipstick:* 3+ protein.

Clinical Reasoning

1. Which data deviate from normal findings, suggesting a need for further investigation?
2. For which additional information should the nurse ask or assess?
3. Based on the data, which risk factors for high-risk pregnancy does this patient have?
4. With which additional health care professionals should you consider collaborating to meet her health care needs?

Assessment of the Older Adult

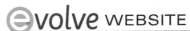
Aging is a normal developmental process that begins at conception. There is no specific age at which one becomes old: everyone ages at a different rate. Biologic, social, and functional ages are more important than chronological age. A suggested classification based on age is shown[1]:

- Young-old: 65-74 years
- Middle-old: 75-84 years
- Older-old: 85 years and older

Approximately 13% of the U.S. population is age 65 years and older, and the percentage will increase to 20% by 2050. The fastest growing age-group in terms of percentage is those ages 60 to 64.[2] Terms related to aging are described:

- *Life expectancy:* The number of years one can be expected to live based on year of birth or current age. In 1900 it was 47 years, while in 1950 it increased to 68 years. In 2005 the life expectancy for women was 80.1

years and for men it was 74.8 years, with an average of 77.5 years. By 2040, life expectancy is predicted to be 91.5 years for woman and 86 years for men.

- *Life span:* The number of years that human beings are probably capable of living is estimated to be about 110 to 120.

Being physically, mentally, and socially active into the 100s is considered normal. High blood pressure, pain, urinary incontinence, and severe memory loss are not a part of healthy aging. Although aging is not a disease, the incidence of chronic health problems increases with advanced age. Therefore nurses must know the difference between healthy aging and disease and not assume that clinical manifestations of disease are caused by age alone. Healthy lifestyle behaviors such as nutrition, regular exercise, and sleep are very important; it is never too late to improve these behaviors.

ANATOMY AND PHYSIOLOGY

As adults grow older, they experience gradual changes in every body system. Thus nurses must recognize the expected anatomic and physiologic changes of older adults and understand how these expected changes may alter the functioning of people in these age-groups. Box 21-1 presents some of the expected changes associated with older adults.

HEALTH HISTORY

Nurses interview patients to collect subjective data about their present health status, past medical history, and personal and psychosocial history. The health history for older adults is similar to that presented in Chapter 2. However, clinical manifestations may be vague and/or different from those that usually occur in younger adults. The most common and important differences that may be noted on assessment of older people are presented in this chapter. Of the IOM Core Competencies, providing patient-centered care and interdisciplinary teamwork apply to older adults. Table 11-1 on p. 196 presents knowledge, skills, and attitudes to use when demonstrating patient-centered care and interdisciplinary teamwork.

BOX 21-1   SELECTED ANATOMIC AND PHYSIOLOGIC CHANGES ASSOCIATED WITH OLDER ADULTS

Skin, Hair, and Nails

- Decreased sebaceous and sweat gland activity causes dry skin and less perspiration.
- The dermis loses elasticity, collagen, and mass, causing folding and wrinkling appearance.[1]
- Loss of subcutaneous fat impairs heat regulation related to hypothermia.[3]
- Reduced blood flow to the dermis accounts for skin pallor and cooler skin temperature.[3]
- Decreased melanin production tends to produce gray hair; and reduced hormonal functioning causes thinning of scalp, axillary, and pubic hair.
- The nails become thicker, brittle, hard, and yellowish; they also develop ridges and are prone to splitting into layers.

Head, Eyes, Ears, Nose, and Throat

- Pupillary response to light is decreased.[4]
- Corneal sensitivity often is diminished so older adults may be unaware of infection or injury.
- Loss of lens elasticity is termed *presbyopia*.
- Night vision and depth perception are decreased.[4]
- Color perception is altered, with difficulty seeing blue, violet, and green.[1]
- A decrease in active sebaceous glands causes the cerumen to become very dry; it may completely obstruct the external auditory canal, resulting in diminished hearing.
- Both conductive and sensorineural hearing losses occur with aging. *Conductive hearing loss* occurs when the tympanic membrane becomes sclerotic. *Sensorineural hearing loss* develops as the hair cells in the organ of Corti begin to degenerate, usually after age 50. Hearing loss first occurs with high-frequency sounds and progresses to lower-frequency tones.
- A decreased sense of smell is caused by a decrease in the number of sensory cells in the nasal lining.
- Gingival tissue is less elastic and more vulnerable to injury. The root surfaces of the teeth are exposed to caries formation. As teeth lose their translucency, they darken and become worn from use.
- Decreased saliva production contributes to a dry mouth.[4]
- Taste perception may diminish as a result of gradual atrophy of the tongue and a decrease in the number of papillae and taste buds.
- Muscle weakness may result in chewing and swallowing difficulties.
- The size of the thyroid decreases as a result of atrophy.
- Increased concave cervical curvature causes forward and downward positioning of the head.
- Lymph nodes may decrease in both size and number with advanced age.

Respiratory System

- Diminished strength of the respiratory muscles results in diminished breath sounds in the bases and reduced maximal inspiratory and expiratory force.

- Kyphoscoliosis, a common finding associated with aging, causes the thorax to shorten and the anteroposterior diameter to increase.
- The chest wall may become stiffer, possibly because of calcification at rib articulation points, resulting in decreased chest wall compliance.
- As the alveoli become less elastic and more fibrous, dyspnea on exertion becomes more frequent.
- Fewer cilia make mucociliary clearance less effective. In addition, mucous membranes become drier and less able to clear retained mucus.[1]

Cardiovascular System

- Increased arterial resistance contributes to hypertension.[4]
- Cardiac output is decreased by 30% to 40%.[4]
- Orthostatic hypotension may contribute to falls.[4]
- An S_4 heart sound can be heard.[4]

Gastrointestinal System

Many of the changes in the function of digestion and absorption of nutrients result from alterations in the cardiovascular and neurologic systems rather than the gastrointestinal (GI) system.

- Motility of the entire GI system is slowed, causing a decrease in transit time through the intestines.
- Decreased motility and lower esophageal pressure increase likelihood of regurgitation.
- Bacterial flora in the intestines become less biologically active, contributing to food intolerance and impaired digestion.
- Decrease in internal sphincter tone and sensation may contribute to occasional fecal incontinence.
- The bladder decreases in size, shape, and muscle tone, which can cause more frequent urination and increase likelihood of stress incontinence.

Musculoskeletal System

- A decrease in bone mass increases the risk for stress fractures. Intervertebral disk space narrows, which results in a loss of height.
- The lordotic or convex curve of the back flattens, and both flexion and extension of the back decrease. Increased flexion of the back changes the posture to a more flexed position, which in turn changes the center of gravity.
- Tendons and muscles decrease in elasticity and tone, with the muscles losing both mass and strength.

Neurologic System

- Speed of fine-motor movement decreases.[4]
- Deep tendon reflexes diminish.[4]
- Functional changes in sensory and motor function, memory, cognition, and proprioception occur at different rates. Short-term memory (e.g., of names and recent events) may decline with age, but long-term memory is usually maintained.
- Older adults have more difficulty falling asleep, spend less time sleeping deeply, and report a greater number of early-morning awakenings.[5]

BOX 21-1 SELECTED ANATOMIC AND PHYSIOLOGIC CHANGES ASSOCIATED WITH OLDER ADULTS—cont'd

Reproductive System

Female Genitourinary System

- After menopause the labia and clitoris become smaller and paler.
- The vaginal introitus may diminish in size, with a shortening and narrowing of the vagina and a thinning and drying of the vaginal mucosa.
- The uterus and ovaries decrease in size; the ovarian follicles gradually disappear.

Male Genitourinary System

- Hyperplasia of the prostate is associated with aging.

Breast

- Before menopause a moderate decrease in glandular breast tissue occurs. After menopause the glandular tissue in the breast continues to atrophy and is replaced by fat and connective tissue.
- Changes to the breast tissue and the relaxation of the suspensory ligaments result in a tendency for the breast to hang more loosely from the chest wall, giving it a flattened appearance.

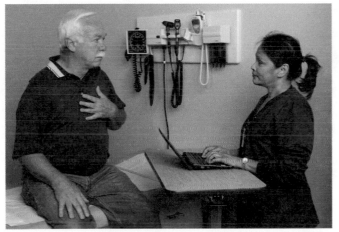

FIG. 21-1 During the interview maintain eye contact and give the patient time to explain symptoms.

When obtaining a health history from an older adult, seek information directly from the patient first, if possible, rather than from relatives who may accompany the patient (Fig. 21-1). During the interview maintain eye contact so the patient can see the movements of the mouth, which helps if there is a hearing problem. Observe for hearing or vision deficits that will affect data collection.

GENERAL HEALTH HISTORY

Present Health Status

Data collected are the same as described in Chapter 2.

Past Health History

Data collected in this section are the same as those described in Chapter 2. Note any chronic illnesses such as diabetes mellitus, osteoarthritis, cardiovascular, and neurologic conditions. Obviously the time span included in the history is longer, and the patient's memory may affect accuracy. Review all medications that the patient is taking. Older adults often take many medications prescribed by more than one health care provider. Specifically ask about allergies and adverse

effects with the medications and if the patient has problems getting access to the drugs (because of financial or transportation restraints). Also ask about immunizations the patient has had such as influenza and pneumococcal vaccines.

Family History

Although the family history provides data about illnesses and the causes of death of relatives, the value of this information for an older adult is questionable. A genogram is not used routinely to document the family history for an older adult.

Personal and Psychosocial History

Many of the aspects of personal and psychosocial history are the same as those previously described for the younger adult. However, a shift in focus in this section reflects changes in roles and perceptions during the retirement years.

Personal Status

Ask the patient for a general statement of feelings about self. Explore the following subjects: work/retirement concerns, reduced/fixed income, moving/selling home, living alone, and role changes.

Family and Social Relationships

Ask about current living arrangements (family members, living alone), satisfaction with living arrangements, sufficient and satisfactory access to family and friends, presence of a pet in the home, participation in family activities and family decisions, presence of conflict with family members, and problems in relationship with the spouse.

Diet/Nutrition

Ask about any decrease in appetite, changes in the taste of food, decrease in saliva, and difficulty chewing or swallowing.

Functional Ability

The functional ability or functional assessment focuses on a person's ability to perform in two areas. The first area is performing self-care activities or *basic activities of daily living*

	Independence (1 point) NO supervision, direction, or personal assistance	Dependence (0 points) WITH supervision, direction, personal assistance, or total care
BATHING Points:_____	(1 point) Bathes self completely or needs help in bathing only a single part of the body, such as the back, genital area, or disabled extremity.	(0 points) Needs help with bathing more than one part of the body, getting in or out of the tub or shower. Requires total bathing.
DRESSING Points:_____	(1 point) Gets clothes from closets and drawers and puts on clothes and outer garments complete with fasteners. May have help tying shoes.	(0 points) Needs help with dressing self or needs to be completely dressed.
TOILETING Points:_____	(1 point) Goes to toilet, gets on and off the toilet, arranges clothes, cleans genital area without help.	(0 points) Needs help transferring to the toilet, cleaning self, or uses bedpan or commode.
TRANSFERRING Points:_____	(1 point) Moves in and out of bed or chair unassisted. Mechanical transferring aids are acceptable.	(0 points) Needs help in moving from bed to chair or requires a complete transfer.
CONTINENCE Points:_____	(1 point) Exercises complete self- control over urination and defecation.	(0 points) Is partially or totally incontinent of bowel or bladder.
FEEDING Points:_____	(1 point) Gets food from plate into mouth without help. Preparation of food may be done by another person.	(0 points) Needs partial or total help with feeding or requires parenteral feeding.

TOTAL POINTS: _____   6 = High (patient independent)   0 = Low (patient very dependent)

FIG. 21-2 Katz Index of Independence in Activities of Daily Living. (From Katz et al., 1970.)

(BADLs), which include skills such as dressing, toileting, bathing, eating, and ambulating. The second area is called *instrumental activities of daily living (IADLs),* which consist of skills that enable the patient to function independently and include preparation of meals, shopping, safe use of medications, management of finances, and ability to travel within the community.[3] Ask the patient (or other family member) to describe his or her ability (independent, partially independent, or dependent) to perform these activities. Fig. 21-2 shows the Katz Index of Independence in Activities of Daily Living, which is one tool used to assess functional ability.

Mental Health

Include a general statement about the patient's ability to cope with stress (you may also want to obtain input from a spouse, adult child, or close friend); recent changes or stresses in the patient's life (e.g., moving, retirement, illness of self or family member, financial stress, death of friend or family member); feelings or symptoms of depression (e.g., insomnia, crying, fearfulness, marked irritability, or anger); changes in personality, behavior, or mood; and use of medications or other techniques during times of anxiety, stress, or depression. Emotional experiences of sadness, grief, response to loss, and

temporary "blue" moods are expected responses in older adults. However, depression is not expected. Those with persistent depression that interferes significantly with ability to function need to be referred for treatment.[6] The Yesavage Geriatric Depression Scale Short Form has been validated for use with this age-group (Fig. 21-3).

Sleep

Ask the patient about the quality of sleep and any problems that he or she may be experiencing. Sleep depth and efficiency decline with age. As a person ages, the proportion of time spent in deep sleep (stages 3 and 4, the most restorative sleep) decreases, whereas the time spent in light sleep (stage 1) increases. The proportion of time spent in rapid eye movement (REM) sleep also decreases slightly. Sleep is less efficient, as evidenced by the need of the older adult to spend more time in bed to achieve the same amount of restorative sleep as when he or she was younger.[5] Sleep complaints of older adults are frequently secondary to chronic health problems, and they often are interrelated: health problems interrupt sleep, and sleep disruptions contribute to health problems. Pain, sleep apnea, shortness of breath, and restless leg syndrome frequently interfere with sleep of older adults.

Yesavage Geriatric Depression Scale, Short Form

Read the following 15 questions. Circle the response *(yes or no)* at the end of the question if it applies to you; that is, if it describes how you are feeling. If the answer given at the end of the question does NOT apply to you, then do not write anything for that question.

1. Are you basically satisfied with your life? (no)
2. Have you dropped many of your activities and interests? (yes)
3. Do you feel that your life is empty? (yes)
4. Do you often get bored? (yes)
5. Are you in good spirits most of the time? (no)
6. Are you afraid that something bad is going to happen to you? (yes)
7. Do you feel happy most of the time? (no)
8. Do you often feel helpless? (yes)
9. Do you prefer to stay home at night, rather than go out and do new things? (yes)
10. Do you feel that you have more problems with memory than most? (yes)
11. Do you think it is wonderful to be alive now? (no)
12. Do you feel pretty worthless the way you are now? (yes)
13. Do you feel full of energy? (no)
14. Do you feel that your situation is hopeless? (yes)
15. Do you think that most persons are better off than you are? (yes)

Score 1 point for each response that matches the yes or no answer after the question.

FIG. 21-3 Yesavage Geriatric Depression Scale, Short Form. (From Yesavage and Brink, 1983.)

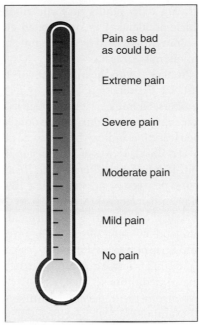

FIG. 21-4 Vertical pain scale. (Used with permission of Keela Herr, PhD, RN, AGSF, FAAN, The University of Iowa.)

Inquire about daytime napping; an increase in the number or length of naps during the day may indicate or contribute to a sleep problem during the night.

Tobacco, Alcohol, and Illicit Drug Use

• Alcohol use: Ask how many alcoholic drinks the patient has in a week. The National Institute on Alcohol Abuse and Alcoholism (NIAAA) recommends that men and women ages 65 and older have no more than seven alcoholic drinks per week.[7] Misuse and abuse of alcohol is becoming a problem among people over the age of 50. Among adults ages 65 and older, 7.6% reported binge drinking (five or more drinks on the same occasion and at least one occasion in the last 30 days). Excessive drinking increases the risk of falls and accidents; depresses mood; and complicates chronic diseases such as diabetes mellitus, hypertension, and gastroesophageal reflux disease.[8]

Environment

Data on environmental safety and comfort should be gathered with a specific focus on problems unique to older adults.

• Hazards in the home: Inadequate heating or cooling, stairs to climb (stairs without handrails, steep stairs), fear of falling, gait or balance problems, slippery or irregular surfaces in home (including throw rugs), inadequate space for maneuvering walker or wheelchair, inadequate lighting in dark hallway/stairs, statement by the patient related to abuse or neglect
• Hazards in the neighborhood: Noise, water, and air pollution; safety concerns; heavy traffic on surrounding streets; overcrowding; isolation from neighbors

Review of Systems

The review of systems is the same as that for the adult; specific components commonly associated with older adults follow.

General Symptoms

• Pain: Questions asked in the pain assessment are the same as those described for the younger adult. Some older adults may perceive pain as an expected aspect of aging that they must endure. They may manifest pain as fatigue, lethargy, or anorexia. For older adults better success has been reported with the use of a numeric rating scale that is vertically oriented (Fig 21-4).[9,10]

Skin, Hair and Nails

• Skin: Excessive dryness or thinning of skin that tears easily
• Hair: Changes in texture or distribution
• Nails: Changes in thickness

Head, Eyes, Ears, Nose, and Throat

• Vision: Recent changes in or problems with near, distant, and peripheral vision and problems with night vision or the ability to recognize colors. These common visual changes among older adults may contribute to falls or motor vehicle accidents. Dry or irritated eyes are a frequent symptom experienced by older adults because of the decrease in quantity of tears.

- Hearing: Problems with hearing; use of hearing aids; date of last ear examination. Asking older patients (or family members) about hearing problems is an effective hearing screening method during periodic health assessments. The Hearing Handicap Inventory for the Elderly—Screening (HHIS-S) is a self-administered instrument effective in identifying patients with hearing impairment.[11] Scores between 0 and 8 indicate a 13% probability of a hearing impairment, scores of 10 to 24 indicate a 50% probability of a hearing impairment, and scores between 26 and 40 indicate an 84% probability of a hearing impairment.[12]
- Nose and mouth: Dry nose and mouth may be an adverse effect of many medications.
- Mouth: Use of prosthetic devices (dentures) and date of last dental examination. Ask specifically if the patient is experiencing difficulty chewing and swallowing. These problems may be caused by a number of things (e.g., ill-fitting dentures, dental pain, neuromuscular conditions, and esophageal motility) and can lead to inadequate nutritional intake aspiration.

Respiratory System

- Fatigue, shortness of breath, cough: Ask about these symptoms of respiratory disorders. The incidence of chronic respiratory disease is higher in older adults.

Cardiovascular System

- Dizziness, blackouts, fainting, palpitations: Atherosclerosis may interfere with blood flow to the brain, causing confusion, dizziness, or fainting.
- Chest pain, fatigue, shortness of breath with exertion or at night, edema in the legs or feet: These symptoms may be associated with coronary artery disease or heart failure; risk of heart disease increases with age.
- Pain, discoloration, coldness, chronic wounds in legs or feet: These symptoms may indicate poor peripheral circulation or heart disease and are more common among older adults.

Gastrointestinal System

- Abdominal pain: Older adults often have nonspecific signs and symptoms of abdominal pain. Frequent manifestations of abdominal disorders may be low-grade fever, tachycardia, and vague abdominal discomfort.
- Constipation: Constipation is a common problem of older adults that may not be reported voluntarily. Ask about frequency of bowel movements and consistency of stool.

Urinary System

- Urgency, frequency, and incontinence: Ask about urine leakage since patient may be reluctant to report it. Ask

when the leakage occurs. Leakage that occurs when sneezing, lifting, or laughing suggests stress incontinence; whereas a strong urge to void more often than every 2 hours suggests urge incontinence. Ask how long the leakage has been experienced. Incontinence for less than 6 months is considered transient and usually reversible.[13]

- Difficulty starting urinary stream: Enlargement of the prostate, which is a common condition among older men, may cause hesitancy, weak urinary stream, and incomplete bladder emptying.

Musculoskeletal System

- Changes in muscle strength, joint pain: Independence in activities of daily living may be interrupted by muscle weakness or joint pain.
- Mobility, gait, balance, use of assistive devices (walker, cane, wheelchair): The degree, ease, and confidence related to mobility and assistive devices provide information about how patients maintain independence or suggest ways that these devices could be used. Mobility aids can prevent falls and improve independence.
- Recent falls and fall prevention, use of assistive devices in home (such as grab bars): Discussing fall prevention with older adults is important. Fall risk is categorized according to intrinsic (illness- or disease-related) or extrinsic (environmental) factors. Inquire about potential hazards in the environment such as steps, throw rugs, inadequate light, and curbs.
- A risk of fall assessment tool is shown in Box 21-2.

Neurologic System

The review of systems for the neurologic system is the same as that for the younger adult.

Reproductive System

- Women: Vaginal itching or dryness: Physiologic changes may cause a decrease in vaginal fluids.
- Women: Vaginal bleeding: Postmenopausal bleeding may have many causes, from friable vaginal tissue to cancer of the uterus. If the patient has postmenopausal bleeding, she should be referred to a health care provider for further evaluation.
- Sexual activity: Sexual activity is normal at any adult age. Ask about any concerns or questions the patient has about fulfilling sexual needs. Also ask how the patient's sexual relationship with the partner has changed with age.[14] If the patient reports physical difficulties that interfere with sexual activity, the nurse assesses what they are, how much they interfere, and what the patient or partner has done to resolve the difficulty. Intercourse may be painful for women because of vaginal dryness secondary to hormonal changes. Older adults may welcome the opportunity to discuss sexual issues; this can be a time of education and encouragement. Some drugs depress sexual function (e.g., antihypertensives, sedatives, tranquilizers, and alcohol).

BOX 21-2 RISK FOR FALLS ASSESSMENT TOOL: FALL ASSESSMENT SCORING SYSTEM

I. Age

65-79 years	1
80 and above	2

II. Mental Status

A. Oriented at all times or comatose	0
Confusion at all times	2
Intermittent confusion	4
B. Agitated/uncooperative/anxious-moderate	2
Agitated/uncooperative/anxious-severe	4

III. Elimination

Independent and continent	0
Catheter and/or ostomy	1
Elimination with assistance	3
Ambulatory with urge incontinence or episodes of incontinence	5

IV. History of Falling Within 6 Months

No history	0
Has fallen one or two times	2
History of multiple falls	5

V. Sensory Impairment

Sensory impairment (blind, deaf, cataracts, not using corrective device)	1

VI. Activity

Ambulation/transfer without assistance	0
Ambulation/transfer with aid of one or assistive devices	2
Ambulation/transfer with aid of two assistive devices	1

VII. Medications

- Narcotics
- Tranquilizers
- Sleeping aids
- Diuretics
- Chemotherapy
- Antiseizure/antiepileptic

For the above medications, check how many the patient is taking currently at home or that the patient will be taking in the hospital.

No medications	0
1 medication	1
2 or more medications	2

Add one more point if there has been a change in these medications or dosages in the past 5 days.

Score _____

A score of 10 or more indicates a high risk for falling. Initiate a high-risk protocol.

If the patient does not meet a score of 10 but in the nurse's judgment is at risk to fall, initiate the high-risk fall protocol.

From MacAvoy S, Skinner T, Hines M: Clinical methods: fall risk assessment tool, *Appl Nurs Res* 9(4):213, 218, 1996.

EXAMINATION

OVERVIEW: THE OLDER ADULT PHYSICAL EXAMINATION

An examination of an older adult proceeds as described for the younger adult. The nurse assesses the patient's level of comfort in different positions needed for the examination. The examination description that follows highlights expected and abnormal findings of the older adult.

VITAL SIGNS AND BASELINE MEASUREMENTS

Vital signs are measured with every visit. The procedures for assessing vital signs are the same as for the younger adult.

Temperature

The expected temperature is usually lower for older adults (97.2° F, 36.2° C) because of decreased metabolism and less physical activity. Older adults are especially prone to hypothermia. If the patient's expected oral temperature is 94° F (34.4° C), a temperature of 98° F (36.6° C) may indicate a fever.

Heart and Respiratory Rates

Heart and respiratory rates are assessed for the same qualities as in the younger adult. Pulse rates do not differ from those of younger adults unless the patient has heart or peripheral vascular disease. Note the pulse rate, rhythm, amplitude, and contour of the radial pulse. Unless the patients have lung disorder, their respiratory rates do not differ from those of other adults, although breathing may be more shallow and rapid.

Blood Pressure

Use the appropriate-size blood pressure cuff for an accurate reading (see Chapter 4).

Expected blood pressure values are the same as for younger adults unless the patient has hypertension or heart disease. Although blood pressure elevations frequently occur in older adults, they are not considered a normal variation. Isolated systolic hypertension (>140 mm Hg) is frequently seen in older adults as a result of atherosclerotic changes.[15]

Height and Weight

Height and weight are measured in the same manner as described for the younger adult. If the scale does not have a handle close by on which to hold, stand close to the scale because some older people may have a problem standing on a small surface off the floor. The height and weight are used to determine the body mass index (BMI) using Table 8-5.

Expected and Abnormal Findings. *Height:* Decreased bone formation reduces height in most older adults, which may cause shortening of the vertebrae and thinning of the vertebral disks. Decreases in height may occur more often in women because of osteoporosis. *Weight:* For those in their eighties and beyond, body weight may decrease because of muscle wasting or chronic diseases. The total body water declines, which contributes to weight loss. Subcutaneous fat distribution shifts from the face and extremities to the abdomen and hips.

EXAMINATION OF THE SKIN, HAIR, AND NAILS

Procedures and techniques for assessing skin, hair, and nails of an older adult are the same as those described in Chapter 9 (Fig. 21-5).

Skin

Two common concerns with the skin of an older adult are sun exposure and signs of abuse. Inspect the sun-exposed areas such as nose, lips, and ears for color and lesions. The American Medical Association recommends screening all older-adult patients for mistreatment.[16] Selected items from the Elder Assessment Instrument (EAI) are included in the skin assessment. Notice bruising or lacerations, pressure ulcers, dehydration, and poor hygiene, which may be indications of mistreatment.[17] More information about geriatric screening and assessment tools is available at www.ConsultGeriRN.org.

Expected and Abnormal Findings. As skin thins it takes on a parchment-like appearance, especially over bony prominences, the dorsal surfaces of the hands and feet, the forearms, and the lower legs (Fig. 21-6). The skin hangs loosely on the frame, secondary to a loss of adipose tissue and elasticity. The skin may be cool because of impaired circulation. Skin tears may occur as a result of thin, fragile texture. Normal variations in the skin of the older adult include findings such as the following:

* *Solar lentigo (liver spots):* Irregularly shaped, flat, deeply pigmented macules that may appear on body surface areas having repeated exposure to the sun (Fig. 21-7).

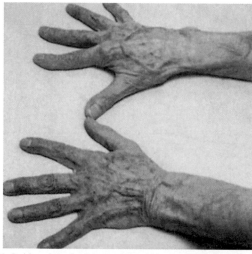

FIG. 21-6 Hands of older adult. Note prominent veins and thin appearance of the skin. (From Seidel et al., 2011.)

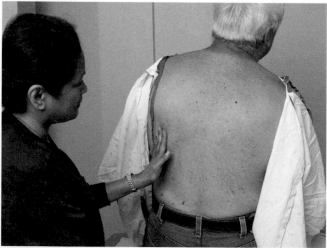

FIG. 21-5 After inspection palpate the skin for texture, temperature, moisture, mobility, turgor, and thickness.

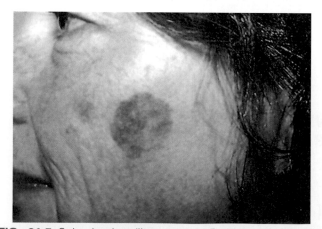

FIG. 21-7 Solar lentigo (liver spots). Brown macules that appear in chronically sun-exposed areas. (From Goldstein and Goldstein, 1997. Courtesy Department of Dermatology, University of North Carolina at Chapel Hill.)

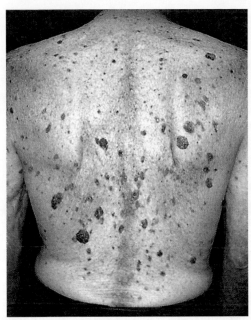

FIG. 21-8 Multiple seborrheic keratosis lesions on the trunk. (From Goldstein and Goldstein, 1997. Courtesy Department of Dermatology, Medical College of Georgia.)

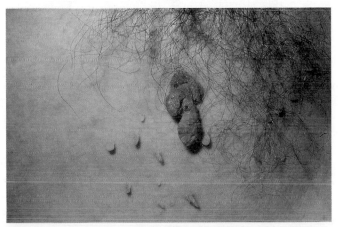

FIG. 21-9 Multiple skin tags. (From Goldstein and Goldstein, 1997. Courtesy Department of Dermatology, University of North Carolina at Chapel Hill.)

- *Seborrheic keratoses:* Pigmented, raised, warty-appearing lesions that may appear on the face or trunk (Fig. 21-8). Differentiate these benign lesions from similar-appearing actinic keratoses, which are premalignant lesions.
- *Acrochordon (skin tag):* Small, soft tag of skin that generally appears on the neck and upper chest (Fig. 21-9). These tags may or may not be pigmented.

Abnormal findings of the skin are the same as those discussed for adults. Dry skin may indicate dehydration or malnutrition. Tenting of the skin may indicate moderate-to-severe dehydration. Edema may indicate fluid retention from cardiovascular or renal disease. Bruising, lacerations, and pressure ulcers require additional follow-up. Refer to Chapter 9 for descriptions of squamous cell and basal cell cancers and malignant melanoma.

Hair

The hair may be thin, gray, and coarse in texture. Symmetric balding may occur in men; a decrease in the amount of body, pubic, and axillary hair occurs in both men and women. Men have an increase in the amount and coarseness of nasal and eyebrow hair, and women may develop coarse facial hair.

Nails

Nails may be thick and brittle, especially the toenails.

EXAMINATION OF THE HEAD, EYES, EARS, NOSE, AND THROAT

Procedures and techniques for assessing the head, eyes, ears, nose, and throat of the older adult are the same as those described in Chapter 10.

Neck

Procedure and Technique. To avoid causing dizziness on movement, assess range of motion of the neck with one movement at a time rather than a full rotation of the neck. Note any pain, crepitus, dizziness, or limited movement.

Abnormal Findings. A stiff neck in the older adult may indicate cervical arthritis.

Eyes and Vision
Eyes

Expected and Abnormal Findings. Eyebrows may be thin along the outer edge, and the remaining brow hair may appear coarse. Pseudoptosis, or relaxed upper eyelid, may be seen, with the lid resting on the lashes. Orbital fat may have decreased so the eyes appear sunken or may herniate, causing bulging on the lower lid or inner third of the upper lid. The lacrimal apparatus may function poorly, giving the eye a lack of luster. Brown spots may appear near the limbus as a normal variation. Bulbar conjunctiva may appear dry, clear, and light pink without discharge or lesions. The cornea is transparent, clear, often yellow; arcus senilis (a gray-white circle around the limbus) is common but not associated with any pathologic condition (Fig. 21-10).

During an ophthalmic examination the retinal structures usually appear dull, with pale blood vessels. The arterioles display a narrower light reflex and are straighter. More defective crossings of arteries and veins are also seen. Benign degenerative hyaline deposits may be noted on the retinal surface (drusen); these do not interfere with vision.

Abnormal findings include ectropion, in which the lower lid drops away from the globe (Fig. 21-11), or entropion, in which the lower lid turns inward (Fig. 21-12).

Vision

Expected and Abnormal Findings. Central and peripheral vision may decrease after age 70. Acuity of 20/20 or 20/30 with corrective lenses is common. Accommodation takes longer. Color perception of blue, violet, and green may be impaired. Presbyopia is decreased near vision that usually

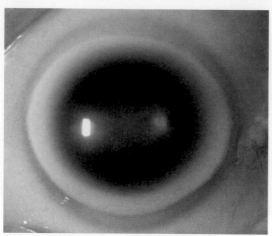

FIG. 21-10 Arcus senilis (a gray-white circle around the limbus). (From Paley and Krachmer, 1997.)

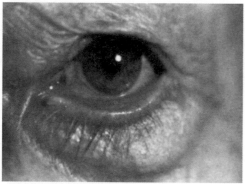

FIG. 21-11 Ectropion. (Courtesy Dr. Ira Abrahamsom, Jr, Cincinnati, Ohio. From Stein, Slatt, and Stein, 1988.)

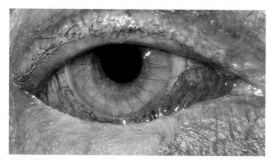

FIG. 21-12 Entropion. (From Paley and Krachmer, 1997.)

occurs after age 40 and is treated with corrective lenses. Abnormal findings include gradual loss of central vision that may be caused by macular degeneration resulting from changes in the retina. The difficulty or inability to visualize the internal structures of the eye may denote cataracts.

Ears and Hearing

Expected Findings. When the patient wears a hearing device, his or her ear should be carefully assessed for any skin irritation or sores that may be secondary to the molded device. There may be the presence of or an increase in wiry hair in the opening of the auditory canal; and the tympanic membrane may appear whiter, opaque, and thickened. If the patient wears a hearing device, there is an increased likelihood of cerumen impaction. Presbycusis is hearing loss associated with aging. Ability to hear high-frequency sounds diminishes first, making high-pitched sounds such as "s" and "th" difficult to hear and tell apart. The speech of others seems mumbled or slurred.

Mouth

Patients with dentures should have an examination with the dental appliance both in and out.

Expected and Abnormal Findings. The surface of the lips may be marked with deep wrinkling. Aging causes the gum line to recede secondary to bone degeneration, causing the teeth to appear longer. The teeth may be darkened or stained. Abnormal findings include fissures at the corners of the mouth (perlèche), which may be associated with overclosure of the mouth or vitamin deficiency. The older patient is at higher risk for squamous cell carcinoma of the lip, especially if he has been a longtime pipe smoker. The gums may be more friable and bleed with slight pressure. Many older adults may have caps or bridges; some may be edentulous. Dental occlusion surfaces may be markedly worn down. Malocclusion of the teeth may be common secondary to the migration of teeth after tooth extraction. A red, edematous tongue with erosions in the corners of the mouth may indicate iron deficiency anemia.

EXAMINATION OF THE RESPIRATORY SYSTEM

Procedures and techniques for assessing an older adult are the same as those described in Chapter 11.

Expected and Abnormal Findings. The thorax and scapulae should be symmetric. The anteroposterior diameter of the chest should be approximately one half the lateral diameter. Older adults may have decreased elasticity and ability to clear the air passages in. Breath sounds are the same as for younger adults. Abnormal findings may include kyphoscoliosis, which is formed by an anteroposterior and a lateral curvature of the spine. It may alter the chest wall configuration and make adequate lung expansion more difficult. It may also increase the anteroposterior diameter. This in turn may result in shallow breathing.

EXAMINATION OF THE CARDIOVASCULAR SYSTEM

Procedures and techniques for assessing an older adult are the same as those described in Chapter 12 (Fig. 21-13).

Expected and Abnormal Findings. Occasional ectopic beats are common and may or may not be significant.

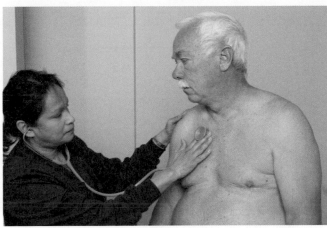

FIG. 21-13 Auscultate for heart sounds using the same procedure as with the younger adult.

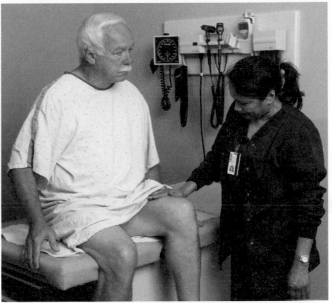

FIG. 21-14 Muscle mass of older adults may be decreased compared to findings in younger adults.

The S₄ heart sound is common in older adults and may be associated with decreased left ventricular compliance. Abnormal findings may include carotid bruits, indicating arteriosclerosis. Cool feet and weak pedal pulses may be noted because of peripheral arterial disease.

EXAMINATION OF THE ABDOMEN AND GASTROINTESTINAL SYSTEM

Procedures and techniques for assessing an older adult are the same as those described in Chapter 13.

Expected Findings. Older adults may have increased fat deposits over the abdominal area, even with decreased subcutaneous fat over the extremities. The abdomen may feel soft because of decreased abdominal muscle tone. Bowel sounds may be hypoactive.

EXAMINATION OF THE MUSCULOSKELETAL SYSTEM

Procedures and techniques for assessing an older adult are generally the same as those described in Chapter 14 (Fig. 21-14). Assess balance and gait when indicated.

Expected and Abnormal Findings. Muscle mass is decreased compared to findings in younger adults. Muscles that are not equal bilaterally may indicate muscle atrophy. Common findings include osteoarthritis changes in joints, which may result in decreased range of motion in affected joints. Many joints may not have the expected degree of movement or range of motion seen in younger adults.

Assess range of motion of the neck with one movement at a time rather than a full rotation of the neck to avoid causing dizziness on movement. A stiff neck in the older adult may indicate cervical arthritis. Note any pain, crepitus, dizziness, or limited movement. Box 21-3 describes the Tinetti Balance and Gait Assessment Tool.

EXAMINATION OF THE NEUROLOGIC SYSTEM

Procedures and techniques for assessing an older adult are the same as those described in Chapter 15. Mental status is assessed while taking the patient's history. Cranial nerves are assessed during the examination of the head, eyes, ears, nose, and throat.

Expected Findings. For indications of the patient's ability to perform activities of daily living, note his or her personal hygiene, appearance, and dress. Be aware that some older adults have slowed responses, move more slowly, or show a decline in function (e.g., the sense of taste). Other expected changes with aging may include deviation of gait from midline; difficulty with rapidly alternating movements; and some loss of reflexes and sensations (e.g., the knee-jerk or ankle-jerk reflexes and light touch and pain sensations). Often a normal flexor response is indistinct, and the plantar reflex may be missing or difficult to interpret.

EXAMINATION OF THE BREASTS

Procedures and techniques for assessing an older adult are the same as those described in Chapter 16. Postmenopausal women and older men should continue to have regular breast examinations.

Expected and Abnormal Findings. The breasts in postmenopausal women may appear flattened and elongated or pendulous secondary to a relaxation of the suspensory ligaments. A normal variation found when palpating the breasts in the older adult is a granular feeling of the glandular tissue of the breast. If the woman had cystic disease earlier in life,

BOX 21-3 FUNCTIONAL ASSESSMENT

Tinetti Balance and Gait Assessment Tool

Balance Tests

Various positions and position changes are evaluated.

Instructions: The patient is seated in a hard, armless chair. The following maneuvers are tested.

1. Sitting balance	Leans or slides in chair	= 0
	Steady, safe	= 1 _____
2. Arises (ask patient to rise without using arms)	Unable without help	= 0
	Able, uses arms to help	= 1
	Able without using arms	= 2 _____
3. Attempts to arise	Unable without help	= 0
	Able, requires more than one attempt	= 1
	Able to arise, one attempt	= 2 _____
4. Immediate standing balance (first 5 seconds)	Unsteady (swaggers, moves feet, trunk sways)	= 0
	Steady but uses walker or other support	= 1
	Steady without walker or other support	= 2 _____
5. Standing balance (once stance balances)	Unsteady	= 0
	Steady but wide stance (medial heels more than 4 inches (10 cm) apart or uses cane or other support	= 1
	Narrow stance without support	= 2 _____
6. Nudged (subject at maximum position with feet as close together as possible; nurse pushes lightly on subject's sternum with palm of hand 3 times)	Begins to fall	= 0
	Staggers, grabs, catches self	= 1
	Steady	= 2 _____
7. Eyes closed (at maximum position, as in 6)	Unsteady	= 0
	Steady	= 1 _____
8. Turning 360 degrees	Discontinuous steps	= 0
	Continuous steps	= 1
	Unsteady (grabs, staggers)	= 0
	Steady	= 1 _____
9. Sitting down	Unsafe (misjudges distance, falls into chair)	= 0
	Uses arm or not a smooth motion	= 1
	Safe, smooth motion	= 2 _____

Balance Score: _____ of 16

Gait Tests

Various components of gait are observed.

Initial instructions: The patient stands with nurse, walks down hallway or across room for at least 10 feet, first at "usual" pace, then back at "rapid but safe" pace (using usual walking aids).

10. Initiation of gait (immediately after being told "go")	Any hesitancy or multiple attempts to start	= 0
	No hesitancy	= 1 _____
11. Step length and height	Right swing foot does not pass left foot with stance	= 0
	Passes left stance foot	= 1
	Right foot does not clear floor completely with step	= 0
	Right foot completely clears floor	= 1
	Left swing foot does not pass right stance foot with step	= 0
	Passes right stance foot	= 1
	Left foot does not clear floor completely with step	= 0
	Left foot completely clears floor	= 1 _____
12. Step symmetry	Right and left step length not equal (estimate)	= 0
	Right and left step length appear equal	= 1 _____
13. Step continuity	Stopping or discontinuity between steps	= 0
	Steps appear continuous	= 1 _____
14. Path (estimated in relation to floor tiles, 12 inches (30.5 cm) square; observe excursion of one of subject's feet over about 10 feet (3 m) of the course)	Marked deviation	= 0
	Mild/moderate deviation or uses walking aid	= 1
	Straight without walking aid	= 2 _____

BOX 21-3 **FUNCTIONAL ASSESSMENT**
Tinetti Balance and Gait Assessment Tool—cont'd

15. Trunk	Marked sway or uses walking aid	= 0
	No sway but flexion of knees or back or spreads arms out while walking	= 1
	No sway, no flexion, no use of arms, and no use of walking aid	= 2 _____
16. Walking stance	Heels apart	= 0
	Heels almost touching while walking	= 1 _____

Gait Score: _____ of 12

Balance and Gait Score: _____ of 28

A score below 19 indicates a high risk for falls. A score of 19 to 24 suggests there is a greater chance of falls but not a high risk.

From Tinetti ME, Williams TF, Mayewski R, Fall Risk Index for elderly patients based on number of chronic disabilities. *Am J Med* 1986:80:429-434.

her breasts are now more likely to feel smoother and less cystic. The inframammary ridge thickness may now be more prominent, and the nipples may be smaller and flatter.

EXAMINATION OF THE REPRODUCTIVE SYSTEM AND PERINEUM

Procedures and techniques for assessing an older adult are the same as those described in Chapter 17.

Female Reproductive System

Procedure and Techniques. Often there is a temptation to defer the routine pelvic examination of the older woman because it may be difficult for her to be positioned in stirrups, she is postmenopausal, or she is no longer sexually active. None of these is a sufficient reason to defer the examination. Instead, older women may have different problems (e.g., urinary incontinence, pelvic relaxation, vaginal irritation, dryness, or rectal problems) that warrant evaluation. The older-adult woman may need assistance to help hold her legs if she is unable to tolerate positioning in the stirrups. In addition, she may need more assistance in assuming a modified lithotomy position and may not be able to stay in the position as long as a younger woman. If the patient is no longer sexually active, a smaller speculum with narrower blades may be necessary to prevent discomfort from the introital constriction. The nurse may also need to lubricate the speculum and the fingers used for palpation to avoid the patient's discomfort because natural vaginal lubrication is decreased.

Expected and Abnormal Findings. The labia and clitoris of the older woman are small and pale. The skin may appear dry and have a shiny appearance. The pubic hair may be sparse, patchy, or absent.

The nurse may find that the patient's vagina is narrower and shorter and that there is an absence of rugation of the vaginal wall. Likewise the cervix may appear smaller and paler, and the fornices may be smaller or absent. The uterus should be small, smooth, firm, freely movable, and nontender. Any uterine enlargement; nodular, irregular, hardened, or indurated areas; areas that are tender on palpation; fixed, nonmobile areas in the pelvis; or masses should be further evaluated.

Because ovaries atrophy with age, they are not usually palpable in aging women. The rectovaginal septum should be thin, smooth, and pliable. The anal sphincter tone may be somewhat diminished; and, because of pelvic musculature relaxation, the patient may have prolapse of the vaginal walls or uterus.

Male Reproductive System

Procedures and techniques for assessing an older adult are the same as those described in Chapter 17.

Expected Findings. Pubic hair tends to be finer and less abundant, sometimes leading to pubic alopecia. The scrotal sac of the patient may appear elongated or pendulous. The patient may have injury or excoriation of the scrotal sac surface secondary to sitting on the scrotum. The testes may feel slightly smaller and softer than in the younger patient.

Perianal Area

Procedures and techniques for assessing an older adult are the same as those described in Chapter 17.

The patient may need assistance getting into an adequate position for the examination. If lying on the back on the examination table, the patient may need assistance turning to a left lateral lying position.

Expected and Abnormal Findings. The examination findings for the older adult are the same as those for the adult. Prostate hyperplasia is a common abnormal finding. The prostate may feel smooth and rubbery; the median sulcus may or may not be palpable. The nurse may also note a relaxation of the patient's perianal muscles and decreased sphincter control when the older adult bears down.

COMMON PROBLEMS AND CONDITIONS

RISK FACTORS

Falls and Malnutrition in Older Adults

Falls

The combination of visual deficits, loss of muscle strength, and slowed reaction time contributes to the increased risk of falls for older adults.

- Gender: Higher risk for males
- Mental status: Confusion, disorientation, depression
- Poor muscle strength and balance, dizziness, vertigo
- Altered elimination
- Adverse effect of medications
- Life style: Alcohol consumption (M)

Malnutrition Older Adults

- Institutionalized (nursing homes or hospitalization)
- Poverty
- Social isolation
- Chronic illnesses
- Alcoholism (M)
- Illness affecting mental capacities (depression, dementia)
- Decreased functional abilities—affecting food purchasing and preparation
- Anorexia
- Feeding problems, including chewing and swallowing problems
- Taking multiple medications

M, Modifiable risk factor.

A list of common problems and conditions of older adults follows. Most of these have been discussed in previous chapters; the chapter number is included beside the category. Those not previously discussed (in *italics*) are described (i.e., macular degeneration, anemia, and urinary incontinence).

Integumentary—See Chapter 9
  Skin cancer
Vision—See Chapter 10
  Cataracts
  Macular degeneration
  Glaucoma
  Diabetic retinopathy
Hearing—See Chapter 10
  Conductive hearing loss
  Sensorineural hearing loss
Respiratory—See Chapter 11
  Asthma
  Chronic obstructive pulmonary disease
  Pneumonia
Cardiovascular—See Chapter 12
  Hypertension
  Angina
  Myocardial infarction
  Valvular heart disease
  Heart failure

  Peripheral arterial disease
  Anemia
Gastrointestinal—See Chapter 13
  Gastrointestinal reflux disease
  Constipation
Genitourinary—See Chapters 13 and 17
  Urinary tract infections—Chapter 13
  Urinary incontinence
  Benign prostatic hyperplasia—Chapter 17
Musculoskeletal—See Chapter 14
  Osteoporosis
  Fractures
  Osteoarthritis
  Gout
Neurologic—See Chapter 15
  Alzheimer's disease
  Cerebrovascular accident (stroke)
  Parkinson's disease

MACULAR DEGENERATION

The macula is an oval yellow spot in the center of the retina that helps provide central vision. As the maculae degenerate, central visual is impaired. Risk factors are age older that 50 years, Caucasian, smoking, hypertension, and cardiovascular disease. **Clinical Findings:** Loss of central vision, decline in visual acuity, a dark spot in the center of vision, and straight lines appear crooked or wavy[15] (Fig. 21-15).

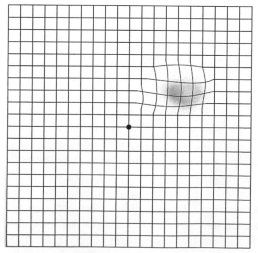

Fig 21-15 Amsler grid used to evaluate central vision as occurs in macular degeneration. (Courtesy Brent A. Bauer, MFA, The Wilmer Institute, The Johns Hopkins University and Hospital, Baltimore, Md. From Seidel et al., 2011.)

ANEMIA

A reduction in the total number of circulating erythrocytes (red blood cells) or a decrease in the quantity or quality of hemoglobin describes anemia. Anemia that affects older adults is caused by lack of nutrients needed to produce erythrocytes or a slow blood loss from a bleeding ulcer or colon cancer, which results in the loss of erythrocytes. Nutrients needed to produce erythrocytes include iron, vitamin B_{12}, and folate. Older adults may lack these nutrients because they cannot afford to purchase them, are not mobile enough to go to the store, do not have the energy to prepare the food containing them, or are unable to chew or swallow food. **Clinical Findings:** Manifestations that may occur regardless of the type of anemia are tachycardia; tachypnea; dyspnea; fatigue; cool, pale skin; light-headedness; and tinnitus. Iron deficiency also causes glossitis; erosions in the corners of the mouth; thin, brittle nails; conjunctiva pallor; and (in older adults) confusion. Folate deficiency produces irritability, memory loss, depression, and sleep deprivation. Vitamin B_{12} deficiency causes neurologic manifestations, including paresthesia of the hands and feet, altered vibratory perception, and ataxia.

URINARY INCONTINENCE

This common urinary disorder occurs when the person is unable to control urination associated with relaxation of the bladder and/or urinary sphincter. Risk factors include multiple pregnancies, abdominal wall weakness, obesity, urinary tract infections, cerebrovascular accident, or multiple sclerosis. **Clinical Findings:** The person may report feeling an immediate urge to void (urge incontinence); leaking of urine when laughing, coughing, or sneezing (stress incontinence); a continuous leakage of urine; or a leakage of urine during sleep (nocturnal enuresis). Consequences of incontinence are skin breakdown, risk for falls, social isolation, and feelings of embarrassment.

CLINICAL APPLICATION AND CLINICAL REASONING

See Appendix D for answers to exercises in this section.

REVIEW QUESTIONS

1. During inspection of the mouth of a 72-year-old male patient, the nurse notices a red lesion at the base of his tongue. What additional datum does the nurse obtain from this patient?
   1. Alcohol and tobacco use
   2. Date of his last dental examination
   3. How well his dentures fit
   4. A history of gum disease

2. On inspection of the eye of an 82-year-old woman, the nurse notes which finding as normal?
   1. Opaque coloring of the lens
   2. Clear cornea with a gray-white ring around the limbus
   3. Dilated pupils when looking at an item in her hand
   4. Impaired perception of the colors yellow and red

3. The nurse notes which finding as abnormal during a thoracic assessment of an older adult?
   1. A skeletal deformity affecting curvature of the spine
   2. Shortness of breath on exertion
   3. An increase in anteroposterior diameter
   4. Bronchovesicular breath sounds in the peripheral lung fields

4. The nurse notes which finding as normal during a cardiovascular assessment of an older adult?
   1. A drop in blood pressure when moving from lying to standing
   2. A loud aortic ejection murmur that radiates to the neck
   3. A radial pulse of 56 beats/min.
   4. A low-pitched blowing sound heard over a carotid artery

5. Which would be an abnormal finding during an abdominal examination of an older adult?
   1. Report of incontinence when sneezing or coughing
   2. Loss of abdominal muscle tone
   3. Bowel sounds every 15 seconds in all quadrants
   4. Silver-white striae and a very faint vascular network

6. Which finding is an expected age-related change for a woman 80 years old?
   1. Kyphosis
   2. Back pain
   3. Loss of height
   4. Crepitation on movement

CASE STUDY

Sara Reinarz is an 80-year-old Caucasian woman who recently developed confusion and urinary incontinence. She lives with her daughter, Megan, who reports that her mother has fallen several times at home. She is admitted to the hospital for assessment for possible fractures and confusion.

Interview Data

The daughter reports that her mother has fallen several times going to the bathroom. This is the first time Sara reported pain after the fall. Megan is concerned about her mother's confusion. Two weeks ago Ms. Reinarz was independent and caring for herself at home. Megan recalled that last year her mother became confused and was diagnosed with a urinary tract infection at the same time. As soon as the urinary tract infection was treated, her mother's confusion stopped. Ms. Reinarz has no allergies to food or medications. She takes calcium with vitamin D for osteoporosis, aspirin for an antiplatelet, and thyroid hormone for hypothyroidism. She does not smoke or drink alcohol.

Examination Data

Vital signs: Blood pressure, 141/86 mm Hg; pulse, 88 beats/min; respiration rate, 22 breaths/min; temperature, 98.3° F (36.8° C). *Weight:* 152 lb (69 kg). Patient confused and oriented to person. Appears anxious. Bruise on her right hip and thigh. Full range of motion of right leg, but movement painful. Muscle strength 4/5. Pedal pulses 1+ and symmetric.

Clinical Reasoning

1. Which data deviate from normal findings, suggesting a need for further investigation?
2. For which additional data should the nurse ask or assess?
3. Based on the data, which risk factors for falls does Ms. Reinarz have?
4. With which health team member would the nurse collaborate to help meet this patient's needs?

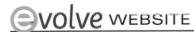

Conducting a Head-to-Toe Examination

Now that you have studied and practiced examining each body system separately, you are ready to put everything together. Although you began with knowledge and techniques specific for each system, the patient is viewed as a whole person. You must organize your techniques to examine the entire person, literally from "head to toe." Therefore, when you begin with the head, you should examine the facial characteristics (i.e., skin, hair, eyes, ears, mouth, throat, and range of motion of the neck) in a systematic, organized manner that incorporates neurologic, integumentary, musculoskeletal, visual, and auditory systems within the head, neck, nose, and mouth regions. You then move on to the next region of the body and repeat the same. After examining all body regions, you document your findings by body system.

Each nurse's approach to a head-to-toe examination is unique. No two nurses do things in exactly the same manner, nor are any two patients exactly the same. As a student you determine which sequence works best for you. Use a systematic method so you do not omit any data. When performing other types of assessment (focused, episodic, shift, or screening), you refer only to regions based on the patient's chief complaint and additional data learned from the history.

PERFORMING A HEAD-TO-TOE EXAMINATION

After cleaning your hands, you begin the examination with the general survey. During this initial meeting observe the patient entering the room, noting gait, posture, and ease of movement. Shake hands with the patient, noting eye contact and firmness of the hand grip. Introduce yourself to him or her and ask what name he or she prefers to be called. Begin data collection by telling the patient what to expect during the examination and asking about the reason for seeking care. Note the language spoken and gross hearing and speech capability. In addition, notice characteristics such as obvious vision impairment or blindness; difficulty standing, sitting, or rising; obvious musculoskeletal difficulties; general affect; appearance of interest and involvement; dress and posture; general mental alertness, orientation, and integration of thought processes; obvious shortness of breath or posture that would facilitate breathing; and obesity, emaciation, or malnourishment.

After the initial observations, obtain the history, assess vital signs, assess vision, and prepare the patient for the examination. Instruct the patient to first empty the bladder (collect specimen if necessary based on patient history) and then remove clothing, put on a gown if needed, and sit on the examination table. You are now ready to conduct an examination that accommodates the patient's needs.

Use the following sequence only as a guide. It was developed to demonstrate how examination of one body system is integrated with other body systems to permit a comprehensive regional assessment. Note in the following example that all relevant body systems in one region are examined. For example, when the nurse is examining the patient's anterior chest, he or she must consider the other body systems in that region that must be assessed simultaneously and incorporate them into an integrated assessment. Body systems that would be assessed during the anterior chest examination include skin; respiratory, lymphatic, cardiovascular, musculoskeletal systems; and breasts. Techniques for a routine examination are listed. Additional techniques that may be indicated are identified by a bullet (•). Advanced practice techniques and procedures are identified by an asterisk (★).

BOX 22-1   EQUIPMENT FOR HEALTH EXAMINATION IN SUGGESTED ORDER OF USE

- Writing surface for nurse
- Scale with height measurement
- Thermometer
- Watch with second hand
- Vision charts—Snellen's or Jaeger card
- Sphygmomanometer
- Stethoscope with bell and diaphragm
- Patient gown
- Drape sheet
- Examination table (with stirrups for female patients)
- Otoscope with pneumatic bulb★
- Tuning fork
- Ophthalmoscope★
- Nasal speculum
- Tongue blade

- Penlight
- Gauze pads
- Nonsterile examination gloves
- Ruler and tape measure
- Marking pen
- Goniometer
- Aromatic items
- Cotton balls
- Sharp and dull testing items
- Objects for stereognosis such as a key or comb★
- Percussion hammer
- Lubricant
- Vagina speculum (for female patients)★
- Pap test materials (for female patients)★
- Gooseneck light

★ Advanced practice.

Tips for success:

- Be organized.
- Develop a routine. This helps with consistency.
- Before you begin the actual examination, have a clear picture in your mind of what you plan to do and in what order.
- Practice, practice, practice so you learn to become systematic and inclusive.
- Imagine yourself as the patient and consider how you would want a nurse to be prepared if he or she were to assess you.

Exactly how the examination proceeds depends on the purpose, the needs of the patient, the nurse's ability, and the policies of the facility where the examination is conducted. Equipment for an examination is listed in Box 22-1.

GUIDELINES FOR ADULT HEAD-TO-TOE EXAMINATION

CLEAN hands.

General Survey (Collected During the History)

Level of consciousness and mental status
Mood or affect
Personal hygiene
Skin color
Posture/position
Mobility
Ability to hear and speak

Assess Vital Signs and Other Baseline Measurements

Nurse is in front of patient who is seated.
Temperature, radial pulse, respirations, and blood pressure
If indicated,
- take blood pressure in both arms
Height, weight, and body mass index
Visual acuity

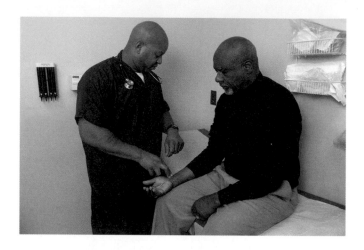

Examine Hands

When taking pulse and blood pressure, inspect skin surface characteristics, temperature, and moisture of hands.
Inspect hands for symmetry.
Inspect and palpate nails for shape, contour, consistency, color, thickness, and cleanliness.
Observe for clubbing of fingers.
Test capillary refill.

Examine Head and Face

Inspect skull for size and shape and hair for color and distribution.
If indicated,
- palpate hair for texture.
- palpate scalp for tenderness and intactness.
- palpate temporal pulses for amplitude.
Inspect for facial features and symmetry.
Inspect bony structures of face for size, symmetry, and intactness.
If indicated,
- ask patient to clench eyes tightly; wrinkle forehead; smile; stick out tongue; and puff out cheeks, noting symmetry.
- evaluate sensitivity of forehead, cheeks, and chin to light touch.
Inspect skin for color and lesions.
If indicated,
- palpate skin for texture, tenderness, and lesions.

- palpate facial bones for size, intactness, and tenderness.
- palpate sinus regions for tenderness and transilluminate sinuses.

Examine Eyes

Assess near and peripheral vision.

Inspect eyebrows for skin characteristics and symmetry.

Inspect eyelids and eyelashes for symmetry, position, closure, blinking, and color.

Inspect conjunctiva and sclera for color and clarity; inspect cornea for transparency.

If indicated,

- inspect anterior chamber for transparency and chamber depth.

Inspect symmetry of eye movements.

If indicated,

- test extraocular eye movements in six cardinal fields of gaze.

Inspect iris for shape and color.

Examine pupillary response, consensual reaction, corneal light reflex, and accommodation.

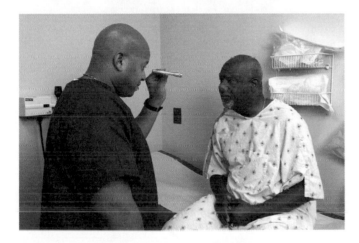

If indicated,

- perform cover-uncover test.

★Ophthalmic examination: Inspect red reflex, disc cup margins, vessels, retinal surface, macula.

Examine Ears

Inspect external ear for alignment, position, size, shape, symmetry, intactness, and skin color.

Inspect external auditory canal for discharge or lesions.

Inspect skin over superficial lymph nodes for edema, erythema, and red streaks.

Palpate lymph nodes of the head for size and tenderness.

Palpate external ear and mastoid areas for tenderness, edema, or nodules.

If indicated,

- perform whisper test to evaluate gross hearing.
- perform Rinne and Weber's tests for conduction and sensorineural hearing losses.

★ Advanced practice.

★ Otoscopic examination: inspect characteristics of external canal, cerumen, eardrum (landmarks).

Examine Nose and Paranasal Sinuses

Inspect nasal structure and septum for symmetry.

Inspect nose for patency, color of turbinates, and discharge.

If indicated,

- evaluate sense of smell.
- palpate nose.
- inspect internal nasal cavity.
- palpate paranasal sinuses.

★ • transilluminate sinuses.

Examine Mouth and Oropharynx

Inspect lips, buccal mucosa, and gums for color, symmetry, moisture, and texture.

Inspect teeth for number, color, stability, alignment, hygiene, and condition.

Inspect floor of mouth and hard and soft palates for color and surface characteristics.

Inspect anterior and posterior pillars, uvula, tonsils, and posterior pharynx for color, surface characteristics, and odor.

If indicated,

- grade tonsils.

Inspect tongue for symmetry, movement, color, and surface characteristics.

If indicated,

- palpate tongue and gums for tenderness and lesions with gloved hands.
- evaluate gag reflex.
- test temporomandibular joint for movement.

Examine Neck

Observe symmetry of neck, trachea, and thyroid.

If indicated,

- palpate trachea for alignment and thyroid for size.

Observe neck for range of motion.

If indicated,

- palpate neck for tenderness and muscle strength.
- test range of motion of head and neck; shrug shoulders against resistance.

Palpate carotid pulses, one at a time, for amplitude.

If indicated,

- auscultate carotid for bruits.

Palpate lymph nodes of neck for size and tenderness.

Observe jugular veins for distention.

Examine Upper Extremities

Inspect patient's arms for skin characteristics and color.

Palpate skin for texture, moisture, mobility, turgor, and thickness.

Palpate arms for temperature.

Palpate elbows, wrists, and fingers for tenderness and deformities.

Palpate brachial or radial pulses for presence and amplitude.

If indicated,
- palpate epitrochlear lymph nodes for size and tenderness.
- palpate ulnar pulse for presence and amplitude.

Observe range of motion of shoulder, elbows, wrists and fingers.

Assess muscle strength of upper and lower arms.

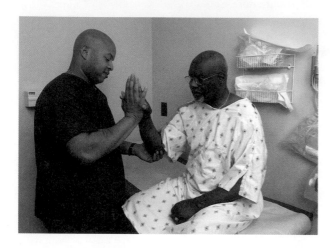

Test deep tendon reflexes.

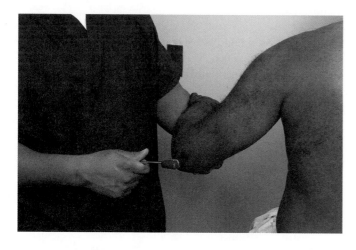

Test for sensation of upper and lower arms.
If indicated,
- perform Phalen's sign or Tinel's sign for carpal tunnel syndrome.
★ • test for rotator cuff damage.

Examine Posterior Chest

Nurse moves behind patient; patient is seated; gown is lowered to waist for men, open in back for women.

Observe posterior and lateral chest for symmetry of shoulders, muscular development, scapular placement, spine alignment, and posture.

★ Advanced practice.

Inspect skin for color, intactness, lesions, and scars.
Palpate vertebrae for alignment and tenderness.
Observe respiratory movement for symmetry, depth, and rhythm of respirations.
If indicated,
- palpate posterior chest and thoracic muscles for tenderness, bulges, and symmetry.
- palpate posterior chest wall for thoracic expansion.
- palpate posterior chest wall for fremitus.
★ • percuss posterior and lateral chest for resonance.
★ • percuss and measure thorax for diaphragmatic excursion.
- percuss with fist along costovertebral angle for tenderness.

Auscultate posterior and lateral chest walls for breath sounds.

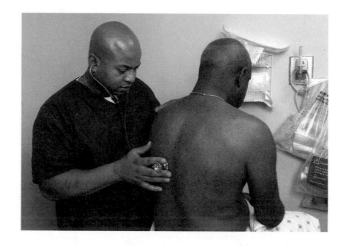

If indicated,
- assess for bronchophony, egophony, and whispered pectoriloquy.

Examine Anterior Chest

Move to front of patient; patient is seated and should lower gown to waist.

Inspect skin for color, intactness, lesions, and scars.
Inspect chest wall for contour, pulsations, lift, heaves, and retractions.
Observe respiratory movement for symmetry, patient's ease with respirations, and posture.
If indicated,
- observe precordium for pulsations or heaving.

Palpate left chest wall to locate point of maximum impulse (PMI).
If indicated,
- palpate chest wall for fremitus, as with posterior chest.
- palpate anterior chest wall for thoracic expansion.
★ • percuss anterior chest for resonance.

Auscultate anterior chest for breath sounds.
Auscultate heart for rate, rhythm, intensity, frequency, timing, splitting of S_1 or S_2 or presence of S_3, S_4, or murmurs.

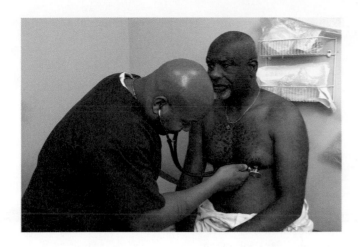

Female Breasts

Inspect for size, symmetry, contour, surface characteristics, and breast or nipple deviation.

Observe for symmetry of breast tissue during movement: arms over head, behind head, behind back; hand pushed together tightly, patient leaning forward.

Male Breasts

Inspect for size, symmetry, breast enlargement, nipple discharge, or lesions.

All Patients

Palpate lymph nodes associated with lymphatic drainage of breasts and axillae.

Examine Anterior Chest in Recumbent Position

Patient is lying. Elevate head of bed 45 degrees.

Inspect for jugular vein pulsations.

If indicated,

- measure jugular venous pressure for height seen above sternal angle.

Palpate anterior chest wall for thrills, heaves, and pulsations.

If indicated,

- measure blood pressure with patient lying to compare with earlier reading.

Female Breasts

Provide chest drape for females; expose abdomen from pubis to epigastric region.

Inspect for symmetry, contour, venous pattern, skin color, areolar area (note size, shape, and surface characteristics), and nipples (note direction, size, shape, color, surface characteristics, and discharge).

Palpate breasts; note firmness, tissue qualities, lumps, areas of thickness, or tenderness. Palpate areolar and nipple areas.

Examine Abdomen

Inspect for skin color, surface characteristics, and venous patterns.

Inspect abdominal contour.

Observe for abdomen movement, peristalsis, and pulsations.

Auscultate abdomen (all quadrants) for bowel sounds, bruits, and venous hums.

Lightly palpate all quadrants for tenderness, guarding, and masses.

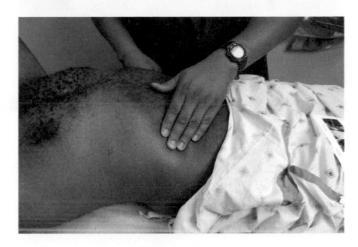

If indicated,

- deeply palpate all quadrants for tenderness, guarding, and masses.
- ★ deeply palpate midline epigastric area for aortic pulsation.
- percuss all quadrants and epigastric region for tone.
- ★ percuss upper and lower liver borders and estimation of liver span.
- ★ percuss left midaxillary line for splenic dullness.
- ★ deeply palpate right costal margin for liver border.
- ★ deeply palpate left costal margin for splenic border.
- ★ deeply palpate abdomen for right and left kidneys.
- ★ test abdominal reflexes.
- ★ assess abdomen for fluid.

Patient raises head to evaluate flexion and strength of abdominal muscles and inspect for umbilical hernia.

If indicated,

- lightly palpate inguinal region for lymph nodes, femoral pulses, and bulges that may be associated with hernia.

Examine Lower Extremities

Patient remains lying; abdomen and chest should be draped.

Inspect legs, ankles, and feet for skin characteristics, vascular sufficiency, hair distribution, and deformities.

Palpate lower legs for temperature.

Palpate lower legs, knees, and feet for tenderness, and deformities.

Palpate dorsalis pedis pulses for presence and amplitude.

Test capillary refill of toes.

★ Advanced practice.

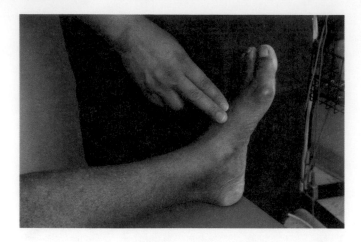

If indicated,
- palpate popliteal and posterior tibial pulses.
- calculate ankle-brachial index.
- measure circumference of each thigh and calf.

Observe range of motion of hips, legs, knees, ankles, and feet.

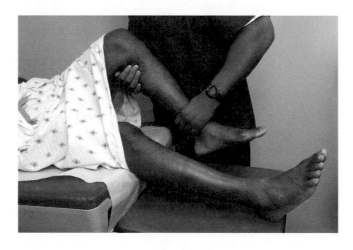

Test motor strength of upper and lower legs.
Test for deep tendon reflexes and ankle clonus.
If indicated,
- test sensation of hips, legs, knees, ankles, and feet.
- palpate hips for stability and tenderness.
- ★ examine for knee effusion with the bulge test or ballottement.
- ★ examine for knee stability with the drawer tests, McMurray's test, or Apley test.
- ★ test for hip flexion contracture with the Thomas test.
- ★ test for nerve root compression with straight leg raises.

Examine Remaining Neurologic System

Observe patient moving from lying to sitting position; note use of muscles, ease of movement, and coordination.

★ Advanced practice.

Examine patient's gait: Observe and palpate patient's spine and posterior thorax for alignment as patient stands and bends forward to touch toes.
If indicated,
- evaluate hyperextension, lateral bending, and rotation of upper trunk.
- ★ test sensory function by using light and deep (dull and sharp) sensation.
- test and compare vibratory sensation bilaterally.
- ★ test proprioception.
- ★ test two-point discrimination.
- ★ test stereognosis and graphesthesia.
- test fine-motor functioning and coordination of upper extremities by observing the patient performing at least two of the following:
  - Alternating pronation and supination of forearm
  - Touching nose with alternating index fingers
  - Rapidly alternating finger movements to thumb
  - Rapidly moving index finger between nose and nurse's finger
If indicated,
- test fine-motor functioning and coordination of lower extremities by instructing patient to run heel down tibia of opposite leg.
- ★ evaluate Babinski's sign.
- assess cerebellar and motor functions by using at least two of the following:
  - Romberg's test (eyes closed)
  - Walking straight heel-to-toe formation
  - Standing on one foot and then other (eyes closed)
  - Hopping in place on one foot and then other
  - Knee bends

Examine Genitalia, Pelvic Region, and Rectum
Males
Patient is lying and adequately draped.
Inspect pubic hair for distribution and general characteristics.
Inspect and palpate penis color, tenderness, discharge, and general characteristics.
Inspect scrotum for texture and general characteristics.
Inspect sacrococcygeal and perianal areas and anus for surface characteristics.
Position patient lying on left side with right hip and knee flexed.
Palpate anal canal and rectum for surface characteristics with lubricated gloved finger. Note characteristics of stool when gloved finger is removed.
If indicated,
- ★ palpate anterior rectal surface for prostate gland size, contour, consistency, mobility, and tenderness.
With patient standing, inspect inguinal canal for bulges.
Palpate testes, epididymides, and vas deferens for location, consistency, tenderness, and nodules.
If indicated,
- ★ transilluminate scrotum for fluid and masses.
- ★ palpate inguinal canal for hernias.

Females

Patient should be lying in lithotomy position; nurse should don gloves.

Inspect pubic hair for distribution.

Inspect and palpate labia majora, labia minora, clitoris, urethral meatus, vaginal introitus, perineum, and anus for surface characteristics.

If indicated,

- palpate Skene's and Bartholin's glands for surface characteristics.
- inspect and palpate muscle tone for vaginal wall tone, rectal muscle, and urinary incontinence.

★ Advanced practice.

★ • insert vaginal speculum and inspect surface characteristics of vagina and cervix.

★ • collect Papanicolaou (Pap) test and culture specimen.

★ • perform bimanual palpation to assess for size and characteristics of vagina, cervix, uterus, and adnexa.

★ • perform vaginal-rectal examination to assess rectovaginal septum and pouch, surface characteristics, and broad ligament tenderness.

- perform rectal examination to assess anal sphincter tone and surface characteristics; note characteristics of stool when lubricated gloved finger removed.

Patient resumes seated position; patient should be wearing gown and be draped across lap.

Documenting the Comprehensive Health Assessment

At the completion of a health assessment, the nurse documents the data so other nurses and health care providers can use the information. The written record serves as a legal document and permanent record of the patient's health status at the time of the nurse-patient interaction. The nurse must record data accurately, concisely, legibly, and without bias or opinion.

As mentioned in Chapter 1, a variety of formats to document assessment findings are used in various health care settings. Both paper and electronic records are common. The amount of information documented reflects the depth and scope of the health assessment. The purpose of this chapter is to provide you with an example of documentation of a comprehensive history and examination for a well patient. At the end of the documentation, the nurse forms a problem list. This provides the basis for determining the plan of care, including education needs of the patient. The actions that follow data collection reflect analysis, clinical judgment, and clinical reasoning (see Fig. 1-2).

HEALTH HISTORY

Biographic Data

Name: Maria S. Griego
Gender: Female
Address: 1000 1st Street, Angus, TX 87123
Telephone numbers: (111) 999-9999, home; (111) 444-4444, work
Birth date: 10-13-54
Birthplace: Houston, Texas
Race/ethnicity: Hispanic
Religion: Catholic
Marital status: Married, 34 years

Occupation: Counselor in a high school
Contact person: Christopher Griego, spouse
Source of interview data: Patient

Reason for Seeking Care

"I need a Pap test."

History of Present Illness

Not applicable.

Present Health Status

Overall health described as "good." *Chronic illnesses*: None. *Medications:* Takes no prescription drugs; does not use herbal preparations; takes one multivitamin each morning. *Allergies:* Reports allergy to penicillin; "give me hives"; no known food allergies.

Past Health History

Childhood illnesses: Measles, mumps, rubella, chickenpox, streptococcal throat, otitis media. *Surgeries and hospitalizations:* 1962 appendectomy; vaginal deliveries 1976, 1980. *Accidents/injuries*: Denies. *Immunizations:* Childhood immunizations for school, tetanus immunization unknown. *Last examinations*: Physical and Pap test 2 years ago. *Dental:* 2 years ago. *Vision:* 2 years ago. *Mammogram:* 2 years ago. *Obstetric history:* G2, P2. Both vaginal deliveries without complications.

Family History

MGM deceased age 70, hypertension and heart failure; MGF deceased age 72, colon cancer; PGM deceased age 84, "old age"; PGF deceased age 81, prostate cancer; mother, age 83, hypertension, arthritis, dementia; father, deceased age 62, myocardial infarction. Patient has no brothers or sisters. Denies family history of stroke, diabetes mellitus, kidney disease, mental disorders, or seizure disorders. Both children in good health.

Personal and Psychosocial History
Personal Status
Patient states that she feels good about herself most of the time. Her cultural affiliation is self-described as middle-class Hispanic female. She has a master's degree in counseling and has been a high school counselor with the same school for 19 years. Overall she enjoys her job but experiences frustration with the social issues of her students. Hobbies include playing piano and gardening.

Family and Social Relationships
Patient lives with husband and mother in a four-bedroom home in a suburban area; both sons live in the same community and remain close. Both sons are married; 3 grandchildren. The patient considers relationship with husband as close; she also speaks of two other very close female friends. Mother is elderly and has moderate dementia and occasional falls, requiring increasing supervision. Patient expresses concerns about meeting her mother's needs in the future and the ongoing physical demands.

Diet/Nutrition
Describes appetite as excellent; no changes in appetite or weight. Reports balanced food intake. 24-hour recall: *Breakfast:* muffin, 1% milk, fruit juice, coffee; *Lunch:* spaghetti, green beans, salad, tea; *Dinner:* chicken, mashed potatoes, applesauce, roll, tea, chocolate cake for dessert; *Snack:* crackers with peanut butter; *Fluid:* 4 glasses of water, 2 cups coffee, and 1 glass tea daily.

Functional Ability
Activities include maintaining a home, working full time, and caring for her mother.

Mental Health
Patient verbalizes frequent episodes of frustration and despair in meeting her mother's needs. She does not feel that husband is supportive of situation and has caused some conflict. She counts on her friends to help her "talk through" stress periods. The patient and her spouse have had marriage counseling on two different occasions, which she believes was beneficial. Also verbalizes stress at work regarding issues with students and administration. Recently she has not been able to find time to exercise; but, when she can, she finds this helpful in coping with the stress. She has had no previous psychiatric or mental health counseling.

Tobacco, Alcohol, and Illicit Drug Use
Denies drug use; 1 to 2 glasses of wine per week; previously a smoker with a 22 pack-year history; has not smoked for over 10 years.

Health Promotion Activities
Reports walking 1.5 miles two to three times per week to stay fit but has not been able to maintain this routine recently. Wears seat belt when in a car.

Environment
Believes that her home and neighborhood environments are safe and without hazards.

Review of Systems
General Symptoms
Considers herself in "good health" but frequently feels fatigued because of obligations of caring for her mother and working full time.

Integumentary System
Skin: Denies lesions, masses, discolorations, or rashes to skin. *Hair:* Denies texture changes or loss, uses hair color monthly to cover gray; no scalp irritation reported from hair coloring. *Nails:* Denies changes in texture, color, shape. *Health promotion:* Uses sunscreen "occasionally" when outside.

HEENT
Denies headache, vertigo, syncope. *Eyes:* Wears glasses/contacts for nearsighted vision. Denies discharge, pruritus, pain, visual disturbances. *Ears:* Denies pain, discharge, tinnitus. *Nose, nasopharynx, paranasal sinuses:* Denies nasal discharge, epistaxis, olfactory deficit, snoring. *Mouth and oropharynx:* Denies sore throat, lesions, gum irritation, chewing or swallowing difficulties, hoarseness, voice changes. *Neck:* Denies tenderness or range-of-motion difficulties. *Health promotion:* Brushes teeth twice daily.

Breasts
No tenderness; denies lumps, masses, or nipple discharge. *Health promotion:* None.

Cardiovascular System
Denies chest pain, shortness of breath, and palpitations; feet frequently feel cold; denies discoloration or peripheral edema. *Health promotion:* Until recently has walked 1.5 miles two to three times a week; has trouble finding time to do this of late.

Respiratory System
Denies breathing difficulties, cough, shortness of breath.

Gastrointestinal System
Denies eating and digestion problems or abdominal pain. Daily bowel movement formed, brown; does not use stool softener or laxatives; denies hemorrhoids.

Urinary System
Describes urine as yellow and clear; voiding frequency four to five times daily; denies problems with voiding, changes in urinary pattern, or pain.

Musculoskeletal System

Denies muscular weakness, twitching, and pain; gait difficulties; and extremity deformities. States that she has occasional joint stiffness but has not experienced pain, edema, or crepitus.

Neurologic System

Denies changes in cognitive function, coordination, and sensory deficits.

Reproductive System

LMP 8 years ago. Denies genital lesions or discharge. States that she is sexually active with husband and satisfied with sexual relationship, although often experiences painful intercourse because of vaginal dryness; denies history of STD. *Health promotion:* Attempts to have Pap test every once in a while but just does not get around to it—"just can't seem to make the time."

PHYSICAL EXAMINATION

General Survey

Cooperative, oriented, alert woman; sitting with erect posture; maintains eye contact; appropriately groomed and dressed. *Vital signs:* BP 110/78; P 78; R 14; T 98° F (36.7° C); wt 137 lb (62 kg); ht 5 ft 3 inches; BMI 24.3.

Skin, Hair, and Nails

Smooth, soft, moist, tanned, warm, intact skin with elastic turgor; hair brown with female distribution, soft texture; nails smooth, rounded, manicured.

Head

Skull symmetric; scalp intact; face and jaw symmetric.

Eyes

Vision 20/20 both eyes with contact lenses; near vision, able to read magazine at 13 inches with contacts. Peripheral vision present; EOM intact; brows, lids, and lashes symmetric; lacrimal ducts pink and open without discharge. Conjunctiva clear; sclera white, moist, and clear; cornea smooth and transparent; iris transparent and flat, PERRLA. Corneal light reflex symmetric. *Ophthalmic examination:* Red reflex present; disc margins distinct, round, yellow; artery-to-vein ratio 2:3, retina red uniformly; macula and fovea slightly darker.

Ears

Hearing intact as noted in general conversation; pinna aligned with eyes, ears symmetric, earlobes pierced once. Cerumen in auditory canal, TM pearly gray, cones of light reflex present.

Nose and Sinuses

Septum midline, nasal passages patent; turbinates pink with no drainage. No pain with sinus palpation.

Mouth and Throat

TMJ moves without difficulty; no halitosis. Lips symmetric, moist, smooth; 28 white, smooth, and aligned teeth; fillings noted in all lower molars. Mucous membranes pink and moist, symmetric pillars, clear saliva. Tongue symmetric, pink, moist, and movable. Hard palate smooth, pale; soft palate smooth, pink, and rises; uvula midline; posterior pharynx pink, smooth; tonsils pink with irregular texture.

Neck

Trachea midline; thyroid smooth, soft, size of thumb pad; full ROM of neck; no palpable lymph nodes.

Chest and Lungs

Breathing quiet and effortless. AP: Lateral diameter 1:2; muscle and respiratory effort symmetric, equal excursion, resonant percussion tones throughout, lungs clear to auscultation throughout lung fields.

Breasts

Moderate size; R slightly > L; no dimpling present. Granular consistency bilaterally but more pronounced in outer quadrants, nipples without discharge, areolas symmetric; symmetric venous pattern; no palpable axillary lymph nodes.

Heart

Apical pulse palpated at fifth LICS, MCL; no lifts, heaves, or thrills or abnormal pulsations, S_1 and S_2 heard without splitting, no murmurs.

Peripheral Vascular

Distal pulses palpable, smooth contour; pulse amplitude 2+ in all pulses; no jugular distention noted; lower extremities warm and pink with symmetric hair distribution, no edema or tenderness; capillary refill <1 second in all nail beds.

Abdomen

Rounded, striae noted; skin smooth; faint 4-inch (10 cm) scar to right lower quadrant; bowel sounds in all quadrants; tympanic percussion tones; abdomen soft, no tenderness, masses, or aortic pulsations noted with light or deep abdominal palpation. Umbilical ring feels round with no irregularities or bulges. Tympany heard over abdomen and spleen and dullness over suprapubic area. Liver spans 3 inches (7.5 cm) at midclavicular line, lower border descends downward 1 inch (2.5 cm). Gallbladder not palpable. No CVA tenderness, no inguinal lymphadenopathy.

Musculoskeletal

Full ROM in all joints without tenderness; muscle strength 5/5 bilaterally, extremities aligned and symmetric, vertebral column straight; coordinated smooth gait.

Neurologic

Oriented to time, place, person; speech understandable and of sufficient volume; cranial nerves I to XII grossly intact;

negative Romberg's sign; peripheral sensation intact, deep tendon reflexes 2+ bilaterally.

Gynecologic

Pubic hair in female distribution; labia smooth and soft; urethral meatus midline; perineum smooth and without lesions; Skene's and Bartholin's glands nontender; vaginal walls smooth, thin, dry; cervix pale pink, midline, parous os, pliable, smooth; no discharge noted; anteverted uterus, smooth, movable, nontender; ovaries smooth, firm, movable. Rectal wall smooth, nontender; sphincter tone tight; two small hemorrhoids. Specimen for Pap test collected.

PROBLEM LIST

- Education regarding health promotion: immunizations, exercise
- Concerned about providing care for mother

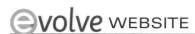

In the previous chapters you have learned which questions to ask to obtain a history and how to perform a head-to-toe assessment. When initially learning how to perform a history and physical examination, students study normal or expected characteristics. Being able to recognize these expected findings is necessary to distinguish them from the abnormal findings. When you assess a patient, you access the knowledge, skills, and attitudes needed for that specific patient.

DIFFERENCES BETWEEN COMPREHENSIVE AND SHIFT ASSESSMENT

This chapter presents examples of adaptations of a comprehensive head-to-toe assessment to a shift assessment in the hospital setting. Nurses perform shift assessments for most patients, regardless of their diagnosis, by collecting the data listed in Box 24-1. A few differences are necessary when conducting an assessment of the hospitalized patient. First, the examination sequence may vary to accommodate patients' limitations. For example, when assessing the lung sounds of a patient who is lying in a supine position, the nurse may delay auscultating lateral and posterior lung sounds until the patient turns to the side or transfers to a chair.

Second, the shift assessment is focused on the immediate needs and potential complications of each patient. For example, when assessing a patient admitted with an exacerbation of heart failure, the nurse's primary focus is the cardiovascular and pulmonary assessment rather than range-of-motion assessment.

A final difference with hospitalized patients is that both the person and the equipment used in the treatment are assessed. As an example, for patients receiving intravenous (IV) fluid therapy, the nurse inspects the IV insertion site for redness and pain and then follows the tubing up to the IV

fluid hanging to make sure that the correct fluid is infusing at the ordered rate and the tubing is labeled with the date that it was hung.

The ability to accurately incorporate ancillary equipment into the assessment requires the nurse to be aware of the equipment that has been ordered, know its purpose, understand how it is used, and be able to recognize if it is not being used properly or functioning correctly. The purpose and use of patient care equipment is beyond the scope of this textbook. The emphasis in this chapter is to remind you of your responsibility to notice the ancillary equipment used by the patients and include it in your assessment.

OBTAINING AND ANALYZING PATIENT DATA

Data about patients are exchanged among nurses in a report at shift change and incorporate information from the medical record, such as the history and physical examination, laboratory data, and radiological reports, in addition to the shift assessment from the previous shift. As an example of a shift assessment consider the following scenario: You are assigned to care for a female patient, Ms. Stone, who was admitted after an automobile accident in which she sustained an open left tibial fracture and a cerebral concussion with loss of consciousness. You start by obtaining a shift report from the nurse who cared for her during the last 12 hours (Fig. 24-1).

Shift Report from the Nurse Who Worked Previous Shift

This is the shift report received from the nurse who cared for Ms. Stone last night from 7 PM to 7 AM.

> Ms. Stone was in an automobile accident 2 days ago in which she sustained an open fracture of the left tibia and a concussion. She had an open reduction and internal fixation of the

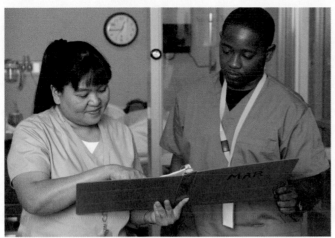

FIG. 24-1 A nurse reports to an oncoming nurse about the status of the patient and data from the care received on the previous shift.

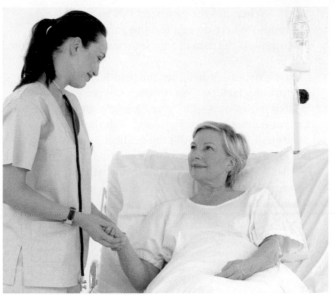

FIG. 24-2 Introduce yourself and tell the patient what you plan to do. (©wavebreakmedia ltd/Shutterstock.com.)

BOX 24-1   COMMON PHYSICAL ASSESSMENT DATA COLLECTED DURING SHIFT ASSESSMENT

- Vital signs: Temperature, pulse, respirations, blood pressure, and oxygen saturation
- Neurologic: Orientation to person, place, time, and situation
- Communication: Speech clear and appropriate
- Cardiac and peripheral vascular system: S_1 and S_2, rate, rhythm, radial and pedal pulse rhythm and amplitude, warmth of extremities, capillary refill
- Lungs and respiratory system: Ease of breathing, skin color, symmetry of thorax, lung sounds
- Abdomen and gastrointestinal system: Appearance of abdomen, bowel sounds, light palpation of the abdomen
- Musculoskeletal system: Compare right and left extremities for symmetry
- Skin: Turgor and intactness
- Drains, catheters, or tubes: Location, patency, and description of drainage, if any

---

left tibia. She lost consciousness at the scene but was conscious at the time of the surgery to realign her leg. She has a history of hypertension; no allergies to drugs or foods. She received pain medication three times during the night for pain of 7 out of 10, with pain relief of 3 to 4 out of 10 after the medication. Her vital signs at 4:00 AM were temperature, 99° F (37.2° C); pulse, 92 beats/min; respirations, 20 breaths/min; oxygen saturation (Sao_2), 96% on room air; and blood pressure, 148/88 mm Hg. The blood pressure was taken just before the last pain medication administration. She is alert and oriented, has regular S_1 and S_2 heart sounds, clear lung sounds, and faint bowel sounds and moves all extremities. Her incision is well approximated, clean and dry; has staples; and is edematous and red. She is able to move her toes and has palpable pedal pulses bilaterally. She has a peripheral IV line in her left arm of D_5NS (5% dextrose in normal saline) at a rate of 100 mL/hr; the IV site is without redness or edema. Physical therapy is coming this morning to assess her for crutch walking.

Current Shift Assessment

You compare and contrast your assessment data for this patient against data from the last 12 hours and your knowledge of expected findings. You apply knowledge, skills, and attitudes that include vital signs; orientation; and assessment of heart, lungs, bowel sounds, movement, peripheral perfusion, and skin integrity, particularly the incision of the left lower leg.

"Good morning, Ms. Stone. My name is Juanita. I will be caring for you today. I want to begin by completing an assessment. Is this a good time?"
Introduce yourself and tell the patient what you plan to do. Get the patient's consent for the assessment at this time (Fig. 24-2).

"Can you tell me your full name and where you are?"
Since this patient had a concussion, this question is asked to determine orientation to person and place.
Procedure: While you are listening to all of the patient's answers to your questions, you are also observing her eye contact, the clarity of her speech, and the symmetry of her head and face. Note any movement of her hands while she talks.
Data: You notice that she maintains eye contact; her speech is clear, and head and face are symmetric. She moves both arms.

"I understand that you had some pain last night. Are you having pain now?"
Procedure: Use the OLD CARTS mnemonic to guide a symptom analysis of her pain.

- Onset—When did the pain start this morning?
- Location—Where do you feel the pain?
- Duration—Is the pain in your leg constant or does it come and go?
- Characteristics—What does the pain feel like?
- Aggravating factors—What makes the pain worse?
- Related symptoms—Do you have any other symptoms such as nausea or sweating along with the pain?
- Treatment—How well did the medication relieve the pain last night? Did you use any other pain-relief methods such as relaxation or distraction to relieve pain?
- Severity—On a scale 0 to 10, using 10 as the worst pain you have had, how would you rate it?

Data: She reports an aching pain in her left leg of 5/10 present since surgery, relieved by distraction and pain medications and aggravated by moving her leg, knee, or ankle.

"I'm going to measure your temperature, pulse, and blood pressure."

Since the patient's peripheral IV line is in her left arm, her blood pressure is taken using her right arm.

Data: Temperature, 100.8° F (38.2° C); pulse, 98 beats/min, easily palpable and regular; respirations, 24 beats/min without effort; blood pressure, 140/86; Sa_{O_2} = 98% on room air.

"Next I'll listen to your heart and lungs."

Procedure: Unsnap her gown so you can place the stethoscope on her anterior chest. Listen at two locations for heart sounds, over the aortic and pulmonic valves. Listen to her anterior lungs and then ask her to lean forward so you can listen to her posterior and lateral thorax for lung sounds.

Data: S_1 an S_2 heart sounds are regular, lungs are clear except for crackles in the bases bilaterally, thoracic movement is symmetric.

"Now I'm going to assess your abdomen by listening and then by pressing lightly with my hands."

Procedure: Inspect her abdomen and then listen for bowel sounds in each quadrant. Lightly palpate the abdomen for tenderness.

Data: Abdomen is flat and a lighter color than extremities, contour is symmetric. Bowel sounds are hypoactive in all quadrants. There is no tenderness to palpation.

"I need to look at your IV site. Does it hurt?"

Inspect the IV site in her left arm. The skin should be without redness or edema, and the IV catheter should be secured. Fig. 24-3 is provided as an example of how an IV insertion site appears. In this figure the IV has been disconnected temporarily from the IV tubing until IV fluids or medications are resumed. This disconnection allows the patient more freedom of movement and is safe for patients who do not require continuous fluid therapy.

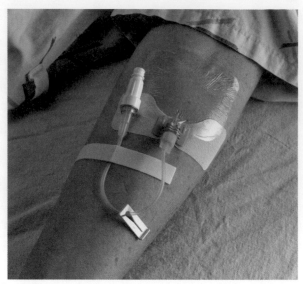

FIG. 24-3 Inspect the intravenous site for redness and edema. (From Ignatavicius and Workman, 2010.)

"I'm going to check the pulses in your arms and feet."

Procedure: Palpate both radial pulses simultaneously and compare them for rhythm and amplitude. Next place the back of your hands on her lower legs simultaneously to compare the temperatures. Then palpate her dorsalis pedis pulses simultaneously for amplitude and compare findings.

Data: Pulses are regular and 2+ bilaterally, legs are equally warm to touch.

"I want to test the strength in your legs. Push against my hands with your feet."

Data: She is able to push her feet against your hands, indicating 5/5 leg strength; but her left leg is not as strong as her right, and she complains of pain in her left leg from the surgical site when pushing against your hand.

"I'm going to look at your incision."

Procedure: Inspect the incision for redness, edema, drainage, and intact staples and measure the length of the incision (Fig 24-4).

Data: The incision has staples, is well-approximated, 17 cm long with redness and edema and no drainage.

Applying the Clinical Judgment Model

After the patient's assessment data are collected, use these data to make decisions about the patient's care.

Notice abnormal findings: Crackles in the bases bilaterally and red, edematous incision.

Interpret data using reasoning patterns: These data differ from data gained from report.

Postsurgical patients are at risk for atelectasis and pneumonia.

Her temperature and heart rate are higher than the last assessment. Her left tibia is red and edematous, which may indicate an infection.

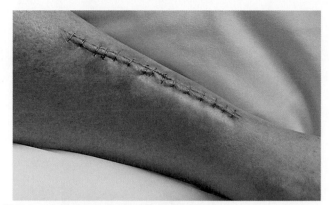

FIG. 24-4 Inspect the incision for redness, edema, drainage, and intact staples and measure the length of the incision. (From Perry, Potter, and Elkin, 2012.)

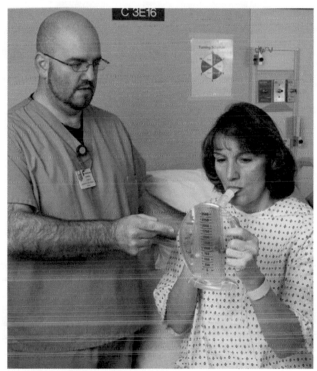

FIG. 24-5 Using an incentive spirometer helps prevent postoperative pulmonary complications. (From Perry, Potter, and Elkin, 2012.)

Action: Document findings. Report changes to the health care provider, encourage patient to cough and deep breathe to prevent pneumonia, encourage fluid intake, and give antimicrobials as ordered. Also encourage her to use the incentive spirometer (IS), which measures the amount of air moved during deep breathing. Typically the patient is asked to use the IS for 10 deep breaths every hour while awake to prevent atelectasis and pneumonia. An example of another patient using an IS is shown in Fig 24-5.

BOX 24-2 **NEVER EVENTS**

The term *Never Events* was developed by the National Quality Forum (NQF) and refers to medical errors that should never occur. Events related to nursing assessment are stage 3 or 4 pressure ulcers acquired after admission to a health care facility and death or serious disability associated with a patient falling while being cared for in a health care facility. See risk factors for falls in Chapter 21. The Centers for Medicare and Medicaid Services (CMS) announced in August 2007 that Medicare would no longer pay for additional costs associated with many preventable errors, including those considered Never Events. Never events are being publically reported, with the goal of increasing accountability and improving the quality of care.

From: Patient Safety Primer: *Never Events,* Agency for Health Care Research and Quality, US Department of Health and Human Services, available at http://psnet.ahrq.gov/primer.aspx?primerID=3, accessed November 14, 2011.

ADAPTING ASSESSMENT SKILLS TO HOSPITALIZED PATIENTS

In assessing other patients in the hospital, you apply your knowledge, skills, and attitudes to perform the shift assessments. What follows are photos of 14 patients who have had different procedures performed that require adaptations to the usual shift assessment procedures shown in Box 24-1. For each of these patients measure vital signs, including pain and oxygen saturation; auscultate heart, lung, and bowel sounds; assess movement of upper and lower extremities and palpate dorsalis pedis pulses. The patients presented require adapted assessment of the following systems: skin, lungs, and respiratory; heart and peripheral vascular; abdomen and gastrointestinal; musculoskeletal; and neurologic.

Adapting Assessment of the Skin

Skin inspection and palpation are essential for all patients on admission and as indicated throughout their hospitalization. Perform a risk assessment for pressure ulcers using a validated tool such as the Braden scale (available at www.bradenscale.com under the heading of "products"). This scale includes risk factors such as the patient's sensory perception, moisture of the skin, activity level, mobility, nutrition, and amount of friction and shear to the skin. When nurses identify patients at risk for pressure ulcers, they initiate plans to prevent their development. When a pressure ulcer is identified, it is documented (in writing and with photographs). Nurses collaborate with health care providers, dietitians, and perhaps wound care nurses to initiate a plan of treatment. Refer to Table 9-5 for staging of pressure ulcers. Development of a pressure ulcer after admission is preventable and is considered a "Never Event" by the National Quality Forum. See Box 24-2 for further discussion of these events.

Patient with a Wound

Patient 1 has a wound that is healing by secondary intention, which means that the edges of the wound are separated; granulation tissue develops to fill in the gap. Examine the wound itself, drainage within the wound, and the dressing. When permitted by the surgeon to remove the dressing, inspect the wound for color, size, and drainage. This wound has red-to-pink granulation tissue, indicating healing of tissue (Fig. 24-6). The lines show how the width and depth of this wound are measured for documentation. Note type of drainage, if present, in the wound or on the dressing. In this case serous drainage is observed. Photographs provide valuable documentation of wounds so healing can be monitored. Because this patient has an open wound, a nutritional assessment may be indicated (see Chapter 8).

Patient with an Infected Incision

Patient 2 had an abdominal surgical procedure, but the wound became infected and the suture line dehisced (rupture of a surgical incision) (Fig. 24-7). Assessment of this wound includes describing the wound and its drainage and measuring the width, length, and depth. A cotton-tipped applicator is placed at various locations in the wound to measure the depth. The location of four previous retention sutures can be seen. There is a small amount of dark necrotic tissue at the lower left side of the incision approximately at the 7 o'clock location using a clock reference. Some granulation (red) tissue and yellow and white exudate are noted within the wound. Health team members with whom you may collaborate are the health care provider, dietitian, and wound care nurse.

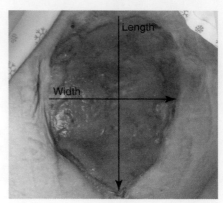

FIG. 24-6 Describe the color of the wound and measure the length and width to document healing. (From Perry, Potter, and Elkin, 2012.)

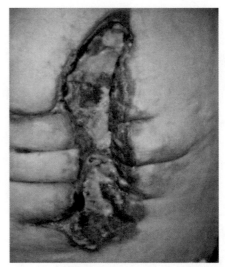

FIG. 24-7 When assessing a dehisced wound, describe the wound and drainage and measure the width, length, and depth. (From Perry, Potter, and Elkin, 2012.)

Adapting Assessment of the Lungs and Respiratory System
Patient Using a Nasal Cannula

Patient 3 has pneumonia requiring oxygen therapy that is delivered by a nasal cannula (Fig. 24-8). In addition to the usual assessment data (see Box 24-1), notice the patient's respiratory effort and the oxygen saturation from the pulse oximeter. Ask the patient about any cough, including the color and amount of sputum expectorated. Ask if the cough is interfering with self-care activities and sleep. Inspect the skin of the nares and behind the helix of her ears for signs of pressure from nasal prongs and oxygen tubing, respectively. Assessment of the respiratory therapy equipment includes inspecting the position of the nasal prongs to ensure that oxygen flow is directed into the nares and examining the oxygen flowmeter to ensure that oxygen is being delivered at the appropriate flow rate.

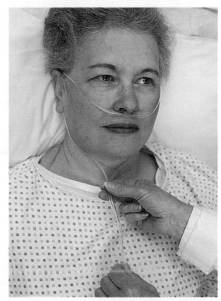

FIG. 24-8 Inspect the nares and behind the ears for pressure from the nasal cannula. (From Perry, Potter, and Elkin, 2012.)

Patient Using an Oxygen Mask

Patient 4 has emphysema and requires oxygen therapy using a ventimask (Fig. 24-9). Assessment of this patient includes noticing the use of accessory muscles to breathe or tripod sitting. Assessing the posterior-to-lateral diameter may be indicated to confirm a barrel chest. Inspect the skin of his face for redness or indentation from the facemask and behind the helix of his ears for signs of pressure from the oxygen tubing. Assessment of the respiratory therapy equipment includes inspecting the ventimask to make sure that it is providing the correct oxygen percentage for this patient.

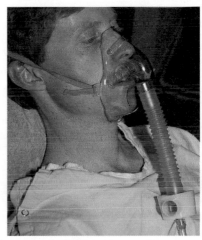

FIG. 24-9 Inspect the face and ears for pressure from the Venturi mask. (From Perry, Potter, and Elkin, 2012.)

Patient with a Tracheostomy

Patient 5 has a tracheostomy that the nurse is suctioning to remove bronchial secretions (Fig. 24-10). The tracheostomy tube is inserted into the trachea as a long-term artificial airway and is held in place by ties that are secured around the patient's neck. Tracheostomy tubes are used for administration of mechanical ventilation, relief of airway obstruction, or clearing of secretions. Patients who have tracheostomy tubes are unable to speak because the air passes through the tube rather than the vocal cords. They may be able to mouth words or write notes to communicate.

After suctioning, place a collar over the tracheostomy tube. The collar delivers humidified oxygen to warm and humidify the air the patient inhales since the nose is bypassed. Patient assessment includes respiratory effort and the amount and color of secretions suctioned from the tracheostomy tube. Also inspect the skin around the tracheostomy tube and the neck for redness, excoriation, or skin breakdown. The gauze square around the tracheostomy tube is changed when it becomes wet from secretions. Assessment of the respiratory equipment includes the oxygen setting on the flowmeter and adequacy of water to provide humidification.

Patient with Chest Tubes

Patient 6 had a thoracotomy (incision into the thoracic cavity) to remove a tumor from the right thorax (Fig. 24-11). Chest tubes are placed in the pleural space to drain blood and secretions after surgery. The chest tubes initially are attached to a drainage system that works with gravity or suction. In addition to the common physical assessment data collected (see Box 24-1), assess this patient's pain from the surgical site, especially when inhaling deeply. When suction is used, it may create a sound that can be heard during chest auscultation, making auscultation more difficult. The sound from the suction may be mistaken for abnormal lung sounds. The dressing around the chest tube is inspected; it should be dry and intact. This dressing is not removed until the surgeon is ready to remove the chest tubes. The color and amount of drainage from the chest tube that collects in the bedside drainage container are noted. Encourage this patient to take deep breaths and cough to prevent atelectasis and pneumonia.

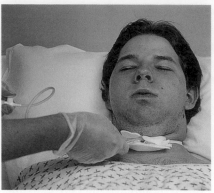

FIG. 24-10 Inspect the skin around the tracheostomy tube and the neck for redness. (From Perry, Potter, and Elkin, 2012.)

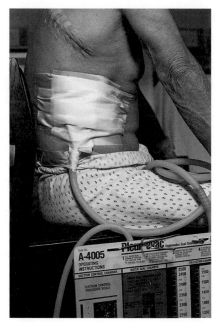

FIG. 24-11 Assess patency of pleural chest tubes attached to suction. (From Elkin, Perry, and Potter, 2008.)

Adapting Assessment of the Heart and Peripheral Vascular System
Patient with Arteriovenous Fistula

Patient 7 has chronic kidney disease, which is treated with hemodialysis three times a week. Hemodialysis is a procedure in which blood is removed through a fistula (abnormal opening between two internal organs) and filtered by a machine that removes wastes and then returns the filtered blood to the patient. A surgical procedure creates an arteriovenous (AV) fistula by suturing together an artery and a vein such as a radial artery and a cephalic vein, shown in Fig. 24-12. For hemodialysis, blood is removed from the arterial side of the fistula and returned to the venous side. Assessing the fistula (Fig. 24-13) is very important to determine if blood flow between the artery and vein is present. Two techniques are used to assess the AV fistula, which indicate blood flow: palpation of the fistula for a thrill and auscultation for a bruit. Absence of the thrill and bruit indicates that the blood flow has slowed or stopped and the fistula cannot be used for hemodialysis without immediate evaluation. You may work collaboratively with a dialysis nurse to coordinate patient care.

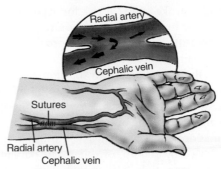

FIG. 24-12 Radial artery and cephalic vein fistula. (From Ignatavicius and Workman, 2010.)

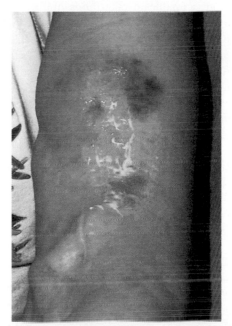

FIG. 24-13 Palpate the fistula for a thrill and auscultate it for a bruit. (From Ignatavicius and Workman, 2010.)

Adapting Assessment of the Abdomen and Gastrointestinal System
Patient with a Gastrostomy Tube

Patient 8 had a stroke and is at risk for aspiration of gastric contents into the lungs, which could cause aspiration pneumonia. To prevent the aspiration and provide nutrition for the patient, a surgeon placed a gastrostomy tube (G tube) through the abdominal wall into the stomach (Figs. 24-14 and 24-15). The tube is used to provide a liquid diet, water, and medications. The diet may be given continuously using a pump at an ordered rate of milliliters (mL) per hour or in bolus feedings on a schedule such as 240 mL of formula every 4 hours followed by 100 mL of water. The patient may not have any fluids by mouth to prevent choking.

Assessment of this patient includes inspection of the skin around the G tube and the oral mucous membranes for moisture since he is unable to take fluids orally. Also aspirate stomach contents as ordered through the G tube to determine the amount of residual feeding in the stomach. When the residual volume is greater than 100 mL, the risk for reflux into the esophagus or trachea increases. Expected findings are intact skin without redness around the G tube. The gingiva and oral mucous membranes are pink and moist. Abnormal findings may include redness, edema and drainage around the G tube, and dry gingival and mucous membranes. Assessment of the equipment includes ensuring administration of the correct formula in the amount and route ordered. Also check the dates on the equipment for currency. For example, the tubing used for continuous feedings through a pump is changed every 24 hours to prevent bacterial growth, and it is dated and timed when hung.

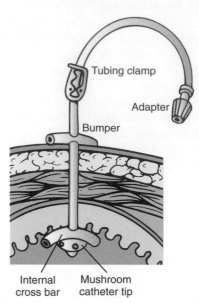

FIG. 24-14 A gastrostomy tube (G tube) is surgically placed through the abdominal wall into the stomach. (From Perry, Potter, and Elkin, 2012.)

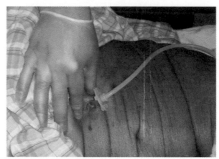

FIG. 24-15 Inspect the skin around the gastrostomy tube. (From Roberts and Hedges, 2009.)

Patient with a Nasogastric Tube and Wound Drain

Patient 9 had a laparotomy to surgically treat a small-bowel obstruction. This procedure involves a surgeon making an incision into the abdomen to locate and repair the cause of the obstruction. After the procedure the patient has a nasogastric tube (NG) to remove gastric contents until peristalsis returns (Fig. 24-16). The NG tube is often attached to intermittent wall suction to decompress the stomach by removing gastric secretions and air. Notice the amount and color of the NG drainage that collects in the container adjacent to the wall suction. A wound drain is placed in the surgical site to prevent accumulation of fluids at the surgical site (Fig. 24-17). The drainage is collected with gentle suction from a bulb-type container. The nurse empties, measures, and discards the drainage. After removing the drainage, the nurse squeezes the bulb and replaces the plug to generate suction. Assessment of this patient begins with inspection of the skin of the naris containing the NG tube for redness from pressure and inspection of the tape attaching the NG tube to the patient's nose to make sure that it is secure. For optimal organization listen to heart and lungs sounds followed by bowel sounds. The sound of the intermittent suction for the NG tube may be heard when listening for bowel sounds, which is an expected deviation. Contrary to common practice, listening to bowel sounds after abdominal surgery is not a good assessment of the recovery of peristalsis[1] (Box 24-3). Next inspect the abdominal dressing, which should be clean and dry. When drainage is found on the dressing, notice the color and measure the approximate area of the drainage. Assessment of the equipment begins by verifying NG tube placement in the stomach by testing the pH of the secretions aspirated (see Fig. 24-16), noticing the volume and color of NG tube drainage, and examining the suction equipment to ensure that it is set as ordered. Expected findings include skin of nares intact without redness, and NG tube to low intermittent wall suction with color and volume of drainage recorded. The expected color of stomach secretions in the tubing is yellow to green. Abdominal dressing dry and intact with serosanguineous drainage in the bulb drain.

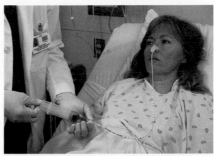

FIG. 24-16 Notice which naris contains the nasogastric tube and inspect the skin of the naris for irritation from the pressure of the tube. (From Perry, Potter, and Elkin, 2012.)

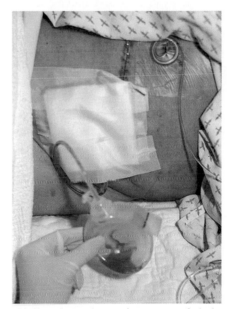

FIG. 24-17 Notice the color and amount of drainage. (From Perry, Potter, and Elkin, 2012.)

BOX 24-3 EVIDENCE-BASED PRACTICE

Best Indicator of Return of Gastrointestinal Motility after Abdominal Surgery

Historically nurses have listened to bowel sounds of patients after abdominal surgery to determine when they can begin drinking fluids. Several studies and systematic reviews revealed that auscultation of the abdomen during early recovery after abdominal surgery is not an effective assessment of the recovery of peristalsis. More useful indicators of returning gastrointestinal motility after abdominal surgery are return of flatus and first bowel movement.

From: Madsen D et al: Listening to bowel sounds: an evidenced-based practice project, *Am J Nurs* 105(12):40-48, 2005.

Patient with an Ostomy

Patient 10 had the descending and transverse colon removed (partial colectomy) to treat a malignancy several days ago. The remaining colon was brought to the abdominal wall to create an artificial anus called a *colostomy,* shown in Fig. 24-18. The colostomy allows stool to be evacuated from the colon into the pouch shown in Fig. 24-19. Assessment of this patient includes inspection of the stoma, the skin around the stoma, the character of the stool, and the colostomy appliance.

The stoma should appear red and moist. The skin around the stoma and under the ostomy appliance should appear intact without lesions, irritation, or areas of excoriation. Abnormal findings are a stoma that is pale from ischemia or brown or black from necrotic tissue and skin around the stoma that is excoriated and tender, with or without exudate.

Describe the color and characteristics of the output from the colostomy. A newly created colostomy will not have stool draining from it until the patient starts eating. If the patient has had a transverse (upper colon)–level colostomy, the stool is mushy. If the patient's colostomy is in the area of the descending or sigmoid (lower) colon, the stool is more solid. When the entire colon is removed, the distal ileum is brought to the abdominal wall to form an ileostomy. The contents from the ileostomy contain digestive enzymes from the small intestine, are a thick liquid consistency, and are secreted continuously. Health team members with whom you may collaborate are a health care provider, dietitian, and enterstomal therapist.

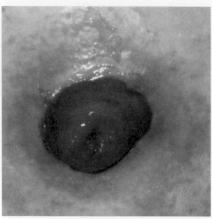

FIG. 24-18 Describe the appearance of the stoma and the skin surrounding it. (From Perry, Potter, and Elkin, 2012.)

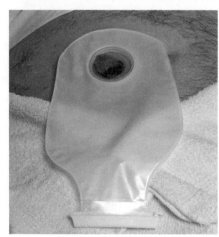

FIG. 24-19 A pouch attached around the stoma. (From deWit, 2009.)

Patient with a Urinary Catheter

Patient 11 has an indwelling urinary catheter to continuously drain the urine into a collection bag hung on the bed frame (Fig. 24-20). Urinary catheters are used to measure urine output, relieve urinary obstruction, after a surgical procedure, or when the bladder empties inadequately as a result of a neurologic condition. Adapt your usual sequence by inspecting the equipment first before the patient's urinary meatus. Inspect the color of the urine in the bedside collection bag in your initial survey of the patient. Inspect the catheter tubing to make sure that the urine is flowing freely without any kinks in the tubing. Some facilities secure the catheter tubing of female patients to the inner thigh to reduce risk of urethral erosion or accidental catheter removal. For male patients the catheter tubing is secured to the upper thigh or lower abdomen.[2] When the bath is given, provide perineal care for the patient during which you clean the external genitalia and surrounding skin. Performing this procedure provides an opportunity to inspect the urinary meatus and surrounding skin. The expected finding for a female is a moist and pink meatus containing a catheter with intact skin surrounding it that is a color consistent with the patient's race. Male patients with urinary catheters also receive perineal care. Abnormal findings are a red and edematous meatus. The surrounding skin may be red or have a scaling red rash with sharply demarcated borders caused by candidiasis, a fungal infection. See Chapter 9, "Common Problems and Conditions." The urine collection bag is emptied at the end of the shift and documented as fluid output.

Adapting Assessment of the Musculoskeletal System
Patient with a Cast

Patient 12 has a cast on the right leg (Fig. 24-21). Assessing circulation, movement, and sensation of the toes distal to the cast is critical. Because of the cast location of this patient, the dorsalis pedis pulse is not accessible to palpation. Instead circulation is determined by assessing capillary refill in the toes and noting the temperature and color of the skin. Ask the patient to move the right toes to assess movement. Place your hand adjacent to the toes so the patient cannot see which toe you touch. Ask him or her to identify which toe you are touching to assess sensation. Expected findings are capillary refill 2 seconds or less and warm temperature and color consistent with the uninjured foot with movement and sensation present.

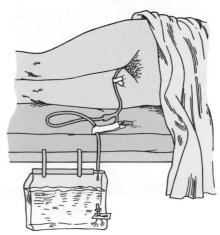

FIG. 24-20 Inspect the color of the urine in the bedside collection bag in your initial survey of the patient. (From Perry, Potter, and Elkin, 2012.)

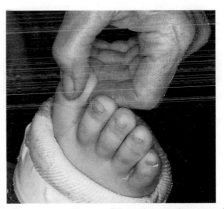

FIG. 24-21 Assess capillary refill to determine arterial circulation to the right toes. (From Perry, Potter, and Elkin, 2012.)

Patient with an External Fixator

Patient 13 has an injury to his left hand requiring an external fixator to hold the bones in place while they heal (Fig. 24-22). Patient assessment includes determining presence of circulation, movement, and sensation of the fingers. Assess capillary refill of the fingers and the radial pulse. Ask the patient to move the fingers to assess motion. Use the same procedures to test sensation as used with Patient 12. Since the external fixator penetrates the skin, the insertion sites are inspected for evidence of infection (i.e., redness, edema, and drainage). Expected findings include that insertion sites of external fixator on right hand are clean without redness. Radial pulse 2+, capillary refill less than 2 seconds, movement and sensation of fingers present. Fingers are edematous with clean, dry dressing of third finger.

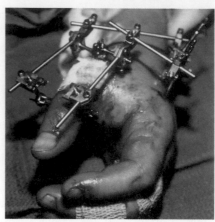

FIG. 24-22 Assess circulation, movement, sensation, and the skin at insertion sites. (From Perry, Potter, and Elkin, 2012.)

Adapting Assessment of the Neurologic System
Patient Who Is Unconscious

Patient 14 had a stroke and is unconscious (Fig. 24-23), which requires a modified neurologic assessment because she cannot actively participate. When interacting with an unconscious patient, *always* assume that he or she can hear *everything* you say; thus tell the patient which actions you are going to perform before you do them. For example, tell the patient, "I'm going to hold your eyelid open and shine a light into your eye to check your pupils."

This patient has an oral endotracheal (ET) tube attached to a ventilator because the patient could not breath adequately on her own when she was admitted. Now that she is able to breathe on her own without using the ventilator, the ET tube will be removed.

As with assessment of any patient, inspection is used first to observe respiratory pattern. For example, Cheyne-Stokes breathing is periods of apnea alternating with hyperventilation (see Fig. 11-13, *F*).

Assess pupillary size and response to determine function of cranial nerve (CN) III (oculomotor), Refer to Table 10-1 in Chapter 10 for pupil abnormalities.

To assess level of consciousness, you need to determine how much stimulation or pain is required to elicit a response from the patient. A response may be the opening of the eyes, an intentional movement, or speech. Begin with a touch and a normal tone of voice. If this does not create a response, shake the patient on the shoulder or leg and shout at him or her. If this does not produce a response, resort to painful stimuli, beginning peripherally and moving centrally. When painful stimuli are used, they should be applied until patients respond in some way or for at least 15 seconds. They should be used for no more than 30 seconds if there is no response. Begin by depressing the nail bed at the cuticle with your fingernail or an object such as the length of a pen or pencil. If this does not elicit a response, squeeze the trapezius muscle very hard and observe for any movement. If this does not yield a response, push upward on the supraorbital notch above the eye. Do not push inward on the eyeball but on the bony orbit above the eyeball. Table 24-1 describes techniques for applying painful stimuli.[3]

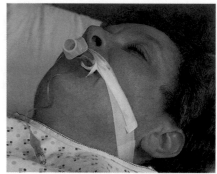

FIG. 24-23 To assess level of consciousness, determine how much stimulation or pain is required to elicit a response from the patient. (From Perry, Potter, and Elkin, 2012.)

TABLE 24-1   TECHNIQUES FOR APPLYING PAINFUL STIMULI

Assessing Peripheral Pain	Technique
Pressing on the nail plate	Apply pressure to only those extremities that did not respond to central painful stimuli. Press in the nail plate (at the cuticle) with the shaft of a pencil or pen. Apply pressure for 15 to 30 seconds and observe for response.

Assessing Central Pain	Technique
Squeezing the trapezius muscle	Squeeze the trapezius muscle by grasping the muscle with the thumb and two fingers, pinching 1 to 2 inches (2.5 to 5 cm) and twisting.
Applying supraorbital pressure	Avoid applying supraorbital pressure if the patient has facial fractures. Palpate the orbital rim beneath the eyebrow until you locate the notch near the center where a sensory nerve is located. With your thumb, push up firmly on the notch. (Do not push inward on the eye globe.)
Applying mandibular pressure	Using your index and middle fingers, push up and inward at the angle of the patient's jaw (just below the earlobe).
Rubbing the sternum	This technique should be used as a last resort because it can cause bruising. Apply pressure downward with your knuckles to the midsternum and turn your knuckles to the left and right without moving them from the sternum.

Since this patient is not able to change her position independently, she is at risk for pressure ulcers. After turning her from her back to a side-lying position, inspect the skin over the areas receiving pressure, such as her sacrum and heels, for redness and moisture. Likewise, after turning her from a side-lying to a supine position, inspect the skin over the areas receiving pressure, such as her trochanter, for redness (see Fig. 9-15). Also she is at risk for developing a venous thrombotic event (VTE), also called deep vein thrombosis (DVT). To prevent this complication, the nurse applies sequential compression devices (SCDs) (Fig. 24-24) to the patient's legs to stimulate circulation and prevent venous stasis. Another device to prevent VTE is the application of thromboembolic deterrent (TED) stockings (Fig. 24-25) to the patient's legs to facilitate the return of venous blood to the heart. When patients wear either of these devices, skin and temperature assessments of the legs must be adapted by removing these devices temporarily to complete the assessment.

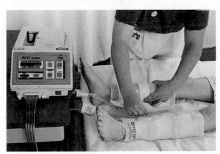

FIG. 24-24 Sequential compression devices (SCDs) help prevent venous thrombus formation. (From Perry, Potter, and Elkin, 2012.)

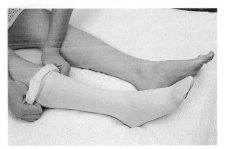

FIG. 24-25 Thrombo Emboli Deterrent (TED) stockings help prevent venous thrombus formation. (From Potter and Perry, 2009.)

Describing Levels of Consciousness

The findings from an assessment of an unconscious patient are described using adjectives with standard definitions or by using a numeric scale such as the Glasgow Coma Scale (GCS). Adjectives used to describe consciousness in decreasing order of consciousness are lethargy, obtunded, stuporous, semicomatose, and comatose. Patients who are *lethargic* can be aroused by saying their name and touching them. Once aroused, they response appropriately but return to "sleep" as soon as the stimuli ceases. Those who are *obtunded* require louder verbal stimuli and vigorous shaking to prompt a response; they carry out requests while awake but return to "sleep" when stimuli stops. Patients who are *stuporous* require painful stimuli to respond, and the response usually is a

Glasgow Coma Scale

Best eye-opening response	Spontaneously	4
	To verbal command	3
	To pain	2
	No response	1
Best verbal response	Oriented, converses	5
	Disoriented, converses	4
	Inappropriate words	3
	Incomprehensible sounds	2
	No response	1
Best motor response	Obeys pain	6
To verbal command	Localizes	5
To painful stimulus	Flexion—withdrawal	4
	Flexion—decorticate	3
	Extension—decerebrate	2
	No response	1
	TOTAL	(3-15)

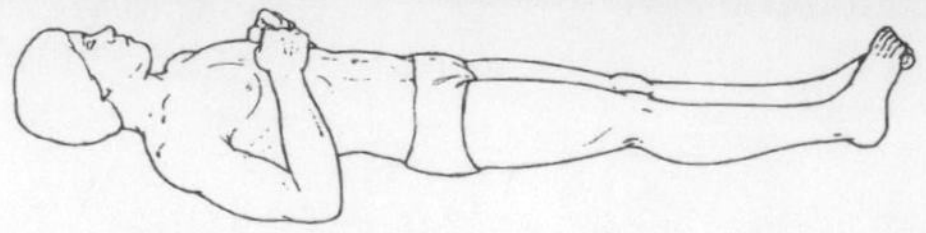

Abnormal flexion (Decorticate) Rigid flexion; upper arms held tightly to the sides of body; elbows, wrists, and fingers flexed; feet are plantar flexed, legs extended and internally rotated; may have fine tremors or intense stiffness

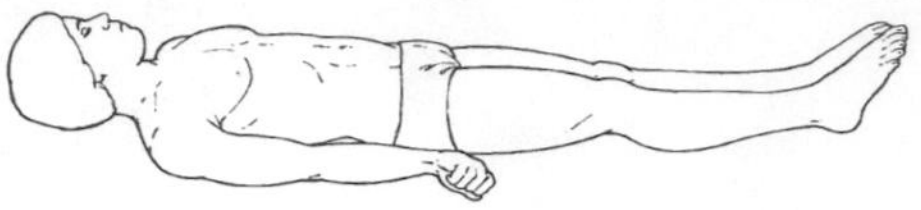

Abnormal extension (Decerebrate) Rigid extension; arms fully extended; forearms pronated; wrists and fingers flexed; jaws clenched, neck extended, back may be arched; feet plantar flexed; may occur spontaneously, intermittently, or in response to a stimulus

FIG. 24-26 Glasgow Coma Scale. (Modified from Chipps, Clanin, and Campbell, 1992.)

withdrawal from the source of pain. *Semicomatose* patients require painful stimuli and respond with abnormal flexion or extension. *Comatose* patients do not respond to any stimuli, even central pain.

Since there may be some overlap in the adjectives used to describe consciousness, some nurses prefer the GCS, which uses a 15-point scale to assess consciousness (Fig. 24-26). This scale is only useful to assess patients with altered consciousness. The patient is assessed for the best response to eye opening, motor response, and verbal response. For example, when assessing the patient who has altered consciousness and is paralyzed on one side as a result of a stroke, use the patient's unaffected side for best motor response. An arbitrary number is assigned to describe the motor response. The response observed from the patient may be a localization of pain (score of 5) when he or she moves as if trying to remove the stimulus, an attempt to withdraw from the stimulus (score of 4), abnormal flexion (formerly called *decorticate posturing*) (score of 3), abnormal extension (formerly called *decerebrate posturing*) (score of 2), or no response at all to any painful stimuli (score of 1). See Fig. 24-26 for examples of abnormal flexion and extension.

When the patient is unable to speak because of an endotracheal or tracheostomy tube placement, the best verbal response of the GCS cannot be assessed. Each institution has its specific way of documenting this. For example, if the patient is comatose, the score may be recorded as 2T, meaning 1 for best eye response, 1 for best motor response, and T for "tube," indicating that verbal response cannot be assessed. A score from 14 to 3 is considered abnormal. The lower the score, the deeper is the coma.

SUMMARY

The patients presented in this chapter provide a few examples of how the head-to-toe assessment of healthy people is adapted to meet the needs of the hospitalized patient. Conducting an assessment at the beginning of each shift provides a baseline for the immediate needs and potential complications of each patient. As you become competent in the knowledge, skills, and attitudes needed for health assessment, you improve your clinical reasoning to help you learn to think like a nurse and provide patient-centered care.

Health History Using Functional Health Patterns

1. Health Perception–Health Management
   - How would you describe your health overall?
   - How would you describe your health at this time?
   - What is the reason for this health care visit? What are your expectations?
   - If ill, describe your illness. What do you think caused it?
   - Which treatments, health care practices, or folk remedies have you used to treat your illness?
   - Are you usually able to follow prescribed instructions given by a health care professional?
   - Do you anticipate problems caring for yourself or others? If so, describe.
   - Describe what you do to keep healthy and prevent disease in yourself and your family, including exercise, leisure activities, regular dental care, routine professional examinations, self-examinations, nutrition, weight control, and immunizations.
   - Which medications (prescribed and over-the-counter) do you take?
   - Do you use tobacco products? Alcohol? If so, how much and how frequently?
   - What safety measures do you take? (Smoke alarms in home? Use of helmets when cycling, skiing, or in-line skating? Weapons in home? Use of seat belt in automobile? Storage of poison in home?)
   - Describe the health of your family (maternal grandparents, mother, paternal grandparents, father, siblings, spouse, children).
   - Are you aware of any risk factors for disease that you have?
2. Nutrition-Metabolic
   - Describe what you usually eat. Breakfast? Lunch? Dinner? Snacks?
   - What is your typical fluid intake? (Name the type of fluids and amounts.)
   - Describe your appetite. Do you have any problems that affect your appetite (e.g., nausea, fullness, indigestion)?
   - Are you following, or have you been following in the past, any specially prescribed diet?
   - Describe your food preferences.
   - Do you take any nutritional supplements (e.g., vitamins or protein)?
   - Do you have any food restrictions? Any food allergies?

   - Have you experienced any difficulties with eating (e.g., chewing or swallowing)?
   - How much do you think you weigh?
   - Have you experienced weight changes (loss or gain) in the last 6 to 9 months?
   - Have you noticed problems with your skin (e.g., dryness, swelling, lesions, or itching)?
   - Do your wounds heal quickly?
   - Do you have any risk factors that make you susceptible to skin ulcers (e.g., decreased circulation, sensory deficits, or decreased mobility)?
3. Elimination
   - How many times a day do you urinate?
   - What color is your urine?
   - Do you have any problems with urination (e.g., pain or burning, dribbling, incontinence, retention, or frequency)?
   - Do you use any assistive devices for urinating (e.g., incontinence pads, intermittent or indwelling catheter, or cystostomy)?
   - Describe your normal bowel elimination pattern, including time and frequency.
   - What does your stool look like (color, consistency)?
   - Do you use any assistive devices for bowel elimination (e.g., laxatives, suppositories, enemas, or colostomy/ileostomy)?
4. Activity Exercise
   - Describe your activity level.
   - Do you exercise? If so, describe the type, frequency, intensity, and duration of exercise.
   - Which leisure activities do you enjoy?
   - Do you experience any of the following: shortness of breath, fatigue or weakness, cough, chest pain, palpitations, leg pain, or pain in muscles or joints? If so, describe.
   - To what extent do you require assistance for the following daily activities:
     - Feeding
     - Bathing
     - Toileting
     - Bed mobility
     - Dressing
     - Grooming
     - General mobility
     - Cooking

- Home maintenance
- Shopping

Level 0: Full self-care
Level I: Requires use of equipment or device
Level II: Requires assistance or supervision from another person
Level III: Requires assistance from another person (and equipment or device)
Level IV: Is dependent and does not participate

5. Sleep-Rest
   - How many hours per night do you generally sleep?
   - What time do you usually go to bed? Wake up?
   - Do you generally feel rested after sleep?
   - Do you have any sleep rituals? If so, describe.
   - Do you experience any problems associated with sleeping (e.g., difficulty falling asleep, difficulty remaining asleep, or early awakening)? If so, describe.

6. Cognitive-Perceptual
   - Are you able to read and write?
   - Which languages do you speak?
   - How do you best learn?
   - Do you experience any problems with hearing? Do you use a hearing aid?
   - Do you wear glasses or contact lenses? Do you experience any problems with vision?
   - When was your last visual examination?
   - Do you experience problems with dizziness? If so, describe.
   - Have you noticed any insensitivity to cold, heat, or pain? If so, describe.
   - Do you experience pain? If so, describe.

7. Self-Perception–Self-Concept
   - How would you describe yourself?
   - Have any recent occurrences made you feel differently about yourself? If so, describe.
   - What concerns you most?
   - Do you frequently have feelings of anger? Anxiety? Depression? Fearfulness? If so, describe.

8. Role-Relationship
   - Describe your living arrangements. Do you live alone? If not, with whom do you live?
   - Do you have a significant other? If yes, is this relationship satisfying?
   - What are the different roles within your family? Do others depend on you? If so, explain.
   - Describe relationships among your family members (close, marital difficulties, or estrangement).
   - How are family decisions made in your family?
   - How are conflicts resolved?
   - Are finances adequate to meet family needs?
   - Outside the family, do you have close friends, or do you belong to any social groups? If so, describe.

9. Sexuality-Reproductive
   - Are you sexually active? If yes, how many partners do you have?
   - Do you routinely use protection against sexually transmitted infections, to prevent pregnancy, or both? If yes, describe.
   - Are you comfortable with your sexual functioning?
   - Are you experiencing any difficulties with sexual activity? If yes, describe.
   - Do you anticipate a change in your sexual activity or relations with illness?
   - Women: Date of last menstruation, description of menstrual flow, age of menarche, age of menopause (if applicable), pregnancy history, problems associated with menstruation.

10. Coping–Stress Tolerance
    - Have there been any major changes in your life within the last couple of years? If so, describe.
    - How do you handle problems that arise in your life? Is this effective most of the time?
    - Is there an individual with whom you can discuss problems? Is this person available to you now?
    - Would you describe yourself as tense or relaxed most of the time? If tense, how do you relieve the tension?
    - Do you use medications, drugs, or alcohol to help you relax? If yes, describe.

11. Value-Belief
    - Do you generally get what you want out of life?
    - Do you have any plans or goals for the future?
    - Do you think that any personal beliefs or values may be compromised?
    - Is religion an important part of your life? If so, describe.

Conversion Tables

TABLE B-1	LENGTH		
IN	**CM**	**CM**	**IN**
1	2.54	1	0.4
2	5.08	2	0.8
4	10.16	3	1.2
6	15.24	4	1.6
8	20.32	5	2
10	25.4	6	2.4
20	50.8	8	3.1
30	76.2	10	3.9
40	101.6	20	7.9
50	127	30	11.8
60	152.4	40	15.7
70	177.8	50	19.7
80	203.2	60	23.6
90	228.6	70	27.6
100	254	80	31.5
150	381	90	35.4
200	508	100	39.4

1 inch = 2.54 cm; 1 cm = 0.3937 inch.

TABLE B-2	WEIGHT		
LB	**KG**	**KG**	**LB**
1	0.5	1	2.2
2	0.9	2	4.4
4	1.8	3	6.6
6	2.7	4	8.8
8	3.6	5	11.0
10	4.5	6	13.2
20	9.1	8	17.6
30	13.6	10	22
40	18.2	20	44
50	22.7	30	66
60	27.3	40	88
70	31.8	50	110
80	36.4	60	132
90	40.9	70	154
100	45.4	80	176
150	66.2	90	198
200	90.8	100	220

1 lb = 0.454 kg; 1 kg = 2.204 lb.

TABLE B-3	TEMPERATURE. FAHRENHEIT AND CELSIUS EQUIVALENTS IN THE BODY TEMPERATURE RANGE								
F°	**C°**	**F°**	**C°**	**F°**	**C°**	**F°**	**C°**	**F°**	**C°**
94	34.44	97	36.11	100	37.78	103	39.44	106	41.11
94.2	34.56	97.2	36.22	100.2	37.89	103.2	39.56	106.2	41.22
94.4	34.67	97.4	36.33	100.4	38	103.4	39.67	106.4	41.33
94.6	34.78	97.6	36.44	100.6	38.11	103.6	39.78	106.6	41.44
94.8	34.89	97.8	36.56	100.8	38.22	103.8	39.89	106.8	41.56
95	35	98	36.67	101	38.33	104	40	107	41.67
95.2	35.11	98.2	36.78	101.2	38.44	104.2	40.11	107.2	41.78
95.4	35.22	98.4	36.89	101.4	38.56	104.4	40.22	107.4	41.89
95.6	35.33	98.6	37	101.6	38.67	104.6	40.33	107.6	42
95.8	35.44	98.8	37.11	101.8	38.78	104.8	40.44	107.8	42.11
96	35.56	99	37.22	102	38.89	105	40.56	108	42.22
96.2	35.67	99.2	37.33	102.2	39	105.2	40.67		
96.4	35.78	99.4	37.44	102.4	39.11	105.4	40.78		
96.6	35.89	99.6	37.56	102.6	39.22	105.6	40.89		
96.8	36	99.8	37.67	102.8	39.33	105.8	41		

To convert Centigrade or Celsius degrees to Fahrenheit degrees: Multiply the number of Centigrade degrees by 9/5 and add 32 to the result.
To convert Fahrenheit degrees to Centigrade degrees: Subtract 32 from the number of Fahrenheit degrees and multiply the difference by 5/9.

A&W	alive and well
AB	abortion
abd	abdomen; abdominal
ADL	activities of daily living
AJ	ankle jerk
AK	above knee
ANS	autonomic nervous system
AP	anteroposterior
BK	below knee
BP	blood pressure
BPH	benign prostatic hyperplasia
BS	bowel sounds; breath sounds
CC	chief complaint
CHD	childhood disease; congenital heart disease; coronary heart disease
CHF	congestive heart failure
CNS	central nervous system
COPD	chronic obstructive pulmonary disease
CV	cardiovascular
CVA	costovertebral angle; cerebrovascular accident
CVP	central venous pressure
Cx	cervix
D&C	dilation and curettage
DM	diabetes mellitus
DOB	date of birth
DOE	dyspnea on exertion
DTRs	deep tendon reflexes
DUB	dysfunctional uterine bleeding
Dx	diagnosis
ECG, EKG	electrocardiogram; electrocardiograph
EENT	eye, ear, nose, and throat
ENT	ear, nose, and throat
EOM	extraocular movement
FB	foreign body
FH	family history
FROM	full range of motion
FTT	failure to thrive
Fx	fracture
G	gravida
GB	gallbladder
GE	gastroesophageal
GI	gastrointestinal
GU	genitourinary
GYN	gynecologic
HA	headache
HCG	human chorionic gonadotropin
HEENT	head, eyes, ears, nose, and throat
HOPI	history of present illness
HPI	history of present illness
Hx	history
ICS	intercostal space
IOP	intraocular pressure
IUD	intrauterine device
IV	intravenous
JVP	jugular venous pressure
KJ	knee jerk
KUB	kidneys, ureters, and bladder
Lat	lateral
LCM	left costal margin
LE	lower extremity
LLL	left lower lobe (lung)
LLQ	left lower quadrant (abdomen)
LMD	local medical doctor
LMP	last menstrual period
LOC	loss of consciousness; level of consciousness
LS	lumbosacral; lumbar spine
LSB	left sternal border
LUL	left upper lobe (lung)
LUQ	left upper quadrant (abdomen)
M	murmur
MAL	midaxillary line
MCL	midclavicular line
MGF	maternal grandfather
MGM	maternal grandmother
MSL	midsternal line
MVA	motor vehicle accident
N&T	nose and throat
N&V	nausea and vomiting
NA	no answer; not applicable
NKA	no known allergies
NKDA	no known drug allergies
NPO	nothing by mouth
NSR	normal sinus rhythm
OM	otitis media
OTC	over the counter
P	para
PE	physical examination
PERRLA	pupils equal, round, react to light, and accommodation
PGF	paternal grandfather
PGM	paternal grandmother
PI	present illness

PID	pelvic inflammatory disease
PMH	past medical history
PMI	point of maximum impulse; point of maximum intensity
PMS	premenstrual syndrome
prn	as necessary
PVC	premature ventricular contraction
RCM	right costal margin
REM	rapid eye movement
RLL	right lower lobe (lung)
RLQ	right lower quadrant (abdomen)
RML	right middle lobe (lung)
ROM	range of motion
ROS	review of systems
RRR	regular rate and rhythm
RSB	right sternal border
RUL	right upper lobe (lung)
RUQ	right upper quadrant (abdomen)

SCM	sternocleidomastoid
Sx	symptoms
T&A	tonsillectomy and adenoidectomy
TM	tympanic membrane
TPR	temperature, pulse, and respiration
UE	upper extremity
URI	upper respiratory infection
UTI	urinary tract infection
WD	well developed
WN	well nourished

Symbols

<	less than
>	greater than
×	times; by (size)
♀	female
♂	male
#	pound

Chapter 1
Review Questions

1. 1
2. 2
3. 2
4. 3
5. 1

Case Study 1

1. *Subjective data:* Abdominal pain in right abdomen. Pain feels like a knife and goes to shoulder. Patient reports nausea, feels exhausted, and has not slept for three nights; pain keeps her awake. Patient hurts too much to move.
2. *Objective data:* Dark circles under eyes. Vital signs: BP, 132/90 mm Hg; pulse, 104 beats/min; RR 22 breaths/min; temperature, 101.8° F (38.8° C). Elevated WBCs. Patient lying in fetal position.

Case Study 2

1. *Subjective data:* Complains of pain in right leg. Pain medication helps only a little bit, and "butt hurts" because he can't move. *Objective data:* Patient has fractured femur. Right leg is in external fixator. Taking Percocet orally for pain every 6 hours.
2. *Subjective data:* No bowel movement for 3 days. Stool looked like "hard, dry rabbit turds." Usual bowel elimination daily. *Objective data:* Patient has limited mobility as a result of external fixator. Fluid intake average ≤1000 mL/day. Eating 30% of meals. Abdomen slightly distended. Active bowel sounds. Taking Percocet for pain.
3. *Subjective data:* "My butt hurts because I can't move around." "The food is horrible." *Objective data:* Patient has limited mobility because of external fixator. Fluid intake average ≤1000 mL/day. Eating 30% of meals. 2 inch (5 cm) diameter redness over sacrum (skin intact).

Chapter 2
Review Questions

1. 2
2. 4
3. 3
4. 1
5. 4

Case Study

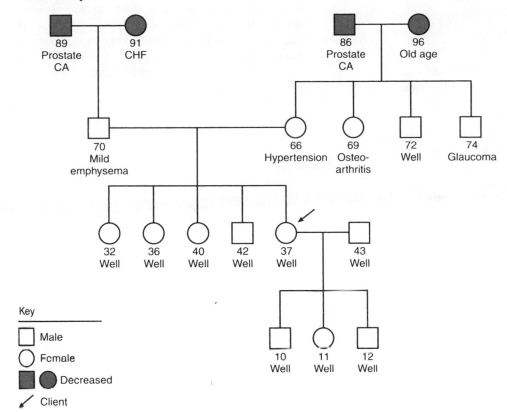

Key

☐ Male

○ Female

■● Decreased

✓ Client

Chapter 3
Review Questions
1. 2
2. 1
3. 4
4. 3
5. 1

Chapter 4
Review Questions
1. 2
2. 3
3. 1
4. 3
5. 4

Chapter 5
Review Questions
1. 2
2. 3
3. 1
4. 2
5. 3

Chapter 6
Review Questions
1. 4
2. 2

3. 2
4. 1
5. 2

Case Study
The patient's description of pain indicates some sort of acute problem, which indicates a need to search for the source of the problem.
1. Data that deviate from expected are signs and symptoms consistent with acute pain. The signs are elevated heart and respiratory rates and diaphoresis. The symptoms are his reports of pain at 12 (on a scale of 10) and nausea.
2. Ask if the pain radiates to any other site and if there are any symptoms associated with urination such as blood in the urine or pain with urination. Ask the patient if he has ever had pain like this before. If so, ask him to describe it. Ask if he has noticed anything that reduces the intensity or if he has taken any medications or tried any self-treatment? Ask him about his past experiences with pain.
3. The team care team member most helpful in this case is the physician who can prescribe pain medication and perform diagnostic tests to determine the cause of the pain and order treatment.

Chapter 7
Review Questions
1. 2
2. 1

3. 3
4. 1
5. 4

Case Study

1. Unkempt general appearance; crying behavior; excessive sleeping; self-deprecating, slow speech with flat affect.
2. Ask about the onset of symptoms and current stressors. Ask about recent changes in her life and identify coping mechanisms. Ask about interpersonal relationships with friends and boyfriend. Consider doing a Holmes stressor scale. Ask her if she takes any medications.
3. Risk factors for depression: She is female and in late adolescence. She may have a distorted perception of her parent's reaction to her performance in school and a pessimistic outlook.
4. Collaborate with a psychiatric nurse practitioner, counselor, or psychologist.

Chapter 8
Review Questions
1. 1
2. 2
3. 4
4. 3
5. 2

Case Study

Subjective data: Fatigue. Shortness of breath. Change in diet. Weight loss. Patient's perception of health.
Objective data: Height for weight. Scaling of skin. Hair findings. Cracks in corner of mouth. Pale conjunctiva.
2. Ask about other symptoms that she may be experiencing; if her appetite has been affected; if weight loss has been intentional; her usual body weight and if she has a history of weight loss. Assess her knowledge regarding a vegetarian diet. Calculate the body mass index (BMI), the desired body weight (DBW), her percent of DBW, and the percent weight change in 4 months from her usual body weight (UBW).
3. Risk factors: Lack of money to buy food. New vegetarian diet.
4. Collaborate with a physician and dietitian.

Chapter 9
Review Questions
1. 3
2. 4
3. 1
4. 1
5. 2
6. 4
7. 4
8. 3

Case Study

1. Foul-smelling odor; loss of appetite; flat affect; 6 feet 2 inches, 153 pounds; skin breakdown; minimal activity.

2. Ask the patient if he is aware of the skin breakdown. Ask about recent weight loss with loss of activity. Assess ulcers to determine stage and presence of infection. Assess other pressure areas for evidence of skin breakdown. Perform a nutritional assessment.
3. Risk factors: He has impaired mobility and no sensation to his skin. He may be poorly nourished, which may also contribute to skin breakdown.
4. Collaborate with a physician, wound care nurse, and dietitian.

Chapter 10
Review Questions
1. 1
2. 1
3. 4
4. 2
5. 1
6. 4
7. 3
8. 2
9. 3
10. 3
11. 1
12. 4

Case Study

1. Fever; complaints of ear pain; presence of drainage in ear canal; tympanic membrane perforation; reduction of hearing in left ear; quiet affect; limited talking.
2. Ask the patient what treatment she has received for the ear pain from the medicine man in the past. Ask if she has ever seen drainage from the ear with past problems. Ask if she has been treated at a hospital or clinic for ear pain in the past. Hearing assessment using an audiometer is indicated.
3. The patient is in pain and has problems with sensory perception (hearing).
4. Collaborate with a physician or nurse practitioner.

Chapter 11
Review Questions
1. 2
2. 4
3. 3
4. 1
5. 3
6. 1
7. 4
8. 1
9. 1
10. 3

Case Study

1. History of shortness of breath; limitation in activity; interrupted sleep (requires pillows); smoking history; labored breathing with tachypnea; presence of cyanosis;

underweight/protruding ribs; increased anteroposterior (AP) diameter; reduced chest wall movement; diminished tactile fremitus; adventitious and diminished breath sounds.

2. Ask about chest pain with shortness of breath and about the presence of a cough. Ask how old the patient was when she started smoking and how long she has been smoking as much as she currently is. Assess oxygen saturation, body weight, and rhythm of breathing pattern. Assess for presence of retraction. Percuss chest for tone and diaphragmatic excursion. Count how many words she can say without taking a breath to assess dyspnea.

3. Risk factor for lung cancer: Her smoking.

4. Collaborate with a physician, a respiratory therapist, and a dietitian to meet her needs.

Chapter 12
Review Questions

1. 4
2. 2
3. 3
4. 2
5. 3
6. 2
7. 3
8. 4
9. 1
10. 3

Case Study

1. Complaint of shortness of breath, fatigue that interferes with routine activities, and sleeping difficulty; labored breathing with elevated respiratory rate, pulse rate, and blood pressure; pitting edema in lower extremities; frothy-looking phlegm.

2. Complete a symptom analysis on the shortness of breath and fatigue. Ask the patient if he has symptoms associated with chest pain, cough, or nocturia. Ask him about cardiovascular history. Perform a precordial assessment, including inspection, percussion, palpation, and auscultation.

3. Risk factors for coronary artery disease: Age, gender, and family history.

4. Collaborate with physician, dietitian, and cardiac rehabilitation personnel.

Chapter 13
Review Questions

1. 4
2. 1
3. 3
4. 1
5. 3
6. 2
7. 3
8. 4
9. 2
10. 3

Case Study

1. Abdominal pain (progressively worse); loss of appetite and nausea; guarded position; hot skin, possibly indicating fever; absence of bowel sounds; pain on palpation and guarding RLQ; positive rebound tenderness in RLQ.

2. Ask if vomiting accompanies her nausea. Ask about her last menstrual period (LMP) and about the possibility of pregnancy. Ask her about bowel elimination (last bowel movement) and appearance of stool. Check vital signs (of particular interest is temperature). Auscultate for arterial bruits and venous hums. Percuss kidney for costovertebral angle (CVA) tenderness.

3. Risk factors (for most cancers of the gastrointestinal system): Smoking.

4. Collaborate with the physician and dietitian.

Chapter 14
Review Questions

1. 1
2. 4
3. 2
4. 4
5. 1
6. 4
7. 3
8. 2

Case Study

1. Significant joint pain; limitations in self-care activities; limitations in socialization; difficulty with posture and gait; deformities to joints; tender, inflamed joints with palpation; subcutaneous nodules at the ulnar surface of the elbows.

2. Ask the patient which medications she is taking for the RA; find out whether she is using any other nonpharmaceutical therapies; ask her whether these things help or make a difference; ask if she uses any assistive devices and if she receives any assistance with self-care activities. Document range of motion (ROM) in various joints. Use of a goniometer would be particularly helpful.

3. Risk factors: Age, gender, race (Asian), family history, and medication (methotrexate).

4. Collaborate with physician, pharmacist, physical therapist, and occupational therapist.

Chapter 15
Review Questions

1. 2
2. 3
3. 1
4. 1
5. 4
6. 2

Case Study

1. The patient was diagnosed with right cerebrovascular accident (CVA); he had a headache preceding incident. He is unable to talk, has absence of sensation and trace-to-no muscle strength on the left arm and leg, requires assistance for mobility, and avoids eye contact and cries.
2. Ask the patient if he feels he can swallow normally and whether he has any pain or discomfort. Ask the patient's wife about medical and family history and medications he may be taking currently. Ask her if her husband lost consciousness or had a seizure with this incident. Assess gag reflex. Test deep tendon reflexes. Assess for drooling.
3. Risk factors: Age, gender, race, and history of diabetes mellitus, hypertension, and smoking.
4. Collaborate with a physician, physical therapist, occupational therapist, speech therapist, and discharge planner.

Chapter 16
Review Questions
1. 3
2. 4
3. 4
4. 3
5. 2
6. 1

Case Study

1. Patient has a history of nontender breast lump, noticeable for about 9 months; mass has increased in size over 9 months; palpable lump is present in left upper outer quadrant; dimpling is noted on left breast; left nipple is retracted; bloody discharge is noted from nipple when squeezed.
2. Ask about personal or family history of breast disease. Ask patient whether she performs breast self-examination (BSE) and whether she has ever had a mammogram. Ask about the location of the lump, whether it is tender now, and whether she has noticed nipple discharge. Ask about changes in the lump size in relation to menstrual cycle. Inspect the areolae. Besides location, the following characteristics must be assessed with a breast mass: size, shape, consistency, tenderness, mobility, and borders. Palpate the axilla. It is especially important to note any lumps or masses in the left axilla.
3. Risk factors: Age, early onset of menarche, and no children. Recommend having mammograms more often than that recommended for women of low risk.
4. Collaborate with a physician or nurse practitioner.

Chapter 17
Review Questions
1. 2
2. 1
3. 4
4. 2
5. 1
6. 3

7. 4
8. 3
9. 3
10. 2

Case Study

1. The history suggests some type of acute inflammation. It also suggests multiple sex contacts, and the primary partner has multiple sex contacts. Mass with inflammation, discharge, and extreme pain on palpation need further evaluation.
2. Discussion is needed regarding past sexual history and associated medical problems, if any. Identification of protection (or lack of it) is also important to discuss. Obtain a culture of the discharge for evaluation. If patient is too uncomfortable for internal examination, it may need to be delayed until the inflammation has resolved.
3. The risk factors are sexual activity and being in a non-monogamous sexual relationship. Use of protection from a sexually transmitted infection (STI) is unknown. Data are unclear about how many sex partners the patient has.
4. Collaborate with a physician or nurse practitioner.

Chapter 18
Review Questions
1. 2
2. 3
3. 1
4. 3
5. 4

Case Study

1. *Subjective data:* Patient recently lost spouse (5 months ago). Son says that his mother has "gone downhill." He indicates that patient is no longer keeping her house clean and is not cooking appropriate meals. He reports significant change in patient's personal hygiene habits (loss of interest in getting hair done or getting dressed for the day). He reports that patient becomes angry when he talks about other living options; patient states, "You think I'm helpless and want to lock me away."
2. *Objective data:* 78-year-old woman; sits quietly during conversation. Overall hygiene—patient appears clean; hair matted; clothes do not match and are badly wrinkled. Speech clear. Overall affect dull; makes no eye contact with her son or nurse. Age-consistent findings with physical examination; no overt physical problems identified.
3. This patient is in Erikson's stage of ego integrity versus despair.
4. She may be struggling with the following developmental tasks: dealing with the death of her spouse; adapting to living arrangements; adjusting to relationships with adult children and grandchildren; adjusting to slower physical and intellectual responses; managing leisure time and remaining active; maintaining physical and mental health; finding the meaning of life.

5. The area of skills of daily living versus mental health/depression needs to be assessed further. Some of the changes noted by the son may indicate physical/cognitive decline, or they may be a result of depression and apathy from the loss of a husband.

Chapter 19
Review Questions

1. 1
2. 1
3. 3
4. 4
5. 3
6. 4
7. 2
8. 1
9. 4
10. 4

Case Study

1. Reported seizure, "shaking all over" lasted 20 minutes. History of seizures, but length of seizure atypical (according to mother).
2. Ask if there was a loss of consciousness; how long ago since the last seizure; if there were any warning signs before the seizure; about change in medication, dose, or adherence; about recent changes (e.g., in health status or appetite, excessive fatigue).
3. Risk for falls, musculoskeletal injury, or head injury.
4. Collaborate with a physician or nurse practitioner. This girl may need a referral to a pediatric neurologist.

Chapter 20
Review Questions

1. 1
2. 4
3. 2
4. 4
5. 1

Case Study

1. *Subjective data:* Symptoms of puffiness to hands and feet. Backache. Fear of excessive labor pain. *Objective data:* Increase in blood pressure. Sudden, excessive increase in weight. 3+ protein in urine.
2. Assess fetal heart tones 1; palpate fetal movement. Assess the extent of the edema, including how far up on the legs and the degree of edema, if pitting. Check her visual acuity. Conduct a neurologic assessment, particularly to check deep tendon reflexes. Ask her about her diet, specifically sodium intake, because this may be contributing to the edema. Get more information about the back discomfort; do a symptom analysis. Determine her knowledge level of the labor and delivery process; assess pain experiences.
3. She has pregnancy-induced hypertension (PIH), excessive weight gain, and evidence of preeclampsia (proteinuria and edema).
4. Collaborate with a physician or nurse practitioner because she is displaying clinical findings associated with PIH, which requires prompt intervention. Collaborate with a dietitian for her dietary needs.

Chapter 21
Review Questions

1. 1
2. 2
3. 4
4. 3
5. 1
6. 3

Case Study

1. The patient is confused, disoriented, and incontinent. She has a history of urinary tract infection (UTI) that has contributed to her confusion. Moving her right hip is painful because of the fall and bruise.
2. A fall risk assessment needs to be completed.
3. Confusion, disorientation, and altered elimination. Collaboration with a physician or nurse practitioner is needed to determine the cause of confusion and disorientation. Incontinence also needs evaluation. Collaboration with a physical therapist may be needed for muscle strengthening and improved balance.

A

abduction   Movement of a limb away from the body.

accommodation   The adjustment of the eye to variations in distance.

active listening   Concentrating on what the patient is saying and the subtleties of the message being conveyed.

adduction   Movement of a limb toward the body.

adnexa   General term meaning adjacent or related structures. *Example:* The ovaries and fallopian tubes are adnexa of the uterus.

adolescent   Refers to a person between 12 and 18 years of age.

adventitious sounds   Breath sounds that are not normal.

adulthood   Stage of life that can be divided into several recognized categories:

Young adult   ages 20 to 35 years

Middle adult   ages 35 to 65 years

Young-old adult   ages 65 to 74 years

Middle-old adult   ages 75 to 84 years

Old-old adult   ages 85 and up

affect   Observable behaviors that indicate an individual's feelings or emotions.

alopecia   Absence or loss of hair.

alveolar ridge   Bony prominences of the maxilla and mandible that support the teeth; in edentulous patient, these structures support dentures.

amblyopia   Reduced vision in an eye not correctable by refraction and with no obvious pathologic or structural cause.

amenorrhea   Absence of menstruation.

anesthesia   Partial or complete loss of sensation.

angina pectoris   Paroxysmal chest pain often associated with myocardial ischemia; pain patterns and severity vary among individuals; pain sometimes radiates to the neck, jaw, or left arm; may be accompanied by choking or smothering sensations.

angle of Louis   Visible and palpable angulation between the sternum and manubrium; also referred to as the *manubriosternal junction*.

ankylosis   Fixation of a joint, often in an abnormal position, usually resulting from destruction of articular cartilage, as in rheumatoid arthritis.

anosmia   Absence or impairment of the sense of smell.

anterior   Referring to the front.

anterior triangle (of the neck)   Landmark area for palpating the submaxillary, submental, and anterior cervical lymph nodes; sectioned by the anterior surface of the sternocleidomastoid muscle, the mandible, and an imaginary line running from the chin to the sternal notch.

anthropometrics   Measurement of body composition and growth; includes measurement of height, weight, body mass index, head circumference, and skinfold thickness.

anular   Type of lesion that forms a ring around a center of normal skin.

anulus   Dense fibrous ring surrounding the tympanic membrane.

anuria   Complete absence of urine production; may also be used to describe situations in which urine output is less than 100 mL per day.

anxiety   A feeling of uneasiness or discomfort experienced in varying degrees, from mild anxiety to panic; anxiety is a response to no specific source or actual object.

apathy   Lack of emotional expression; indifference to stimuli or surroundings.

aphakia   Absence of the crystalline lens of the eye.

aphasia   A neurologic condition in which language function is absent or severely impaired.

aphthous ulcer (canker sore)   Painful ulcer on the mucous membrane of the mouth.

apical   Refers to the top portion (apex) of an organ or part.

apnea   Absence of breathing.

apocrine sweat glands   Secretory dermal structures located in the axillae, nipples, areolae, scalp, face, and genital area; they develop at puberty and respond to emotional stimulation.

arcus senilis   Gray ring composed of lipids deposited in the peripheral cornea; commonly seen in older adults. Also called *arcus cornealis*.

areola   Circular, darkly pigmented area around the nipple of the breast.

arteriosclerosis   General term denoting hardening and thickening of the arterial walls.

ascites   Accumulation of serous fluid in the peritoneal cavity.

assessment   First step in the nursing process involving collection of comprehensive data pertinent to the patient's health or situation.

asthma   Paroxysmal dyspnea that is accompanied by wheezing and caused by spasm of the bronchial tubes or swelling of their mucous membranes.

astigmatism   Visual distortion resulting from an irregular corneal curvature that prevents light rays from being focused clearly on the retina.

ataxia   Inability to coordinate muscular movement.

atelectasis   Shrunken, airless alveoli or collapse of lung tissue.

atherosclerosis   Formation of plaques within arterial walls that results in thickening of the walls and narrowing of the lumen; end organs supplied by these vessels receive diminished circulation.

atrophy   Wasting or decrease in size or physiologic activity of a part of the body because of disease or other influences.

auricle   The external ear; also called the *pinna*.

auscultatory gap   Phenomenon sometimes noted by a nurse listening for blood pressure sounds; temporary silent interval between systolic and diastolic sounds that may cover a range of 40 mm Hg; commonly occurs with hypertensive patients with a wide pulse pressure.

B

balano   Prefix that denotes the glans penis. *Example: Balanitis* means inflammation of the glans penis.

ballottement   Technique of palpating a floating structure in the abdomen by bouncing it gently and feeling it rebound.

Bartholin's glands   Two mucus-secreting glands located within the posterolateral vaginal vestibule.

bilateral   Relating to or referring to two sides.

Biot breathing   Breathing characterized by several short breaths followed by long, irregular periods of apnea.

bipolar disorder   A mood disorder characterized by episodes of mania, depression, or mixed moods.

blepharitis   Inflammation of the eyelid.

blocking   Interruption in a train of thought, a loss of an idea, or a repression of a feeling or idea from conscious awareness; can be a normal behavior or in extreme form indicative of abnormality.

body mass index (BMI)   Method to evaluate height-weight ratio; calculated by dividing the weight (kilograms) by the height (meters).

borborygmi   Abdominal sounds produced by hyperactive intestinal peristalsis that is audible at a distance.

boutonniere deformity   Common deformity of the hands seen in patients with rheumatoid arthritis; involves flexion of the proximal interphalangeal joint and hyperextension of the distal interphalangeal joint.

bradycardia   Abnormally slowed heart rate, usually under 60 beats/min.

bradykinesia   Abnormal slowness of movement.

bradypnea   Breathing that is abnormally slow.

bronchial breath sounds   High-pitched breath sounds normally heard over the trachea and the area around the manubrium; considered abnormal if heard anywhere over the posterior or lateral chest.

bronchitis   Inflammation of the bronchi.

bronchophony   An abnormality in vocal resonance. When lungs are auscultated, the patient says "ninety-nine" or "one, two, three." If there is lung consolidation, the sounds are clear; without consolidation, the sounds are muffled.

bronchovesicular breath sounds   Refers to breath sounds at a moderate pitch heard in the posterior chest over the outer center of the back on either side of the spine between the scapulae and in the anterior chest around the sternal border.

Brudzinski's sign Examination technique used to detect meningeal irritation by flexing the neck of a supine patient forward.

bruit Audible murmur (a blowing sound) heard when auscultating over a peripheral vessel or an organ.

buccal Pertaining to the inside of the cheek, the surface of a tooth, or the gum beside the cheek.

bulbar conjunctiva Thin, transparent mucous membrane that covers the sclera and adjoins the palpebral conjunctiva, which lines the inner eyelid.

bulla Elevated, circumscribed, fluid-filled lesion greater than 1 cm in diameter.

bunion Abnormal prominence on the inner aspect of the first metatarsal head with bursal formation; results in lateral or valgus displacement of the great toe.

bursa Fibrous, fluid-filled sac found between certain tendons and the bones beneath them.

bursitis Inflammation of a bursa.

C

cachexia Severe malnutrition and wasting of muscles associated with a chronic illness such as cancer.

callus Hyperkeratotic area caused by pressure or friction; usually not painful.

canthus Outer or inner angle between the upper and lower eyelids.

carpal tunnel syndrome Painful disorder of the wrist and hand induced by compression of the median nerve between the inelastic carpal ligament and other structures within the carpal tunnel.

cataract Opacity of the crystalline lens of the eyes.

cauliflower ear Thickened, disfigured ear caused by repeated trauma such as blows to the ear.

cellulitis Diffuse spreading infection of the skin or subcutaneous or connective tissue.

cerumen Waxy secretion of the glands of the external acoustic meatus; earwax.

chalazion Small, localized swelling of the eyelid caused by obstruction and dilation of the meibomian gland.

circumduction Circular movement of a limb.

circumoral Pertaining to the area around the mouth.

circumscribed Well-defined, limited, and encircled.

clonus Abnormal pattern of neuromuscular functioning characterized by rapidly alternating involuntary contraction and relaxation of skeletal muscles.

clubbing Broadening and thickening of the fingernails or toenails associated with an increased angle of the nail greater than 180 degrees; associated with chronic hypoxia.

coarctation Stricture or narrowing of the wall of a vessel as the aorta.

cochlea Conical bony structure of the inner ear; perforated by numerous apertures for passage of the cochlear division of the acoustic nerve.

cognitive functioning Appraisal of an individual's perception of his or her intellectual awareness, potential for growth, and recognition by others for his or her mental skills and contributions.

coherency Conversation and behavior that conveys thoughts, feelings, ideas, and perceptions in a logical and relevant manner.

compulsive behavior Repetitive act that usually originates from an obsession; extreme anxiety emerges if the act is not completed.

condyloma acuminatum (wart) Soft, warty, papillomatous projection that appears on the labia and within the vaginal vestibule; viral in origin and sexually transmitted.

condyloma latum Slightly raised, moist, flattened papules that appear on the labia or within the vaginal vestibule; a sign of secondary syphilis; sexually transmitted.

confabulation Fabrication of events or sequential experiences often recounted to cover up memory gaps.

confluent Describes lesions that run together.

consensual reaction The constriction of the iris and pupil of one eye when a light is shone in the opposite eye.

consolidation Increasing density of lung tissue caused by pathologic engorgement.

contusion (bruise) Swelling, discoloration, and pain without a break in the skin.

Cooper ligaments Suspensory ligaments of the breast.

corn Hyperkeratotic, slightly raised, circumscribed lesion caused by pressure over a bony prominence.

costal angle Costal margin angle formed on the anterior chest wall at the base of the xiphoid process where the ribs separate.

crackles Abnormal respiratory sound heard during auscultation, characterized by discontinuous bubbling sounds; heard over distal bronchioles and alveoli that contain serous secretions; formerly called *rales*.

crepitus Dry, crackling sound or sensation heard or felt as a joint is moved through its range of motion.

cricoid cartilage Lowermost cartilage of the larynx.

crust Dried serum, blood, or purulent exudate on the skin surface.

cryptorchism Failure of one or both of the testicles to descend into the scrotum.

cyanosis Bluish-gray discoloration of the skin resulting from the presence or abnormal amounts of reduced hemoglobin in the blood.

cycloplegia Paralysis of the ciliary muscle resulting in a loss of accommodation and a dilated pupil; usually induced with medication to allow for examination or surgery of the eye.

cystocele Bulging of the anterior vaginal wall caused by protrusion of the urinary bladder through relaxed or weakened musculature.

D

Darwinian tubercle Blunt point projecting up from the upper part of the helix of the ear.

database Collection or store of information.

deciduous teeth Twenty teeth that appear normally during infancy: four incisors, two canines, and four molars in the upper and lower jaw.

delirium An acute, reversible organic mental disorder characterized by confusion, disorientation, restlessness, anxiety, and excitement.

delusion Persistent belief or perception that is illogical or improbable.

dementia Broad term that indicates impairment of intellectual functioning, memory, and judgment.

depersonalization Sense of being out of touch with one's environment; loss of a sense of reality and association with personal events.

depression An abnormal mood state in which a person characteristically has a sense of sadness, hopelessness, helplessness, worthlessness, and despair resulting from some personal loss or tragedy.

desquamation Sloughing process of the cornified layer of the epidermis; when accelerated, the process can cause peeling, scaling, and loss of the deeper layers of the skin.

diaphoresis Sweating.

diaphragmatic excursion Extent of movement of the diaphragm with maximum inspiration and expiration.

diarthrotic joint Joint that permits relatively free movement; types of diarthrotic joints include hinge joints, pivot joints, condyloid joints, ball-and-socket joints, and gliding joints.

diastole Period of time within the cardiac cycle in which ventricles are relaxed and filling with blood.

diffuse Spread out, widely dispersed, copious.

diplopia Double vision.

distal Refers to the area farthest away from a point of reference.

dizziness Sensation of faintness.

dorsal Refers to the back or posterior part of an anatomic structure. *Example:* Dorsal aspect of the hand.

dorsiflexion Upward or backward bending or flexion of a joint.

dysarthria Speech disorder involving difficulty with articulation and pronunciation of specific sounds; results from loss of control over the muscles of speech.

dysesthesia Sensation of something crawling on the skin or pricks of pins and needles.

dyskinesia Refers to a reduced ability to perform voluntary movements.

dysmenorrhea Abnormal pain associated with the menstrual cycle. Mild, self-limiting premenstrual pain is considered normal. Pain becomes abnormal when it is severe; disabling; or accompanied by other severe symptoms such as nausea, vomiting, fainting, or intestinal cramping.

dyspareunia   Pain associated with sexual intercourse; most often used to describe female conditions, including vaginal spasms, lack of lubrication, or genital lesions.

dysphagia   Difficulty swallowing.

dysphasia   A neurologic condition in which language function is absent or severely impaired.

dysphonia   Difficulty in controlling laryngeal speech sounds; can be a normal event such as male vocal changes occurring at puberty.

dyspnea   Breathing that is labored or difficult.

dysuria   Difficulty, pain, or burning sensation associated with urination.

E

ecchymosis   Discoloration of skin or a mucous membrane caused by leakage of blood into the subcutaneous tissue; can also be a bruise.

eccrine sweat glands   Secretory dermal structures distributed over the body that secrete water and electrolytes and regulate body temperature; heat, emotional reactions, and physical exercise are the primary stimulants for secretion from these glands.

ectopic   An event that occurs away from its usual location such as a premature ventricular contraction.

ectropion   Abnormal outward turning of the margin of the eyelid.

eczematous   Superficial inflammation characterized by scaling, thickening, crusting, weeping, and redness.

edema   Excessive accumulation of fluid within the interstitial space.

effacement   The shortening of the vaginal portion of the cervix and the thinning of its walls as it is stretched and dilated by the fetus during labor.

egophony   Abnormality in vocal resonance; when lungs are auscultated, the patient says "e-e-e," but the nurse hears "a-a-a"; suggests pleural effusion.

embolus   Foreign object (composed of air, fat, or clustered cellular elements) that circulates through the blood and usually lodges in a vessel, causing some degree of occlusion.

emesis   Vomit.

emphysema   Chronic pulmonary disease characterized by permanent enlargement of air spaces caused by destruction of alveolar walls.

enophthalmos   Abnormal backward placement of the eyeball.

entropion   Abnormal inward turning of the margin of the eyelid.

enuresis   Any involuntary urination, especially during sleep.

epicondyle   Round protuberance above the condyle (at the end of a bone).

epididymitis   Inflammation of the epididymis (tightly coiled, comma-shaped structure overlying the posterolateral surface of the testis).

epiphysis   End of a long bone that is cartilaginous during early childhood and becomes ossified during late childhood.

epispadias   Congenital defect in which the urinary meatus opens on the dorsum of the penis.

epistaxis   Bleeding from the nose.

erosion   Wearing away or destruction of the mucosal or epidermal surface; often develops into an ulcer.

erythematous   Redness (of the skin).

erythroplakia   Red lesion of the oral mucous membrane that may be precancerous.

euphoria   Sense of elation or well-being; can be a normal feeling or exaggerated to the extent of distorting reality.

eustachian tube   Tube lined with mucous membrane that joins the nasopharynx and the tympanic cavity.

eversion   Outward turning as with a foot, or an inside-out position as with an eyelid.

exacerbation   Increase in intensity of signs or symptoms.

excoriation   Scratch or abrasion on the skin surface.

exophthalmos   Abnormal forward placement of the eyeball.

extension   Movement that brings a joint into a straight position.

external rotation   Turning a limb outward or away from the midline of the body.

extrapyramidal system   Motor pathways lying outside the pyramidal tract that help to maintain muscle tone and control body movements such as walking; includes nerve pathways between the cerebral cortex, the basal ganglia, the brainstem, and the spinal cord.

F

fasciculation   Localized, uncoordinated, uncontrollable twitching of a single muscle group innervated by a single motor nerve fiber.

fifth vital sign   Assessment of pain, including location, quality, quantity, chronology, and setting.

fissure   Linear crack in the skin.

flaccid   Referring to muscles that lack tone.

flail chest   Unstable, flapping chest wall caused by fractures of the sternum and ribs.

flank   Part of the body between the bottom of the ribs and the upper border of the ilium; it overlies the kidneys.

flatulence   Presence of excessive amounts of gas in the stomach or intestines.

flexion   Movement that brings a joint into a bent position.

fontanel   Unossified space or soft spot lying between the cranial bones of an infant.

Fordyce spots   Small yellow spots on the buccal membrane that are visible sebaceous glands; a normal phenomenon seen in many adults that is sometimes mistaken for abnormal lesions. Also called *Fordyce granules*.

fornix (plural: fornices)   General term designating a fold or an archlike structure. The vaginal fornix is the ringed recess (pocket) that forms around the cervix as it projects into the vaginal vault; although continuous, this fornix is anatomically divided into the anterior, posterior, and lateral fornices.

fourchette   Small fold of membrane connecting the labia minora in the posterior part of the vulva.

frenulum (lingual)   Band of tissue that attaches the ventral surface of the tongue to the floor of the mouth.

friction rub   Sound produced by the rubbing of the pleura around the lung or the pericardium around the heart.

functional assessment   Appraisal of an individual's perception of his or her capacity to maneuver within a defined environment.

G

gallop rhythm   Audible extra heart sound produced by an abnormal third or fourth heart sound.

gate (referring to pain)   An area in the dorsal horn of the spinal cord that controls the stimulation of spinothalamic sensory tracts within the spinal cord.

gate theory of pain   When A-delta or C sensory nerve fibers stimulate (open) the "gate," pain impulses enter the spinal cord and ascend in the spinothalamic tract to the thalamus.

gingiva   Pertaining to the gum.

glaucoma   Eye disease characterized by abnormally increased intraocular pressure caused by obstruction of the outflow of aqueous humor.

glossitis   Inflammation of the tongue.

goiter   Hypertrophy of the thyroid gland, usually evident as a pronounced increase in its size.

gout   Metabolic disease associated with abnormal uric acid metabolism that is a form of acute arthritis; marked by inflammation of the joints.

graphesthesia   Ability to recognize symbols, numbers, or letters traced on the skin.

gravida   Denotes number of pregnancies. *Example: Multigravida* indicates more than one pregnancy.

guarding   Protective withdrawal or positioning of a body part during an injury.

gynecomastia   Abnormally large mammary glands in the male.

H

hallucination   Sensory perception that does not arise from an external stimulus; can be auditory, visual, tactile, gustatory, or olfactory.

health history   Collection of subjective data by interview from a patient as a component of health assessment.

heave   Palpable, diffuse, sustained lift of the chest wall or a portion of the wall.

helix   Margin of the external ear.

hemangioma   Benign tumor found predominantly in subcutaneous tissue or skin; caused by newly formed blood vessels.

hematuria   Presence of blood in the urine.

hemoptysis   Coughing up blood or referring to bloody sputum.

hernia   Abnormal opening in a muscle wall or cavity that permits protrusion of its contents.

herpetiform   Describes a cluster of vesicles resembling herpes lesions.

hirsutism   Excessive body hair, usually in a masculine distribution, owing to heredity, hormonal dysfunction, porphyria, or medication.

Homans' sign   Calf pain associated with rapid dorsiflexion of the foot, indicative of thrombophlebitis in 10% of patients.

hordeolum (stye)   Infection of a sebaceous gland at the margin of the eyelid.

hydramnios   Excess formation of amniotic fluid during pregnancy.

hydrocele   Nontender, serous fluid mass located within the tunica vaginalis (layered, hollow membrane adjacent to the testis).

hymenal remnants   Small, irregular, fleshy projections that are remnants of a ruptured hymen; a normal phenomenon that may or may not be present at the vaginal introitus in varied sizes and shapes.

hyoid   U-shaped bone suspended from the styloid process of the temporal bone.

hyperesthesia   Abnormally increased sensitivity to sensory stimuli such as touch or pain.

hyperextension   Refers to the extension of a body part beyond normal limits of extension.

hyperkinesis   Hyperactivity or excessive muscular activity.

hyperkinetic   Hyperactive.

hyperopia (farsightedness)   Refractive error in which light rays focus behind the retina.

hyperplasia   Increase in the number of cells of a body part that results from an increased rate of cellular metabolism.

hyperresonance   Sound elicited by percussion; very loud intensity and very low pitch with a booming quality; heard over lungs when air is trapped in emphysema.

hypertension   Blood pressure above 120 mm Hg systolic or 80 mm Hg diastolic on two or more readings taken at two or more visits.

hypoesthesia   Decreased or dulled sensitivity to stimulation.

hyposmia   Decreased sense of smell.

hypospadias   Congenital defect in which the urinary meatus opens on the ventral aspect of the penis; opening may be located in the glans, penile shaft, scrotum, or perineum.

hypotension   Refers to abnormally low blood pressure.

hypoxemia   Abnormal reduction of oxygen content in the arterial blood.

hypoxia   Abnormal reduction of oxygen delivery to body tissue.

hypovolemic   Pertaining to decreased blood volume; usually refers to a state of shock resulting from massive blood loss and inadequate tissue perfusion.

I

illusion   Perceptual distortion of an external stimulus. *Example:* A mirage in a desert.

"inching"   Recommended method for moving the stethoscope over the precordium while listening for heart sounds; small, sliding movements (rather than lifting and lowering the stethoscope from side to side) may enable the listener to hear more sounds.

incus   One of three ossicles in the middle ear; resembling an anvil, it communicates sound vibrations from the malleus to the stapes.

induration   Hardening of the skin, usually caused by edema or infiltration by a neoplasm.

infancy   First year of life.

infarct   Localized area of tissue necrosis caused by prolonged anoxia.

inferior   Lower surface of an organ; refers to a position that is lower in relation to another.

infection   Redness, heat, edema, and fever secondary to pathogenic microorganisms.

intermittent claudication   Condition characterized by symptoms of pain, aching, cramping, and localized fatigue of the legs that occur while walking but that can be relieved by rest (2 to 5 minutes); discomfort occurs most often in the calf but may arise in the foot, thigh, hip, or buttock.

internal rotation   Inward turning of a limb.

introitus   General term denoting an opening or the orifice of a cavity or hollow structure.

inversion   Turning inside out or upside down.

inverted nipple   Nipple that is turned inward.

ischemia   Diminished supply of blood to a body organ or surface; characterized by pallor, coolness, and pain.

isthmus glandulae thyroideae   Narrow portion of the thyroid gland connecting the left and right lobes.

J

jaundice   A yellow discoloration of the skin, mucous membrane, and sclera caused by increased bilirubin in the blood.

K

keloid   Hypertrophic scar tissue; prevalent in nonwhite races.

keratosis   Overgrowth and thickening of the cornified epithelium.

Kernig's sign   Diagnostic sign of meningeal irritation characterized by pain and inability of a supine patient to completely extend the leg when the knee and hip are flexed on the abdomen.

kinesthetic sensation   Ability to detect muscle movement and position.

Koplik spots   Lesions that appear in the prodromal stage of measles; they appear as small bluish-white lesions with irregular borders on the buccal mucosa opposite the molar teeth.

Korotkoff sounds   Sounds heard during the taking of blood pressure.

Kussmaul respiration   Rapid deep respiration often associated with ketoacidosis.

kyphosis   Abnormal convexity of the posterior curve of the spine.

L

labile emotions   Unpredictable, rapid shifting of expression of feelings.

labyrinth   Complex structure of the inner ear that communicates directly with the acoustic nerve by transmitting sound vibrations from the middle ear through the fluid-filled network of three semicircular canals that join at a vestibule connected to the cochlea.

lateral   Referring to the side; position away from the middle.

Leopold's maneuvers   Series of palpation techniques used to determine fetal presentation, position, and lie.

lesion   A pathologically or traumatically altered area of tissue.

leukoplakia   Thickened, white, well-circumscribed patch that can appear on any mucous membrane; sometimes precancerous; often a response to chronic irritation such as pipe smoking.

leukorrhea   White vaginal discharge; can be a normal phenomenon that occurs (or increases) with pregnancy, the use of birth control medication or as a postmenstrual phase; can also be an abnormal sign indicating malignancy or infection.

lichenification   Thickening of the skin characterized by accentuated skin markings; often the result of chronic scratching.

light reflex   Triangular landmark area on the tympanic membrane that most brightly reflects the nurse's light source.

lordosis   Abnormal anterior concavity of the spine.

lower motor neurons   Nerve cells that originate in the anterior horn cells of the spinal column and travel to innervate the skeletal muscle fibers; injury or disease of this area results in decreased muscle tone, reflexes, or strength.

lymphadenitis   Inflammation of the lymph nodes.

lymphadenopathy   Enlargement of lymph nodes greater than 1.5 cm.

lymphedema   Swelling caused by obstruction of the lymphatic system and accumulation of interstitial fluid.

lymphoma   General term for the growth of new tissue in the lymphatic area; generally refers to malignant growth.

M

macule   Flat, circumscribed lesion of the skin or mucous membrane that is 1 cm or less in diameter.

malleus   Innermost ossicle of the middle ear; resembling a hammer, it is connected to the tympanic membrane and transmits sound vibrations to the incus.

mastitis   Inflammation of the breast.

mastoid process   Conical projection of the temporal bone extending downward and forward behind the external auditory meatus.

McBurney point   Point of specialized tenderness in acute appendicitis that is situated on a line between the umbilicus and the right anterosuperior iliac spine about 1 or 2 inches above the latter.

medial   Referring to the middle; the median plane of the body.

mediastinum   Space within the thoracic cavity positioned behind the sternum, in front of the vertebral column, and between the lungs.

menarche   Onset of menstruation.

menopause   The period that marks the cessation of menstrual cycles.

menorrhagia   Abnormally heavy or extended menstrual periods.

metrorrhagia   Menstrual bleeding at irregular intervals, sometimes prolonged, but of expected amount.

Mini Mental State Examination (MMSE)   A standardized screening tool used to estimate cognitive function and detect organic brain disease.

midaxillary line   Vertical line extending downward from the midaxillary fold; used in assessment as an anatomic reference point.

midclavicular line   Vertical line extending downward from the middle of the clavicle; used in assessment as an anatomic reference point.

miosis   Condition in which the pupil is constricted; usually drug induced.

modulation   Fourth step in the pain process when the body releases endogenous opioids to inhibit transmission of nociceptive impulses to reduce pain perception.

Montgomery tubercles   Small sebaceous glands located on the areola of the breast.

Murphy's sign   Sign of gallbladder disease consisting of pain when taking a large breath when the nurse's fingers are pressing on the approximate location of the gallbladder.

myalgia   Tenderness or pain in the muscle.

mydriasis   Dilation of the pupil; usually drug induced.

myoclonus   Twitching or clonic spasm of a muscle group.

myopia (nearsightedness)   Refractive error in which light rays focus in front of the retina.

N

nabothian cyst (retention cyst)   Small white or purple firm nodule that commonly appears on the cervix; forms within the mucus-secreting nabothian glands, which are present in large numbers on the uterine cervix.

narcolepsy   Sudden onset of excessive daytime sleepiness that lasts from 10 to 30 minutes.

nares (singular: naris)   Nostrils; anterior openings of the nose.

necrosis   Localized death of tissue.

neonate   Newborn infant during the first 28 days of life.

neurosis   Ineffective or troubled coping mechanism stemming from anxiety or emotional conflict.

nevus   Congenital pigmented area on the skin. *Example:* Mole, birthmark.

nicking   Abnormal condition showing compression of a vein at an arteriovenous crossing; visible through an ophthalmoscope during a retinal examination.

nociceptor   Free nerve endings that are located at the ends of small, thinly myelinated or unmyelinated nerve fibers and initiate an action potential.

nocturia   Excessive urination during the night.

nodule   Solid skin elevation that extends into the dermal layer and that is 1 to 2 cm in diameter.

nystagmus   Involuntary rhythmical movement of the eyes; oscillations may be horizontal, vertical, rotary, or mixed.

O

objective data   Data obtained from examination, measurements, or diagnostic tests; observable by the nurse.

obsession   Persistent thought or idea that preoccupies the mind; not always realistic and may result in compulsive behavior.

obsessive-compulsive disorder   An anxiety disorder that develops when the patient tries to resist an obsession or compulsion.

odynophagia   A severe sensation of burning, squeezing, pain while swallowing.

oligomenorrhea   Abnormally light or infrequent menstruation.

oliguria   Inadequate production or secretion of urine (usually less than 400 mL in a 24-hour period).

orchi   Combining form that denotes the testes. *Example: Orchitis* means inflammation of one or both of the testes.

orthopnea   Difficulty breathing in any position other than an upright one.

osteoarthritis   Form of arthritis in which one or many of the joints undergo destruction of cartilage.

otalgia   Pain in the ear.

otitis externa   Infection of the external canal or auricle of the ear.

otitis media   Infection of the inner ear.

P

Paget's disease of the nipple   Condition characterized by an excoriating or scaling lesion of the nipple extending from an intraductal carcinoma of the breast.

palmar   Relating to the palm of the hand.

palpebral conjunctiva   Thin, transparent mucous membrane that lines the inner eyelid and adjoins the bulbar conjunctiva, which covers the sclera.

palpebral fissure   Opening between the upper and lower eyelids.

palpitation   Sensation of pounding, fluttering, or racing of the heart; can be a normal phenomenon or caused by a disorder of the heart.

papilla   General term for a small projection; dorsal surface of the tongue is composed of a variety of forms of papillae that contain openings to the taste buds.

papule   Solid, elevated, circumscribed, superficial lesion 1 cm or less in diameter.

paradoxical pulse   Diminished pulse amplitude on inspiration with increased amplitude on expiration; an exaggeration of a normal response to respiration.

paralysis   Loss of muscle function, loss of sensation, or both.

paranoia   Sense of being persecuted or victimized; suspicion of others.

paraphimosis   Condition characterized by the inability to pull the foreskin forward from a retracted position.

paresis   Motor weakness.

paresthesia   Abnormal sensation such as numbness or tingling.

parity   Denotes the number of viable births.

paronychia   Inflammation of the skinfold that adjoins the nail bed.

paroxysmal nocturnal dyspnea (PND)   Periodic acute attacks of shortness of breath that awaken a person, usually after several hours of sleep in a recumbent position.

pars flaccida   Small portion of the tympanic membrane between the mallear folds.

pars tensa   Larger portion of the tympanic membrane.

patch   Flat, circumscribed lesion of the skin or mucous membrane that is more than 1 cm in diameter.

peau d'orange   Dimpling of the skin that resembles the skin of an orange.

pectoralis major muscle   One of the four muscles of the anterior upper portion of the chest.

pectus carinatum   Abnormal prominence of the sternum.

pectus excavatum   Abnormal depression of the sternum.

perception of pain   The third step in the pain process that occurs when the parietal lobe is stimulated, causing a conscious experience of pain.

periodontitis (pyorrhea)   Inflammation and deterioration of the gums and supporting alveolar bone; occurs in varying degrees of severity; if neglected, this condition results in loss of teeth.

peristalsis   Alternating contraction and relaxation of the smooth muscles of the intestinal tract to propel contents forward.

perlèche (cheilosis, cheilitis)   Fissures at the corners of the mouth that become inflamed; caused by overclosure of the mouth in an edentulous patient, marked loss of the alveolar ridge, or riboflavin deficiency; saliva irritates the area, and moniliasis is a common complication.

petechiae   Tiny, flat purple or red spots on the surface of the skin resulting from minute hemorrhages within the dermal or submucosal layers.

phimosis   Tightness of the foreskin that results in an inability to retract it.

phobia   Uncontrollable and often unreasonable intense fear of a specific object or event.

photophobia Ocular discomfort caused by exposure of the eyes to bright light.

physical functioning Appraisal of an individual's perception of his or her ability to control and manipulate the physical environment and judgment of the ability of his or her inner resources to control and use his or her body effectively.

pilonidal fistula (or sinus) Abnormal channel containing a tuft of hair that is situated most frequently over or close to the tip of the coccyx; may also occur in other regions of the body.

pinna Auricle or projected part of the external ear.

plantar flexion A toe-down motion of the foot at the ankle.

plantar Referring to the bottom surface of the foot.

plaque Solid, elevated, circumscribed, superficial lesion more than 1 cm in diameter.

plaque (dental) Film that accumulates on the surface of the teeth; made up of mucin and colloidal material from saliva; subject to bacterial invasion.

pleximeter Finger placed on the skin surface to receive the taps from the percussion hammer or plexor; used in percussion.

point of maximum impulse (PMI) Specific area of the chest where the heartbeat is palpated strongest; usually the apical impulse, located in the fourth or fifth intercostal space along the midclavicular line.

polyuria Excessive urine excretion.

posterior Referring to the back.

posterior triangle (of neck) Landmark area for palpating the posterior cervical chain, the supraclavicular chain, and the occipital lymph chain; sectioned along the anterior border by the sternocleidomastoid muscle, the posterior border by the trapezius muscle, and the bottom by the clavicle.

precipitating factor Event or entity that hastens the onset of another event.

precordium Area of the chest that overlies the heart and adjacent great vessels.

predisposing factor (risk factor) Event or entity that contributes to the cause of another event. *Example:* A family history of obesity increases a patient's risk for obesity.

prehypertension An elevated blood pressure of 120 to 139 mm Hg systolic or 80 to 89 mm Hg diastolic on two or more readings taken at two or more visits.

presbycusis Impairment of hearing in older adults.

presbyopia Loss of accommodation (ability to focus on near objects) associated with older adults.

preschool age Refers to children between 3 and 5 years of age.

problem list Compilation of findings that appear at the end of a database; may be diagnoses (medical or nursing), clusters of interrelated findings, or isolated findings that the nurse wishes to pursue but cannot label or attach to other findings.

pronate To turn the forearm so the palm faces downward or to rotate the leg or foot inward.

proprioception Awareness of body posture, movement, and changes in equilibrium originating from sensory nerve endings (proprioceptors) within muscles and tendons.

pruritus Itching.

psychosis Any major mental disorder characterized by greatly distorted perceptions and severe disorganization of the personality.

psychosocial functioning Appraisal of an individual's capacity to attain and maintain satisfactory intimate and social relationships with others.

ptosis Drooping of the upper eyelid; can be unilateral or bilateral.

ptyalism Excessive salivation.

pudendum Collective term denoting the external genitalia; for the female it includes the mons pubis, labia majora, labia minora, vaginal vestibule, and vestibular glands; for the male it includes the penis, scrotum, and testes.

pulse deficit Discrepancy between the ventricular rate auscultated over the heart and the arterial rate palpated over the radial artery.

pulse pressure Difference between systolic and diastolic pressures, usually within the range of 30 to 40 mm Hg; tends to increase as systolic pressure rises with arteriosclerosis of the large vessels (specifically the aorta).

pulsus alternans Alternating pulse; abnormal pulse characterized by a regular rhythm in which a strong beat alternates with a weaker one.

purpura Hemorrhage into the tissue, usually circumscribed; lesions may be described as petechiae, ecchymoses, or hematomas, according to size.

pustule Vesicle or bulla that contains pus.

pyramidal tract Bundle of upper motor neurons that coordinate voluntary movements originating in the motor cortex of the brain; nerve fibers travel from the frontal lobe through the brainstem and the spinal cord, where they synapse with anterior horn cells; responsible for the coordinated response of voluntary movements.

pyrosis Burning sensation in the epigastric and sternal region with the raising of acid liquid from the stomach; also called *heartburn.*

pyuria Presence of white cells (pus) in the urine.

R

rebound tenderness Sign of inflammation in the peritoneum in which pain is elicited by a sudden withdrawal of a hand pressing on the abdomen; often found in patients with appendicitis.

rectocele Bulging of the rectum and posterior vaginal wall through relaxed or weakened musculature of the vagina.

red reflex Red glow over the pupil created by light illuminating the retina.

refraction Deviation of light rays as they pass from one transparent medium into another of different density.

remission Disappearance or diminishment of signs or symptoms.

reticular Describes a netlike pattern or structure of veins on a tissue surface.

retraction Shortening or drawing the skin backward.

rheumatoid arthritis Chronic, autoimmune inflammatory disease of connective tissue characterized by localized inflammation, thickening, and edema of the joints and systemic symptoms such as fatigue.

rhino Combining form that denotes the nose.

rhonchus Loud, low-pitched, coarse sound similar to a snore heard on auscultation of an airway obstructed by thick secretions, muscular contraction, neoplasm, or external pressure; also called a *sonorous wheeze.*

Romberg's test Test of cerebellar function that evaluates an individual's ability to maintain a given position when standing erect with feet together and eyes closed.

S

scale Small, thin flake of epithelial cells.

schizoid Exhibiting behaviors or having characteristics that resemble schizophrenia.

school age Refers to children between 6 and 12 years of age.

scoliosis Lateral curvature of the spine.

scotoma Defined area of blindness within the visual field; can involve one or both eyes.

sebaceous glands Secretory dermal structures that produce sebum, an oily substance; puberty stimulates production of sebum; the primary areas for secretion are in the face, chest, and upper part of the back.

seborrhea Group of skin conditions characterized by noninflammatory, excessively dry scales or excessive oiliness.

sensorium Status of level of consciousness and orientation to surroundings.

shifting dullness Change in the dull sounds heard with palpation; at first the dull sound is heard in one location and then in a different location.

shotty node Small lymph node that feels hard and nodular; generally movable and nontender; may show evidence of having been infected many times in the past.

sign Objective finding perceived by the nurse.

Skene's glands (periurethral) Mucus-secreting glands that lie just inside the urethral orifice of women; not visible during examination.

sleep apnea Breathing abnormalities that occur during sleep, ranging from a reduction in airflow to complete cessation of airflow.

smegma Secretion of sebaceous glands, especially the cheesy, foul-smelling secretion sometimes found under the foreskin of the penis and at the base of the labia minora near the glans clitoris.

spasticity Increased tone or contractions of muscles causing stiff and awkward movements; seen with upper motor neuron lesions.

spermatocele (epididymal cyst) Painless, fluid-filled epididymal mass that contains spermatozoa.

spinothalamic tract Sensory nerve tract that carries impulses of pain, pressure, and temperature from the spinal cord to the thalamus.

spiritual state Individual's version of his or her effectiveness in developing and sustaining a belief and value system that assists in self-acceptance and in his or her relationship to others and to a higher being.

spondylitis Inflammation of one or more of the spinal vertebrae; usually characterized by stiffness and pain.

sprain Traumatic injury to the tendon; characteristics are pain, swelling, and discoloration of the skin over the joint.

stapes One of the ossicles in the middle ear; resembles a tiny stirrup and transmits sound vibrations from the incus to the internal ear.

stereognosis Ability to recognize objects by the sense of touch.

sternocleidomastoid muscle Major muscle that rotates and flexes the head; originates by two heads from the sternum and clavicle and inserts on the mastoid process and the occipital bone.

stoma General term that means opening or mouth.

strabismus Condition in which the eyes are not directed at the same object or point.

strain Temporary damage to the muscles usually caused by excessive physical effort.

striae Streaks of linear scars that often result from rapidly developing tension in the skin; also called *stretch marks*.

stridor Shrill, harsh sound heard during inspiration and caused by laryngeal obstruction.

subjective data Data obtained from a health history or provided to the nurse by the patient.

subluxation Partial or incomplete dislocation of a joint.

superior Upper surface of an organ; also refers to a position that is higher in relation to another.

supernumerary nipple Extra nipple.

supinate To turn the forearm so the palm faces upward or to rotate the foot and leg outward.

symptom Subjective indicator or sensation perceived by the patient.

syncope Sudden, temporary loss of consciousness; fainting.

systole Period of time within the cardiac cycle in which the ventricles contract and eject blood into the aorta and pulmonary arteries.

T

tachycardia Rapid heart rate (more than 100 beats/min).

tachypnea Rapid breathing; a respiratory rate that is faster than 20 breaths/min.

tactile fremitus Vibratory sensations of the spoken voice felt through the chest wall on palpation.

tail of Spence Upper outer tail of the breast that extends into the axillary region.

telangiectasia Dilation of a superficial capillary or network of small capillaries that produces fine, irregular, red lines on the skin surface.

tendinitis Inflammation of a tendon.

thrill Palpable murmur; feels like the throat of a purring cat.

thrombophlebitis Inflammation of a vein; often associated with clot formation.

thrombus Blood clot attached to the inner wall of a vessel; usually causes some degree of occlusion.

tic Spasmodic muscular contraction most commonly involving the face, head, neck, or shoulder muscles.

tinnitus Tinkling or ringing sound heard in one or both ears.

toddlerhood Refers to 12 to 36 months of age.

tophus Calculus that contains sodium urate deposits; develops in periauricular fibrous tissue; associated with gout.

torsion (of spermatic cord) Twisting of the spermatic cord that results in an infarction of the testis.

tragus Cartilaginous projection in front of the exterior meatus of the ear.

transduction The first step in the pain process involving the conversion of mechanical, thermal, chemical, or electrical stimuli that damage tissues.

transmission The second step in the pain process that begins with stimulation of one of the four types of afferent nerves by the nociceptors and ends by closing or opening the "gate" (substantia gelatinosa).

trapezius muscle Major muscle that rotates and extends the head; originates along the superior curved line of the occiput and the spinous processes of the seventh cervical and all thoracic vertebrae and inserts at the clavicle, acromion, and base of the scapula.

tremor Continuous involuntary trembling movement of a part or parts of the body.

trimester Refers to a period of time during pregnancy. There are three trimesters during pregnancy; each trimester lasts a period of 3 months.

tumor Solid skin elevation that extends into the dermal layer and is more than 1 cm in diameter.

turbinates Extensions of the ethmoid bone located along the lateral wall of the nose; these fingerlike projections are covered with erectile mucosal membranes that become swollen or inflamed in response to allergy or viral invasion.

turgor Normal resiliency of the skin.

two-point discrimination Ability to identify being touched by two sharp objects simultaneously.

tympany Low-pitched note heard on percussion of a hollow organ such as the stomach.

U

ulcer Circumscribed crater on the surface of the skin or mucous membrane that leaves an uncovered wound.

umbo Central depressed portion of the concavity of the lateral surface of the tympanic membrane; marks the spot where the malleus is attached to the inner surface.

unilateral Relating to or referring to one side.

upper motor neurons Nerve cells that originate in the frontal lobe of the cerebral cortex and project downward; make up the corticobulbar and pyramidal tracts and end in the anterior horn of the spinal cord; responsible for fine and discrete conscious movements.

urticaria (hives) Pruritic wheals; often transient and allergic in origin.

uvula A small, cone-shaped tissue suspended midline from the soft palate.

V

vaginitis Inflammation of the vaginal vault; has various causes.

valgus Bending outward.

varicocele Abnormal tortuosity and dilation of spermatic veins; spermatic cord is described as feeling like a bag of worms; condition is not painful but involves a pulling or dragging sensation.

varus Turning inward.

vellus hair Soft nonpigmented hair that covers the body.

verge (anal) External ring at the opening of the anus.

vermilion border Demarcation point between the mucosal membrane of the lips and the skin of the face; common site for recurrent infections such as herpes infections and carcinoma; blurring of this border may be an early sign of lesion development.

vertigo Sensation of moving around in space (whirling motion; subjective vertigo) or of objects moving about themselves (objective vertigo); results in disturbance of the individual's equilibrium.

vesicle Fluid-filled, elevated, superficial lesion 1 cm or less in diameter.

vesicular breath sounds Normal breath sounds heard over most of the lungs.

vestibule Middle part of the inner ear located behind the cochlea and in front of the semicircular canals.

vocal fremitus Vibratory sensations of the spoken voice felt through the chest wall on palpation; also known as tactile fremitus.

volar Referring to or denoting the palmar aspect of the hand or the plantar aspect of the foot.

vulva External female genitalia; also referred to as the *pudendum*.

W

wheal Elevated, solid, transient lesion; often irregularly shaped but well demarcated; an edematous response.

wheeze High-pitched, musical noise that sounds like a squeak; heard during auscultation of a narrowed airway.

whispered pectoriloquy Transmission of whispered words through the chest wall, heard during auscultation; indicates solidification of the lungs.

X

xerostomia Dryness of the mouth.

American Academy of Dermatology and Institute of Dermatologic Communication and Education, Schaumburg, Ill.

American College of Rheumatology: *Clinical slide collection of the rheumatic diseases*, Atlanta, 1991, 1995, 1997, American College of Rheumatology.

Baran R, Dawber RR, Levene GM: *Color atlas of the hair, scalp, and nails*, St Louis, 1991, Mosby.

Barkauskas VH, et al: *Health and physical assessment*, ed 3, St Louis, 2002, Mosby.

Beaven DW, Brooks SE: *Color atlas of the nail in clinical diagnosis*, ed 2, London, 1994, Times Mirror International Publishers.

Bedford MA: *Color atlas of ophthalmological diagnosis*, ed 2, London, 1986, Wolfe.

Belcher AE: *Cancer nursing*, St Louis, 1992, Mosby.

Bingham BJG, Hawke M, Kwok P: *Atlas of clinical otolaryngology*, St Louis, 1992, Mosby.

Black J, Hawks J: *Medical-surgical nursing*, ed 7, St Louis, 2005, Saunders.

Black J, Hawks J: *Medical-surgical nursing*, ed 8, St Louis, 2009, Saunders.

Bluestone C, et al: *Pediatric otolaryngology*, ed 4, Philadelphia, 2003, Saunders.

Bonewit-West K: *Clinical procedures for medical assistants*, ed 8, 2012, Saunders.

Bowden VP, et al: *Children and their families: the continuum of care*, Philadelphia, 1998, Saunders.

Butcher G: *Gastroenterology*, St Louis, 2004, Churchill Livingstone.

Canobbio MM: *Cardiovascular disorders*, St Louis, 1990, Mosby.

Chipps EM, Clanin NJ, Campbell VG: *Neurologic disorders*, St Louis, 1992, Mosby.

Christensen B, Kockrow E: *Adult health nursing*, ed 6, St Louis, 2011, Mosby.

Cohen BA: *Atlas of pediatric dermatology*, London, 1993, Wolfe.

Cummings NH, Stanley-Green S, Higgs P: *Perspectives in athletic training*, St Louis, 2009, Mosby.

deWit SC: *Fundamental concepts and skills for nursing*, ed 3, St Louis, 2009, Saunders.

Diagnostic picture tests in clinical medicine, St Louis, 1984, Mosby.

Doughty DB, Jackson DB: *Gastrointestinal disorders*, St Louis, 1993, Mosby.

Drake RL, Vogl W, Mitchell AWM: *Gray's anatomy for students*, ed 2, Philadelphia, 2010, Churchill Livingstone.

Elkin MK, Perry AG, Potter PA: *Nursing interventions and clinical skills*, ed 4, St Louis, 2008, Mosby.

Farrar WE, et al: *Infectious diseases: text and color atlas*, ed 2, London, 1992, Gower.

Forbes CD, Jackson WF: *Color atlas and text of clinical medicine*, ed 3, St Louis, 2003, Elsevier.

Fortunato N, McCullough SM: *Plastic and reconstructive surgery*, St Louis, 1998, Mosby.

400 Self-assessment picture tests in clinical medicine, London, 1984, Wolfe.

Frazier M, Drzymkowski J: *Essentials of human diseases and conditions*, ed 4, St Louis, 2008, Saunders.

Francis CC, Martin AH: *Introduction to human anatomy*, ed 7, St Louis, 1975, Mosby.

Gallager HS, et al: *The breast*, St Louis, 1978, Mosby.

Goldstein BG, Goldstein AO: *Practical dermatology*, ed 2, St Louis, 1997, Mosby.

Gould B, Dyer R: *Pathophysiology for the health professions*, ed 4, St Louis, 2011, Saunders.

Greenberger NJ, Hinthorn DR: *History taking and physical examination*, St Louis, 1993, Mosby.

Grimes DE: *Infectious diseases*, St Louis, 1991, Mosby.

Habif TP: *Clinical dermatology: a color guide to diagnosis and therapy*, ed 3, Philadelphia, 1996, Mosby.

Habif TP: *Clinical dermatology: a color guide to diagnosis and therapy*, ed 5, St Louis, 2010, Mosby.

Harkreader H, Hogan M, Thobaben M: *Fundamentals of nursing: caring and clinical judgment*, ed 3, St Louis, 2007, Mosby.

Herlihy B: *The human body in health and illness*, ed 4, St Louis, 2011, Mosby.

Hill MJ: *Skin disorders*, St Louis, 1994, Mosby.

Hockenberry MJ, Wilson D: *Wong's essentials of pediatric nursing*, ed 8, St Louis, 2009, Mosby.

Hockenberry MJ, et al: *Wong's nursing care of infants and children*, ed 7, St Louis, 2003, Mosby.

Hockenberry MJ, et al: *Wong's nursing care of infants and children*, ed 9, St Louis, 2011, Mosby.

Huether S, McCance K: *Understanding pathophysiology*, ed 4, St Louis, 2008, Mosby.

Ignatavicius D, Workman L: *Medical-surgical nursing*, ed 6, Philadelphia, 2010, Saunders.

Jachmann-Jahn U: *Clinical symptoms guide to differential diagnosis*, 2009, Urban and Fischer.

Jellinek MS, et al: Screening 4- and 5-year-old children for psychosocial dysfunction: a preliminary study with the pediatric symptom checklist, *J Dev Behav Pediatr* 15:191, 1994.

Kamal A, Brocklehurst JC: *Color atlas of geriatric medicine*, London, 1991, Wolfe.

Katz S, et al: Progress in development of the index of ADL, *Gerontologist* 10(1):20, 1970.

LaFleur Brooks M: *Exploring medical language*, ed 7, St Louis, 2009, Mosby.

Lehne R: *Pharmacology for nursing care*, ed 7, Philadelphia, 2010, Saunders.

Lemmi F, Lemmi C: *Physical assessment findings CD-ROM*, Philadelphia, 2000, Saunders.

Lewis SL, Heitkemper MM, Dirksen SR: *Medical-surgical nursing: assessment and management of clinical problems*, ed 5, St Louis, 2000, Mosby.

Lewis SL, Heitkemper MM, Dirksen SR: *Medical-surgical nursing: assessment and management of clinical problems*, ed 6, St Louis, 2004, Mosby.

Lewis SL, Heitkemper MM, Dirksen SR: *Medical-surgical nursing: assessment and management of clinical problems*, ed 7, St Louis, 2007, Mosby.

Lewis SL, et al: *Medical-surgical nursing: assessment and management of clinical problems*, ed 8, St Louis, 2011, Mosby.

Lloyd-Davies RW, et al: *Color atlas of urology*, ed 2, London, 1994, Wolfe.

Lowdermilk DL, Perry SE: *Maternity and women's health care*, ed 9, St Louis, 2007, Mosby.

Lowdermilk DL, Perry SE, Cashion MC: *Maternity nursing*, ed 8, St Louis, 2011, Mosby.

Mansel R, Bundred N: *Color atlas of breast disease,* St Louis, 1995, Mosby-Wolfe.

Marshall WA, Tanner JM: Variations in pattern of pubertal changes in girls, *Arch Dis Child* 44:291, 1969.

Marx J, et al: *Rosen's emergency medicine,* ed 7, Philadelphia, 2010, Mosby.

Mashburn J, Scharbo-DeHaan M: A clinician's guide to Pap smear interpretation, *Nurse Pract* 22(4):115, 1997.

McCaffery M, Pasero C: *Pain: clinical manual,* ed 2, St Louis, 1999, Mosby.

McCance KL, Huether SE: *Pathophysiology: the biologic basis for disease in adults and children,* ed 4, St Louis, 2002, Mosby.

McCance KL, Huether SE: *Pathophysiology: the biologic basis for disease in adults and children,* ed 6, St Louis, 2010, Mosby.

McKenry LM, Salerno E: *Mosby's pharmacology in nursing,* ed 21, St Louis, 2003, Mosby.

McLaren DS: *A colour atlas and text of diet-related disorders,* ed 2, St Louis, 1992, Wolfe.

Melzack R, Katz J: Pain measurement in persons with pain. In Wall PD, Melzack R, editors: *Textbook of pain,* ed 3, New York, 1994, Churchill-Livingstone.

Monahan F, et al: *Phipps' medical-surgical nursing,* ed 8, St Louis, 2007, Mosby.

Montelcone JA: *Recognition of child abuse for the mandated reporter,* ed 2, London, 1996, GW Medical Publishing.

Mourad LA: *Orthopedic disorders,* St Louis, 1991, Mosby.

National Institute on Alcohol Abuse and Alcoholism (NIAAA): *Helping patients who drink too much: a clinician's guide,* 2005, Patient Education Materials, *What's a standard drink,* www.niaaa.nih.gov.

Newell FW: *Ophthalmology: principles and concepts,* ed 7, St Louis, 1992, Mosby.

Newell FW: *Ophthalmology: principles and concepts,* ed 8, St Louis, 1996, Mosby.

Paley D, Krachmer J: *Ophthalmology for the primary care physician,* St Louis, 1998, Mosby.

Pasero C, McCaffery M: *Pain assessment and pharmacologic management,* St Louis, 2011, Mosby.

Patton K, Thibodeau G: *Anatomy and physiology,* ed 7, St Louis, 2010, Mosby.

Perry A, et al: *Nursing interventions and clinical skills,* ed 4, St Louis, 2008, Mosby.

Perry AG, Potter PA, Elkin MK: *Nursing interventions and clinical skills,* ed 5, St Louis, 2012, Mosby.

Perry S, et al: *Maternal child nursing care,* ed 4, St Louis, 2010, Mosby.

Potter PA, Perry AG: *Basic nursing: theory and practice,* ed 2, St Louis, 1991, Mosby.

Potter PA, Perry AG: *Fundamentals of nursing,* ed 7, St Louis, 2009, Mosby.

Potter PA, et al: *Fundamentals of nursing,* ed 8, St Louis, 2013, Mosby.

Price S, Wilson L: *Pathophysiology,* ed 6, St Louis, 2003, Mosby.

Prior JA, Silberstein JS, Stang JM: *Physical diagnosis: the history and examination of the patient,* ed 6, St Louis, 1981, Mosby.

Rakel R, Bope E: *Conn's current therapy 2004,* Philadelphia, 2004, Saunders.

Regezi JA, Sciubba JJ, Jordan RC: *Oral pathology: clinical pathologic correlations,* ed 6, Philadelphia, 2012, Saunders.

Roberts J, Hedges J: *Clinical procedures in emergency medicine,* ed 5, Philadelphia, 2009, Saunders.

Salvo SG: *Mosby's pathology for massage therapists,* ed 2, St Louis, 2009, Mosby.

Sanders M: *Mosby's paramedic textbook,* ed 3, St Louis, 2007, Mosby.

Scully C, Welbury R: *Color atlas of oral diseases in children and adolescents,* London, 1994, Wolfe.

Seeley RR, Stephens TD, Tate P: *Anatomy and physiology,* ed 3, St Louis, 1995, Mosby.

Seidel HM, et al: *Mosby's guide to physical examination,* ed 4, St Louis, 1999, Mosby.

Seidel HM, et al: *Mosby's guide to physical examination,* ed 5, St Louis, 2003, Mosby.

Seidel HM, et al: *Mosby's guide to physical examination,* ed 6, St Louis, 2006, Mosby.

Seidel HM, et al: *Mosby's guide to physical examination,* ed 7, St Louis, 2011, Mosby.

Shade B, et al: *Mosby's EMT-intermediate textbook,* ed 3, St Louis, 2012, Mosby.

Sorrentino SA, Gorek B: *Mosby's textbook for long term care assistants,* ed 5, St Louis, 2007, Mosby.

Stein HA, Slatt BJ, Stein RM: *The ophthalmic assistant: fundamentals and clinical practice,* ed 5, St Louis, 1988, Mosby.

Stenchever M, et al: *Comprehensive gynecology,* ed 4, St Louis, 2001, Mosby.

Stoy W, et al: *Mosby's EMT-basic textbook,* ed 2, St Louis, 2012, Mosby.

Swartz MH: *Textbook of physical diagnosis: history and examination,* ed 5, Philadelphia, 2006, Saunders.

Swartz MH: *Textbook of physical diagnosis: history and examination,* ed 6, Philadelphia, 2010, Saunders.

Symonds EM, MacPherson MBA: *Color atlas of obstetrics and gynaecology,* London, 1994, Mosby-Wolfe.

Tanner C: Thinking like a nurse: a research-based model of clinical judgment in nursing, *Nurs Educ* 45:204, 2006.

Tanner JM: *Growth at adolescence,* ed 2, Oxford, England, 1962, Blackwell Scientific Publications.

Taylor PK: *Diagnostic picture tests in sexually transmitted diseases,* London, 1995, Mosby.

Thibodeau GA, Patton KT: *Anatomy and physiology,* ed 4, St Louis, 1999, Mosby.

Thibodeau GA, Patton KT: *Anatomy and physiology,* ed 5, St Louis, 2003, Mosby.

Thibodeau GA, Patton KT: *Anatomy and physiology,* ed 6, St Louis, 2007, Mosby.

Thibodeau GA, Patton KT: *The human body in health and disease,* ed 5, St Louis, 2010, Mosby.

Thompson JM, et al: *Mosby's clinical nursing,* ed 3, St Louis, 1993, Mosby.

Thompson JM, et al: *Mosby's clinical nursing,* ed 4, St Louis, 1997, Mosby.

Thompson JM, et al: *Mosby's clinical nursing,* ed 5, St Louis, 2002, Mosby.

Townsend CM, et al: *Sabiston textbook of surgery,* ed 18, Philadelphia, 2008, Saunders.

Urden LD, Stacy KM, Lough ME: *Critical care nursing: diagnosis and management,* ed 6, St Louis, 2010, Mosby.

US Department of Agriculture: http://www.choosemyplate.gov/. Accessed July 5, 2012.

Van Wieringen JC, et al: *Growth diagrams 1965 Netherlands. Second national survey on 0-24-year-olds,* Groningen, Netherlands, 1971, Wolters-Noordhoff.

Weston WL, Lane AT, Morelli JG: *Color textbook of pediatric dermatology,* ed 2, St Louis, 1996, Mosby.

Weston WL, Lane AT, Morelli JG: *Color textbook of pediatric dermatology,* ed 3, St Louis, 2002, Mosby.

White G: *Color atlas of dermatology,* ed 3, Edinburgh, 2004, Elsevier.

White GM: *Color atlas of regional dermatology,* St Louis, 1994, Mosby-Wolfe.

White GM, Cox N: *Diseases of the skin: a color atlas and text,* St Louis, 2000, Mosby.

Yanoff M, Duker JS: *Ophthalmology,* ed 3, St Louis, 2009, Mosby.

Yesavage JA, Brink TL: Development and validation of a geriatric depression screening scale: a preliminary report, *J Psychiatr Res* 17:37, 1983.

Young AP: *Kinn's the administrative medical assistant,* ed 7, St Louis, 2011, Saunders.

Zitelli BJ, McIntire SC, Nowalk AJ: *Zitelli and Davis' atlas of pediatric physical diagnosis,* ed 6, 2012, Mosby.

CHAPTER 1

1. American Nurses Association: *Nursing: scope and standards of practice*, ed 2, Washington, DC, 2010, Author, *www.nursebooks.org*.
2. Finkelmann A, Kenner C: *Teaching the IOM: Implications of the Institute of Medicine reports for nursing education*, ed 2, Silver Springs, Md, 2009, American Nurses Association.
3. National Institute of Health: Electronic health records overview, 2006, available at http://www.ncrr.nih.gov/publications/informatics/ehr.pdf, accessed November 21, 2010.
4. Giddens JF: A survey of physical assessment techniques performed by RNs: lessons for nursing education, *J Nurs Educ* 46:83, 2007.
5. Secrest JA, Norwood BR, duMont PM: Physical assessment skills: a descriptive study of what is taught and what is practiced, *J Prof Nurs* 21(2):114, 2005.
6. Barbarito C, Carney L, Lynch A: Refining a physical assessment course, *Nurse Educ* 22:6, 1997.
7. Tanner C: Thinking like a nurse: a research-based model of clinical judgment in nursing, *J Nurs Educ* 45:204, 2006.
8. Pender NJ, Murdaugh CL, Parsons MA: *Health promotion in nursing practice*, ed 6, Upper Saddle River, NJ, 2011, Prentice Hall.
9. US Department of Health and Human Services: Healthy people 2020, available at http://www.healthypeople.gov/2020/, Accessed March 5, 2012.

CHAPTER 2

1. Smith RC: *Patient-centered interviewing*, Philadelphia, 2002, Lippincott Williams & Wilkins.
2. Riley JB: *Communication in nursing*, ed 6, St Louis, 2008, Mosby.
3. Calvillo E, et al: Cultural competency in baccalaureate nursing education, *J Transcultural Nurs* 20:137, 2009.
4. Dunn AM: Culture competence and the primary care provider, *J Pediatr Health Care* 16:105, 2002.
5. American Nurses Association: *Essentials of genetic and genomic nursing: competencies, curricula guidelines, and outcome indicators*, ed 2, Silver Springs, Md, 2006, ANA.
6. North American Nursing Diagnosis Association: *Nursing diagnosis: definitions and classification 2007-2008*, Philadelphia, 2007, North American Nursing Diagnosis Association.
7. Gordon MJ: *Nursing diagnosis: process and application*, ed 3, St Louis, 1994, Mosby.

CHAPTER 3

1. World Health Organization (WHO): WHO guidelines on hand hygiene in health care, 2009, available at http://whqlibdoc.who.int/publications/2009/9789241597906_eng.pdf, accessed March 5, 2012.
2. Siegel JD, et al and the Healthcare Infection Control Practices Advisory Committee: 2007 Guideline for isolation precautions: preventing transmission of infectious agents in health care settings, 2007, available at http://www.cdc.gov/hicpac/pdf/isolation/Isolation2007.pdf, accessed March 5, 2012.
3. National Institute for Occupational Safety and Health (NIOSH): *NIOSH alert preventing allergic reactions to natural rubber latex in the workplace*, NIOSH pub no 97-135, Cincinnati, Ohio, 1997, NIOSH.
4. American Latex Allergy Association: Latex allergy statistics (n.d.), available at http://www.latexallergyresources.org/statistics, accessed March 5, 2012.
5. El-Rahdi AS: An evaluation of tympanic thermometry in a paediatric emergency department, *Emerg Med J* 23:40, 2006.
6. Farnell S: Temperature measurement: comparison of non-invasive methods used in adult critical care, *J Clin Nurs* 14:632, 2005.
7. Leon C: Infrared ear thermometry in the critically ill patient: an alternative to axillary thermometry, *J Crit Care* 20:106, 2005.
8. Titus MO, et al: Temporal artery thermometry utilization in pediatric emergency care, *Clin Pediatr* 48:90, 2009.
9. Lawson L, et al: Accuracy and precision of non-invasive temperature measurement in adult intensive care patients, *Am J Crit Care* 16:485, 2007.
10. Heinemann M, et al: Automated versus manual blood pressure measurement: a randomized crossover trial, *Int J Nurs Pract* 14:296, 2008.
11. National Institutes of Health, National High Blood Pressure Education Program, National Heart, Lung, and Blood Institute: *The 7th report of the Joint National Committee on Prevention, Detection, Evaluation and Treatment of High Blood Pressure*, NIH pub no 03-5233, Bethesda, Md, 2003, National Institutes of Health.
12. Pinkering TG, et al: Recommendations for blood pressure measurement in humans and experimental animals. Part 1: Blood pressure measurement in humans, *Hypertension* 45:142, 2005.
13. Armstrong RS: Nurses' knowledge of error in blood pressure measurement technique, *Int J Nurs Pract* 8:118, 2002.
14. Anderson, DJ, Anderson MA, Hill P: Location of blood pressure measurement, *MedSurg Nurs* 19(5):287, 2010.

CHAPTER 4

1. Lockwood C, Conroy-Hiller T, Page T: Vital signs, *JBI Rep* 2:207, 2004.
2. Braun CA: Accuracy of pacifier thermometers in young children, *Pediatr Nurs* 32:413, 2006.
3. Lawson L, et al: Accuracy and precision of non-invasive temperature measurement in adult intensive care patients, *Am J Crit Care* 16:485, 2007.
4. Titus MO, et al: Temporal artery thermometry utilization in pediatric emergency care, *Clin Pediatr* 48:90, 2009.
5. Jensen B, et al: Accuracy of digital tympanic, oral, axillary and rectal thermometers compared with standard rectal mercury thermometers, *Eur J Surg* 166:848, 2002.
6. Thomas K, et al: Axillary and thoracic skin temperatures poorly comparable to core body temperature circadian rhythm: results from 2 adult populations, *Biol Res Nurs* 5:187, 2004.
7. Walsh K: How to acclimate to altitude, 2010, available at http://www.ehow.com/how_7620894_acclimate-altitude.html, accessed March 5, 2012.
8. Archer LJ, Smith AJ: Blood pressure measurement in volunteers with and without padding between the cuff and the skin, *Anaesthesia* 56(9):847, 2001.

9. Ma G, Sabin N, Dawes M: A comparison of blood pressure measurement over a sleeved arm verses a bare arm, *Can Med Assoc J* 178:585, 2008.

10. Moore C, et al: Comparison of blood pressure measured at the arm, ankle and calf, *Anaesthesia* 63:1327, 2008.

11. Schell K: Evidence-based practice: noninvasive blood pressure measurement in children, *Pediatr Nurs* 32:263, 2006.

12. Bern L, et al: Differences in blood pressure values obtained with automated and manual methods in medical inpatients, *Med Surg Nurs* 16:356, 2007.

13. Heinemann M, et al: Automated versus manual blood pressure measurement: randomized crossover trial, *Int J Nurs Pract* 14:296, 2008.

14. Pinkering TG, et al: Recommendations for blood pressure measurement in humans and experimental animals. Part 1: Blood pressure measurement in humans, *Hypertension* 45:142, 2005.

15. Anderson DJ, Anderson MA, Hill P: Location of blood pressure measurement, *MedSurg Nurs* 19(5):287, 2010.

16. Armstrong RS: Nurses' knowledge of error in blood pressure measurement technique, *Int J Nurs Pract* 8:118, 2002.

17. Dickson BK, Hajjar I: Program improves measurement accuracy in community-based nurses: a pilot study, *J Am Acad Nurse Pract* 19:93, 2007.

18. Howell M: Pulse oximetry: an audit of nursing and medical staff understanding, *Br J Nurs* 11:191, 2002.

CHAPTER 5

1. Lowe J, Struthers R: A conceptual framework of nursing in Native American culture, *J Nurs Scholarsh* 33:279, 2001.

2. Narayan M: Culture's effects on pain assessment and management, *Am J Nurs* 110(4):38, 2010.

3. Office of Minority Health: *National standards for culturally and linguistically appropriate services in health care*, Washington, DC, 2001, US Department of Health and Human Services.

4. Spector RE: *Cultural diversity in health and illness*, ed 7, Upper Saddle River, NJ, 2009, Pearson Prentice Hall.

5. Galanti G: *Caring for patients from different cultures*, ed 4, Philadelphia, 2008, University of Pennsylvania Press.

6. Purnell L, Paulanka B: *Guide to culturally competent care*, Philadelphia, 2005, FA Davis.

7. Unruh, AM, Versnel J, Kerr N: Spirituality unplugged: a review of commonalities and contentions, and a resolution, *Can J Occup Ther* 69:5, 2002.

8. Puchalski CH, Ferrell B: *Making health care whole: integrating spirituality into patient care*, West Conshohocken, Pa, 2010, Templeton Press.

9. The Joint Commussion: Spiritual assessment, 2008, available at www.jointcommission.org/standards_information/jcfaqdetails. aspx?StandardsFaqId=290&ProgramId=1, accessed April 21, 2011.

10. Saha S, Beach M, Cooper L: Patient centeredness, cultural competency and healthcare quality, *J National Med Assoc* 100(11):1275, 2008.

11. Finkelmann A, Kenner C: *Teaching the IOM: implications of the Institute of Medicine reports for nursing education*, ed 2, Silver Springs, Md, 2007, American Nurses Association.

12. Fagan A: *The spirit catches you and you fall down: a Hmong child, her American doctors and the collision of two cultures*, New York, 1997, Farrar, Straus and Giroua.

13. Huber L: Making community health care culturally correct, *Am Nurse Today* 4(5):13, 2009.

14. Puchalski CH, Romer AL: Taking a spiritual history allows clinicians to understand patients, *J Palliative Med* 3:129, 2000.

CHAPTER 6

1. Herr K, et al: Pain assessment in the non-verbal patient: Position statement with clinical practice recommendations, *Pain Manage Nurs* 7(2):44, 2006.

2. Merskey H, Bugduk N: *Classification of chronic pain: descriptions of chronic syndromes and definitions of pain terms*, ed 2, Seattle, 1994, IASP Press.

3. McCaffery M: *Nursing practice theories related to cognition, bodily pain, man-environment interactions*, Los Angeles, 1968, University of California at Los Angles Students' Store.

4. Chapman CR, Okifuji A: Pain mechanisms and conscious experience. In Dworkin RH, Breitbart WS, editors: *Psychosocial aspects of pain: a handbook for health care providers*, Seattle, 2004, IASP Press, p 3.

5. Charlton JE, editor: *Psychosocial and cultural aspects of pain: core curriculum for professional education in pain*, Seattle, 2005, IASP Press.

6. Pasero C, Portenoy RK: Neurophysiology of pain and analgesia and pathophysiology of neurologic pain. In Pasero C, McCaffery M, editors: *Pain assessment and pharmacologic management*, St Louis, 2011, Mosby, p 1.

7. Huether S: Pain, temperature regulation, sleep and sensory function. In McCance K, Huether S, editors: *Pathophysiology: the biologic basis for disease in adults and children*, ed 6, St Louis, 2010, Mosby, p 481.

8. The Joint Commission (TJC): *Approaches to pain management: an essential guide for clinical leaders*, ed 2, Oak Brook Terrace, Ill, 2010, TJC.

9. American Pain Society: Assessment of pain, available at www.ampainsoc.org/ce/enduring/downloads/npc/section_2.pdf, accessed October 11, 2010.

10. D'Arcy Y: Pain management survey report, *Nursing 2008* 38(6):42, 2008.

11. Narayan M: Culture's effects on pain assessment and management, *Am J Nursing* 110(4):38, 2010.

12. Melzack R, Wall PD: Pain mechanisms: a new theory, *Science* 150(699):971, 1965, doi:10.1126/science.150.3699.971. PMID 5320816.

13. Davidhizar R, Giger JN: A review of the literature on care of patients in pain who are culturally diverse, *Int Nurs Rev* 51:47, 2004.

14. Melzack R: The McGill Pain questionnaire: major properties and scoring methods, *Pain* 1:277, 1975.

15. National Center for Complimentary and Alternative Medicine: Chronic pain and CAM: At a glance, 2010, available at www.nccam.nih.gov/health/pain/chronic.htm, accessed April 28, 2011.

16. Pasero C, McCaffery M: *Pain assessment and pharmacologic management*, St Louis, 2011, Mosby, p 49.

17. Jacox AK, et al: *Acute pain management operative or medical procedures and trauma clinical practice guideline No. 1*, Rockville, Md, 1992, US Department of Health and Human Services, Agency for Health Care Policy and Research, AHCPR Publication 92-0032.

18. Jacob E: Pain assessment and management in children. In Hockenberry M, Wilson D, editors: *Wong's nursing care of infants and children*, ed 8, St Louis, 2007, Mosby, p 205.

CHAPTER 7

1. World Health Organization: Mental health: Strengthening our response, 2010, Available at www.who.int/mediacentre/factsheets/fs220/en, September, 2010, accessed September 5, 2011.
2. Schirmer J, Campbell P, Cyr PR: *It never hurts to ask. You may save a life: screening, assessment, and management of domestic violence in the primary health care setting* (training video), Portland, Maine, 2003, National Child Welfare Resource Center for Organizational Improvement.
3. Murphy K: Shedding the burden of depression and anxiety, *Nursing 2008* 38(4):34, 2008.
4. Flitcraft A, et al: American Medical Association Diagnostic and Treatment Guidelines on Domestic Violence, *Arch Fam Med* (1):39, 1992.
5. Mayo Clinic: Depression in women: Understanding the gender gap, 2010, available at www.mayoclinic.com/health/depression/MH00035, September 1, 2010, accessed September 5, 2011.
6. Varcarolis E, Halter M: *Foundations of psychiatric mental health nursing: a clinical approach*, ed 6, Philadelphia, 2010, Saunders.
7. Bernsein K: Clinical assessment and management of depression, *MedSurg Nurs* 15(6):333, 2006.
8. American Foundation for Suicide Prevention: Facts and figures, 2012, available at http://www.afsp.org/index.cfm?fuseaction=home.viewpage&page_id=050fea9f-b064-4092-b1135c3a70de1fda, accessed April 16, 2012.
9. Folstein M, Folstein SE, McHugh PR: "Mini mental state" a practical method for grading the cognitive state of patients for the clinician, *J Psych Res* 12(3):189, 1975.
10. Lussier-Cushing M, et al: Is your medical/surgical patient withdrawing from alcohol? *Nursing 2007* 37(10):50, 2007.
11. Savage C: How to screen patients for alcohol use disorders, *Am Nurse Today* 3(12):7, 2008.
12. National Institute on Alcohol Abuse and Alcoholism: Helping patients who drink too much, 2005, available at http://pubs.niaaa.nih.gov/publications/Practitioner/ClinicansGuide2005/clinicians_guide.htm, accessed March 15, 2012.
13. Screening for drug use in general medical setting: a resource for providers, available at www.nida.nih.gov/NIDAMED/screening, accessed July 2, 2011.

CHAPTER 8

1. Institute of Medicine: *Dietary reference intakes for energy, carbohydrate, fiber, fat, fatty acids, cholesterol, protein and amino acids*, Washington, DC, 2002, National Academies Press.
2. Dietary Guidelines Advisory Committee: US Department of Health and Human Services and US Department of Agriculture: Dietary guidelines for Americans, 2010, available at http://www.cnpp.usda.gov/DGAs2010-DGACReport.htm, accessed March 15, 2012.
3. Fletcher J: Identifying patients at risk of malnutrition: nutrition screening and assessment, *Gastrointest Nurs* 7(5):12, 2009.
4. Pender N, Murdaugh C, Parsons MA: *Health promotion in nursing practice*, ed 6, Upper Saddle River, NJ, 2011, Prentice Hall.
5. Helder SG, Collier DA: The genetics of eating disorders, *Curr Top Behav Neurosci* 6:157, 2011.
6. US Department of Agriculture: MyPlate, available at http://www.choosemyplate.gov/, accessed March 15, 2012.
7. Grodner M, Roth, SL, Walkingshaw B: *Nutritional foundations and clinical applications: a nursing approach*, ed 5, St Louis, 2012, Mosby.
8. Centers for Disease Control and Prevention: Adult obesity, available at www.cdc.gov/obesity/data/adult.html, accessed March 15, 2012.
9. Nixon JV: Cholesterol management and the reduction of cardiovascular risk, *Prev Cardiol* 7(1):34, 2004.
10. Scheinfeld NS: Protein energy malnutrition, 2011, Medscape, available at http://emedicine.medscape.com/article/1104623-overview, accessed March 15, 2012.
11. National Center for Health Statistics: National health and nutrition examination survey 2007-2008, available at http://www.cdc.gov/nchs/nhanes.htm, accessed March 15, 2012.

CHAPTER 9

1. American Cancer Society (ACS): *Cancer facts & figures 2011*, Atlanta, 2011, ACS.
2. Perez OA, English JC: Internal medicine and dermatology: what's new? *Dermatol Nurs* 22(3):12, 2010.
3. Centers for Disease Control and Prevention: Skin exposures and effects, 2011, available at http://www.cdc.gov/niosh/topics/skin/, accessed March 15, 2012.
4. Etter L, Meyers SA: Pruritus in systemic disease: mechanisms and management, *Dermatol Clin* 20:459, 2002.
5. Finlayson K, Edwards H, Courtney M: The impact of psychosocial factors on adherence to compression therapy to prevent recurrence of venous leg ulcers, *J Clin Nurs* 19:1289, 2010.
6. Iblher N, Stark B: Cupping treatment and associated burn risk: a plastic surgeon's perspective, *J Burn Care Res* 28(2):355, 2007.
7. Leonhardt JM, Heymann WR: Thyroid disease and the skin, *Dermatol Clin* 20:473, 2002.
8. Ferringer T, Miller OF: Cutaneous manifestations of diabetes mellitus, *Dermatol Clin* 20:483, 2002.
9. Sperling LC: Hair and systemic disease, *Dermatol Clin* 19:711, 2002.
10. Kumar G, Vaidyanathan M, Stead L: Koilonychia associated with iron-deficiency anemia, *Ann Emerg Med* 49(2):243, 2007.
11. National Pressure Ulcer Advisory Panel: Updated staging system, 2007, available at www.npuap.org.
12. Milstein A: Ending extra payment for "never events"—stronger incentives for patients' safety, *N Engl J Med* 360(23):2388, 2009. doi:10.1056/NEJMp0809125.
13. Centers for Disease Control and Prevention: Group A streptococcal (GAS) disease, 2011, available at http://www.cdc.gov/ncidod/dbmd/diseaseinfo/groupastreptococcal_g.htm, accessed March 15, 2012.
14. Centers for Disease Control and Prevention: Lyme disease data and statistics, 2011, available at http://www.cdc.gov/lyme/stats/index.html, accessed March 15, 2012.
15. Monteleone JA: *Child abuse: quick reference for health care professionals, social services, and law enforcement*, St Louis, 2003, Mosby.
16. Giardino AP, Giardino ER: *Recognition of child abuse for the mandated reporter*, ed 3, St Louis, 2002, STM Learning.
17. Centers for Disease Control and Prevention: Parasites—lice, 2011, available at: http://www.cdc.gov/parasites/lice/, accessed March 15, 2012.
18. Ekback M, Wijma K, Benzein E: It is always on my mind: women's experiences of their bodies when living with hirsutism, *Healthc Women Int* 30(5):358. 2009.

19. Gulcan A, et al: Prevalence of toenail onychomycosis in patients with type 2 diabetes mellitus and evaluation of risk factors, *J Am Podiatr Assoc* 101(1):49, 2011.
20. Watkins J: Ingrown toenail, *Pract Nurs* 21(8):397. 2010.

CHAPTER 10

1. Agrup C: Immune-mediated audiovestibular disorders in the paediatric population: a review, *Int J Audiol* 47(9):560, 2008.
2. Fausti SA, et al: Hearing health and care: the need for improved hearing loss prevention and hearing conservation practices, *J Rehabil Res Dev* 42(4(suppl 2):45, 2005.
3. Occupational Safety and Health Administration: Occupational noise exposure standards, (nd) available at http://www.osha.gov/SLTC/noisehearingconservation/standards.html, accessed March 22, 2012.
4. Sandhaus S: Stop the spinning: diagnosing and managing vertigo, *Nurse Pract* 27:11, 2002.
5. Kennedy V: Causes of tinnitus and approaches to treatment, *Pract Nurs* 21(12):650, 2010.
6. Tickle J, Sewell C: Managing allergic rhinitis, *Pract Nurse* 33(8):15, 2007.
7. Cooper BC, Kleinberg I: Examination of a large patient population for the presence of symptoms and signs of temporomandibular disorders, *CRANIO: J Craniomandibular Pract* 25(2):114, 2007.
8. Yueh B, et al: Screening and management of adult hearing loss in primary care, *JAMA* 289:1976, 2003.
9. Bryan RH: Are we missing vitamin B12 deficiency in the primary care setting? *J Nurse Pract* 6(7):519, 2010.
10. Schlenker E, Roth SL: *Williams' Essentials of nutrition and diet therapy*, ed 10, St Louis, 2011, Mosby.
11. Beckmann YY, et al: Chronic migraine: a prospective descriptive clinical study in a headache center population, *Pain Practice* (5):380, 2009.
12. Evans RW, Krymchantowski AV: Cluster and other nonmigraine primary headaches with aura, *Headache: J Head Face Pain* 51(4):604, 2011.
13. Watkinson S: Visual impairment in older people, *Nurs Older People* 21(8):30, 2009.
14. Gallichan M: Managing long-term health risks in diabetes, *Practice Nurse* 31:29, 2006.
15. Kanner E, Tsai JC: Glaucoma medications: use and safety in the elderly population, *Drugs Aging* 23:321, 2006.
16. Rovers MM, et al: Antibiotics for acute otitis media: a meta-analysis with individual patient data, *Lancet* 368:1429, 2006.
17. Ko J: Presbycusis and its management, *Br J Nurs* 19(3):160, 2010.
18. Melia L, McGarry GW: Epistaxis: update on management, *Curr Opin Otolaryngol Head Neck Surg* 19(1):30, 2011.
19. Ivker RS: Chronic sinusitis. In Rakel D, editor: *Integrative medicine*, ed 2, Philadelphia, 2007, Saunders.
20. Patel AR, et al: Treatment of herpes simplex virus infection: rationale for occlusion, *Adv Skin Wound Care* 20(7):408, 2007.
21. Cope G, Cope A: Gingivitis: symptoms, causes and treatment, *Dent Nurs* 7(8):436, 2011.
22. Mayo Clinic: Tonsillitis, available at http://www.mayoclinic.com/health/tonsillitis/DS00273, accessed March 24, 2012.
23. Crispian S: Aphthous ulcers, available at http://emedicine.medscape.com/article/867080-overview, accessed March 24, 2012.
24. American Cancer Society (ACS): *Cancer facts and figures 2011*, Atlanta, 2011, ACS.
25. Weeks BH: Graves disease: the importance of early diagnosis, *Nurse Pract* 30:34, 2005.
26. Braverman L, Utiger R: *The thyroid*, ed 9, Philadelphia, 2005, Lippincott Williams & Wilkins.

CHAPTER 11

1. Healthy People.gov: Tobacco use, available at www.healthypeople.gov/2020/topicsobjectives2020/default.aspx?topicid=41 [pg 11], accessed April 3, 2012.
2. U.S. Deperment of Labor: Respiratory protect6ion, available at www.osha.gov/SLTC/respiratoryprotection/index.html, accessed August 30, 2011.
3. Mayo Clinic: Chronic cough, available at www.mayoclinic.com/health/chronic-cough/DS00957/DSECTION=causes, accessed April 9, 2012.
4. Swartz MH: *Textbook of physical diagnosis: history and examination*, ed 5, Philadelphia, 2006, Saunders.
5. Seidel H, et al: *Mosby's guide to physical examination*, ed 7, St Louis, 2011, Mosby.

CHAPTER 12

1. National Heart Lung and Blood Institute: What are the signs and symptoms of heart disease? 2011, available at www.nhlbi.nih.gov/health/health-topics/topics/hdw/signs.html, accessed August 17, 2012.
2. Heart disease in women: understanding symptoms and risk factors, January 12, 2011, available at www.mayoclinic.com/health/heart-disease/HB00040, accessed September 23, 2011.
3. Warning signs of heart failure, available at www.heart.org/HEARTORG/Conidtions/HeartFailure/WarningSignsforHeartFailure_UCM_002045article.jsp, 2011, accessed September 23, 2011.
4. Swartz MH: *Textbook of physical diagnosis: history and examination*, ed 5, Philadelphia, 2006, Saunders.
5. Glover AG: How to detect and defend against DVT, *Nursing* 35(10):32hn1, 2005.
6. Vascular Disease Foundation: ABI, available at http://www.vdf.org/diseaseinfo/pad/anklebrachial.php, last updated December 21, 2010, accessed September 27, 2011.
7. Bucher L, Castellucci D: Nursing management: Coronary artery disease and acute coronary syndrome. In Lewis S, et al, editors: *Medical-surgical nursing: Assessment and management of clinical problems*, ed 8, St Louis, 2011, Mosby, p 760.
8. Wipke-Tipke D, Rich K: Nursing management: vascular disorders. In Lewis S, et al, editors: *Medical-surgical nursing: assessment and management of clinical problems*, ed 8, St Louis, 2011, Mosby, p 866.

CHAPTER 13

1. Martin JL, et al: Systematic review and meta-analysis of methods of diagnostic assessment for urinary incontinence, *Neurourol Urodyn* 15(4):674, 2006.
2. Swartz MH: *Textbook of physical diagnosis: history and examination*, ed 5, Philadelphia, 2006, Saunders.

CHAPTER 14

1. Swartz MH: *Textbook of physical diagnosis: history and examination*, ed 5, Philadelphia, 2006, Saunders.

2. Rourke K: Nursing management: musculoskeletal trauma and orthopedic surgery. In Lewis S, et al, editors: *Medical-surgical nursing: assessment and management of clinical problems*, ed 8, St Louis, 2011 Mosby, p 1583.

3. Wilson D, Curry M, DeBoer S: The child with musculoskeletal or articular dysfunction. In Hockenberry M, Wilson D, editors: *Wong's Nursing care of infants and children*, ed 8, St Louis, 2007, Mosby, p 1730.

CHAPTER 15

1. National Institute on Deafness and other Communication Disorders (NIDCD): Balance, 2009, available atwww.nidcd.nih.gov.health/balance, accessed October 23, 2011.

2. Swartz M: *Textbook of physical diagnosis: history and examination*, ed 5, Philadelphia, 2006, Saunders.

3. Seidel H, et al: *Mosby's guide to physical examination*, ed 7, St Louis, 2011, Mosby.

4. Hickey JV: *Clinical practice of neurological and neurosurgical nursing*, ed 6, Philadelphia, 2008, Lippincott Williams & Wilkins.

CHAPTER 16

1. McCance K, Huether, S: *Pathophysiology: the biologic basis for disease in adults and children*, ed 6, St Louis, 2010, Mosby.

2. Chase C, Wells J, Eley S: Caffeine and breast pain, *Nurs Women's Health* 15(4):286, 2011.

3. American Cancer Society: What are the risk factors for breast cancer? 2012, available at http://www.cancer.org/Cancer/BreastCancer/DetailedGuide/breast-cancer-risk-factors, accessed April 16, 2012.

4. US Preventive Services Task Force: Screening for breast cancer recommendation statement, 2009, available at http://www.uspreventiveservicestaskforce.org/uspstf09/breastcancer/brcanrs.htm, accessed April 16, 2012.

5. Eberl MM, et al: Characterizing breast symptoms in family practice, *Ann Fam Med* 6(6):528, 2008.

6. Hussain AN, Policarpio C, Vincent MT: Evaluating nipple discharge, *Obstet Gynecol Surv* 61:278, 2006.

7. Morrough M, King TA: The significance of nipple discharge of the male breast, *Breast J* 15(6):632, 2009.

8. Lee E: Evidence-based management of benign breast diseases, *Am J Nurse Pract* 13:22, 29, 2009.

9. Rahal RM, de Freitas-Júnior R, Paulinelli R: Risk factors for duct ectasia, *Breast J* 11:262, 2005.

10. PubMed Health: Intraductal papilloma, 2011, ADAM Health, available at http://www.ncbi.nlm.nih.gov/pubmedhealth/PMH0002218/, accessed April 16, 2012.

11. American Cancer Society (ACS): *Cancer facts and figures 2012*, Atlanta, 2012, ACS.

12. Noonan M: Lactational mastitis: recognition and breastfeeding support, *Br J Midwifery* 18(8):503, 2010.

CHAPTER 17

1. Centers for Disease Control and Prevention: Ovarian cancer risk factors, 2010, available at http://www.cdc.gov/cancer/ovarian/basic_info/risk_factors.htm, accessed April 16, 2012.

2. American Cancer Society (ACS): *Cancer facts and figures 2011*, Atlanta, 2011, ACS.

3. Centers for Disease Control and Prevention: Sexually transmitted diseases treatment guidelines 2010, *MMWR* 59(RR12), 2010.

4. Ward KD, et al: Testicular cancer awareness and self-examination among adolescent males in a community-based youth organization, *Prev Med* 41:386, 2005.

5. US Preventive Services Task Force: Screening for cervical cancer, 2012, available at http://www.uspreventiveservicestaskforce.org/uspstf/uspscerv.htm, accessed April 16, 2012.

6. Lewis JA, Black JJ: Sexuality in women of childbearing age, *J Perinat Educ* 15:29, 2006.

7. Monroe LM, et al: The experience of sexual assault: findings from a statewide victim needs assessment, *J Interpers Violence* 20:767, 2005.

8. Katz VL, et al: *Comprehensive gynecology*, ed 5, St Louis, 2007, Mosby.

9. Lloyd TD, et al: Women presenting with lower abdominal pain: a missed opportunity for *Chlamydia* screening? *Surgeon* 4:15, 2006.

10. Saigal CS, Wessells H, Wilt T: Predictors and prevalence of erectile dysfunction in a racially diverse population, *Arch Intern Med* 166:207, 2006.

11. Zheng H, et al: Predictors for erectile dysfunction among diabetics, *Diabetes Res Clin Pract* 71:313, 2006.

12. Barry MJ, et al: The American Urologic Association symptom index for benign prostatic hyperplasia, *J Urol* 148(11):1549, 1992.

13. Clayton AH, et al: Exploratory study of premenstrual symptoms and serotonin variability, *Arch Womens Ment Health* 9:51, 2006.

14. Koci A, Strickland O: Relationship of adolescent physical and sexual abuse to perimenstrual symptoms (PMS) in adulthood, *Issues Ment Health Nurs* 28:75, 2007.

15. Schneck F, Bellinger M: Abnormalities of the testes and scrotum and their surgical management. In Wein A, editor: *Campbell-Walsh Urology*, ed 9, Philadelphia, 2007, Saunders.

16. Nickel JC: Inflammatory conditions of the male genitourinary tract: prostatitis and related conditions, orchitis, and epididymitis. In Wein A, editor: *Campbell-Walsh Urology*, ed 9, Philadelphia, 2007, Saunders.

17. Bostwick DG, Quian J, Schlesinger C: Contemporary pathology of prostate cancer, *Urol Clin North Am* 30:181, 2003.

CHAPTER 18

1. Erickson EH: *Childhood and society*, ed 2, New York, 1963, Norton.

2. Boeree CG: Erik Erikson, 2006, available at http://webspace.ship.edu/cgboer/erikson.html, accessed October 28, 2011.

3. Piaget J, Inhelder B: *The psychology of the child*, New York, 1969, Basic books (Translated by H Weaver).

4. Shaie KW: Intellectual development in adulthood. In Birren JE, Shaie KW, editors: *Handbook of the psychology of aging*, ed 2, Orlando, Fla, 1996, Academic Press.

5. Cafferella RS, Baumgartner LM: *Learning in adulthood: a comprehensive guide*, ed 3, San Francisco, 2007, Josey-Bass.

6. Sternberg RJ: *The triarchic mind: a new theory of human intelligence*, New York, 1988, Viking Press.

7. Duvall EM, Miller BC: *Marriage and family development*, ed 6, New York, 1985, Harper & Row.

8. Denver II Developmental Screening: available at http://www.acf.hhs.gov/programs/opre/ehs/perf_measures/reports/resources_measuring/res_meas_cdij.html, updated 2002, accessed October 28, 2011.

9. Saewyc EM: Health promotion of the adolescent and family. In Hockenberry MJ, Wilson D, editors: *Wong's nursing care of infants and children*, ed 8, St Louis, 2007, Mosby, p 811.
10. Touhy TA: Gerontological nursing and an aging society. In Ebersole P, et al, editors: *Toward healthy aging: human needs & nursing response*, ed 7, St Louis, 2008, Mosby, p 1.

CHAPTER 19

1. American Medical Association: Guidelines for adolescent preventive services (GAPS), available at http://www.ama-assn.org/ama/pub/physician-resources/public-health/promoting-healthy-lifestyles/adolescent-health/guidelines-adolescent-preventive-services.page? Accessed April 23, 2012.
2. Reference deleted in proofs.
3. Jellinek MS, et al: Use of the pediatric symptom checklist to screen for psychosocial problems in pediatric primary care: a national feasibility study, *Arch Pediatr Adolesc Med* 153:254, 1999.
4. Riddell A, Eppich W: Should tympanic temperature measurement be trusted? *Arch Dis Child* 85:433-434, 2001.
5. Paes BF, et al: Accuracy of tympanic and infrared skin thermometers in children, *Arch Dis Child* 95(12):974, 2010.
6. US Department of Health and Human Services, National Institute of Health: The 4th report on the diagnosis, evaluation, and treatment of high blood pressure in children and adolescents, National Institute of Health Publication No. 05-5267, 2005, available at http://www.nhlbi.nih.gov/health/prof/heart/hbp/hbp_ped.pdf, accessed April 23, 2012.
7. Hockenberry MJ, Wilson D: *Wong's nursing care of infants and children*, ed 9, St Louis, 2011, Mosby.
8. McGee S, Burkett KW: Identifying common pediatric neurosurgical conditions in the primary care setting, *Nurs Clin North Am* 35:61, 2000.
9. US Preventive Services Task Force: Universal screening for hearing loss in newborns: US Preventive Services Task Force Recommendation Statement, AHRQ Publication No. 08-05117-EF-2, 2008, http://www.uspreventiveservicestaskforce.org/uspstf08/newbornhear/newbhearrs.htm.
10. Pena KS, Rosenfeld JA: Evaluation and treatment of galactorrhea, *Am Fam Physician* 63:1763, 2001.
11. Giardino AP, Giardino ER: *Recognition of child abuse for the mandated reporter*, ed 3, St Louis, 2002, Mosby.
12. Selway J: Case review in adolescent acne: multifactorial considerations to optimizing management, *Dermatol Nurs* 22:1, 2010.
13. Tanner JM: *Growth at adolescence*, ed 2, Oxford, England, 1962, Blackwell Scientific Publications.
14. Harlan WR, Harlan EA, Grillo GP: Secondary sex characteristic of girls 12-17 years of age: the U.S. health examination survey, *J Pediatr* 96:1074, 1980.
15. Rovers MM, et al: Antibiotics for acute otitis media: a meta-analysis with individual patient data, *Lancet* 368:1429, 2006.

CHAPTER 20

1. Tillett J, Kostich LM, VandeVusse L: Use of over-the-counter medications during pregnancy, *J Perinat Neonatal Nurs* 17:3, 2003.
2. Lee AI, Okam MM: Anemia in pregnancy, *Hematol Oncol Clin North Am* 25(2):241, 2011.
3. Young SL: Pica in pregnancy: new ideas about an old condition, *Annu Rev Nutr* 30:403, 2010.
4. Eisenhauer E, et al: Establishment of a low birth weight registry and initial outcomes, *Matern Child Health J* 15(7):921, 2011.
5. Ma Y, et al: Predictors of smoking cessation in pregnancy and maintenance postpartum in low-income women, *Matern Child Health J* 9:393, 2005.
6. Muckle G, et al: Alcohol, smoking, and drug use among Inuit women of childbearing age during pregnancy and the risk to children, *Alcoholism: Clin Exper Res* 35(6):1081, 2011.
7. Harrison PA, Sidebottom AC: Alcohol and drug use before and during pregnancy: an examination of use patterns and predictors of cessation, *Matern Child Health J* 13(3):386, 2009.
8. Watanabe H, et al: A review of inadequate and excessive weight gain in pregnancy, *Curr Womens Health Rev* 5(4):186, 2009.
9. Wells CS, et al: Factors influencing inadequate and excessive weight gain in pregnancy: Colorado, 2000-2002, *Matern Child Health J* 10:55, 2006.
10. Cunningham F, et al: *Williams obstetrics*, ed 23, New York, 2010, McGraw-Hill.
11. Uthman OA: Effect of low birth weight on infant mortality: analysis using Weibull Hazard Model, *Internet J Epidemiol* 6(1):8, 2008.
12. Pariente G, et al: Placental abruption: critical analysis of risk factors and perinatal outcomes, *J Matern Fetal Neonat Med* 24(5):698, 2011.
13. Magann EF, et al: A review of idiopathic hydramnios and pregnancy outcomes, *Obstet Gynecol Surv* 62(12):795, 2007.
14. Sibai BM: Caring for women with hypertension in pregnancy, *JAMA* 298:1566, 2007.
15. DiRenzo GC, et al: Guidelines for the management of spontaneous preterm labor: identification of spontaneous preterm labor, diagnosis of preterm premature rupture of membranes, and preventive tools for preterm birth, *J Matern Fetal Neonat Med* 24(5):659, 2011.

CHAPTER 21

1. Meiner S, Lueckenotte AG: *Gerontologic nursing*, ed 3, St Louis, 2006, Mosby.
2. US Census: Age and sex composition, available at www.census.gov/prod/cen2010/briefs/c2010br-03.pdf, updated May 2011, accessed November 12, 2011.
3. Ebersole P, et al: *Toward healthy aging: Human needs & nursing response*, ed 7, St Louis, 2008, Mosby.
4. Gray-Vickrey P: Gathering "pearls" of knowledge for assessment older adults, *Nursing* 40(3):34, 2010.
5. Cole C, Richards K: Sleep disruption in older adults: harmful and by no means inevitable, it should be assessed and treated, *Am J Nurs* 107(5):40, 2007.
6. National Institute of Mental Health: Older adults: depression and suicide fact sheet, available at www.nimh.nih.gov/publicat/elderlydepsuicide, accessed November 2, 2011.
7. National Institute on Alcohol Abuse and Alcoholism: *Helping patients who drink too much: a clinician's guide*, Bethesda, Md, 2005, US Department of Health and Human Services, National Institutes of Health, National Institute on Alcohol Abuse and Alcoholism, available at http://pubs.niaaa.nih.gov/publications/Practitioner/CliniciansGuide2005/guide.pdf, accessed November 4, 2011.

8. Naegle MA: Screening for alcohol use and abuse in older adults, *Am J Nurs* 108(11):50, 2008.

9. Hadjistavropoulos T, Fine P: Chronic pain in older persons: prevalence, assessment and management, *Rev Clin Gerontol* 16:231, 2006.

10. D'Arcy Y: Overturning barriers to pain relief in older adults, *Nursing* 39(10):32, 2009.

11. Yueh B, et al: Screening and management of adult hearing loss in primary care, *JAMA* 289:1976, 2003.

12. Lichstenstein MJ, Bess FH, Logan SA: Validation of screening tools for identifying hearing impaired elderly in primary care, *JAMA* 259:2875, 1988.

13. Dowling-Castronovo A, Specht JK: Assessment of transient urinary incontinence of older adults, *Am J Nurs* 109 (2): 62, 2009.

14. Wallace MA: Assessment of sexual health in older adults, *Am J Nurs* 108 (7):52, 2008.

15. Tabloski PA: *Clinical handbook for gerontological nursing*, Upper Saddle River, NJ, 2007, Pearson Prentice Hall.

16. Fulmer T, et al: Progress in elder abuse screening and assessment instruments, *J Am Geriatr Soc* 52(2):297, 2004.

17. Fulmer T: Screening for mistreatment of older adults, *Am J Nurs* 108(12):52, 2008.

CHAPTER 24

1. Madsen D, et al: Listening to bowel sounds: an evidenced-based practice project, *Am J Nurs* 105(12):40, 2005.

2. Perry AG, Potter PA, Elkin MK: *Nursing interventions & clinical skills*, ed 5, St Louis, 2012, Mosby.

3. Lower J: Using pain to assess neurologic response, *Nursing* 33:56, 2003.

Note: Page numbers followed by b, f, and t indicate boxes, figures, and tables, respectively.

586

SPECIAL FEATURES